CASEBOOK FOR
HERFINDAL & GOURLEY'S
TEXTBOOK OF THERAPEUTICS
DRUG AND DISEASE
MANAGEMENT

6TH EDITION

EDITORS

DONNA J. SCHROEDER, PHARM.D.
Manager, Healthcare Management
Axion HealthCare Inc.
San Bruno, California

Assistant Clinical Professor
Division of Clinical Pharmacy
University of California
San Francisco, California

DICK R. GOURLEY, PHARM.D.
Dean
College of Pharmacy
Professor
Department of Pharmacy and Pharmacoeconomics
University of Tennessee
Memphis, Tennessee

ERIC T. HERFINDAL, PHARM.D., M.P.H.
Senior Vice President
Axion HealthCare Inc.
San Bruno, California

Professor Emeritus
School of Pharmacy
University of California
San Francisco, California

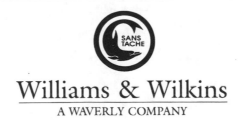

Williams & Wilkins
A WAVERLY COMPANY

BALTIMORE • PHILADELPHIA • LONDON • PARIS • BANGKOK
BUENOS AIRES • HONG KONG • MUNICH • SYDNEY • TOKYO • WROCLAW
1996

Editor: Donna Bolado
Managing Editor: Victoria Rybicki Vaughn
Production Coordinator: Danielle Santucci
Book Project Editor: Robert D. Magee
Cover Designer: Tom Scheuerman
Typesetter: Port City Press
Printer: Port City Press
Binder: Port City Press

Copyright © 1996 Williams & Wilkins

351 West Camden Street
Baltimore, Maryland 21201-2436 USA

Rose Tree Corporate Center
1400 North Providence Road
Building II, Suite 5025
Media, Pennsylvania 19063-2043 USA

Accurate indications, adverse reactions and dosage schedules for drugs are provided in this book, but it is possible that they may change. The reader is urged to review the package information data of the manufacturers of the medications mentioned.

Printed in the United States of America

First Edition,

The publishers have made every effort to trace the copyright holders for borrowed material. If they have inadvertently overlooked any, they will be pleased to make the necessary arrangements at the first opportunity.

To purchase additional copies of this book, call our customer service department at **(800) 638-0672** or fax orders to **(800) 447-8438.** For other book services, including chapter reprints and large quantity sales, ask for the Special Sales department.

Canadian customers should call **(800) 268-4178,** or fax **(905) 470-6780.** For all other calls originating outside of the United States, please call **(410) 528-4223** or fax us at **(410) 528-8550.**

Visit Williams & Wilkins on the Internet: **http://www.wwilkins.com** or contact our customer service department at **custserv@wwilkins.com.** Williams & Wilkins customer service representatives are available from 8:30 am to 6:00 pm, EST, Monday through Friday, for telephone access.

96 97 98 99
1 2 3 4 5 6 7 8 9 10

CASEBOOK FOR
HERFINDAL & GOURLEY'S
TEXTBOOK OF THERAPEUTICS
DRUG AND DISEASE MANAGEMENT
6TH EDITION

PREFACE FOR CASEBOOK

The purpose of this Casebook, like the previous edition, is to help the student develop skills in therapeutics. While the textbook, *Textbook of Therapeutics: Drug and Disease Management,* as well as other sources, provides the facts and knowledge to make therapeutic decisions; students must develop their analytical skills before they attain competence. The Workbook, when used with the sixth edition *Textbook of Therapeutics: Drug and Management* under the guidance of a clinical educator, will help the student develop skills in therapeutics and in making patient-specific decisions.

As with the previous edition, the case format is used. Many of the cases are written by the authors of the chapters of the textbook. The introduction to the Casebook presents the problem-oriented approach to therapy. This approach, used extensively by healthcare providers, is a comprehensive and organized method for assessing and treating problems.

The cases are organized in sections that correspond to the 20 sections of *Textbook of Therapeutics: Drug and Management.* The cases in the beginning are simple, to allow development of the problem-oriented approach. The cases become more complicated and cumulative later in the book. This helps the student continually review previous material.

There are three types of cases in this edition of the Casebook. The first cases within each section have been fully analyzed and discussed by the authors in SOAP (S = subjective, O = objective, A = assessment, P = plan) notes. These are followed by approximately five questions that are likely to be asked about this patient by a preceptor during discussions. These are often "what if" questions. The answers to these questions are provided in the Appendix of the Workbook. These first cases are considered practice cases. The second type of case is not followed by SOAP notes. Icons have been placed where the student needs to write a SOAP note. A blank SOAP note sheet is provided in the introduction for the student to copy for writing these notes. The student is encouraged to write these notes in order to actually make therapeutic decisions and to practice writing SOAP notes.

These cases are then followed by approximately five "what if" questions. The answers for these questions can be found in the sixth edition *Textbook of Therapeutics: Drug and Disease Management.* Occasionally other sources may also be required to answer these questions. The final cases in each section have neither SOAP notes nor questions. The student must write the SOAP notes and develop the questions that are likely to be asked during discussions. Previous course material and current literature sources may be necessary to write SOAP notes or answer some of the questions.

The student should not memorize the SOAP notes that are provided, since each is patient-specific and may not apply to other patients. Information in the Casebook may become incorrect as new discoveries are made or new drugs become available. The cases in the Casebook do not cover all of the material in the textbook. Based on personal interpretation of the literature or clinical experience, practitioners frequently argue over the best way to treat a patient, and some may disagree with the approach taken by the authors. This is expected and is one of the lessons all students must learn; there are often several correct answers to any clinical problem. The student should try to develop the most patient-specific therapeutic plan by carefully weighing the risk versus benefit for the patient.

This edition of the Casebook includes 200 cases. This number of cases allows repetition of the problem-oriented approach to drug therapy. The student can practice on these patients, and no error can result in harm to these patients. Thus, the authors have provided the opportunity for the student to assess current therapy, to recommend new therapy, to monitor therapy, and to provide patient education.

Our thanks to the authors for their contributions to the Casebook.

D.J.S
D.R.G
E.T.H.

Special Acknowledgment

We would like to express our sincere appreciation to Dr. Shalini Lynch who served as a consulting editor for this edition of this casebook. Her assistance during the casebook compilation process was invaluable. Dr. Lynch is also a consulting editor for the Textbook; her dedication to the book is greatly appreciated.

CONTRIBUTORS

TERESA R. F. K. ALLARD, Pharm.D.
Clinical Pharmacist/Assistant Clinical Professor
of Pharmacy
Pharmaceutical Services
San Francisco General Hospital
San Francisco, California

BRIAN K. ALLDREDGE, Pharm.D.
Associate Professor of Clinical Pharmacy and Neurology
Departments of Clinical Pharmacy and Neurology
University of California, San Francisco
San Francisco, California

ANN B. AMERSON, Pharm.D.
Professor
Division of Pharmacy Practice and Science
College of Pharmacy
University of Kentucky
Lexington, Kentucky

ROBERT J. ANDERSON, Pharm.D.
Professor
Department of Pharmacy Practice
Mercer University
Atlanta, Georgia

ILENE K. AUER, Pharm.D.
Associate Clinical Professor of Pharmacy
University of California
San Francisco, California

FRANCESCA T. AWEEKA, Pharm.D.
Associate Clinical Professor
Department of Pharmacy Practice
School of Pharmacy
San Francisco, California

SANDRA BALDINGER, Pharm.D.
Resident in Pharmacy Practice
University of California, San Francisco
San Francisco, California

JOSEPH A. BARONE, Pharm.D., FCCP
Associate Professor & Chair
Department of Pharmacy Practice and Administration
Rutgers University College of Pharmacy
Piscataway, New Jersey

STEVEN L. BARRIERE, Pharm.D.
Associate Director, Anti-Infectives
Clinical Research and Development
Rhône-Poulenc Rorer
Collegeville, Pennsylvania

ROSEMARY R. BERARDI, Pharm.D., FASHP
Professor of Pharmacy
College of Pharmacy
University of Michigan
Ann Arbor, Michigan

PAUL M. BERINGER, Pharm.D.
Assistant Professor of Clinical Pharmacy
Department of Clinical Pharmacy
University of Southern California
Los Angeles, California

KIMBERLY A. BERGSTROM, Pharm.D.
Director, Disease Management
Axion HealthCare Inc.
San Bruno, California

ERIC G. BOYCE, Pharm.D.
Associate Professor of Clinical Pharmacy
Department of Pharmacy Practice and
Pharmacy Administration
Philadelphia College of Pharmacy and Science
Philadelphia, Pennsylvania

MARY E. BRADLEY, Pharm.D.
Director of External Professional Programs
Department of Pharmacy Practice and Administration
Rutgers University College of Pharmacy
Piscataway, New Jersey

REX O. BROWN, Pharm.D., BCNSP
Professor of Clinical Pharmacy
College of Pharmacy
University of Tennessee
Memphis, Tennessee

R. KEITH CAMPBELL, B.Pharm., CDE, MBA
Associate Dean/Professor of Pharmacy
College of Pharmacy
Washington State University
Pullman, Washington

JANNET M. CARMICHAEL, Pharm.D., BCPS, FCCP
Clinical Pharmacy Coordinator
Department of Pharmacy
VA Medical Center
Associate Professor of Medicine
Department of Internal Medicine
University of Nevada
Reno, Nevada

LOAN CAT, Pharm.D.
Resident in Pediatrics Pharmacy Practice
School of Pharmacy
University of Southern California
Los Angeles, CA

BETTY CHAN, Pharm.D.
Specialty Resident in Oncology
University of California
San Francisco, California

JUDY L. CHASE, Pharm.D.
Clinical Pharmacy Specialist
Division of Pharmacy
UT University of Texas Cancer Center
Houston, Texas

BRUCE D. CLAYTON, B.S., Pharm.D.
Associate Dean and Professor of Pharmacy Practice
Department of Pharmacy Practice
Butler University College of Pharmacy and Health Sciences
Indianapolis, Indiana

STEPHANIE E. COOKE, Pharm.D.
Clinical Pharmacy Specialist
Department of Pharmacy
Methodist Hospitals of Memphis
Memphis, Tennessee

ROBIN L. CORELLI, Pharm.D.
Assistant Clinical Professor
Division of Clinical Pharmacy
University of California
San Francisco, California

CATHI DENNEHY, Pharm.D.
Specialty Resident in Pharmacy Administration
University of California
San Francisco, California

BETH DEVINE, Pharm.D., BCPS
Assistant Director, Department of Pharmaceutical Services,
Pharmacoeconomics and Clinical Outcomes
Assistant Clinical Professor
Division of Clinical Pharmacy
University of California
San Francisco, California

MICHELLE DISHON, Pharm.D.
Resident in Pharmacy Practice
University of California
San Francisco, California

BETTY J. DONG, Pharm.D.
Professor of Clinical Pharmacy and Family
Community Medicine
Division of Clinical Pharmacy
Department of Family and Community Medicine
University of California
San Francisco, California

A. C. DREYER, B.SC. (Pharm.), D.SC.
Professor
Department of Pharmacy Practice
Potchefstroom University for Christian Higher Education
Potchefstroom, South Africa

KIRSTEN DUNCAN, Pharm.D.
Specialty Resident in Pediatrics
University of California
San Francisco, California

REBECCA S. FINLEY, Pharm.D., M.S.
Associate Professor
Pharmacy Practice and Science
University of Maryland School of Pharmacy
Baltimore, Maryland

CARLA B. FRYE, Pharm.D., BCPS
Assistant Professor and Director, Pharmacy Practice
College of Pharmacy and Health Science
Butler University
Indianapolis, Indiana

JOHN FRYE, Pharm.D.
Assistant Clinical Professor
Division of Clinical Pharmacy
University of California
San Francisco, California

DARLENE F. FUJIMOTO, Pharm.D.
Assistant Clinical Professor
Pharmaceutical Services
University of California, Irvine
Orange, California

STEPHEN FULLER, Pharm.D., BCPS
Associate Professor
Department of Pharmacy Practice
Campbell University
Fayetteville, North Carolina

STACEY FUNG, Pharm.D.
Resident in Pharmacy Practice
University of California
San Francisco, California

MARK W. GARRISON, Pharm.D.
Associate Professor of Pharmacy
College of Pharmacy
Washington State University at Spokane
Spokane, Washington

KRISTIN R. GERICKE, Pharm.D.
Assistant Clinical Professor
Division of Clinical Pharmacy
University of California
San Francisco, California

DENISE GOMEZ, Pharm.D.
Medical Student
University of California, Irvine
Irvine, California

DICK R. GOURLEY, Pharm.D.
Dean
College of Pharmacy
Professor
Department of Pharmacy and Pharmacoeconomics
University of Tennessee
Memphis, Tennessee

ANDRIES G. GOUS, Pharm.D.
Clinical Pharmacist
Baragwanath Hospital
Johannesburg, South Africa

EMILY B. HAK, Pharm.D., BCNSP
Associate Professor of Clinical Pharmacy
College of Pharmacy
The University of Tennessee
Memphis, Tennessee

MARY F. HEBERT, Pharm.D.
Associate Professor
Department of Pharmacy
University of Washington
Seattle, Washington

RICHARD HELMS, Pharm.D., BCNSP
Professor, Clinical Pharmacy and Vice Chair
Department of Clinical Pharmacy
College of Pharmacy
LeBonheur Children's Medical Center
The University of Tennessee
Memphis, Tennessee

ERIC T. HERFINDAL, Pharm.D., M.P.H.
Senior Vice President
Axion HealthCare Inc.
San Bruno, California
Professor Emeritus
School of Pharmacy
University of California
San Francisco, California

SHERMAN HO, Pharm.D.
Resident in Pharmacy Practice
University of California
San Francisco, California

VALERIE W. HOGUE, Pharm.D., CDE
Associate Professor
Department of Clinical and Administrative
Pharmacy Sciences
College of Pharmacy and Pharmaceutical Sciences
Howard University
Washington, DC

JOHN M. HOLBROOK, PH.D.
Professor
Pharmaceutical Sciences
School of Pharmacy
Mercer University
Atlanta, Georgia

MARTIN L. JOB, Pharm.D., M.A., BCPS, FASHP, FCCP
Professor and Vice Chair
Department of Pharmacy Practice
Mercer University School of Pharmacy
Atlanta, Georgia

ARCELIA JOHNSON-FANNIN, Pharm.D.
Associate Professor
Clinical Pharmacy Division
College of Pharmacy
Florida A&M University
Tallahassee, Florida

MARK S. JONES, Pharm.D.
Clinical Pharmacist/Assistant Clinical Professor
Department of Pharmaceutical Services
San Francisco General Hospital
San Francisco, California

SUZANNE M. FIELDS JONES, Pharm.D.
Outpatient Infusion Center
Tyler Hematology-Oncology
Tyler, Texas

LESLIE FLOREN, Pharm.D.
Resident in Pharmacy Practice
University of California
San Francisco, California

MAHTAB JAFARI-FESHARAKI, Pharm.D.
Resident in Pharmacy Practice
University of California
San Francisco, California

JOAN KAPUSNIK-UNER, Pharm.D.
Associate Clinical Professor
Division of Clinical Pharmacy
University of California
San Francisco, California

STEVEN R. KAYSER, Pharm.D.
Clinical Professor of Pharmacy
Director, Anticoagulation Clinic
Division of Clinical Pharmacy
University of California, San Francisco
San Francisco, California

PETER J. S. KOO, Pharm.D.
Associate Clinical Professor
School of Pharmacy
University of California
San Francisco, California

LISA KROON, Pharm.D.
Resident in Pharmacy Practice
University of California
San Francisco, California

S. CASEY LAIZURE, Pharm.D., BCPS
Associate Professor of Clinical Pharmacy
Department of Clinical Pharmacy
College of Pharmacy
University of Tennessee, Memphis
Memphis, Tennessee

MICHELLE L. LAUDERMAN, Pharm.D.
Clinical Oncology Pharmacist
Pharmaceutical Services
University of California
Los Angeles, California

IVY LEE, Pharm.D., BCPS
Clinical Pharmacist/Assistant Clinical Professor
Division of Clinical Pharmacy
University of California
San Francisco, California

ANDREW LUBER, Pharm.D.
Resident in Pharmacy Practice
University of California, San Francisco
San Francisco, California

SHALINI LYNCH, Pharm.D.
Drug Experience Associate
Medical and Safety Services
Alza Corporation
Palo Alto, California

JANELLE M. MAHONEY, Pharm.D.
Medical Services Manager
Bristol-Myers Squibb
Leawood, Kansas

GAIL W. McSWEENEY, Pharm.D.
Clinical Pharmacy Consultant
San Francisco, California

SUSAN W. MILLER, Pharm.D., FASCP
Professor
Department of Pharmacy Practice
Mercer University School of Pharmacy
Atlanta, Georgia

ROBERT M. MOWERS, Pharm.D., BCPS
Coordinator, Drug Information Service
Associate Clinical Professor
University of California
Davis, California

Assistant Clinical Professor
University of California
San Francisco, California

ESMAIL MOZAFFARI, Pharm.D.
Pharmacoeconomics Research Scientist
Clinical Research and Development
Alza Corporation
Palo Alto, California

GARY M. ODERDA, Pharm.D., M.P.H.
Professor and Chair
Department of Pharmacy Practice
University of Utah College of Pharmacy
Salt Lake City, Utah

PATTI ORMA, Pharm.D.
Assistant Professor
Department of Pharmacy Practice
University of Colorado Health Sciences Center
Pediatric Clinical Pharmacist
Department of Pharmacy
The Children's Hospital
Denver, Colorado

MICHAEL A. OSZKO, Pharm.D., BCPS
Associate Professor
Department of Pharmacy Practice
The University of Kansas School of Pharmacy
Kansas City, Kansas

DAVID J. QUAN, Pharm.D.
Clinical Pharmacist/Assistant Clinical Professor
Division of Clinical Pharmacy
University of California
San Francisco, California

LORI A. REISNER-KELLER, Pharm.D.
Assistant Clinical Professor
Division of Clinical Pharmacy
University of California
San Francisco, California

TED L. RICE, B.S., M.S.
Clinical Assistant Professor and Clinical Pharmacist
Department of Pharmacy Services
University of Michigan Medical Center
Ann Arbor, Michigan

MARJORIE ROBINSON, Pharm.D.
Infectious Disease Fellow
University of California, San Francisco
San Francisco, California

KEVIN M. RODONDI, Pharm.D.
Director, Corporate Operations
OnCare Inc.
San Bruno, California
Associate Clinical Professor
University of California
San Francisco, California

RONALD J. RUGGIERO, Pharm.D.
Clinical Professor
Division of Clinical Pharmacy and Department of
Obstetrics, Gynecology and Reproductive Sciences
University of California
San Francisco, California

GORDON S. SACKS, Pharm.D.
Nutrition Support Specialist
Clinical Pharmacy
Huntsville Hospital
Huntsville, Alabama

CHARLES F. SEIFERT, Pharm.D., FCCP, BCPS
Director of Clinical Pharmacy Services
Rapid City Regional Hospital
Adjunct Professor of Clinical Pharmacy
College of Pharmacy
South Dakota State University
Rapid City, South Dakota

ELIZABETH A. SHLOM, Pharm.D.
Director, Clinical Pharmacy Services
GNYHA Services, Inc.
New York, New York

DONNA J. SCHROEDER, Pharm.D.
Manager, Health Care Management
Axion HealthCare Inc.
San Bruno, California
Assistant Clinical Professor
University of California
San Francisco, California

JANICE L. STUMPF, Pharm.D.
Clinical Pharmacist and Clinical Assistant Professor
Department of Pharmacy Services
University of Michigan Center and College of Pharmacy
Ann Arbor, Michigan

DAVID S. TATRO, Pharm.D.
Consultant Pharmacist
San Carlos, California

KEVIN A. TOWNSEND, Pharm.D.
Clinical Pharmacist—Internal Medicine and Clinical
Assistant Professor of Pharmacy
University of Michigan
Ann Arbor, Michigan

CANDY TSOUROUNIS, Pharm.D.
Resident in Drug Information
University of California
San Francisco, California

TOBY TRUJILLO, Pharm.D.
Resident in Pharmacy Practice
University of California
San Francisco, California

SHAWN WEDWORTH, Pharm.D.
Resident in Pharmacy Practice
University of California
San Francisco, California

BARBARA G. WELLS, Pharm.D.
Professor and Dean
College of Pharmacy
Idaho State University
Pocatello, Idaho

MICHELE WHEELER, Pharm.D.
Specialty Resident in Pharmacokinetics
University of California
San Francisco, California

JOHN R. WHITE, Pharm.D.
Assistant Professor
Washington State University/Sacred Heart Medical Center
Drug Studies Unit
Spokane, Washington

WENDY O. WIEHL, Pharm.D.
Assistant Clinical Professor
Division of Clinical Pharmacy
University of California, San Francisco
Clinical Pharmacist
Haight-Ashbury Free Medical Clinics, Inc.
San Francisco, California

JOANNE YASUDA, Pharm.D.
Resident in Pharmacy Practice
University of California
San Francisco, California

WINNIE YU, Pharm.D.
Resident in Pharmacy Practice
University of California
San Francisco, California

CONTENTS

GUIDELINES FOR USING THIS BOOK

This Casebook was designed to accompany the sixth edition of *Textbook of Therapeutics Drug and Disease Management;* it is organized in sections that correspond to the 20 sections in the textbook. The cases within each section illustrate patients with diseases that are discussed in that section of the textbook. In addition, the patients frequently also have diseases that were discussed earlier in the textbook. The cases are realistic and represent those that would likely be encountered in a hospital or clinic.

CASES: THREE TYPES IN EACH SECTION

Some cases are fully analyzed using the SOAP method (the SOAP method will be discussed later in this introduction). In these cases, the authors have assessed the patient's current therapy and recommended appropriate therapy. These cases are followed by questions that are likely to be asked about the therapy. Some of the questions are "what if" questions, e.g., "What if the patient develops a rash while using your recommended therapy?" These questions help the student anticipate changes that may be necessary during the course of the disease. Other questions test understanding and ability to utilize information presented in the textbook. The answers to the questions are presented in the Appendix of the Casebook. The answers that are provided are not meant to be complete discussions of the topic; for more information the student should refer to the corresponding section in the sixth edition of the textbook.

Other cases are not fully analyzed but are followed by questions. The student should fully analyze such cases prior to answering the questions to avoid giving incorrect or incomplete responses. Answers are not provided for these questions; the student is referred to the corresponding section of the sixth edition of *Textbook of Therapeutics Drug and Disease Management.* With a few of the questions, the answers will not be discussed in the textbook and the students should rely on previous coursework or consult other references for the answers.

The final type of case has not been analyzed and has neither questions nor answers. It is important for the student to practice with these cases because he or she needs to begin to anticipate the types of questions that will be asked in a clinical setting. The student needs to identify the questions that need to be asked about a patient's therapy.

Cases that are fully analyzed and are followed by questions and answers are considered a study case. The other two case types are considered practice cases. Every aspect of each disease and every potential therapeutic problem cannot be discussed in cases in this Casebook. Therefore, the Casebook cannot be used to ensure understanding of all of the material in a section of the textbook. However, it is likely that a student who is able to analyze and to answer or to pose and answer questions bout the cases in the Casebook has a good grasp of the material in the textbook. The cases will become more difficult as the student progresses through the Casebook. The cases will also become more integrated and require review of material from previous sections.

PROBLEM-ORIENTED APPROACH

In order to use the Casebook, it is necessary to become familiar with the Problem-Oriented Medical Record. In 1964, Lawrence E. Weed published the problem-oriented approach to medical records, patient care, and medical education. The method differed from the previous method in which health care providers approached the patient from the point of view of their medical specialties. Prior to 1964, a physician would write a note in the chart about one of the patient's diseases. The note usually stated the condition of the patient at that time, or if a procedure was performed, the note would describe the procedure and its results. The note usually did not summarize previous data and rarely outlined a thought process about how a diagnosis was made or how a particular treatment was chosen. Many notes were contradictory. The "source method," as this method was called, was cited as a cause of fragmented patient care, and Dr. Weed suggested that this form of record keeping was inappropriate for more sophisticated health care where the medical record was used as a means of communication between health care providers. The problem-oriented method, in addition to being comprehensive due to better communication among all persons contributing to health care, allows auditing of care to assure quality. Today, nearly all health care providers follow some form of the problem-oriented method of patient care and the medical record.

Clinicians should learn the problem-oriented method of health care so that a systematic, disciplined approach to each patient is used and no important therapeutic considerations are missed. The approach should always be the same regardless of the simplicity or complexity of the problem.

TWO MAIN COMPONENTS OF PROBLEM-ORIENTED METHOD

Problem List

A problem is defined as a patient concern, a health professional concern, or a concern of both. Many problems are diseases that have been fully worked up and diagnosed, but all problems are not diagnoses. A problem may be a patient complaint (i.e., a symptom), abnormal results from a laboratory test or an abnormal finding from a physical examination (i.e., a sign), a social or financial situation, a psychological concern, or a physical limitation. A problem is identified as generally or as specifically as possible, based on available information. A symptom may result in a sign after the physical examination is completed; this may lead to a diagnosis after the completion of the appropriate diagnostic tests. The diagnosed disease may then be cured by treatment. For example, a patient may complain of cough, fever, and sputum production. A physician hears rales and rhonchi on chest auscultation and orders a sputum culture and chest radiograph, which leads to the diagnosis of pneumococcal pneumonia. Penicillin is administered and the pneumonia is cured. Thus, problems are dynamic: problems are resolved and new problems develop. Patients frequently have some stable and some inactive problems, but they usually have one problem that is the most severe or that demands attention before the others.

The problem list is developed from the data in a medical record, which would typically include the chief complaint, history of the present illness, past medical history, social history, family history, drug history, review of systems, results of laboratory tests and diagnostic procedures such as electrocardiogram and radiographs, and the physical examination. Healthcare providers gather information to contribute to the data and organize the data to develop the problem list (see Fig. 1). However, each health care provider may not interpret the data in exactly the same manner, nor will he or she consider each problem in the same rank of importance; ranking

will depend upon the perspective of the health care provider. The problem list is the table of contents of the medical record and the framework for patient care.

Each of the cases in the casebook has a problem list that is considered complete for the medical problems. However, therapeutic problems such as adverse drug reactions or drug interactions are not always identified. All problems must be considered in the treatment of any other problem and the treatment of a given problem is affected by all other problems and their therapies.

SOAP Note

The second component of the problem-oriented medical record is the organization of the data into the SOAP (subjective, objective, assessment, and plan) note. Each chart entry is recorded in this format. For each problem, the subjective and objective data are recorded and the data are usually also recorded. The plan may be to order more tests or procedures to obtain more data, to initiate treatment, to continue or discontinue previous treatment, or to wait for further development. All the analyzed cases in this Casebook are analyzed in the SOAP format. In addition, the student should analyze the other cases using this format; markers show where the student should write SOAP notes following each case. A blank SOAP sheet follows the introduction. **Students should make copies of this sheet** for writing each of their SOAP notes.

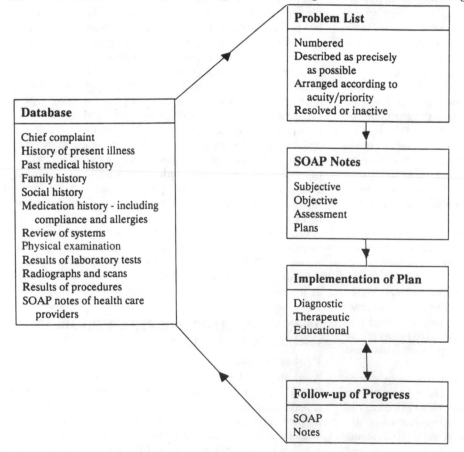

Figure 1.

Each component of the SOAP note is discussed next, and an example case follows the discussion.

SUBJECTIVE (S)

Subjective data record how the patient feels or what can be observed about the patient. Subjective data are descriptive in nature and usually cannot be confirmed by procedures or tests. The primary way to obtain subjective data is to listen to the patient's descriptions of complaints or symptoms and responses to questions that are asked in a systematic fashion as a review of systems (ROS). Subjective data are also obtained by observing how the patient looks, talks, acts, responds, etc. Other health care providers may have also recorded subjective information about this problem in the medical record.

OBJECTIVE (O)

Objective data include the history as documented in the medical record and the results of various tests, procedures, and assessments. Objective data may include vital signs, findings on physical examination, results of laboratory tests, and findings for diagnostic procedures such as radiographs, CT scans, and electrocardiograms. Current medications are listed under objective data. This is to remind the clinician what the patient is receiving for each problem. Every medication that the patient is receiving should correspond to a problem. If a patient is receiving medications for an unidentified problem, the problem list is incomplete. Note that some drugs may treat more than one problem.

ASSESSMENT (A)

The clinician uses the subjective and objective data to assess therapy or to develop a therapeutic plan. A systematic method for assessing each problem should be developed so that the assessment is complete. There are three components to the assessment of each problem.

1. **Etiology:** The clinician should first assess whether this is a drug-induced problem. Many problems are not diseases but are adverse reactions to drugs. Under etiology, the clinician should also identify any risk factors or predisposing factors for a problem in the patient. Modification or reduction of these factors may be a part of the treatment plan and may be as important as drug therapy.

2. **Assessment if therapy is indicated:** Problems may be mild, moderate, or severe; they may be acute or chronic; and they may be stable or progressing. Obviously, the need and urgency of treatment varies with each of these. For acute, severe problems, emergency aggressive therapy may be required, while for mild stable problems, a wait-and-watch approach may be more appropriate. Some problems may not be severe enough for drug treatment, and non-drug therapy may be more appropriate for some problems. At times, the diagnosis may not yet be established; more data may be required for diagnosis or an isolated abnormal value may not be a rational basis for drug therapy.

3. **Assessment of current therapy and/or new therapy:** Patients frequently have multiple chronic problems and are therefore already receiving drug therapy. However, this therapy may not be the best possible choice for this patient. New therapy may be initiated for new or old problems. The clinician must systematically evaluate the patient's current therapy as well as the new therapy. The same process applies to both situations. The SOAP note should list all of the reasons for the current assessment. The reasons are important for all health care providers to understand why therapy was changed, for auditing the quality of care, and for helping the healthcare professional remember the reasons for the changes.

   a. The clinician should determine that this is the best (i.e., drug of choice) for this patient. This does not necessarily mean that it is the usual "drug of choice" for this disease. There may be patient-specific reasons why the usual "drug of choice" would be contraindicated or inappropriate for this patient. The drug should be chosen considering the patient's other problems (drug-disease interactions), other drugs (drug-drug interactions), age, renal and hepatic function, allergies (considering cross-sensitivities), risk factors for adverse reactions or side effects, convenience, compliance, and cost.

   b. The clinician should determine the correct dose of the drug for this patient considering the patient's age, sex, weight, renal and hepatic function, other drugs that the patient is taking, and any other pertinent factors. The pharmacist on the team should always perform pharmacokinetic calculations based on population parameters or previous drug levels.

   c. The correct dosage form, route, and schedule of administration should be determined. Patient-specific factors, convenience, compliance, costs, and lifestyle should be considered.

   d. The correct duration of therapy should be determined. Patient-specific factors may require that therapy be longer or shorter than what is usually recommended for this problem. Some problems require that therapy be continued for lifetime or until circumstances change, while other problems are cured by a single course of therapy. Unfortunately, patients are frequently started on therapy that is never discontinued, although the problem has resolved. Some patients need to be treated longer because the disease is severe or they have certain predisposing factors. Other patients may need to be treated only during an acute exacerbation of their disease. Thus, the duration of therapy is patient specific.

   e. A determination should be made as to whether or not all the drugs that the patient is taking are required. All drugs taken by the patient should be for problems identified on the problem list. The patient should not be taking additional drugs; if there are additional drugs, the problem list is incomplete.

Duplication of drugs from the same therapeutic category frequently occurs, and some of these drugs may be discontinued. A higher dose of a single agent may be preferred to two drugs for the same problem. At times, a single drug may be used to treat more than one problem. Some problems do not require drug therapy. Health Care Professionals should always try to minimize the number of drugs that a patient is taking.

f. For current therapy, in addition to the above the following should be determined.

(1) if the patient is responding appropriately to therapy. Patient-specific factors should be considered and include the items discussed under goals and monitoring parameters below.

(2) if the patient is having any adverse reactions, side effects, or drug interactions. Obviously, the plan will be influenced by the occurrence of any of these.

(3) if the medications have been taken as prescribed. Drugs that are not taken as prescribed are usually not effective. The plan for treatment of a noncompliant patient is different from the plan for a patient who is compliant but not responding. Serious consequences can occur in a noncompliant patient when therapy is altered based on the assumption of compliance. Questions must be phrased carefully to obtain accurate information about compliance.

PLAN (P)

After the assessment of the subjective and objective data and therapy, a plan is developed.

a. **Therapeutic:** Current therapy must be either continued or discontinued. The reasons for continuing or discontinuing current therapy should have been stated in the assessment portion of the SOAP note. If new therapy is initiated, the clinician should state the drug, dose, dosage form, route, schedule, duration, and exactly how therapy will be initiated. Therapy may be initiated at full doses or the dose may be titrated, depending on the drug and the patient or problem. If the drug is to be titrated, the size and frequency of dosage changes should be stated. Precise instructions for drug administration should be included. The reasons for selecting the drug, dose, dosage form, route, schedule, and duration should have been stated in the assessment portion of the SOAP note.

b. **Drugs to be avoided:** The clinician should list all drugs that could potentially be used to treat this problem but that should be avoided in this patient for patient-specific reasons. If the patient is likely to receive a drug for another problem which would interact with the therapy for this problem, it should be stated that it, too, should be avoided. If these drugs are not documented in the POMR as ones to avoid, other health care providers may inadvertently prescribe them. The clinician should list the reasons why these drugs are being avoided, such as allergies, age, drug-disease interactions, drug-drug interactions, renal or hepatic dysfunction, risk factors for adverse reactions or side effects, convenience, compliance, or cost, if these reasons were not already stated in the assessment portion of the SOAP note.

c. **Goals:** Each treatment plan should have a long-term goal that should be both problem- and patient-specific. Some problems are cured, while others are controlled or relieved. In some patients, the subjective and objective evidence of the problem will return to normal; in other patients with severe problems the subjective and objective evidence will only return toward normal. Other appropriate goals include preventing acute complications, preventing long-term morbidity and mortality, avoiding adverse drug reactions or drug interactions, improving compliance, improving quality of life, and decreasing health care costs.

d. **Therapeutic and toxicity monitoring parameters:** Each therapeutic plan should be monitored by specific parameters to assess response and to document that no adverse drug reactions or side effects are occurring.

(1) **Therapeutic monitoring parameters:** The clinician must select the appropriate subjective and objective data that will be followed to assess response to therapy. These parameters should be chosen carefully, considering cost, invasiveness, risks of the procedure, sensitivity, and reliability. Usually the same subjective and objective data that were used to diagnose the disease are used to monitor therapy, except expensive or invasive tests are not always repeated as monitoring parameters. The frequency for monitoring these parameters should be stated. Some critically ill patients should be monitored every 5 minutes, while other tests may be performed only yearly in stable patients. End points should be established for each therapeutic plan. The end points should be patient-, drug-, and problem-specific. Like the goals, the monitoring parameters may return to normal or toward normal, depending upon the patient, drug, or problem. The end point may indicate that therapy is complete or has been inadequate. If the end point shows that therapy is complete, then it should be stated that the drugs will be discontinued. If the end point shows that therapy is inadequate, additional or alternative therapy may be prescribed.

(2) **Toxicity monitoring parameters:** Each therapeutic plan should be monitored for adverse drug reactions, side effects, and drug interactions. The clinician must select the appropriate

subjective and objective data that will be observed for assessment of toxicity. The intervals for monitoring these data should be stated. Any abnormalities that would be revealed by routine screening tests and that would indicate a drug-induced problem should also be identified in the plan along with the frequency of these observations. The plan should include how serious or frequently encountered adverse effects should be handled.

e. **Patient education:** The plan will be useless unless it is implemented correctly. All patients should know the names(s), dose, indication, schedule, storage, precautions, duration, and side effect/adverse reactions of the drugs that they are using. Some plans involve nondrug therapy or lifestyle changes as well as drug therapy. Some dosage forms require more detailed instruction for administration than others. Specific information or techniques to enhance compliance should be discussed and documented in the POMR. Any patient concerns about the medication should be addressed. Any information required for the safe and proper use of the drug should be discussed.

f. **Future plans:** It is likely that the patient will be seen again, so some plans should be made for follow-up. Another clinic visit may be scheduled, additional tests may be required to establish a baseline before treatment is initiated, or contingency plans may be made in case the patient does not respond to therapy or develops a drug-induced problem. The clinician should document what future plans are needed for this patient.

In conclusion, using the SOAP format is a systematic way to critique or plan drug therapy for a patient. Because it is a systematic approach if it is employed in a disciplined way for each patient, only patient-specific treatment decisions will be made. Just as a pharmacist has learned a systematic and disciplined way to check each prescription, each pharmacist should have a similar way of analyzing a case.

An example case will be analyzed using the SOAP format to illustrate the method that is used in this Workbook. The information is obtained from the medical record. For the sake of saving space in this Workbook, all information from the chart has been abbreviated and condensed. The laboratory data have been reported in SI units followed by standard units in parentheses. Abbreviations have been used less frequently than they are used in medical charts, but common abbreviations are used to save space and familiarize the student with these abbreviations.

EXAMPLE CASE

CC: RJ is a 74-year-old man who comes to clinic today with a complaint of weakness and lethargy for 2 months.

Past Medical History (PMH)

RJ has seizures as a result of a motor vehicle accident 2 years ago. The seizures have been well controlled, and RJ suffers one seizure about every 6 months.

RJ has had hemorrhoids for 12 years.

RJ has degenerative joint disease in his knees and hips. His complaints are slight pain and stiffness that do not interfere with his activities.

Medication History

Phenytoin 300 mg p.o. q.h.s.
Aspirin 650 mg p.o. q.i.d.
Over-the-counter (OTC) hemorrhoid ointment applied p.r.n.
RJ is a complaint patient.

Social History

Tobacco-negative
Alcohol-heavy in the last 6 months since his wife's death

Physical Examination (PE)

GEN (general): Well-developed, well-nourished (WDWN) male in no distress

VS (vital signs): BP 120/80 RR 20 T 37 Wt 62 kg (70 kg 6 months ago) Ht 180 cm

HEENT (head, eyes, ear, nose, and throat): Pale mucous membranes and skin, no nystagmus

COR (coronary): Normal S1 and S2, no murmurs, rubs, or gallop

CHEST: Clear to auscultation and percussion

ABD (abdomen): Soft, nontender, with no masses or organomegaly

GU (genitourinary): WNL (within normal limits)

RECTAL: Guaiac-positive, large inflamed hemorrhoids

EXT (Extremities): Pale nail beds, tenderness of both knees but no signs of inflammation, limited range of motion of both hips

NEURO (neurological): Oriented to time, place, and person (oriented × 3); cranial nerves intact (CNI); normal deep tendon reflexes (DTRs)

Results of Laboratory Tests

Hct 0.32 (32)	Serum Fe 6.8 (38)
Hgh 100 (10)	TIBC 91 (510)
RBC 4 × 10^{12} (4 × 10^6)	
Plts 320 × 10^9 (320 × 10^3)	
MCV 80 (80)	
MCHC 280 (28)	

Peripheral blood smear: microcytic and macrocytic RBCs

PROBLEM LIST

1. Degenerative joint disease
2. Hemorrhoids
3. Seizures
4. Mixed anemia

Use | **SOAP** | for the above problems.

The student analyzing this case should first rearrange the problem list into the appropriate order for this clinic visit. RJ's complaint today is consistent with the problem of anemia, and this problem should be discussed first. The hemorrhoids are contributing to the anemia and should be discussed second. The other two problems appear to be well controlled and are stable. Remember that the number of the problem does not change although the order does. The student then needs to analyze each of the problems using the SOAP format and following the systematic approach outlined previously.

Problem 4. Mixed Anemia

S: RJ complains of weakness and lethargy. The physician noted pale mucous membranes and pale nail beds.

O: Hct, Hgh, MCHC, RBC, and serum Fe are decreased. The TIBC is increased, while iron saturation is decreased. MCV is normal, but the smear shows microcytic and macrocytic cells. Stool is guaiac-positive.

A: RJ is suffering from iron deficiency anemia and is likely to have folate deficiency as well. The iron deficiency is due to his blood loss secondary to his bleeding hemorrhoids and perhaps due to gastrointestinal (GI) blood loss secondary to bleeding caused by aspirin and alcohol. His diet may be low in iron and folate because of his drinking, and his recent weight loss may indicate inadequate intake. He may not be eating appropriately since his wife died. In addition, both the phenytoin and the alcohol decrease the absorption of folate. However, because treating a B_{12} deficiency anemia with folate can correct the anemia but will allow the nervous system damage to progress, a B_{12} deficiency must be ruled out prior to treating the folate deficiency. The suspicion of folate deficiency must be confirmed. Because RJ is not in acute distress, the oral route may be used for iron replacement. Ferrous sulfate is the cheapest form of oral iron. The dose of iron required to reverse the signs and symptoms and to replete his iron stores is about 40 mg/day of elemental iron for 6 months. This may be achieved with 325 mg $FeSO_4$ t.i.d. RJ should avoid aspirin and alcohol. Acetaminophen may be effective for treating his degenerative joint disease (DJD) inasmuch as no inflammation is present (see below).

P: Begin $FeSO_4$ 325 mg p.o. t.i.d. for 6 months. Obtain a folate and a B_{12} level and a reticulocyte count. Monitor weakness, lethargy, pallor, and reticulocyte count (expect an increase in 7 days and return to normal in 2–3 weeks), Hct (expect a 0.6 (6) increase in 3 weeks and a return to normal in 6 weeks), Hgb (expect a 20 (2) increase in 3 weeks and a return to normal in 6 weeks), and peripheral blood smear. RJ should take the iron on an empty stomach, if possible. If this causes too much GI distress, he may take the iron with food, but the duration of treatment may need to be longer. He should not take the iron with milk or antacids. The iron may cause his stools to turn black, but this may be distinguished from tarry-looking stools that would indicate GI bleeding. The iron may cause constipation, so he should increase the fiber in his diet and he should take a bulk laxative such as psyllium 1 teaspoonful t.i.d., but not at the same time as the iron. The iron must be kept away from children; iron poisoning in children may be fatal. RJ should also increase the iron in his diet by eating more red meat, liver, and other sources of iron. If the suspicion of folate deficiency is confirmed, RJ should begin folic acid 1 mg p.o. q.d. for 2–3 weeks to reverse thesigns and symptoms of anemia and to replete his body stores. Because RJ is taking phenytoin, he may require folate supplementation for as long as he requires phenytoin. RJ should decrease his alcohol consumption and should be referred for appropriate counseling. The social worker should evaluate RJ's need for help with cooking and housekeeping. In 2 weeks, RJ should have another stool guaiac test to rule out other sources of GI bleeding.

Problem 2. Hemorrhoids

S: None

O: Large inflamed hemorrhoids noted on physical examination. Guaiac-positive stool.

A: His hemorrhoids should be treated to stop the bleeding. The drugs for treating hemorrhoids are only useful for treating the symptoms and the inflammation. Over-the-counter preparations do not contain steroids needed for effective treatment of the inflammation.

P: Refer RJ to a proctologist. Discontinue the topical hemorrhoidal ointment: Begin Anusol hydrocortisone (HC) suppositories, 1 rectally b.i.d. RJ should remove the foil from the suppository and insert the suppository into the rectum in the morning and at bedtime for 3–6 days until the inflammation subsides. If the suppositories cause staining, the stains may be removed from the fabric by washing. Begin the bulk laxative as in problem 4 to decrease straining at stool.

Problem 1. Degenerative Joint Disease

S: RJ complains of slight pain and stiffness in his knees.

O: Pain in both knees without evidence of inflammation but with limited range of motion in both hips was noted on physical examination.

A: RJ has pain and stiffness that does not interfere with his activities, and he has no signs of inflammation. The aspirin may be contributing to his iron deficiency anemia and should be discontinued. Because the degenerative joint disease (DJD) does not appear to involve an inflammatory process at this time, acetaminophen may be adequate to treat the DJD. However, large doses of acetaminophen would be hepatotoxic in the patient with a heavy alcohol intake. If acetaminophen is ineffective or causes an adverse reaction, then ibuprofen in analgesic doses is likely to cause less GI blood loss than aspirin.

P: Obtain liver function test results. Discontinue the aspirin. Begin acetaminophen 650 mg p.o. q.i.d. Do not exceed 4 g/day of acetaminophen. Avoid any other products that might contain either acetaminophen or aspirin. Discontinue or limit the ingestion of alcohol to no more than two drinks per day. Monitor liver function test results every month for 3 months. If RJ is unable to tolerate acetaminophen or it is ineffective, begin ibuprofen 400 mg q.i.d. and monitor stool guaiac and renal function test results.

Problem 3. Seizures

S: None

O: RJ has only one seizure every 6 months. Nystagmus was not present on physical examination.

A: RJ's seizure disorder appears to be well controlled, and he is not suffering any adverse effects from his phenytoin therapy other than the contribution of the phenytoin to his anemia. If RJ is given folic acid therapy, his phenytoin dose may have to be adjusted due to decreased serum concentrations from this drug interaction.

P: Obtain a serum phenytoin concentration. Monitor for an increase in seizure frequency or a decrease in serum concentration if folate therapy is begun. Monitor for adverse drug reactions to phenytoin including nystagmus, ataxia, GI distress, skin reactions, liver function tests, CBC, and signs and symptoms of hypothyroidism, lymphadenopathy, and intoxication. Explain the need for good oral hygiene and for regular dental appointments to avoid gingival hyperplasia. Explain that all healthcare providers should know about his phenytoin therapy because of the numerous drug interactions with phenytoin.

The student who has analyzed this case in this manner is now in a position to answer specific questions concerning the case. For example, the student could answer questions about how this patient's anemia should be treated or what monitoring parameters should be followed to assess the efficacy of the treatment of the anemia. Likewise, the student could also answer questions about the treatment of RJ's DJD or the efficacy of the treatment of his seizures. The student should anticipate the questions that are likely to be asked in a clinical setting concerning this patient's therapy, such as what should be used to treat his DJD if acetaminophen causes an adverse reaction. These questions may also include predicting a phenytoin level for RJ. The student who has analyzed the case in the suggested fashion is unlikely to give inaccurate or incomplete answers to these questions, because no important therapeutic considerations have been omitted.

Conclusion:

The SOAP format allows a systematic approach to therapy and is widely used in medical education and practice. However, each practitioner would analyze a case slightly differently. In many cases, the correct therapy for an individual patient will be agreed upon by all who analyze the case, because in these situations there is only one possible therapy based upon the contraindications or other patient variables. In other cases, the correct therapy is not so straightforward, and two or three alternatives may be equally acceptable. In these cases, the choice of therapy frequently rests with the individual practitioner's preference. In other cases, there may be one therapy that would be the best for the patient, but other alternatives may be acceptable because of extenuating circumstances such as a history of noncompliance. Therefore, the student should use the cases in the Casebook to learn the method of analyzing cases rather than to learn specific facts. The answers given in these cases are usually not the only acceptable answers, and other available alternatives would be equally efficacious and safe. The therapy and information given in these cases may become incorrect as new knowledge is accumulated. In some cases, the available literature is conflicting or controversial, and two practitioners may have different opinions based on the available information. In all cases, the case analysis and answers to the questions pertain only to the patient involved. The information may or may not be applicable to other patients with the same problem. Therefore, the student is warned against memorizing these cases and thinking that he or she knows the material and will then be able to pass examinations. This Workbook allows the student to practice analyzing cases and making decisions concerning therapeutics in a situation that cannot harm a patient. By this process, the student should develop skill in therapeutics. If this Casebook is used as intended, the student will make a commitment to a method of analyzing the patient's case. This will be useful in developing the skills that are necessary for performance in a clinical setting. Thus, the student is encouraged to write the SOAP notes. A single book cannot be responsible for the development of a critical evaluation skills, but this Workbook, in conjunction with the sixth edition of *Textbook of Therapeutics: Drug and Disease Management* and with the guidance of faculty in appropriate courses, will serve in preparing students for a career healthcare.

SAMPLE SOAP CHART

Case _____ Problem _____

S:

O:

A: Etiology:

    Indication for therapy:

    Assessment of therapy:

P: Therapeutic plan:

Drugs to be avoided:

Goals:

Therapeutic monitoring:

Toxicity monitoring:

Education plan:

Future plan:

GENERAL

CASE 1

CC: BL is a 70 year-old female inpatient who was admitted for treatment of a syndrome of Inappropriate antidiuretic hormone (SIADH). She presents now with a maculopapular rash on her abdomen.

History of Present Illness

Two days prior to the development of this rash, BL presented to her primary physician with complaints of weakness and general malaise. Laboratory results and clinical symptoms led to a diagnosis of SIADH. She was admitted to the hospital and started on a treatment regimen which included fluid therapy, furosemide, and demeclocycline.

Past Medical History

BL was diagnosed with major depression three months prior to this admission. She had been treated with amitriptyline and developed anticholinergic side effects of dry mouth and constipation. The amitriptyline was gradually discontinued and fluoxetine started. She was started at a dose of 20mg/day and has been taking this agent for two weeks.

Medication History

Fluoxetine 20mg daily

Allergies

Trimethoprim/Sulfamethoxazole, Contrast dye

Social History

Tobacco - 1 ppd
Alcohol - negative

Physical Examination

GEN:	Thin female appearing tired and somewhat confused
VS:	BP 120/86, HR 80, T 99, Wt 110 lb., Ht 5'3"
HEENT:	PERRLA, EOMI
COR:	Regular rate and rhythm, no murmurs
CHEST:	Clear to auscultation and percussion
ABD:	Maculopapular rash, soft, nontender, positive bowel sounds
RECT:	Deferred
EXT:	No clubbing, cyanosis, or edema
NEURO:	Some mild confusion

Results of Laboratory Tests

Na 137 (137)	HCO₃ 23 (23)	Hct 0.35 (35)
K 3.0 (3.0)	BUN 4.3 (12)	Hgb 130 (13)
Cl 90 (90)	CR 88.4 (1.0)	Lkes $8.0\times10^9 (8\times10^3)$
		Plts $210\times10^9 (210\times10^3)$

Serum Osmolality: 258 (258)
Urine Osmolality: 390 (390)
Urine Na: 45 (45)
Thyroid function studies: WNL
Urine drug screen: N/C

Problem List

1. Drug-induced SIADH
2. Allergic reaction
3. Depression

CASE 1 SOAP NOTES
Problem 1. Drug-induced SIADH

S: BL complained of fatigue and general malaise. She was slightly confused on presentation to her physician.
O: Hyponatremia, decreased serum osmolality, increased urine osmolality, and increased urinary sodium
A: Given this patient's clinical presentation in combination with the above laboratory results, a diagnosis of SIADH is made. Causes of SIADH such as hypothyroidism, adrenal insufficiency, malignancy, and psychogenic polydipsia were ruled out. Drug-induced SIADH secondary to fluoxetine remains a possible etiology.
P: Discontinue the fluoxetine. Fluid intake should be restricted to 1000 cc/day or less. If rapid correction of fluids and electrolytes is required, the treatment may include furosemide in conjunction with hypertonic saline. Agents which block the action or secretion of vasopressin may be required in patients who do not respond to fluid therapy alone. Demeclocycline in doses of 600-1200 mg/day had been shown to be effective. Lithium may also be used, however it has been shown to be generally less effective than demeclocycline and more toxic.

Problem 2: Allergic reaction

S: BL complains of pruritis of her abdomen and arms.
O: BL has a history of sulfa allergy and has recently received furosemide and presents with a maculopapular rash over her abdomen and upper extremities.
A: Given BL's recent exposure to furosemide, a diuretic which is structurally similar to sulfonamides, and her history of allergy to sulfa drugs, it appears that the allergic reaction is likely due to furosemide.
P: All of the thiazide diuretics (e.g. hydrochlorothiazide, met-

olozone, etc.), the sulfonamide diuretics (eg. indapamide), and the loop diuretics (except ethacrynic acid), are associated with cross-sensitivity in patients with sulfonamide allergies. The incidence of cross sensitivity is unknown, therefore the clinical situation must dictate the individual risk/benefit ratio associated with the administration of these agents to patients with such reported allergies. The risk of BL's hyponatremia, and its sequelae, were weighed against the risk of allergic reaction to furosemide. It was decided to administer the furosemide and monitor the patient for adverse effects. Corticosteroids may be administered to suppress the immune response. Antihistamines (eg. diphenhydramine) may ameliorate the associated symptomatology

Problem 3: Depression

S: BL complained of dry mouth and constipation while receiving amitriptyline. She also complained of fatigue, malaise, and confusion (later found to be SIADH) secondary to fluoxetine.

O: BL was diagnosed with depression three months prior to this admission. She has since been treated with amitriptyline and fluoxetine, both of which caused intolerable side effects.

A: Patient's diagnosis of major depression requires treatment with an antidepressant. Adverse reactions to amitriptyline and fluoxetine indicate need for careful drug monitoring.

P: No firm algorithm is available for antidepressant drug selection, and the choice of agent is based on prior history of positive response to a particular agent or differences in side effect profiles. The anticholinergic adverse effects experienced by BL do not necessarily indicate that all TCAs are contraindicated. The secondary amines (ie. desipramine; nortriptyline) and amoxapine are less likely to cause these effects than the tertiary amines such as amitriptyline. Trazodone and the monamine oxidase inhibitors have rarely been associated with anticholinergic adverse effects, however each class of agents has its own unique adverse effect profile which must be considered. Bupropion may also be an option due to its low level of anticholinergic side effects. The selective serotonin reuptake inhibitors (SSRIs) also have a low incidence of anticholinergic effects, however, BL developed SIADH secondary to fluoxetine. The SIADH caused by fluoxetine may or may not recur upon reexposure to this agent or with administration of another agent from this class, therefore the SSRIs remain an option for treatment in this patient.

QUESTIONS FOR CASE 1

1. What is the mechanism by which furosemide facilitates the treatment of SIADH?
2. Although hypersensitivity reactions are most commonly noted in association with sulfonamide antimicrobials, other classes of agents are similar in structure and cause similar reactions. Which drug classes contain agents having sulfonamide structure, and what types of reactions may occur?

CASE 2

CC: PH is a 40 year-old female inpatient who was admitted for treatment of infective endocarditis. After her first dose of penicillin, she complains of "throat tightening," difficulty breathing, and generalized pruritis.

History of Present Illness

PH has a history of mitral valve prolapse with regurgitation. She had a tooth extracted 1 month prior to this admission for which she received antibiotic prophylaxis with erythromycin. One week prior to this presentation, she developed symptoms consisting of low grade fever, fatigue, arthralgia, and an unintentional weight loss of 6 lbs. She was admitted for work-up of these nonspecific symptoms. After positive blood cultures identifying alpha-hemolytic streptococcus, she was diagnosed with infective endocarditis. Therapy with intravenous penicillin G and gentamicin was initiated. One hour after her first dose of penicillin, she presents with symptoms of laryngospasm, dyspnea, and pruritis with a generalized rash.

Past Medical History

PH was diagnosed at the age of 25 with mitral valve prolapse with regurgitation. Since that time she has received chemoprophylaxis for all dental procedures. She has not undergone any other procedure which has required antibiotic prophylaxis (i.e. genitourinary or gastrointestinal procedures). Erythromycin has been the agent of choice for PH since she developed a rash during therapy with amoxicillin. Dental procedures, prior to this recent extraction, were without complications.

Medication History

Erythromycin ethylsuccinate 800mg 2 hours before dental procedures and 6 hours after the initial dose.
Ibuprofen 400mg q6h p.r.n. pain after tooth extraction

Allergies

Amoxicillin - patient reports rash

Social History

Tobacco - negative
Alcohol - negative
IVDA - negative

Physical Examination

GEN: Thin, apprehensive, anxious female who appears to be diaphoretic and in respiratory distress
VS: BP 90/70, HR 100, T 100.9, Wt 123 lb., Ht 5'4"
HEENT: PERRLA, conjunctival petechiae, oral cavity without signs of infection or inflammation
COR: sinus tachycardia, grade III/VI diastolic murmur with mitral regurgitation

CHEST: Clear to auscultation and percussion bilaterally
ABD: Soft, nontender without organomegaly
RECT: Guaiac negative
EXT: Erythematous papules on pads of toes (Osler nodes)
SKIN: Generalized maculopapular rash

Results of Laboratory Tests (on admission)

Na 130 (130)	Hct 0.36 (36)	AST 0.5 (30)	Glu 5.3 (95)
K 4.1 (4.1)	Hgb 137 (13.7)	ALT 0.2(12)	Ca 2.37(9.5)
Cl 103 (103)	Lkes 18.3×10⁹(18.3×10⁵)	LDH 2.0(120)	PO₄ 1.36(4.2)
HCO₃ 23(23)	Plts 220×10⁹(220×10⁵)	AlkPhos 1.5 (87)	Mg1.2 (2.9)
BUN 5.4 (15)	MCV 68 (68)	Alb 38 (3.8)	ESR 66 (66)
CR 88.4 (1.0)	T Bili 17.1 (1.0)		

Urinalysis: microscopic hematuria

Blood cultures: Two positive cultures for alpha-hemolytic strep. Further identification of organism pending.

Chest X-ray: WNL

PROBLEM LIST

1. Allergic reaction/Anaphylaxis
2. Bacterial endocarditis
3. Mitral valve prolapse with regurgitation

CASE 2 SOAP NOTES

Problem 1. Anaphylaxis

S: PH is apprehensive and anxious. She is diaphoretic and is having difficulty breathing. She complains of generalized pruritis.

O: T: 100.9, RR: 26, BP: 110/70, HR: 100 History of rash with amoxicillin and recent administration of penicillin G.

A: Given this patient's history of rash associated with amoxicillin and the recent administration of penicillin G, it is likely that the symptoms of respiratory distress, hypo-tension, tachycardia, and pruritis are manifestations of an anaphylactic (Type I, IgE mediated) reaction. Although amoxicillin associated rash is not necessarily an indication of a penicillin class allergy, this history, in combination with the current reaction's temporal relationship to penicillin administration, indicates a probable hyper-sensitivity to this class of agents.

P: Immediately discontinue the penicillin. Establish an airway if necessary and start an IV line. Administer epinephrine 1:1000 subcutaneously and if vascular collapse occurs, give epinephrine 1:10,000 by rapid intravenous injection. Put patient in Trendelenburg position and administer IV fluids and pressors (ie. dopamine, norepinephrine) if required to maintain blood pressure. Methylprednisone or another corticosteroid may be administered until symptoms of hypersensitivity subside. H_1 and H_2 antagonists (e.g. diphenhydramine, cimetidine) may provide symptomatic relief of cutaneous reactions such as urticaria, pruritis, and angioedema.

Problem 2. Endocarditis

S: PH complained of fatigue, arthralgia, weight loss and fever

on admission.

O: T: 100.9, two blood cultures positive for alpha-hemolytic streptococcus, diastolic murmur with mitral insufficiency.

A: PH's mitral valve prolapse with regurgitation and recent dental procedure indicate that this patient's clinical symptoms may be secondary to endocarditis. Nonspecific complaints such as fatigue, weight loss, fever and arthralgia are consistent with endocarditis. Fever, as demonstrated by PH, tends to be low grade. Cardiac murmurs are present in more than 85% of patients with endocarditis, and a diastolic murmur with mitral insufficiency is consistent with *Streptococcus viridans*. A definitive diagnosis of endocarditis was made with positive blood cultures identifying alpha hemolytic streptococcus. Although PH received antibiotic prophylaxis, endocarditis has been reported to develop even after apparently appropriate prophylaxis.

P: *Streptococcus viridans* is the most common cause of endocarditis involving native valves. Viridans refers to a number of alpha hemolytic streptococcus species which are normal inhabitants of the oral cavity. Based on the blood cultures positive for alpha-hemolytic streptococcus, therapy was initiated with high dose IV penicillin and gentamicin. This therapy would have been continued for two weeks. Other options, which also include penicillin, are 4 weeks of high dose penicillin alone, or 2 weeks of combination penicillin and an aminoglycoside followed by two weeks of penicillin alone. Because of the diagnosis of penicillin allergy, this patient should receive therapy with vancomycin. The recommended adult dose of vancomycin is 30mg/kg IV daily in 2 or 4 equally divided doses (maximum dose is 2g/24 hours unless dosing is adjusted by serum levels). Vancomycin therapy is continued for 4 weeks. Cephalothin and cefazolin are also recommended for penicillin allergic patients except for those with immediate-type (anaphylactic) hypersensitivity such as in this patient.

Problem 3: Mitral Regurgitation

S: None

O: History of mitral regurgitation without prior incidence of complications, Penicillin allergy

A: PH requires chemoprophylaxis with agents prior to any oral, upper respiratory, genitourinary, or gastrointenstinal procedure.

P: The American Heart Association, in conjunction with the American Dental Association, has published recommendations for the prevention of bacterial endocarditis. Although no prospective study has proven the effectiveness of prophylaxis, the use of antibiotics prior to procedures which may result in bacteremia, and, subsequently, endocarditis, has become routine. Specific agents are suggested for use in penicillin allergic patients. For dental, oral, or upper respiratory tract procedures, erythromycin or clindamycin may be given orally to those who can take medications by mouth. Clindamycin may be given intravenously for those who cannot take p.o.. Vancomycin is recommended for patients considered to be at high risk. For genitourinary procedures, vancomycin is recommended for those with penicillin allergies. These joint guidelines may be consulted for specific dosing recommendations: Prevention of Bacterial Endocarditis: *Recommendations by the American Heart Association* by the Committee on Rheumatic Fever, Endocarditis, and Kawasaki Disease. *JAMA* 1990; 264:2919-2922.

QUESTIONS FOR CASE 2

1. What is the rationale for using a penicillin/aminoglycoside combination in patients with endocarditis secondary to *Streptococcus viridans*?
2. In a non-penicillin allergic patient, what are the considerations in deciding which of the three penicillin containing regimens to use?
3. Is a history of rash associated with amoxicillin considered to be a contraindication to penicillin therapy?
4. Should echocardiograpy have been used as a diagnostic tool in this patient?

CASE 3

CC: CS is a 32-year-old female who returns to the gynecology clinic one hour after seeing her doctor with complaints of shortness of breath, flushing, itching, swollen lips and tongue, wheezing, dizziness, confusion, abdominal pain, and diarrhea.

History of Present Illness

CS has a history of seasonal allergies (allergic rhinitis) that responds well to over-the-counter antihistamines. Three months ago, she was treated with oral penicillin for five days for a dental abscess. She took the penicillin as directed without complaints and her dental problem resolved. She went in to see her gynecologist today because she has noticed a sore on her labia minor. Her physician's diagnosis was syphilis; she was treated with an intramuscular shot of slow-release penicillin.

Social History

Tobacco - negative
Alcohol - one glass of wine per night
New sex partner for 3 weeks

Past Surgical History

Noncontributory

Medication History

Ortho-Novum 777, used as directed
Penicillin G Benzathine 2.4 Million Units IM × 1

Allergies

Bee stings- shortness of breath

Physical Examination

Gen: Patient appears to be in acute distress with labored breathing

VS: BP 70/40, HR 89, RR 12, T 37°C
Wt 63 kg, Ht 162cm
HEENT: Swollen lips, tongue, and eyes
COR: Within normal limits
CHEST: Wheezing
ABD: Crampy abdominal pain; excessive bowel sounds (+) guarding
EXT: Itchy wheal at injection site and pruritus/urticaria appearing on the neck, back, and shoulders; (+) facial flushing
NEURO: Alert and oriented x 2, (+) dizziness

Results of Laboratory Tests

Na 138 (138)	Hct 0.39 (39)
K 4.3 (4.3)	Hgb 139 (13.9)
Cl 102 (102)	BUN 3.2 (9)
Cr 97 (1.1)	

PROBLEM LIST

Type I Hypersensitivity reaction
Acute anaphylaxis

CASE 3 SOAP NOTES

Problem: Anaphylaxis

S: CS has symptoms of: shortness of breath; wheezing; labored breathing; swollen lips, eyes, and tongue; itching; facial flushing; pruritus; urticaria; abdominal pain; diarrhea; excessive bowel sounds; (+) guarding; and dizziness.

O: CS has hypotension (BP 70/40), and is alert and oriented x 2.

A: CS is suffering from acute anaphylaxis from the parenteral administration of penicillin G benzathine, and is in need of immediate treatment. CS's signs and symptoms indicate that she is suffering from three potentially fatal complications of anaphylaxis: cardiovascular collapse, lower respiratory obstruction, and cerebral hypoperfusion. In addition, CS has symptoms of angioedema which, if left untreated, may progress into an upper airway obstruction. Because the patient is hypotensive, IV fluids need to be administered in order to stabilize her blood pressure. The duration of penicillin G benzathine may last as long as one to four weeks; because a relatively large dose (2.4 million units) was given, prolonged treatment may be necessary to prevent relapse.

P: Treatment should be divided into initial and secondary drug regimens. The initial drug treatment includes epinephrine 0.3-0.5mg SQ q 10-20 min, as needed, to maintain airway, normal saline IV at a rate of 1L every 20-30 minutes, as needed, to maintain systolic blood pressure 80-100 mmHg, oxygen to maintain a PO2 > 60mmHg, and nebulized metaproterenol 0.3mL in 2.5mL of normal saline to reverse lower respiratory obstruction. Secondary treatment should include methylprednisolone 50mg IV q6h in order to prevent late-phase reactions, and diphenhydramine 25mg IV q6h p.r.n. for pruritis/urticaria. Monitoring parameters should include vital signs, cardiac rhythm, and pulmonary function, as well as resolution of CS's presenting signs and symptoms. Furthermore, CS should be monitored for signs of drug treatment side effects. Epinephrine and metaproterenol may cause nervousness, hypertension, and arrhythmias. Rapid infusion of normal saline may cause pulmonary edema, congestive heart failure, and fluid overload if not adjusted properly. In addition, methylprednisolone may lead to fluid overload and hyperglycemia. Upon hospital discharge, CS should be given a prescription for EpiPen to use in the event of a bee sting, and instructed to wear a Medilert bracelet to warn medical professionals of her history of anaphylactic reaction to penicillin.

QUESTIONS FOR CASE 3

1. Why did CS have this serious reaction to IM penicillin, but not to PO penicillin?
2. What is the pathogenesis of anaphylaxis?
3. What other types of reactions can occur as a result of drug-induced hypersensitivity?
4. What other agents are associated with a high risk of anaphylaxis?
5. What is the incidence of severe penicillin-related anaphylaxis?

CASE 4

CC: FL, a 43-year-old woman, complains of a 5- to 7-day history of crampy, right upper quadrant pain. She woke up this morning and discovered that the whites of her eyes were yellow, as were the palms of her hands. She has been feeling quite bloated and having a lot of flatulence after she eats. She has also had diarrhea in which the stools have been clay colored and more foul smelling than usual. Her urine is the color of tea.

Past Medical History

Noncontributory

Medication History

She uses occasional acetaminophen for headaches.

Social History

She drinks approximately 12-24 cans of beer a day and has done so for the last 8-10 months.

Physical Examination

GEN: Obese female in no acute distress
VS: BP 156/100, HR 100, RR 28, T 37.8°C, Wt 113.6 kg, Ht 157 cm
HEENT: Scleral icterus
ABD: Obese with tenderness in the RUQ
RECTAL: Stools are pasty, light colored, and guaiac-negative.
SKIN: Jaundiced

Results of Laboratory Tests

Na 140 (140)	K 3.1 (3.1)
Cl 114 (114)	HCO3 14 (14)
BUN 12.5 (35)	CR 140 (1.6)
ALT 4.9 (294)	AST 3.67 (220)
Alk Phos 18.67 (1120)	LDH 2.67 (160)
D Bili 56 (3.2)	T Bili 144 (8.2)
Amylase 9.9 (320)	GGTP 18.34 (1100)
Urinalysis: 4+ bilirubin	Lipase 4.6 (1.0)

Problem List

1. Obstructive jaundice
2. Dehydration
3. Metabolic acidosis
4. Hypertension

Problem 1. Obstructive Jaundice

S: FL has crampy, right upper quadrant pain. Whites of her eyes and palms of her hands are yellow. She experiences flatulence after eating, has light, clay-colored, foul-smelling diarrhea, and tea-colored urine.

O: She is obese, has scleral icterus, jaundice, and pasty and light-colored stools. Laboratory findings included T Bili 144 (8.2), D Bili 56 (3.2), AST 3.67 (220), ALT 4.90 (294), Alk Phos 18.67 (1120), GGTP 18.34 (1100), LDH 2.67 (160), and U/A 4+ bilirubin.

A: FL is the classic patient who is predisposed to choledocholithiasis. A mnemonic of the five F's describes the typical patient: fat, forty, female, flatulent, and foul-smelling stools. She has the enzyme pattern typical of obstructive jaundice with higher elevations of Alk Phos and GGTP than transaminases and LDH. She also has the characteristic clay-colored stools and dark urine caused by obstruction of the biliary tract. Because they are not secreted in the bile to color the stool, bilinogen pigments are reabsorbed and excreted in the urine.

P: One should obtain abdominal ultrasound. Surgery should be performed, if it were indicated. One should encourage a low-fat diet, and monitor the patient for scleral icterus, jaundice, stool character, urinalysis, RUQ pain, bilirubin, AST, ALT, Alk Phos, GGTP, and LDH.

Problem 2. Dehydration

S: Diarrhea.

O: HR 100, K 3.1 (3.1), BUN 12.5 (35), SCr 140 (1.6).

A: Due to this patient's obstructive jaundice, bile cannot reach the gastrointestinal tract and emulsify dietary fat. Free fatty acids after bacterial breakdown cause the foul smell of the stool and steatorrhea, which causes the pasty appearance of the stool. Continued steatorrhea causes diarrhea and fluid and electrolyte loss. The patient is volume depleted as evidenced by tachycardia and elevated BUN:SCr ratio. She is also moderately hypokalemic because she is acidotic and probably has a greater intracellular potassium depletion than that reflected by serum potassium.

P: One should administer intravenous 0.9% saline with 40 mmol/liter of KCl at 150 ml/hr for a total of 3 liters, and monitor vital signs, K, BUN, and SCr.

Problem 3. Metabolic Acidosis

S: Diarrhea.

O: Na 140, Cl 114, CO2 14.

A: This patient's anion gap is 12, which is normal. This indicates a bicarbonate loss which, in this patient, is most likely due to diarrhea. This is otherwise known as hyperchloremic metabolic acidosis. This patient needs approximately 300 mEq of bicarbonate to correct to a normal serum bicarbonate of 25: $(25 - 14) \times 0.5 \times IBW = 300$. Commercial preparations of sodium citrate and citric acid are converted hepatically in vivo to bicarbonate. Each 1 ml of solution is converted to approximately 1 mmol of bicarbonate.

P: One should administer 30 ml of sodium citrate and citric acid diluted in water with meals t.i.d. for three days, and monitor serum electrolytes.

Problem 4. Hypertension

S: None.

O: BP 156/100, HR 100.

A: After the acute episode is resolved, this patient must be evaluated for hypertension. She is dehydrated, yet has a blood pressure of 156/100 in light of intravascular depletion. Because she is an obese woman, the correct size blood pressure cuff is extremely important in evaluation of her blood pressure.

P: One should reevaluate blood pressure after surgery.

QUESTIONS FOR CASE 4

1. This patient has three potential causes of hyperbilirubinemia: acetaminophen, alcohol, and choledocholithiasis. What are the typical enzymatic patterns for each of the three causes of hyperbilirubinemia?

2. Describe the origin of amylase isoenzymes and conditions in which they are elevated. Why is this patient's elevation in amylase not due to acute pancreatitis?

3. In obstructive jaundice, why do Alk Phos and GGTP increase greater and faster than do transaminases or LDH?

4. What condition should be considered if this patient's enzyme pattern were changed to the following?

AST 16.37 (920)	ALT 13.86 (830)
Alk Phos 3.84 (230)	GGTP 20.88 (1250)
LDH 2.67 (160)	Amylase 9.92 (320)
Lipase 4.63 (1.0)	

5. What condition should be considered if this patient's enzyme pattern were changed to the following?

AST 1.67 (100)	ALT 1.40 (84)
Alk Phos 0.80 (48)	GGTP 0.75 (45)
LDH 1.84 (110)	Amylase 19.59 (632)
Lipase 101.86 (22.0)	

CASE 5

CC: TT is a 58-year-old male who presents to the general medicine clinic for follow-up and a refill of his nitroglycerin SL tablets.

History of Present Illness

TT has a history of HTN and CAD. At his last appointment, TT reported occasional chest pain and a dry cough. His chest pain is often associated with exertion and is relieved by 1 or 2 nitroglycerin SL tablets. Today he complains that his cough is annoying him; he wants to know what he can do to stop it because dextromethorphan hasn't helped. He states that the frequency and severity of his chest pain has not changed since his last appointment. He reports that he is trying to cut down on his fat and salt intake, but he continues to eat a bowl of his favorite ice cream every evening. He walks about 20 blocks, in approximately 40 minutes, a few times a week. He denies having muscle weakness, fatigue, nausea, vomiting, and headache. He is compliant with his medications.

Past Medical History

HTN x 14 years
CAD x 6 years
Hyperlipidemia x 12 years

Medication History

Isosorbide Dinitrate 40mg po t.i.d.
Nitroglycerin 0.4mg SL p.r.n. chest pain
Enalapril 10mg po b.i.d. (started 3 months ago)
Simvastatin 40mg po qHS

Allergies

No known drug allergies

Social History

Tobacco - negative
Alcohol - approximately six beers per week

Family History

Father died of MI at age 55
Mother died of a stroke at age 62

Physical Examination

GEN: elderly-appearing male in no acute distress
VS: BP 134/86, HR 74, RR 16, T 37.0°C, Wt 94 kg, Ht 180 cm
HEENT: PERRLA
COR: normal S1 and S2
CHEST: clear to auscultation and percussion
ABD: soft, nontender with bowel sounds
GU: unremarkable
RECT: guaiac-negative
EXT: moves all extremities, no signs of edema
NEURO: oriented to person, place, and time; cranial nerves intact

Results of Laboratory Tests

Na 134 (134)	Hct 0.41 (41)	ALT 0.67 (40)	Ca 2.25 (9)
K 5.7 (5.7)	Hgb 152 (15.2)	LDH 4.37 (169)	PO4 1.3 (4)
Cl 98 (98)	Lkcs 6×10^9 (6×10^3)	Alk Phos 2.53 (152)	Mg 1.1 (2.2)
HCO3 23 (23)	Plts 340×10^9 (340×10^3)	Alb 40 (4.0)	Uric Acid 297 (5)
BUN 5.4 (15)	MCV 96 (96)	T bili 18 (1.0) PT 11.5	
CR 115 (1.3)	AST 0.75 (45)	Glu (Random): 6.1 (110)	

WBC differential: WNL
Urinalysis: WNL
Chest Radiography: WNL
ECG: normal sinus rhythm

PROBLEM LIST

1. Hypertension
2. Coronary artery disease
3. Hyperkalemia
4. Increased LFTs

CASE 5 SOAP NOTES

Problem 1. Hypertension

S: None.
O: History of high blood pressure.
A: TT has blood pressure within normal limits while taking enalapril. However, TT is experiencing a bothersome, nonproductive cough and has an increased potassium level, both most likely secondary to enalapril use. Alternative agents for treating TT's HTN include, but are not limited to: beta-blocker, calcium channel blocker, HCTZ, alpha blocker, and clonidine. Using an agent that could treat HTN and CAD without adversely affecting TT's lipid profile would be ideal. HCTZ should be avoided because of the potential to adversely affect TT's lipid profile and CAD. Beta-blockers are useful in the management of CAD; however, they too may adversely affect TT's lipid profile. A calcium channel blocker appears to be the best alternative for TT. It should help to maintain BP within normal limits, decrease myocardial oxygen demand, increase myocardial blood supply, and should not adversely affect lipid profile.
P: One should discontinue enalapril, and start a calcium channel blocker (i.e., Nifedipine 10mg po t.i.d. or Diltiazem 30mg po t.i.d.). This dose can be titrated to achieve a desired blood pressure and then DS may be switched to a once-daily preparation (i.e. Nifedipine XL or Diltiazem CD) for ease of administration. TT should return to clinic in two weeks for a follow-up visit and reevaluation.

Problem 2: Coronary Artery Disease

S: Occasional chest pain, DOE.
O: None.
A: TT appears to have stable CAD at present. His chest pain is relieved with 1 or 2 nitroglycerin SL tablets. He appears to tolerate his medications with minimal side effects.
P: One should continue isosorbide dinitrate and nitroglycerin SL

Problem 3: Hyperkalemia

S: None.
O: Increased potassium (5.7).
A: TT has an elevated potassium level that is most likely due to enalapril. He is asymptomatic and has no changes on ECG; therefore, he can be managed by discontinuing enalapril.
P: One should discontinue enalapril (see problem 1: HTN), and monitor potassium levels.

Problem 4. Increased LFT's

S: None.
O: Increased alkaline phosphatase, increased AST.
A: TT has increased LFT's most likely secondary to simvastatin. Elevations in liver enzymes, particularly alkaline phosphatase AST, may occur during therapy with HMG CoA reductase inhibitors, but patients usually remain asymptomatic. These elevations have been reported to resolve with continued therapy and usually reverse when therapy is discontinued.
P: One should continue simvistatin treatment; however, one should monitor LFT's periodically and discontinue simvastatin if liver enzyme levels were three times normal values or if TT were to develop any signs of hepatotoxicity.

QUESTIONS FOR CASE 5

1. What major risk factors does TT have for CAD? Which of these factors can be altered?
2. TT shows you an advertisement he saw in a magazine about a new nitrate drug, isosorbide mononitrate. He wants to know if he should take this instead of isosorbide dinitrate.
3. What are the incidence and proposed mechanism(s) of ACE-inhibitor-induced cough?
4. You give TT a prescription for more nitroglycerin SL tablets. Counsel TT on proper storage and usage of nitroglycerin SL.

CASE 6

CC: RH is a 52-year-old male who was brought to the emergency room late in the evening from a company party. He is confused, weak, dizzy, and complains of sudden onset of nausea.

Past Medical History

RH was diagnosed with diabetes 15 years ago. He checks his urine for glucose once a week and it is usually negative. RH has had hypertension for five years.

Medication History

Tolbutamide 500 mg p.o. t.i.d.
Propranolol 60 mg p.o. t.i.d.
Multivitamin 1 p.o. q.d.
Vitamin C 1 g p.o. q.d.

Allergies

NKDA

Social History

Tobacco - 1-2 PPD for 29 years
Alcohol - 1-2 drinks per day plus socially at parties

Physical Examination

GEN: Well-developed, well-nourished male who is intoxicated

VS: BP 125/85, HR 66, RR T 37.0°C, Wt 68 kg, Ht 172 cm

HEENT: WNL

CHEST: Clear to A&P

ABD: Soft, nontender, without masses or organomegaly

GU: WNL

RECTAL: Guaiac-negative

EXT: Unremarkable

NEURO: Oriented to person and place, otherwise normal

Results of Laboratory Tests

Na 139 (139)
K 3.9 (3.9)
Cl 102 (102)
Glu 1.6 (30)
Blood alcohol 190 mg/dl

Problem List

1. Alcoholism
2. Hypertension
3. Hypoglycemia

Problem 1. Alcoholism

S: RH usually has one to two drinks per day, plus drinking socially at parties. Currently, patient has been drinking all evening and is confused and disoriented.

O: Blood alcohol 190 mg/dl.

A: Patient is intoxicated and must stop drinking because it can complicate diabetes causing both hypo- and hyperglycemia. Alcohol interacts with his medication therapy.

P: One should recommend that the patient stop drinking and seek professional help.

Problem 2. Hypertension

S: Five-year history of hypertension.

O: BP 125/85, HR 66 RR.

A: Hypertension is currently under control with propranolol.

P: Propranolol interacts with RH's diabetes by masking the sympathomimetic s/sx of diabetes (see description above). One should recommend another antihypertensive agent, such as an ACE inhibitor or calcium channel blocker.

Patient education should include:
1. Low-sodium diet
2. Stop smoking
3. Compliance

Problem 3. Hypoglycemia

S: RH is confused, weak, dizzy, and nauseated. He has been drinking for hours and probably has not eaten since lunch.

O: Serum glucose is 1.6 (30), and no glucose or ketones are in urine.

A: RH is hypoglycemic. He has been socializing for hours and has probably had quite a few drinks. He is confused, not

oriented to time, weak, dizzy, and nauseated. The concurrent propranolol treatment masks the initial sympathomimetic signs of hypoglycemia (perspiration, tachycardia, and tremors). Alcohol has additive effects with insulin, which can cause hypoglycemia.

P: One should begin treatment to prevent further complications of hypoglycemia: orange juice, sugar, and/or carbohydrates (orally, if tolerated; intravenous glucose or dextrose if not). Tolbutamide can interact with alcohol and give a disulfiramlike reaction. Because he has a drinking problem, it would be better to change to another sulfonylurea. Second-generation sulfonylureas do not have this reaction with alcohol. Vitamin C can interact with some urine glucose tests, giving a false-negative result. One should recommend that the patient begin blood glucose monitoring.

Patient education should include:
1. Diet
2. Exercise
3. S/Sx hypo- and hyperglycemia and how to handle
4. Stop drinking

QUESTIONS FOR CASE 6

1. Would thiazide diuretics be a good choice to treat RH's hypertension?
2. What other drugs cause an Antabuse type reaction?
3. Are there urine glucose tests that do not react with vitamin C?
4. RH takes ibuprofen occasionally to relieve his headaches. Will this interact with his oral hypoglycemic regimen?
5. What additional laboratory tests may help to monitor RH's DM?

CASE 7

CC: JK is a 67-year-old female patient who has been in the hospital for three weeks secondary to exacerbation of congestive heart failure (CHF) and development of nosocomial pneumonia (resolved) and atrial fibrillation. Presently, her chief complaint is a three-day history of nausea and vomiting, which has become increasingly severe in the last 24 hrs.

Past Medical History

JK was diagnosed with CHF three years ago and has been treated for mild hypertension for five years.

Medication History

Digoxin 0.25 mg q. day (for the last six months)
Quinidine 300 mg q8h (started five days ago)
Hydrochlorothiazide 25 mg q. day
Temazepam 15 mg HS p.r.n. for sleep
Prochlorperazine 5 mg q4h p.r.n. for nausea (started four days ago)

Social History

She lives alone; husband died seven years ago. She smoked two packs of nonfilter cigarettes a day for 35 years and quit smoking two years ago. She does not drink alcoholic beverages. She maintains an active driver's license and drives regularly to the store and church. She has immediate family members willing to provide support, who live 12 miles from her home.

Physical Examination (three weeks postadmission)

GEN:	Well-developed, well-nourished female who looks younger than her stated age, suffering from increasingly severe nausea
VS:	BP 135/75, HR 62, T 37.0°C, Wt 61 kg, Ht 165 cm
HEENT:	WNL
COR:	Slow, irregular rhythm
ABD:	Soft, nontender, with no masses or organomegaly
GU:	WNL
RECTAL:	WNL
EXT:	WNL
NEURO:	Oriented to place and person, cranial nerves intact, normal deep tendon reflexes

Results of Laboratory Tests

Na 141 (141)
CR 88.4 (1.0)
Hgb 110 (11)
Plts 320×10⁹ (320×10⁵)
Mg 0.699 (1.7)

K 2.9 (2.9)
Hct 0.38 (38)
Lkcs 5.7×10⁹ (5.7×10⁵)
Ca 2.44 (9.8)

Serum Drug Concentrations

Quinidine 9.86 nmol/liter (3.2 μg/ml) (collected 7 hr postdose)

Digoxin 3.7 nmol/liter (2.9 ng/ml) (collected 23 hr postdose)

Digoxin 2.7 nmol/liter (2.1 ng/ml) (collected 48 hr postdose)

Problem List

1. Hypertension
2. Atrial fibrillation
3. Status post (S/P) nosocomial pneumonia
4. Digoxin toxicity (CHF)
5. Hypokalemia

CASE 7 SOAP NOTES

Problem 1. Hypertension

S: The patient is asymptomatic.

O: The patient has documented hypertension, with BP 145/95 before treatment with thiazide diuretic. Presently, BP is well controlled (135/75).

A: Hypertension is well controlled only by hydrochlorothiazide.

P: No change in therapy is recommended.

Problem 2. Atrial Fibrillation

S: The patient is asymptomatic.

O: ECG demonstrates irregular R-R intervals with no P waves. QRS complex is normal.

A: The patient has developed atrial fibrillation, possibly secondary to the added stress of her present illness. She is presently being treated with quinidine.

P: No change in therapy is recommended.

Problem 3. S/P Pneumonia

S: Patient had mild SOB after resolution of CHF.

O: The patient had a temperature of 39°C and Lkcs of 13.5 × 109 (13,500). Presently, the patient has no SOB, chest radiography is clear, Lkcs are normal, and patient remains afebrile.

A: Patient had bacterial pneumonia that responded to antibiotic therapy.

P: None.

Problem 4. Digoxin Toxicity (CHF)

S: The patient complains of new-onset nausea and vomiting.

O: This patient has been taking digoxin (0.25 mg p.o. q. day) for three weeks and has a number of signs and symptoms consistent with digoxin intoxication: (a) nausea and vomiting, (b) bradycardia, (c) mild confusion, and (d) high digoxin trough concentration. The patient is taking quinidine. The patient's dose was held after an SDC of 3.7 nmol/liter (2.9 ng/ml) was reported by the laboratory.

A: JK's digoxin dose should be held until the concentration decreases below 2.56 nmol/liter (2.0 ng/ml) and all signs and symptoms secondary to digoxin intoxication subside. This may be difficult because many of the clinical symptoms of digoxin intoxication (nausea, vomiting, mental confusion) are nonspecific. If the digoxin concentration were to decrease to 1.92 nmol/liter (1.5 ng/ml), one could be fairly confident that the continuing symptoms were not secondary to digoxin.

P: One should calculate the time required for this patient's digoxin concentration to decrease from 3.7 nmol/liter (2.9 ng/ml) to 1.92 nmol/liter (1.5 ng/ml) and determine a new digoxin dose to maintain digoxin SDC about 1.92 nmol/liter (1.5 ng/ml). One can calculate $t_{1/2}$ and time for concentration to decrease to 1.5 ng/ml by the following:

26 hr (post time of digoxin SDC of 2.1 ng/ml)

One can estimate new digoxin dose by the following:

0.129 mg/day

One should recommend holding the dose for 24 hrs and checking digoxin SDC. If digoxin were close to 1.92 nmol/liter (1.5 ng/ml), one should restart digoxin dosing the next morning at 0.125 mg q. day. Recheck digoxin SDC in two weeks, when clinical symptoms warrant, or when quinidine administration is stopped or changed.

Problem 5. Hypokalemia

S: None.

O: Potassium concentration 2.9.

A: The low potassium level is most likely due to the potassium-wasting effect of the thiazide diuretic. It is prudent to correct the potassium concentration, which reduces the risk for development of cardiac arrhythmias.

P: One should recommend giving potassium chloride oral supplements (8 mEq) b.i.d. as long as the patient remains on thiazide diuretics.

QUESTIONS FOR CASE 7

1. How would your dosing recommendation be altered if the postdose time of the toxic SDC 3.7 nmol/liter (2.9 ng/ml) had been 1 hr?
2. What is the benefit of digoxin in the treatment of atrial fibrillation?
3. Assuming JK's digoxin half-life is as previously estimated (54 hr), what would the steady-state concentration be if an SDC collected four days after the start of therapy were 2.3 nmol/liter (1.8 ng/ml)?
4. What are the symptoms of digoxin toxicity and how do you distinguish the cardiotoxic effects of digoxin from the patient's underlying heart disease?

CASE 8

CC: AG is an 18-month-old boy who ingested 15 ferrous sulfate tablets (325 mg) 2 hr ago. He vomited twice prior to arrival in the emergency department. On presentation he was lethargic and irritable. He was lavaged with 1 liter of 0.45 NS. Samples for baseline laboratory tests, including a serum iron level, were drawn, and he was admitted to the pediatric intensive care unit. Intravenous deferoxamine therapy was initiated at a dose of 90 mg/kg given at a rate of 15 mg/kg/hr.

Past Medical History

AG has had two episodes of otitis media treated with amoxicillin. Immunizations are up-to-date.

Medication History

None.

Social History

Lives with parents and an older sibling.

Physical Examination

      GEN: Lethargic, irritable male
       VS: BP 60 systolic, HR 160, RR 35, T 37.2°C, Wt 12 kg
   HEENT: Pupils equal and reactive to light
     COR: WNL
   CHEST: Clear to auscultation and percussion
     ABD: Soft, minimal tenderness
      GU: Deferred
  RECTAL: Guaiac-positive
     EXT: Clammy skin, pale
   NEURO: Lethargic, responsive, DTRs intact

Results of Laboratory Tests

Na 140 (140)	Hgb 120 (12)
K 4.6 (4.6)	Lkcs 17×10⁹ (17×10³)
Cl 98 (98)	AST .40 (24)
HCO₃ 16 (16)	ALT .45 (27)
BUN 12.5 (35)	T Bili 9 (0.5)
CR 53 (0.6)	Glu 9.7 (175)
Hct 0.38 (38)	PT 11

ABGs pH 7.28, P_{CO_2} 4.0 kPa (30 mmHg), P_{O_2} 13.3 kPa (100 mmHg)

Serum iron level (2.5 hr postingestion) 122.5 μmol/liter (684 μg/100 ml)

TIBC pending

Abdominal flatplate: negative

Problem List

1. Iron overdose

Problem 1. Iron Overdose

S: AG ingested iron tablets.

O: AG ingested 81.25 mg/kg of elemental iron, and has lethargy, tachycardia, hypotension, hyperglycemia, leukocytosis, and serum iron level 122.5 μmol/liter (684 μg/100 ml).

A: AG has ingested a large overdose of iron and is experiencing toxicity. Hyperglycemia and leukocytosis correlate with an elevated serum iron level. A serum iron level of 122.5 μmol/liter (684 μg/100 ml) is clearly toxic and requires treatment. Normal serum iron levels are generally in the range of 9.0-26.9 μmol/liter (50-150 μg/100 ml). The minimal iron levels that would be expected to produce toxicity are generally In one series, 69% of children with iron levels below 53.7 μmol/liter (300 μg/100 ml) were mildly poisoned or asymptomatic, while 64% of patients with iron levels 53.7-89.6 μmol/liter (300-500 μg/100 ml) were moderately or severely poisoned, compared with 75% who were moderately or severely poisoned at > 89.6 μmol/liter (500 μg/100 ml).

P: In the emergency department, the patient was lavaged with 0.45 NS. It is no longer recommended to use phosphate or bicarbonate lavage solutions to form iron phosphate or iron carbonate and to reduce iron absorption and GI irritation because of limited effectiveness. Administration of large amounts of phosphate salts can also cause hyperphosphatemia and hypocalcemia. The use of oral deferoxamine is controversial because the complex, ferrioxamine, is absorbable from the GI tract and its potential toxicity and efficacy in reducing morbidity and mortality is unclear. One should administer 20 ml/kg of an isotonic solution (normal saline or Ringer's lactate) intravenously over 1-2 hrs to increase BP to a systolic pressure of 80-100 mm Hg, then administer D5 0.2 NS to maintain hydration and blood pressure. Administer deferoxamine at a rate of 15 mg/kg/hr. When the rate exceeds this, hypotension is a potential adverse effect. Although this limit is appropriate in many patients, those with severe, life-threatening iron poisoning, may require the administration of deferoxamine at a more rapid rate. If hypotension were to occur, decreasing the rate should rapidly improve BP. One should monitor BP, heart rate, and serum iron level, and continue deferoxamine until symptoms resolve and serum iron level decreases below 62.7 μmol/liter (350 μg/100 ml).

QUESTIONS FOR CASE 8

1. How does the timing of the serum iron level influence interpretation of the level, especially when delayed?
2. When an iron level cannot be readily obtained, do methods exist to estimate the iron level? Could they be used in this patient?
3. What are the toxicities and complications of iron overdose?
4. What are possible methods of gastric emptying if ipecac and/or lavage were ineffective?
5. What does urine color change after deferoxamine administration indicate? Is it an effective way to monitor therapy?

CASE 9

CC: JS is a 29-year-old male who presents to the emergency room with shaking chills and sweats. He stated that he has turned yellow over the last week and a half, and his urine is similar in color to a cola.

Past Medical History

Unknown

Medication History

None

Social History

JS has been homeless since the 1989 San Francisco earthquake. He abuses crack and heroin intravenously and also drinks approximately 1 pint of whiskey or vodka a day.

Physical Examination

GEN: Very ill appearing male with intermittent chills and shakes, coughing up greenish-yellow sputum

VS: BP 90/30, HR 140, RR 32, T 39.6°C, Wt 60 kg, Ht 180 cm

HEENT: Scleral icterus, with normal funduscopic examination

CHEST: Scattered rales with dullness to percussion in the bases

COR: NL S1, S2 with a loud III/VI systolic murmur over the RSB which was heard throughout the precordium.

ABD: Tenderness in the RUQ with no rebound

RECTAL: Negative for blood

EXT: Cold and cyanotic; without evidence of Osler's nodes or Janeway lesions

SKIN: Jaundiced with multiple fresh needle tracks

Results of Laboratory Tests

HCO3 29 (29)	AST 208.75 (12,500)
BUN 13.0 (36.4)	ALT 254.15 (15,220)
CR 120 (1.4)	LDH 17.51 (1048)
Hct 0.258 (25.8)	Alk Phos 21.46 (1285)
Hgb 5.34 (8.6)	Alb 14 (1.4)
Lkcs 3.24×10^9 (3.24×10^3)	T Bili 335.16 (19.6)
Plts 35×10^9 (35×10^3)	D Bili 174.42 (10.2)
MCV 78 (78)	GGTP 19.15 (1147)
Retic 0.10 (10)	CK 18.37 (1100)

Chest radiography: multiple, small cavitary lesions with pulmonary edema

Lkcs differential: 0.88 Segs, 0.08 Bands, 0.04 Lymphs

Blood cultures: positive for Staphylococcal aureus

Arterial blood gases on room air: pH 7.36, Pco₂, 50 Po₂ 54

Problem List

1. Sepsis
2. Infective endocarditis
3. Viral hepatitis
4. Anemia

CASE 9 SOAP NOTES

Problem 1. Sepsis

S: Shaking chills and sweats.

O: Findings include BP 90/30, HR 140, T 39.6°C, Lkcs 3.24 × 10^9/liter (3.24 × 10^3) with left shift, positive blood cultures for Staphylococcus aureus, and Alb 14 (1.4). Extremities are cold and cyanotic.

A: JS is clearly hypotensive and in a state of shock. He needs aggressive support with fluids and broad-spectrum antibiotics; however, administering fluid too rapidly could be dangerous because albumin is low and the patient already has pulmonary edema. The administration of fluids in this patient should be approached cautiously.

P: One should implement volume expansion with 250 ml of either 0.9% saline or Hetastarch 6%, and begin antibiotics as described in problem 2. One should monitor vital signs, blood cultures and sensitivities, Lkcs, BUN, SCr, urine output, and serum gentamicin concentrations.

Problem 2. Infective Endocarditis

S: Shaking chills and sweats. Intravenous drug abuser.

O: BP 90/30, HR 140, RR 32, T 39.6°C. Scattered rales with dullness. III/VI systolic murmur over the tricuspid area. Cold and cyanotic extremities. Elevated Lkcs with left shift. Positive blood culture with S. aureus.

A: Intravenous drug abusers are prone to develop infective endocarditis especially of the tricuspid valve. The vegetations on this valve usually embolize to the lungs, creating microabscesses with resultant pneumonitis. These vegetations are most commonly infected with Staphylococcus aureus, Pseudomonas aeruginosa, and enterococcal species. Further definition of the murmur and size of the vegetation is indicated with echocardiogram or transesophageal echocardiogram (TEE). S. aureus in these patients is usually sensitive to nafcillin. When the organism is sensitive to nafcillin, gentamicin should be continued for approximately two weeks for a synergistic effect then discontinued. Nafcillin should be continued for a full four-to-six-week course depending on lesion size, location, embolization, and organism sensitivity. The organism should be saved for testing of serum bactericidal titers. Valvulotomy is not usually performed unless fever or bacteremia persists despite adequate antibiotics.

P: One should begin nafcillin 2 g IV q4h plus gentamicin 120 mg IV q8h, and obtain culture and sensitivities of the organism. TEE should be used to evaluate the size of the vegetation and valvular obstruction. Monitor vital signs, cough, shaking chills, chest examination, characteristics of murmur, Lkcs, blood cultures, serial TEEs, BUN, SCr, urine output, serum bactericidal titers, and serum gentamicin concentrations.

Problem 3. Viral Hepatitis

S: Skin has turned yellow and urine has turned dark. JS is an intravenous drug abuser.

O: Scleral icterus. Tenderness in the RUO. Jaundiced skin. T Bili 335.16 (19.6), D Bili 174.42, (10.2), AST 208.75 (12.500), ALT 254.15 (15.220), Alk Phos 21.46 (1285), GGTP 19.15 (1147), and LDH 17.51 (1048).

A: Patient is a candidate for both hepatitis B and alcoholic hepatitis; however, the enzyme pattern is indicative of severe hepatocellular injury. Drug therapy is not effective for these types of hepatitis.

P: One should obtain viral hepatitis panel, and monitor vital signs, scleral icterus, jaundice, abdominal pain, bilirubin, ALT, AST, GGTP, Alk Phos, and LDH.

Problem 4. Anemia

S: None.

O: No blood on rectal examination. LDH 18 (1048), Hb 5.34 (8.6), Hct 0.258 (25.8), MCV 78 (78), reticulocyte count 0.10 (10), and platelet count 35×10^9 (35×10^3).

A: The patient is anemic but has no evidence of gross blood loss. The reticulocyte count is high with a low MCV. This indicates increased Erc destruction or loss. In this septic patient, disseminated intravascular coagulation (DIC) is a distinct possibility, especially with a decreased platelet count. Increased Erc destruction should cause an elevation of LDH with $LDH_1 > LDH_2$; however, hepatic disease will mask this due to elevations in LDH_5.

P: One should obtain values for PT, aPTT, fibrin degradation products, fibrinogen, and LDH isoenzymes. Type and cross-match two units of fresh-frozen plasma and packed Ercs, but hold them in reserve. The peripheral smear should be investigated for anisocytosis. Monitor Hb, Hct, platelet count, PT, aPTT, stools, and other sites for bleeding.

QUESTIONS FOR CASE 9

1. This patient is hypoalbuminemic probably due somewhat to malnutrition, but mainly due to sepsis. How are his vascular hemodynamics altered from normal levels?

2. What is this patient's absolute neutrophil count? What is meant by a "shift to the left"?
3. Why does this patient's enzyme pattern indicate viral hepatitis and not alcoholic hepatitis
4. What is this patient's corrected reticulocyte count? How does this predict increased Erc destruction?
5. It does not appear that this patient has bled extensively, but the platelet count is low. At what platelet count is clinically important bleeding a potential problem?

CASE 10

CC: CF is a 71-year-old male with a 5-year history of chronic myelogenous leukemia who presents to his medical oncologist with complaints of weakness and fatigue.

Past Medical History

Diagnosed with CML in 1990
Hypertension × 15 years
Mild, acute myocardial infarct in 1981

Medications

Busulfan 4mg p.o. daily
Furosemide 20mg p.o. daily
Aspirin 81 mg p.o. daily
Multiple vitamins 1 p.o. daily

Allergies

Penicillin

Physical Examination

GEN: Thin, frail-appearing male in no distress
VS: BP 130/82, supine; 110/65 standing; HR 128, RR 32, T 37.0°C, Wt 62 Kg, Ht 178 cm
HEENT: Bruised right cheek, dentures appear to be ill-fitting
CHEST: Scattered rales with dullness to percussion throughout
COR: RRR, nl S1, S2
ABD: Soft, nontender, no masses
GU: WNL
Rect: (-) for blood on stool guaiac
EXT: Full range of motion, some edema in the lower extremities
SKIN: WNL
NEURO: Oriented x 3

Results of Laboratory Tests

Na 138 (138)			
K 4.0 (4.0)	Hgb 10 (10)	Blasts 8%	Alk Phos 1.8 (110)
CL 102 (102)	Retic 2.6 (26)	AST 0.58 (35)	Alb 31 (3.1)
BUN 12 (12)	MCV 84 (84)	ALT 0.7 (42)	T Bili 18 (1)
CR 71 (0.7)	Lkcs 3×10^9	LDH 1.6 (100)	Erythropoietin level 150

Chest radiography: consistent with pulmonary fibrosis

Cardiac ejection fraction: < 35% on the left

Problem List

1. Busulfan-induced pulmonary fibrosis
2. Anemia (normocytic) with fatigue and shortness of breath
3. H/O Myocardial Infarction
4. Coronary Artery Disease
5. Orthostatic Hypotension (probably anemia induced)
6. Chronic Myelogenous Leukemia (stable disease)

Problem 1. Busulfan-induced Pulmonary Fibrosis

S: No complaints.

O: Chest radiography consistent with pulmonary fibrosis; busulfan is known to cause pulmonary fibrosis.

A: Even though CF has no complaints, it is likely that his pulmonary fibrosis will worsen with continued use of busulfan.

P: One should discontinue busulfan, and begin either hydroxyurea 500mg p.o. daily or α-interferon 3-9 MU sq daily. One should have CF return to clinic in one month to check blood counts and repeat chest radiography.

Problem 2. Anemia (normocytic)

S: CF is complaining of fatigue and shortness of breath. Signs of bruising may indicate internal blood loss.

O: Postural hypotension, Hgb 9, reticulocyte count 2.6, MCV 84, erythropoietin level 150 mU/mL, and HR 128.

A: CF is probably suffering from anemia of chronic disease or anemia of cancer. Stool guaiac was negative; however, one may want to consider endoscopy to rule out blood loss. In light of other normal blood counts, it would not be wise to perform bone marrow biopsy at present to look for bone marrow disorder. CF has symptomatic anemia and with a low erythropoietin level he is a candidate for erythropoietin.

P: One should begin erythropoietin 100 U/kg sq TIW, monitor Hgb in four weeks, and titrate dose to Hgb increase of > 1gm/dL over four weeks. If Hgb were not to increase at least 1gm/dl with a dosage increase after four weeks, one should check ferritin level. If ferritin level were normal, one should increase erythropoietin again. Continue to monitor blood pressure; if blood pressure were to remain low, one should consider discontinuing furosemide. If blood pressure were to increase, consider thrombosis effect of erythropoietin as a contributing factor. Erythropoietin may cause an increase in blood pressure secondary to a too rapid increase in hemoglobin.

Problem 3. H/O Myocardial Infarction

S: Fatigue.

O: Ankle swelling.

A: It is important to prevent future MIs through continued BP control, aspirin prophylaxis, and control of coronary artery disease.

P: One should treat coronary artery disease, continue aspirin, and continue BP monitoring and control.

Problem 4. Coronary Artery Disease

S: Fatigue, shortness of breath.

O: Ankle swelling, cardiac ejection fraction: < 35% (on the left), H/O MI.

A: Even though CF has no subjective complaints of CAD, he is at risk for vessel closure with poor left-sided ejection fraction.

P: Percutaneous transluminal coronary angioplasty should be performed to improve vessel patency. CF should have lipid status evaluated. All preventative measures to decrease his risks for furthering his CAD should be employed.

Problem 5. Orthostatic Hypotension

S: None.

O: BP 130/82 supine, 110/65 standing, ankle swelling, HR 128.

A: CF has moderate orthostatic hypotension, probably anemia-induced.

P: One should treat underlying anemia and consider discontinuing furosemide if blood pressure were not to improve.

QUESTIONS FOR CASE 10

1. The medical oncologist takes CF off of busulfan and begins α-interferon 3MU SQ daily. In reviewing this new medication with the patient, what side effects would you warn him about?
2. What factors are contributing to this patient's anemia? How would you treat and monitor the anemia?
3. Is CF a candidate for abciximab (ReoPro®) during coronary angioplasty? Why or why not?

CASE 11

CC: SD is a 48-year-old, obese, depressed female who has adult-onset diabetes. She came to the ambulatory care clinic with the chief complaint of intense right arm pain, which began after she fell trying to get out of the bathtub. She also complained of having a bad cold that began two days ago.

Past Medical History

Diabetes was diagnosed 10 years ago. SD monitors her blood glucose three times a week. She has been depressed for two months after gaining 10 kg on a "lose-weight-quick" diet.

Medication History

Chlorpropamide 250 mg p.o. b.i.d.
Phenelzine 15 mg p.o. t.i.d.

Allergies

NKDA

Social History

Tobacco - neg
Alcohol - neg

Physical Examination

GEN: Obese, depressed female who is experiencing se-
vere pain
VS: BP 135/85, HR 70, T 37.0°C, Wt 101 kg, Ht 160
cm
HEENT: Nasal congestion
CHEST: Clear to A&P
ABD: Obese, soft, nontender
GU: WNL
RECTAL: WNL
EXT: Right forearm swollen, red, and warm; otherwise
unremarkable
NEURO: Normal

Results of Laboratory Tests

Glu 8.3 (150)
UA ketones: neg
Glucose: neg
Radiography: Fractured right ulnar

Problem List

1. Diabetes
2. Cold/congestion
3. Depressed
4. Fractured arm

QUESTIONS FOR CASE 11

1. What antidepressant would you recommend for SD if you
were concerned that she might try to commit suicide by
ingesting an overdose of medication?
2. Are there any OTC products that SD could use to help her
lose weight?
3. If SD were allergic to codeine, what alternative analgesic
could be prescribed?
4. Can SD take cold products containing antihistamines?

CASE 12

CC: TE is a 55-year-old female who complains of short
of breath (SOB), cough, nausea, jitters, and insomnia.

Past Medical History

She has a long history of asthma that is often poorly controlled,
with many past ER admissions for asthma attacks.

Medication History

Aminophylline 30 mg/hr IV continuous infusion (started 32
hrs ago)

Erythromycin 500 mg IV q6h
Tobramycin 80 mg q8h (30-min infusion)
Metaproterenol 5% solution 0.3 ml in 2.5 ml saline by nebu-
lizer
Methylprednisolone 125 mg IVP every morning
O_2 2 liter/min BNC

Social History

Nonsmoker

Physical Examination

GEN: Well-developed, well-nourished female suffering
from SOB and increasingly severe nausea and
jitters
VS: BP 135/80, HR 125, T 39.0°C, Wt 72 kg, Ht
162.5 cm
HEENT: Chest: labored respirations, wheezing, rhonchi,
bilateral rales; chest radiography: bilateral infil-
trates
COR: Tachycardia (120 beats/min)
ABD: Soft, nontender, with no mass or organomegaly
GU: WNL
RECTAL: WNL
EXT: WNL
NEURO: Oriented to time, place, and person; cranial
nerves intact; normal deep tendon reflexes

Results of Laboratory Tests

Lkcs 15.6×10⁹ (15,600)
SCr 88.4 (1.0 mg/dl)
ABG pH 7.45 Po₂ 61, Pco₂ 31, O₂ sat 91%

Serum Drug Concentrations
Theophylline 172 μmol/liter (31 μg/ml) (32 hrs
post start of infusion)
Tobramycin peak: 4.7 μg/ml (1.2 hrs postdose)
Trough: 0.7 μg/ml (7.7 hrs postdose)

Problem List

1. Asthma
2. Pneumonia
3. Theophylline toxicity
4. Subtherapeutic tobramycin concentrations

Problem 3. Theophylline Toxicity

S: TE complains of nausea, jitters, and insomnia.
O: TE has a high theophylline concentration, and the physical
examination demonstrates tachycardia.
A: TE suffers from theophylline toxicity, and the dose should
be reduced to achieve a SDCss of 83.25 nmol/liter (15
μg/ml.) The high theophylline concentration is secondary
in part to the concomitant administration of erythromycin,
which inhibits the clearance of theophylline.
P: One should calculate how long to hold the dose and a
new IV continuous-infusion administration rate to achieve
the target theophylline concentration:
Hold dose 8 hr
New dose 15 mg/hr

One should hold the aminophylline infusion for 8 hrs and check theophylline SDC. If the rate were below 99.9 nmol/liter (18 μg/ml), one should restart aminophylline infusion at 15 mg/hr.

Problem 4. Subtherapeutic Tobramycin Concentrations

S: TE continues to have SOB.

O: TE has bilateral rales, infiltrates on chest radiography, and high Lkcs and temperature.

A: Broad-spectrum coverage is implemented to treat the pneumonia, but the aminoglycoside therapy is subtherapeutic. The tobramycin dose should be adjusted to achieve steady-state peak and trough SDCs of 8 and 1 μg/ml, respectively.

P: One should calculate the new dose, half-life, and steady-state peak and trough using the Sawchuk/Zaske equations. Calculated pharmacokinetic parameters include the following:

$t\frac{1}{2}$ = 2.37 hr

V = 14.3 liter

C_{max} 5.8 mg/L

C_{min} 0.6 mg/L

New estimated dose and interval:

7.6 hr

Dose 110.9 mg (based on interval of 8 hr)

Recommendation:

  110 mg q8h

Predicted peak and trough:

C_{ss-max} = 7.9 mg/L

C_{ss-min} = 0.9 mg/L

Tobramycin dose should be increased to 110 mg q8h and one should check peak and trough concentrations around the third dose of this new regimen.

Problem 1. Asthma

S: On admission, she had moderately severe shortness of breath, but presently she complains only of mild shortness of breath.

O: Past ER evaluations demonstrated increased respiratory rate with wheezing and use of accessory muscles for breathing. On this occasion, the patient had a FEV_1 (forced expiratory volume in 1 sec) < 30% of predicted, requiring admission to the hospital and IV aminophylline, β-agonist, and steroids. Subsequently, the patient improved, and the most recent FEV1 was 70% of predicted.

A: TE had acute asthma exacerbation that improved with aggressive therapy.

P: One should maintain present therapy until shortness of breath completely resolves.

Problem 2. Pneumonia

S: TE complains of shortness of breath and chills.

O: TE has bilateral infiltrates on radiography, increased temperature, and increased Lkcs.

A: TE suffers from acute asthma attack brought on by the onset of pneumonia.

P: One should continue treatment with erythromycin and tobramycin.

QUESTIONS FOR CASE 12

1. At high SDCs, it is not uncommon for theophylline to exhibit nonlinear elimination. If TE's SDC of 172 nmol/liter (31 μg/ml) were in the range of nonlinearity, what error would be incurred in our calculation of a new dose using equation (1.38)?

2. How would you determine whether this patient has clinical toxicity?

3. If TE had a theophylline SDC of 88.8 nmol/liter (16 μg/ml) while receiving 20 mg/hr of aminophylline (not on concomitant erythromycin), what dose and interval of TheoDur would you recommend?

4. How would the SDCs compare between the constant IV infusion and the TheoDur 200 mg given every 12 hrs?

CASE 13

CC: ST is a 23-year-old female who presented to the ER at 3:15 AM after taking an unknown number of adult acetaminophen tablets at 1:50 AM that morning in a suicide attempt. Samples for baseline laboratory tests, including a plasma acetaminophen level, have been drawn, and she has been lavaged.

Past Medical History

ST has been in good general health.

Medication History

Ortho Novum 1/50 1 q.d.

Allergies

Developed a rash while taking ampicillin

Physical Examination

GEN: Well-developed, well-nourished white female who is emotionally upset

VS: BP 132/84, HR 84, RR 22, T 37.0°C, Wt 72 kg, Ht 173 cm

HEENT: WNL

COR: WNL

CHEST: Clear to percussion and auscultation

ABD: Soft with no masses or tenderness

GU: WNL

RECT: WNL

EXT: WNL

NEURO: Oriented X three, cranial nerves intact, and deep tendon reflexes normal

Results of Laboratory Tests

Acetaminophen 3182 μmol/liter (481 μg/ml) approximately 2 hrs postingestion)

ALT 0.41 (25)
AST 0.47 (28)
LDH 2.92 (175)
PT 12 sec

Problem List

1. Acetaminophen overdose

QUESTIONS FOR CASE 13

1. The 4-hr plasma acetaminophen level is 1687 μmol/liter (255 μg/ml). Is this a toxic level? Should the N-acetylcysteine be continued?
2. Thirty minutes after administration of the loading dose of N-acetylcysteine, the patient vomits. The vomitus has a strong sulfide smell. Should the dose be repeated? What can be done to prevent further vomiting?
3. Is cimetidine effective as an acetaminophen antidote?
4. If ST were pregnant, would her fetus be at risk of developing hepatic injury? Is pregnancy a contraindication to using N-acetylcysteine?
5. How does the time between the acetaminophen overdose and administration of N-acetylcysteine affect the outcome?

CASE 14

CC: SL, a 57-year-old woman presented to the urgent care center with a history of a gradual onset of SOB over the previous 18 hrs. Prior to her arrival at the urgent care center, she had no respiratory complaints. She now has dyspnea at rest.

Past Medical History

Type II diabetes mellitus for 10 years
Coronary artery disease for 6 years

Medication History

Verapamil SR 120 mg b.i.d.
Glyburide 10 mg b.i.d.
Nitroglycerin 0.4 mg SL p.r.n.

Family History

Mother and grandmother had diabetes mellitus

Social History

The patient smokes one pack per day and has done so for 20 years

Physical Examination

GEN: The patient is in moderate respiratory distress
VS: BP 132/68, HR 110, RR 28, T 37.2°C, Wt 79.2 kg, Ht 165 cm

HEENT: Funduscopic examination reveals mild nonproliferative retinopathy.
CHEST: Bibasilar rales
COR: NL S1 & S2, +S3 with II/VI systolic murmur heard loudest at the LSB
EXT: 3+ pretibial and ankle edema

Results of Laboratory Tests

Na 120 (120)	AST 6.67 (400)
K 4.2 (4.2)	LDH 30.84 (1850)
Cl 92 (92)	Alb 38 (3.8)
HCO3 25 (25)	T Bili 21 (1.2)
BUN 12.5 (35)	D Bili 5 (0.3)
CR 140 (1.6)	Glu 9.0 (162)
Hct 0.327 (32.7)	CK 1.83 (110)
Hgb 109 (10.9)	Chol 7.55 (292)
Lkcs 0.92×10^9 (0.92×10^3)	

Chest radiography: cardiomegaly, fluffy infiltrates with vascular redistribution

Lkcs differential: 0.60 segs, 0.38 lymphs, 0.02 monos

Arterial blood gases on room air: pH 7.48, Paco$_2$ 32, Pao$_2$ 52

ECG: NSR, rate 75, Q waves in leads I & AVL, and ST-segment depression in V1-V3. Q waves are new since previous ECG two months ago.

CK isoenzymes: MM 1.83, MB 0, BB 0

LDH isoenzymes: LDH$_1$ 17.67

LDH$_2$ 11.84

LDH$_3$ 0.83

LDH$_4$ 0.25

LDH$_5$ 0.25

Problem List

1. Type II diabetes mellitus
2. Coronary artery disease
3. Congestive heart failure
4. Silent myocardial infarction
5. Hypercholesterolemia

CASE 15

CC: AA is a 37-year-old female who has epilepsy and is an alcoholic. Two weeks prior to her present clinic visit, she began treatment for alcoholism. She also began taking cimetidine for a duodenal ulcer at that time. Today, she complains of ataxia and is experiencing nystagmus.

Past Medical History

AA has had epilepsy for eight years. She has been without seizures for six months. She has experienced multiple episodes of gastritis over the past three years.

Medication History

Phenytoin 300 mg p.o. q. HS
Valproic acid 250 mg p.o. q.i.d.

Disulfiram 500 mg p.o. q.d.
Cimetidine 800 mg p.o. q. HS

Allergies
NKDA

Social History
Tobacco - 1 PPD for 15 years
Alcohol - stopped two weeks ago; 1 pint whiskey per day prior to that. She began drinking alcohol as a teenager.

Physical Examination
GEN: Cachexic female not in acute distress
VS: BP 120/80, HR 60, RR, T 37.0°C, Wt 50 kg, Ht 165 cm
HEENT: Nystagmus
CHEST: Clear
ABD: Soft, nontender
GU: Normal
RECTAL: Guaiac-negative
EXT: Normal
NEURO: Ataxia

Results of Laboratory Tests
DPH 162.5 μmol/liter 41 (μg/ml)
Valproic acid 492 μmol/liter (71 μg/ml)

Problem List
1. Alcoholism
2. Epilepsy
3. Duodenal ulcer

CASE 16
CC: RM is a 32-year-old female who was found unconscious after ingesting an unknown amount of desipramine and alcohol. A suicide note was discovered by her side. On presentation to the emergency department she developed seizures that were treated with diazepam and hypotension that was treated initially with intravenous fluids. She was intubated and placed on a ventilator; lavage was performed and a dose of activated charcoal and a cathartic was administered.

Past Medical History
RM has a history of depression and has attempted suicide twice in the past five years.

Medical History
Desipramine 200 mg/day

Social History
Tobacco - negative
Alcohol - social drinker

Physical Examination
GEN: Well-developed, well-nourished female, unconscious
VS: BP 70 systolic, HR 140, RR 12 and shallow (prior to intubation and placement on ventilator), T 37.0°C, Wt 58 kg, Ht 163 cm
HEENT: Pupils 5 mm and minimally reactive to light
COR: WNL
CHEST: Clear to auscultation and percussion
ABD: Diminished bowel sounds
GU: WNL
RECTAL: WNL
EXT: WNL
NEURO: Comatose, unresponsive to painful stimuli, DTRs diminished

Results of Laboratory Tests

ABGs on presentation: pH 7.2, P_{CO_2} 6.7 kPa (50 mmHg), P_{O_2} 9.3 kPa (70 mmHg)
After intubation (FiO_2 25%): pH 7.38, P_{CO_2} 6.7 kPa (40 mmHg), P_{O_2} 13.1 kPa (98 mmHg)
ECG: Sinus tachycardia, PR 0.21 sec, QRS 0.16 sec, RBBB
Blood alcohol level: 33 mmol/liter (150 mg/100 ml)

Problem List
1. History of depression
2. Overdose of desipramine and ethanol

FLUIDS AND ELECTROLYTES AND NUTRITION

CASE 17

CC: HR is a 56-year-old male brought to the emergency room after being found unconscious at home. Ten minutes later, the neighbor who called the paramedics arrives with HR's suicide note, an empty bottle of aspirin, and an unopened container of phenobarbital 30 mg tablets from HR's medicine cabinet.

Past Medical History

Unknown seizure disorder

Social History

The neighbor reports that HR began to drink heavily after the death of his wife three months ago and has also lost at least 18 kg (40 lbs) in that time.

Past Surgical History

The neighbor says that HR had some sort of "brain operation" 10 years ago, but has no further information.

Medication History

Phenobarbital 30 mg p.o. q.i.d.
No other information available

Allergies

No information

Physical Examination

GEN: Thin, well-developed man who moans when shaken, but who is otherwise unresponsive
VS: BP 130/70, HR 100, T 37.1°C, RR 25, Wt 60 kg (132 lbs), Ht 188 cm (6'2")
HEENT: Dry mucous membranes, sunken eyes; well-healed craniotomy scar
EXT: Cool fingers and toes, dry skin, decreased skin turgor without tenting, slightly depressed reflexes
Remainder of the physical examination is normal

Results of Laboratory Tests

Na 145 (145)	Hct 0.53 (53)	AST 0.3 (18)	Glu 5 (90)
K 4 (4)	Hgb 160 (16)	ALT 0.3 (17)	Ca total 2.5 (10)
Cl 107 (107)	Lkcs 5.5 × 10⁹ (5.5 × 10³)	LDH 2 (150)	PO₄ 1.3 (4)
HCO₃ 15 (15)	MCV 83 (83)	Alk Phos 1 (60)	Mg 1 (2)
BUN 10 (27)		Alb 40 (4.0)	
CR 120 (1.3)		T Bili 9 (0.5)	

Urinalysis: WNL
Chest x-ray: WNL
ECG: WNL
ABGs: pH 7.25, Po2 98, Pco₂ 35
Toxicology Screen:
　Salicylate level 0.45 g/liter (45 mg/dl)
　Ethanol level 2.5 g/liter (0.25%)
　Phenobarbital level 0
Urine output 15 ml/hr
Stool: guaiac-negative

PROBLEM LIST

1. Seizure disorder
2. Suicide attempt
3. Metabolic acidosis
4. Respiratory alkalosis
5. Dehydration
6. Electrolyte abnormalities
7. Malnutrition

CASE 17 SOAP NOTES

Problem 2. Suicide Attempt

S: Suicide note; history of recent weight loss.
O: Salicylate level 0.45 g/liter (45 mg/dl); ethanol level 2.5 g/liter (0.25%).
A: This appears to be a suicide attempt that would have been successful if HR had not been found by his neighbor.
P: One should take precautions so that HR will not attempt suicide again. He will need psychiatric evaluation/counseling and a follow-up plan developed prior to discharge from the hospital.

Problem 3. Metabolic Acidosis

S: Somnolence.
O: pH 7.25, HCO₃ 15 mmol/liter (15 mEq/liter), Pco₂ 35, RR 25, and anion gap 23 mmol/liter (23 mEq/liter).
A: This is primary metabolic acidosis with some respiratory compensation and positive anion gap. The abnormal anions present are salicylate (level is 0.45 g/liter) and lactate (inferred from ethanol level of 2.5 g/liter). Serum bicarbonate level is low as the result of increased renal excretion of HCO₃

to maintain electrical neutrality. This is not a true bicarbonate deficit but rather a compensatory response to accumulated salicylate and lactate anions. Metabolism and excretion of these substances results in correction of the plasma pH as HCO_3 is regenerated by the kidneys. HR has good hepatic and renal function, so the acidosis should resolve spontaneously over the next 3–4 hrs, along with improvement in level of consciousness. At the moment, HR is hemodynamically stable and has good oxygenation; his plasma pH is above 7.2 and salicylate and ethanol levels are not life-threatening. One should not give IV Na bicarbonate to rapidly correct plasma pH or alkalinize urine; the risk of causing metabolic alkalosis outweighs any benefit. If pH were to decrease to below 7.2, one should calculate a dose and give $NaHCO_3$ (refer to Chapter 8 for this therapy). One should also not begin hemodialysis to remove salicylate ions from the blood; this procedure is invasive and HR is currently hemodynamically stable.

P: One should give a total of 100 g of activated charcoal mixed with 1 liter of water in 300–350 ml increments by gastric lavage to remove any remaining aspirin from the stomach. A saline cathartic, such as 30–45 ml of 20% sorbitol, is also indicated to speed elimination of aspirin from the lower GI tract. Recheck ABGs in 1 hr, and salicylate and ethanol levels in 3–4 hrs. Monitor vital signs and mental status every 15 min until pH is > 7.3 or HR revives.

Problem 4. Respiratory Alkalosis

S: None.

O: P_{CO_2} 35, RR 25.

A: HR has respiratory alkalosis secondary to central nervous system stimulation by salicylates and as a compensation for metabolic acidosis. Although HR does have an increased respiratory rate, oxygenation is good and he is not showing signs of impending respiratory failure. His breathing rate and P_{CO_2} will normalize as his salicylate level decreases and plasma pH normalizes.

P: One should monitor RR and ABGs.

Problem 5. Dehydration

S: Dry mucous membranes, sunken eyes, cool extremities, decreased skin turgor.

O: Hct 0.53 (53%), BUN/Cr ratio >20, and urine output (UO) 15 ml/hr.

A: HR has dehydration (a total body salt and water deficit), probably as the result of decreased intake of fluids, but no signs of hypovolemia (tachycardia, orthostatic changes). The elevated BUN/Cr ratio, dry mucous membranes, and sunken eyes indicate a decrease in the volume of interstitial and intracellular compartments. His hematocrit is slightly elevated, UO is < 0.5 ml/kg/hr, and extremities are cool; these findings indicate some decrease in the size of the intravascular fluid compartment and compromised whole body perfusion but are not severe enough to cause cardiopulmonary difficulties. The first goal of therapy is to normalize HR's intravascular volume to prevent ischemic injury to his kidneys and other tissues. This involves rapid replacement with fluid that is isotonic with plasma at an infusion rate that increases UO to at least 0.5 ml/kg/hr. As HR is unconscious and is getting gastric lavage, this therapy will have to be given intravenously. The total amount of fluid to be given over the next 24 hrs is a combination of the amount needed to replace his current total body salt and water deficit along with his maintenance fluid and electrolyte requirement; for a person of HR's size, this will probably be 5–6 liters.

P: One should begin D5 lactated Ringer's solution IV at 250 ml/hr. In 1 hr, one should reassess the patient's status to see that UO is >30 ml/hr; if UO were to remain at or go below 15 ml/hr, increase the rate of D5LR to 300–500 ml/hr. D5LR is chosen because it contains less Na and Cl than NS—HR's serum Na and Cl are currently at the upper limits of normal—and lactate is converted to bicarbonate in the body. When UO is adequate and extremities are warm, adjust IV infusion rate to maintain perfusion. One should also check BP, HR, and UO hourly until HR is stable, and monitor serum Na, Cl, Cr, BUN, Hct, and warmth of extremities every 4–6 hrs.

Problem 6. Electrolyte Abnormalities

S: None.

O: Depressed reflexes, HCO_3 15 mmol/liter (15 mEq/liter), Ca 2.5 mmol/liter (10 mg/dl), and K 4 mmol/liter (4 mEq/liter).

A: The low HCO_3 is the result of decreased generation of bicarbonate by the kidneys. When the positive anion gap metabolic acidosis resolves, it will be normalized by bicarbonate manufactured in the kidneys. Serum potassium is currently within the normal range, but a compensation in acidosis is to shift potassium ions into the extracellular space in exchange for H^+ ions moved into the intracellular space; serum potassium decreases to 3.1 mmol/liter when the pH becomes 7.4. One should give potassium acetate 10 mmol/hr IV for 4 hr, recheck serum K level, and continue to give potassium to keep the serum level between 4 and 5 mmol/liter. With the pH at 7.25, the total serum calcium of 2.5 mmol/liter (10 mg/dl) "corrects" to an effective concentration of 3.2 mmol/liter (12.5 mg/dl). In acidosis, calcium is displaced from protein-binding sites by hydrogen ions. The "total" amount of calcium in the blood has remained the same, but the active, ionized concentration is increased by 0.42 mmol/liter (1.68 mg/dl) for each 0.1 decrease in plasma pH. HR's ionized calcium now is 1.76 mmol/liter (3.5 mEq/liter) and may be contributing to his mental status changes and depressed reflexes. The therapy for hypercalcemia now is correction of acidosis. When this is done, HR's ionized calcium will be 1.12 mmol/liter (2.2 mEq/liter). The incidence and severity of the mental status changes seen with hypercalcemia are not directly related to the serum concentration. If HR were to remain unresponsive when his ionized calcium, ethanol, and salicylate levels were normal, it would be necessary to lower his serum calcium by one of the methods discussed in Chapter 8.

Problem 1. Seizure Disorder

S: Phenobarbital tablets were prescribed for HR.

O: Craniotomy scar, phenobarbital level = 0.

A: The current state of unconsciousness does not appear to be the result of seizures because HR's EEG is normal. Because he had some kind of neurosurgical procedure 10 years ago, HR may have been given phenobarbital as treatment or prophylaxis for seizures, but one has no way of determining that now. When he regains consciousness, a medication history and possibly a neurology consultation will help to determine the value of reinstituting phenobarbital.

P: One should not begin any seizure prophylaxis while HR has altered mental status and no signs of seizure activity. Because his phenobarbital level is zero, HR will need to have loading and maintenance doses determined if therapy with phenobarbital were indicated. Assuming a bioavailability (F) of 100% and a volume of distribution (VD) of 0.7 liter/kg, HR's loading dose of phenobarbital to achieve a level of 20 mg/liter (the midpoint of the therapeutic range) is found by multiplying the VD by the desired serum concentration. At 60 kg, HR has a VD for Pb of 42 liters and will require 840 mg to reach a serum level of 20 mg/liter. HR has no significant renal or hepatic dysfunction; therefore, normal population parameters can be used to calculate the initial maintenance dose. Using a clearance (Cl) of 5.76 liter/day (from 0.096 liter/day/kg), a half-life ($t_{1/2}$) of 5 days, and a dosing interval of 1 day, HR's maintenance dose is 115 mg. Given practical considerations and the assumptions inherent in the PK equations, HR should receive 800 mg as a loading dose and 100 mg/day maintenance therapy. Before he is discharged, HR should be educated about the importance of taking his medications as prescribed.

Problem 7. Malnutrition

S: Thin, history of recent weight loss.

O: Albumin 40 g/liter (4 g/dl), 15–20 kg below ideal body weight for height.

A: HR has decreased fat stores, but the normal Alb level indicates that deficits in the visceral protein mass are mild. Nevertheless, intervention is indicated before significant malnutrition develops. If HR were not to improve in the next 24 hrs to the point that he could take in protein and calories at 30–40% above his basal energy expenditure, he should be started on tube feeding. Parenteral nutrition is not indicated because HR has a functioning GI tract and his recent weight loss seems to indicate acute depression and anorexia since his wife's death.

P: One should add thiamine 100 mg and a multivitamin preparation to HR's first liter of D5LR; his alcoholism and recent weight loss put him at significant risk for vitamin deficiencies. Based on his age, sex, height, and weight, HR needs 1800–2000 kcal/day to begin to repair his current deficit. He does not require a predigested tube-feeding formula, but the tube itself should be beyond the pyloric sphincter because altered mental status increases the risk of aspiration of stomach contents. HR should be evaluated for iron and folic acid deficiency by means of a red blood cell smear; the MCV of 83 fl may be masking mixed anemia. Consultation with a dietitian is important before HR is discharged.

QUESTIONS FOR CASE 17

1. HR had been on phenobarbital 30 mg p.o. q.i.d. Why do you suggest giving 100 mg once daily?

2. How do you know that HR's fluid requirement over the next 24 hrs will be 5–6 liters? Why should you begin therapy at 250 ml/hr?

3. HR's hematocrit is slightly elevated. Why is an anemia workup and vitamin repletion indicated?

4. It is now 24 hrs after admission and HR's serum Alb level has decreased to 31 g/liter (3.1 g/dl). Does this alter your initial goal of 1800–2000 kcal/day for nutritional repletion?

5. At the same time, salicylate and ethanol levels have decreased to zero, EEG remains normal, and HR's pH is 7.4, but he remains unresponsive. The total serum calcium level is 2.5 mmol/liter (10 mg/dl); is specific treatment for hypercalcemia indicated?

CASE 18

CC: JR is a 31-year-old male who sustained a severe closed-head injury following a motor vehicle accident. No other significant injuries were present. He underwent an emergent left parietal craniotomy for removal of a large subdural hematoma. He had an intraventricular catheter placed for monitoring intracranial pressure. Soon after admission, JR developed an ileus; thus, he needed to receive nutritional support by the parenteral route. He has received 9 days of parenteral nutrition and his physicians state that his bowel function is now returning. They would like to begin long-term enteral nutrition support in light of prolonged neurologic recovery.

Past Medical History

None

Medication History

Ticarcillin IV 3 g q4h

Phenytoin 200 mg IV q 12 hrs

Heparin 5000 units SQ q 12 hrs

Ranitidine 150 mg/250 ml NS @ 10 ml/hr

Acetaminophen suppositories 650 mg q 6h prn temp > 38.3°C

Parenteral nutrition final concentrations (6% Novamine, 20% dextrose, 3% intralipid) @ 125 ml/hr

Allergies

No known drug allergies

Physical Examination

GEN: Well-developed, well-nourished male in no apparent distress

VS: BP 116/76, HR 85, RR 20, T 37.0°C, Wt 100 kg, Ht 194 cm

HEENT: Craniotomy site healing well, no visible redness, minimal swelling and tenderness
COR: Normal S1 and S2, no murmurs, rubs, or gallops
CHEST: Clear to auscultation and percussion
ABD: Soft, nontender, nondistended, no masses or organomegaly, positive bowel sounds
GU: WNL
RECTAL: WNL
NEURO: Withdraws to pain, no verbal rsponse, no eye opening

Results of Laboratory Tests

Na 144 (144)	AST 0.3 (18)	Glu 7.8 (140)
K 4.5 (4.5)	ALT 0.32 (20)	Ca 2.22 (8.9)
Cl 100 (100)	LDH 1.0 (60)	PO₄ 1.25 (3.9)
HCO₃ 28 (28)	Alk Phos 0.9 (56)	Mg 0.9 (2.2)
BUN 6.0 (17)	Alb 36 (3.6)	Uric Acid 190 (3.2)
CR 80 (0.9)	T Bili 12 (0.7)	TG 0.96 (85)
	T. Prot 65 (6.5)	

PROBLEM LIST

1. Severe closed-head injury
2. Ileus
3. Nutrition

Problem 2. Ileus

S: None.
O: JR developed an ileus, probably related to acute head injury and trauma. JR now has positive bowel sounds.
A: JR's bowel function is returning.
P: One should continue to monitor the patient.

Problem 3. Nutrition

S: None.
O: JR has received parenteral nutrition for 9 days, and his physicians now want him changed to enteral nutrition. He has positive bowel sounds, and has minimal gastric output.
A: JR will require long-term enteral nutrition because he cannot take nutrition by mouth.
P: One should schedule JR for a percutaneous endoscopic gastrostomy (PEG), and begin enteral nutrition 6 hrs after placement of the PEG. JR's nonprotein calorie and protein goals while hospitalized are as follows:
BEE = 66.473 + 13.7516(100) + 5.0033(194) − 6.755(31) = 2203 kcal/day
Nonprotein caloric goal: 1.4 × BEE = 3084 kcal/day
Protein goal: 1.8 g protein/kg/day × 100 kg = 180 g protein/day
JR receives 180 g protein/day and 2940 kcal/day (1.33 × BEE) from the PN solution. JR should be started on a standard enteral regimen @ 25 ml/hr and increased by 25 ml/hr/day to a goal rate as tolerated. The hospital has Jevity® (44.4 g protein/liter, 1.06 kcal/ml) on its formulary as the standard enteral product. JR should be started on Jevity with 20 g protein powder supplement/liter, which will provide 3053 kcal/day and 185 protein/day at a goal rate of 120 ml/day.

Problem 1. Severe Closed-head Injury

S: None.
O: JR received a severe closed-head injury to the face 12 days ago. He has had a craniotomy for removal of a subdural hematoma. His Glasgow Coma Scale (GCS) Score was 6 on admission, and is presently 8–9.
A: His neurologic condition is stable and slowly improving.
P: One should consult physical therapy for assistance with rehabilitation, and continue to monitor for improvements in neurologic function.

QUESTIONS FOR CASE 18

1. JR is now receiving his full rate of enteral nutrition. His 24-hr urine collection results are UUN 1000 mg/dl, urine volume 2600 ml/24 hr. You should assume that he received his full rate of prescribed enteral feeding; what is his nitrogen balance? Does his enteral formula need to be changed to attempt to achieve nitrogen balance, or has he attained it already?
2. JR develops hyponatremia and his laboratory parameters are consistent with the syndrome of inappropriate antidiuretic hormone (SIADH) secretion. What changes, if any, can be made in the enteral regimen?
3. Why should JR be changed to enteral nutrition support if he were tolerating parenteral feedings without problems?

CASE 19

CC: CB is a 36-year-old woman who presents to the ER complaining of weakness, extreme fatigue, and intermittent fevers to 38.5°C. She says that she has been consuming only orange juice, ice cream, and Mylantà for the past three days to help her nausea and vomiting. She had not taken any of her medications and many of her co-workers have recently been sick with the flu.

Past Medical History

Polycystic kidney disease
CB's last clinic visit was six days ago. At that time, serum creatinine was 270 μmol/liter (3 mg/dl), BUN was 17 mmol/liter (46 mg/dl), and all electrolytes were normal.

Medication History

Al(OH)₃ 1 cap q.i.d.
Calcitriol 100 μg daily
Calcium carbonate 1250 mg (500 mg of elemental Ca) q.i.d.
Al(OH)₃/Mg(OH)₂ with simethicone 30 ml t.i.d./p.r.n.

Allergies

NKDA

Physical Examination

GEN: Thin woman who responds appropriately to questions but is quite lethargic

VS: BP 140/85, HR 85, T 38.2°C, RR 20 Urine output 20 ml/hr (normal finding for CB) Wt 53 kg (usual weight 55 kg) Ht 173 cm (5'8")

HEENT: Dry, cool skin, parched lips, and sunken eyes

CHEST: Few rales, no rhonchi

EXT: Cool hands and feet, slightly depressed reflexes, some peripheral muscle wasting

Remainder of the physical examination is normal

Results of Laboratory Tests

Na 132 (132)   Ca ionized 1.3 (2.6)
K 5.2 (5.2) PO_4 1.8 (5.6)
Cl 90 (90)   Mg 2 (4)
HCO_3 29 (29)   Alb 34 (3.4)
BUN 20 (57)
CR 280 (3.1)

PROBLEM LIST

1. Chronic renal insufficiency
2. Fever and GI disturbances of unknown origin
3. Dehydration
4. Electrolyte abnormalities
5. Malnutrition

CASE 19 SOAP NOTES
Problem 3. Dehydration

S: CB has a history of nausea, vomiting, fever, and decreased intake of food and fluids; she has cool hands and feet, and dry lips, skin, and eyes.

O: Na 132 mmol/liter (132 mEq/liter), Cl 90 mmol/liter (90 mEq/liter) HCO_3 29 mmol/liter (29 mEq/liter), 2-kg weight loss.

A: CB has dehydration without evidence of hypovolemia. Her hands and feet are slightly cool, but UO, BP, and heart rate are normal for her. It is extremely important to avoid hypovolemia in CB because a slight decrease in renal perfusion could precipitate complete renal shutdown.

P: One should give 3 liters of normal saline IV over the next 4–6 hrs. This will replace CB's salt and water deficits and give her a maintenance fluid requirement of 1200-1400 ml/day (insensible loss plus fixed UO of 480 ml/day). The slightly hypertonic solution is indicated because she has low Na and Cl values. One should check serum Na, Cl, and HCO_3 after the NS infusion, and monitor for correction of signs and symptoms of dehydration. Before she leaves the ER, one should tell CB to drink Gatoradè, bouillon, or canned soft drinks (good sources of sodium) rather than fruit juices. This should help to keep her serum sodium in the normal range without causing hyperkalemia again. One should also reinforce to CB the importance of keeping herself hydrated and tell her to return if she were to have trouble taking in (and keeping down) 1500–2000 ml in the next 24 hrs.

Problem 4. Electrolyte Abnormalities

S: CB has weakness, lethargy, and a history of taking in orange juice, ice cream, and antacid. She states that she has not taken calcitriol and $Al(OH)_3$ capsules for the past three days.

O: Na 132 (132), K 5.2 (5.2), Ca 1.3 (2.6), Cl 90 (90), HCO_3 29 (29), PO4 1.8 (5.6), and Mg 2 (4).

A: CB's electrolyte disturbances indicate the impact that minor changes in intake and output of fluids and electrolytes can have on a person with her degree of renal dysfunction. Her weakness and lethargy are attributable to low Na and high Mg and Ca levels. A reduction in fluid intake combined with fever and vomiting has given her hyponatremia, hypochloremia, and contraction alkalosis. A few days of consuming antacid and orange juice have resulted in hyperkalemia and hypermagnesemia. The combination of $CaCO_3$ and ice cream has been enough to cause hypercalcemia even though she has not been taking calcitriol. The calcitriol has continued to exert a hypercalcemic effect because its half-life is three to five days. She is exhibiting no adverse effects attributable to K of 5.2 mmol/liter (5.2 mEq/liter); therefore, discontinuing the orange juice is sufficient intervention at present. If she were to stop taking antacid and $CaCO_3$ tablets and were to avoid ice cream for the next few days, CB's Ca and Mg levels should also return to normal. After missing three days of $Al(OH)_3$, her serum PO_4 level is 1.8 mmol/liter (5.6 mg/dl), but this is not a problem. Hyperphosphatemia does not cause any hemodynamic problems, and the Ca/PO_4 product is not high enough to cause calcium deposition in soft tissue.

P: One should administer NS in combination with the recommendations about Gatorade, bouillon, and soft drinks to treat the dehydration; this should be enough to return and keep CB's Na, Cl, and HCO_3 levels in the normal ranges. One should check K, Mg, and Ca levels in 4–6 hrs, and monitor for resolution of the signs and symptoms of her electrolyte abnormalities. To treat hyperphosphatemia, one should instruct CB to take $Al(OH)_3$ as prescribed.

Problem 5. Malnutrition

S: Thin, weak, some muscle wasting.

O: Usual Wt = 55 kg (121 lb), Alb 34 g/liter (3.4 g/dl).

A: Renal insufficiency results in continuous metabolic stress that causes a daily protein loss approaching 1.5 g/kg. It also increases the need for calories to levels above those required by healthy individuals. "Renal failure" diets that restrict patients to a protein intake of 1 g/kg/day can add an iatrogenic component to protein malnutrition. CB is 8–10 kg (18–22 lb) below the ideal body weight for her height; this, combined with some muscle wasting and serum Alb 34 g/liter (3.4 g/dl), indicates a moderate degree of protein-calorie malnutrition.

P: CB's protein intake should be increased to 1.2–1.5 g/kg/day along a with total caloric intake that results in a weight gain of 0.5-1 kg (1-2 lb) per week.

Problem 1. Chronic Renal Insufficiency

S: History of polycystic kidney disease.

O: Cr 280 µmol/liter (3.1 mg/dl), BUN 20 mmol/liter (57 mg/dl)

A: CB's serum creatinine is stable, but situations that can decrease renal perfusion must be treated quickly. Even minor changes in perfusion can cause complete renal shut-down and necessitate hemodialysis.

P: One should reinforce to CB the importance of keeping herself well-hydrated and returning to the ER within 24 hrs when she has any trouble maintaining this level.

Problem 2. Fever and GI Disturbances of Unknown Origin

S: Weakness, lethargy, history of nausea and vomiting.

O: T 38.2°C.

A: The patient probably has influenza which was caught from co-workers. Self-medication with antacid has had no impact on the cause of CB's GI symptoms and is making her serum magnesium increase.

P: One should discontinue the antacid, and give acetamino-phen 650 mg q4-6h p.r.n. for treatment of fever. One should also suggest to CB that she get an influenza vaccine before the next flu season.

QUESTIONS FOR CASE 19

1. CB's repeat serum potassium level is 6 mmol/liter (6 mEq/liter) but cardiac function remains normal. Which treatment for hyperkalemia is indicated?

2. When told to take in more protein, CB is afraid her renal function will deteriorate and that she will then need hemo-dialysis. What is your response to these concerns?

3. CB's hematocrit result is 0.25 (25%). What are the likely nutritional deficiencies that can lead to anemia in CB?

4. After your discussion with CB about her risks of developing vitamin and mineral deficiencies, she asks you to recom-mend a vitamin supplement. What would you recommend?

5. CB will be taking calcitriol indefinitely unless she receives a kidney transplant. She asks for a listing of significant drug reactions or side effects associated with its long-term use. What would your response be?

CASE 20

CC: GM is a 45-year-old female who is being seen in the ambulatory care clinic today with a complaint of dry skin and skin patches that are scaling and itching.

Past Medical History

Peptic ulcer disease one year ago

Medication History

Famotidine 40 mg b.i.d.

Vitamin A 10,000 units, 5 caps q. AM & PM

Surbex-750 (multivitamin with minerals, without vitamin A or D).

Calcium carbonate 500 mg b.i.d.

Allergies

No known allergies

Physical Examination

GEN: Pale, thin female with complaints of being tired, chronic dermatitis, and loss of hair

VS: BP 120/80, HR 74, T 98.0°F, Wt 59 kg, Ht 167.6 cm (66 inches)

COR: WNL

CHEST: Clear

HEENT: Loss of hair, lip fissures (cheilosis)

RECTAL: WNL, guaiac-negative

SKIN: Dry, cracking skin covering both arms and legs; patchy, scaly lesions on elbow of right arm and on both upper arms

Results of Laboratory Tests

Na 142 (142)	BUN 10 (3.57)
K 4.0 (4.0)	Cr 0.9 (79.56)
Cl 96 (96)	Ca 6 (1.497)
HCO$_3$ 26 (26)	Fe 80 (14.128)

PROBLEM LIST

1. PUD
2. Hypervitaminosis A

QUESTIONS FOR CASE 20

1. Define the term "megadose."
2. What are the symptoms of vitamin D toxicity?
3. Explain the drug/food interaction between famotidine and meals.

CASE 21

CC: CM is a 61-year-old male who comes to the clinic today with complaints of loss of appetite and significant weight loss.

Past Medical History

CM was diagnosed with esophageal cancer six months ago. His malignant tumor has been deemed inoperable by his physicians, and he is being treated with intermittent radiation therapy as a palliative measure. Over the past several months, he has had a progressive weight loss (20 kg in six months). He has extreme difficulty swallowing solid food and usually vomits any solid food he ingests. CM has a long history of epilepsy (tonic-clonic seizures), but he has not had any recent seizures on his current dose of antiepileptic medication.

Social History

Alcohol—40-year history of ingestion, heavy ingestion last 10 years since wife's death

Tobacco—40 pack/year history

Medication History
Theophylline elixir 400 mg po t.i.d.
Phenytoin suspension, 150 mg b.i.d. (9 AM, 9 PM)
Ensure, 1 can t.i.d.
OTC aspirin, as needed, for headaches

Allergies
No known drug allergies

Physical Examination
GEN: Malnourished male in no apparent distress
VS: BP 135/85, HR 60, RR 12, T 36.9°C, Wt 75 kg (95 kg 6 months ago), Ht 188 cm
HEENT: Hoarseness, difficulty swallowing
COR: Normal S1 and S2, no murmurs, rubs, or gallops
CHEST: Clear to auscultation and percussion
ABD: Soft, nontender, with no masses or organomegaly; vomiting with eating; positive bowel sounds
GU: WNL
RECTAL: Guaiac-negative
EXT: Normal skin turgor
NEURO: Oriented to time, place, and person; cranial nerves intact; normal deep tendon reflexes

Results of Laboratory Tests

Na 139 (139)	AST 0.66 (40)	Glu 5.0 (90)
K 3.7 (3.7)	ALT 0.76 (45)	Ca 2.0 (8.0)
Cl 97 (97)	LDH 2.5 (150)	Po$_4$ 0.8 (2.5)
HCO$_3$ 26 (26)	Alk Phos 2.3 (140)	Mg 0.74 (1.8)
BUN 6.5 (18)	Alb 28 (2.8)	Uric Acid 390 (6.5)
CR 100 (1.1)	T Bili 13.7 (0.8)	

PROBLEM LIST
1. Esophageal cancer
2. Epilepsy (tonic-clonic seizures)
3. COPD
4. Malnutrition: severe weight loss, loss of appetite

CASE 21 SOAP NOTES
Problem 3. Malnutrition
S: CM states he has lost his appetite, vomits with eating, and has lost "a lot" of weight. CM appears thin. He cannot swallow solid food without vomiting.
O: CM has lost 20 kg in six months (21% of his usual body weight). He is now 91% of his IBW. Alb concentration is 28 g/liter (2.8 g/dl), suggesting moderate protein depletion. His abdomen was soft and nontender on examination, with positive bowel sounds.
A: This patient is moderately malnourished. CM requires long-term enteral nutrition.
P: One should place a gastrostomy tube and begin enteral nutrition by it. CM should be started on standard enteral feeding. His protein and nonprotein caloric goals may be calculated as follows:

$$BEE = 66.4730 + 13.7516(75) + 5.0033(188)$$
$$6.755(61) = 1626 \text{ kcal/day}$$

Nonprotein caloric goal: 1.5 BEE = 2439 kcal/day
Required protein dose: 1.2 g protein/kg/day 75 kg = 90 g protein/day

Because CM desires unrestricted activity during the daytime, he should be started on nocturnal feedings. The home healthcare company that will supply his feeding formula supplies Enrich as its standard enteral feeding. CM should be started on full-strength Enrich at 50 ml/hr for 14 hr each night (8 PM to 10 AM). The enteral rate should be increased by 25 ml/hr/day, as tolerated, until a goal of 160 ml/hr over the 14-hr period is attained.

CM must undergo some patient education sessions taught by his home healthcare company. He should be taught how to operate his enteral feeding pump and how to check blood glucose via accuchecks two times a day. He should record his stool frequency and consistency daily. CM must sleep with his head elevated at a 30° angle to promote stomach emptying. He also must record any symptoms of stomach bloating. A registered nurse should visit CM daily for the first week at home after he is trained to continue to observe him closely.

CM's therapy should be monitored by scheduling twice-monthly clinic visits during the first two months, then monthly thereafter. At his clinic visits, CM should be weighed, have laboratory work and nutritional assessments done, and have any changes in his clinical condition recorded.

Problem 1. Esophageal Cancer
S: CM is unable to swallow solid food and has difficulty swallowing in general.
O: CM has had esophageal cancer for six months. He has a malignant esophageal tumor that has been declared inoperable. He receives periodic radiation therapy.
A: CM requires continued radiation therapy to attempt to decrease or control the size of his malignant tumor. CM is not a candidate for surgery because his tumor is large and has spread beyond the esophageal wall. Surgery would be extremely invasive, and his physicians believe that the risks of this surgery for CM (e.g., sepsis, anesthesia, morbidity, mortality) would outweigh the benefits. Similarly, CM is not a candidate for chemotherapy because he is elderly, and again the risks outweigh the benefits in his case.
P: One should continue radiation therapy. The goals are to prevent the tumor from increasing in size any further and, if possible, to decrease tumor size. Progress of therapy will be monitored by measuring the tumor via endoscopy or radiography.

Problem 2. Epilepsy (Tonic-clonic Seizures)
S: None.
O: CM has had no recent seizures on his current dose of phenytoin.
A: CM's epilepsy is not an active problem at present.
P: One should continue the present medication (phenytoin) with no dosage change. Due to changes in absorption when phenytoin suspension is administered with tube feedings, CM should take phenytoin 2 hrs before and 2 hrs after tube feedings. Alternatively, he may be changed to the intravenous form of phenytoin given undiluted via gastrostomy tube.

QUESTIONS FOR CASE 21

1. What potential complications may CM experience due to tube feedings?
2. CM develops a respiratory infection and is hospitalized. While in the hospital, serum glucose and accuchecks remain elevated, despite insulin therapy [Accuchecks mostly 12.5–18 (225–325)]. CM is to be changed to a lower carbohydrate formula. Which one should he receive, and for how long?
3. CM is moderately malnourished. As CM's enteral nutrition therapy is started, what syndrome must be monitored for, and what adjunct therapies (if any) may he require?
4. After three months of radiation therapy, the size of CM's tumor has decreased enough that he may ingest liquids. He begins taking three cans of Ensurè daily (8 oz can: 8.8 g protein and 250 kcal) and tolerates this without a problem. His enteral regimen can now be changed so that he may continue to receive overall the same daily protein and nonprotein caloric doses as when he was receiving the enteral formula alone (goals: 90 g protein/ day and 2439 kcal/day). His physician wants to simplify matters for CM; therefore, he wants the rate left the same as before (160 ml/hr). Over how many hours should CM's enteral formula be given now?

CASE 22

CC: MM is a 20-year-old male with cystic fibrosis who was admitted to the hospital two days ago with recurrent upper respiratory infection.

Past Medical History

Cystic fibrosis (recurrent URIs)

Medication History

Tobramycin 2.5 mg/kg q6h
Pancrease 4 caps q.d. with meals
Vitamin A 5000 units q. day
Vitamin E 400 units q. day
Vitamin D 800 units q. day
Stress tabs 1 cap q. GM
Vitamin K 5 mg two times a week

Results of Laboratory Tests

Na 142 (142)	BUN 10 (3.57)
K 3.1 (3.1)	Cr 0.9 (79.56)
Cl 96 (96)	PT 36 sec (36)
HCO₃ 26 (26)	

Sputum: *Pseudomonas aeruginosa*
Infiltrates on chest radiography

Physical Examination

GEN: 20-year-old male, small in stature, with productive cough, SOB, diarrhea, abnormal pain, and no appetite

VS: HR 100, BP 120/80, T 38.0°C, RR 28, Ht 170.2 cm (67 inches), Wt 56 kg
HEENT: Productive cough, wheezing
COR: Rales, tachycardia
ABD: Tender, distention

Social History

Denies use of alcohol

PROBLEM LIST

1. Upper respiratory infection
2. Malabsorption
3. Hypokalemia, dehydration

CASE 23

CC: JF is a 53-year-old hospitalized female who has had surgery for small-bowel adhesions (surgery: lysis of adhesions and breakup of mechanical obstruction). She developed a postoperative ileus, and was started on parenteral nutrition support seven days ago. She also developed catheter sepsis and was prescribed intravenous vancomycin (she has received the drug for one day thus far).

Past Medical History

None—previously healthy

Medication History

Vancomycin IV 500 mg q12h X 10 days
Acetaminophen suppositories 650 mg q6h p.r.n. for T > 38.3°C

Allergies

Morphine, bee stings

Physical Examination

GEN: Well-developed female in mild distress, complains of chills
VS: BP 104/70, HR 110, RR 26, T 39.4°C, Wt 73 kg, Ht 173 cm
HEENT: Unremarkable
COR: Tachycardic, normal sinus rhythm
CHEST: Clear to auscultation and percussion
ABD: Abdomen distended and tender, no bowel sounds; surgical wound site healing well without redness, swelling, or tenderness
RECTAL: WNL
EXT: Redness, swelling, and tenderness around catheter site
NEURO: Oriented to place, person

Results of Laboratory Tests

Na 138 (138)	CR 90 (1.0)	Alk Phos 0.9 (53)	Po_4 0.95 (2.9)
K 4.0 (4.0)	Lkcs 17×10^9 (12×10^3)	Alb 29 (2.9)	Mg 0.82 (2.0)
Cl 97 (97)	AST 0.5 (30)	T Bili 22 (1.3)	Uric Acid 240 (4.0)
HCO_3 21 (21)	ALT 0.42 (25)	Glu 12.5 (225)	
BUN 6 (17)	LDH 1.66 (100)	Ca 2.14 (8.6)	

PROBLEM LIST

1. Small-bowel obstruction
2. Postoperative ileus
3. Catheter sepsis

DISEASES OF THE BLOOD

CASE 24

CC: SB is a 40-year-old male admitted to the ICU with a fever of 39.1°C, altered mental status, BP 85/55, and UO 250 cc over the last six hours.

Past Medical History/History of Present Illness

SB presented with a one-week history of fatigue, bruising, and sore throat. Leukocyte count was 54×10^9 (54×10^3) with 50% blasts. Bone marrow biopsy revealed acute myelocytic leukemia (AML). SB then underwent induction chemotherapy with daunorubicin $45mg/m^2$ on days one to three and cytarabine $100mg/m^2$ on days one to seven. Induction chemotherapy was completed nine days ago. The leukocyte count has decreased since induction therapy. SB has no other significant medical history.

Review of Systems

As described above

Medication History

As described above for hospital course; no medications prior to admission

Allergies

NKDA

Physical Examination

> GEN: Well-developed male; obtunded, but arousable
> VS: BP 85/55, HR 125, RR 40, T 39.1°C(rectal), Wt 80 kg, Ht 177.8 cm
> HEENT: Mouth ulcerations, no evidence of oral thrush, PERRLA
> CHEST: Diffuse rales through both lung fields
> COR: Regular rate and rhythm, no murmurs or gallops
> ABD: Soft, nontender, active bowel sounds; liver and spleen enlarged and palpable
> GU: WNL
> RECT: Guaiac negative
> EXT: Extremities warm bilaterally, no petechiae, IV sites clean without tenderness
> NEURO: AxOx2, confused

Results of Laboratory Tests

Na 136 (136)	Hct .28 (28%)	Alk Phos 1.8 (110)	Glu 6.1 (120)
K 4.5 (4.5)	Hgb 95 (95)	AST .58 (35)	Ca 2.27 (9.1)
Cl 97 (97)	MCV 82 (82)	ALT .5 (30)	Po$_4$ 1.58 (4.9)
CO$_2$ 13 (13)	WBC 2×10^9 (2×10^3)		Mg 1.05 (2.1)
BUN 21 (60)	Plts 25×10^9 (25×10^3)		Uric acid 357 (6)
Cr 185 (2.1)			

WBC differential: not available due to low white count

Prothrombin time: 13.0 sec/12.5 sec control

Fibrinogen: 3.3 (330)

Urinalysis: No RBC, no WBC, no organisms on Gram stain

Chest radiography: Diffuse infiltrates in both lung fields

Arterial blood gases: pH 7.26, Pco$_2$ 27 mm Hg, Po$_2$ 58 mm Hg, 83% saturation on 50% O$_2$ via facemask.

Sputum gram stain: Few WBC, many GNR, culture pending

Blood cultures: Pending

PROBLEM LIST

1. Septic shock
2. Neutropenia—probable pneumonia
3. Adult respiratory distress syndrome (ARDS)
4. AML—status postinduction with daunorubicin and cytarabine; chemotherapy-induced mucosal ulceration

CASE 24 SOAP NOTES

Problem 1. Septic Shock

S: Patient is confused and has altered mental status.

O: BP 85/55, HR 125, T 39.1, decreased UO, pH 7.26.

A: Early and rapid intervention is necessary to prevent complications and death. Support for cardiovascular, pulmonary, and metabolic systems must be instituted immediately. Due to ongoing capillary leakage, the most important initial therapy is adequate support of BP with replacement of intravascular volume. The choice between crystalloids (normal saline, Ringer's lactate), colloids (albumin, hetastarch), and various blood products remains controversial. Cyrstalloids are usually administered first and colloids reserved unless the patient requires large amounts of fluids. Antibiotic therapy should be initiated after obtaining appropriate cultures. Vasoactive agents may be instituted along with fluid challenges to maintain adequate BP and cardiac output. Dopamine is usually the initial vasoactive agent used, although epinephrine and norepinephrine may also be used. Dobutamine may be used if low cardiac output were contributing to low BP.

P: One should administer antibiotic therapy per neutropenia problem: 500 ml to 1 liter normal saline over 30 minutes for volume support. If needed, albumin or hetastarch may be administered. Dopamine should be started at a rate of 5 µg/kg/min and titrated upwards, as needed, to maintain adequate BP and tissue perfusion.

Problem 2. Neutropenia and Probable Pneumonia

S: None.

O: T 39.1°C, sepsis, diffuse rales, infiltrates on chest radiography, urinalysis clear, blood and sputum cultures pending, IV sites clean, sputum gram stain: (+) gram-negative rods.

A: Patients undergoing chemotherapy are at high risk for infection due to the myelosuppressive properties of chemotherapy. SB is nine days postinduction therapy and his decrease in white count corresponds to the typical nadir of 7–10 days for many chemotherapy agents. SB needs immediate antibiotic therapy because infection is the likely etiology for sepsis. Empiric choice of an antimicrobial agent should be directed at gram-negative rods, particularly *Pseudomonas aeruginosa*. Because SB is neutropenic and septic, he should receive two drugs with antipseudomonal activity. Coverage for gram-positive organisms should be added when evidence exists, such as an infected IV site. Therapy should be continued for four to seven days after the patient becomes afebrile and the ANC > 500. SB's serum creatinine is currently elevated due to volume depletion. Antimicrobial dosages should be adjusted for the elevated serum creatinine. Renal function should improve as septic shock is treated; doses of all agents should be adjusted as renal function improves.

P: One should start ceftazidime 2 g IV q8h and tobramycin 2mg/kg/dose IV q12h (160 mg IV q12h), and obtain tobramycin peak and trough after third dose to ensure adequate therapy.

Problem 3. ARDS

S: None.

O: RR 40, P_{CO_2} 27, P_{O_2} 58, O_2 saturation 83% on 50% O_2 facemask, infiltrates in both lung fields on chest radiography, sepsis.

A: ARDS results from altered pulmonary capillary permeability leading to exudation of fluid and protein into the pulmonary interstitium. This may result in alveolar collapse and perfusion of unventilated alveoli leading to severe hypoxemia, and respiratory failure. The general principle of therapy is to maintain O_2 delivery while minimizing O_2 consumption. The mainstay of therapy is intubation and mechanical ventilation. The use of high O_2 concentrations has limited effect and may cause lung damage. Oxygen concentrations above 50% should be avoided. The use of positive end-expiratory pressure (PEEP) or continuous positive airway pressure (CPAP) will further support adequate blood oxygenation. Maintenance of adequate BP and cardiac output as discussed in Problem 1 ensures adequate O_2 delivery to the tissues. Correction of body temperature elevations may help to stabilize the O_2 demand. Unless contraindicated, acetaminophen should be used to keep body temperature below 37.5°C. Specific pharmacologic interventions for ARDS at present are unproved.

P: One should intubate and ventilate the patient using PEEP or CPAP, set O_2 at 50%, and maintain BP and cardiac output as in Problem 1. Acetaminophen should be given 650mg po/pr p.r.n. for T > 38.5°C.

Problem 4. AML

S: None.

O: SB was diagnosed with AML on bone marrow biopsy: status postinduction therapy one week ago. Currently, examinations determined the patient to be leukopenic (WBC = 0.2 × 10^9), thrombocytopenic (Plts = 25 × 10^9), and to have mouth ulcerations.

A: SB is now status postinduction therapy. On day 14 following induction therapy, SB should undergo bone marrow biopsy to ascertain whether any residual leukemia exists. If leukemic cells were still present, an additional course of cytarabine 100mg/m^2 IV × 5 days and daunorubicin 45 mg/m^2 for 2 days should be given. Postremission therapy is indicated because of a high rate of relapse for patients with AML. Treatment of chemotherapy-induced mucositis includes adequate pain relief and antimicrobial prophylaxis. Platelet transfusions should be given to keep platelets > 20 × 10^9 and packed red blood cells to keep hematocrit > 0.3 (30%).

P: One should administer viscous lidocaine 1–2% 5–15 ml po q4-6h (swish/spit) and chlorhexidine gluconate 30 ml po t.i.d. (swish/spit), as well as intravenous narcotics, as needed, for further pain control; PCA may be useful. Platelet and PRBC transfusions should be administered as needed. Postremission chemotherapy includes cytarabine 2–3 g/m2 IV q12h for 4–12 doses every two months for two to four courses when the patient can tolerate it.

QUESTIONS FOR CASE 24

1. What is the role of monotherapy in the treatment of febrile neutropenia?
2. When should empiric antifungal therapy with amphotericin B be initiated in the treatment of febrile neutropenia and fever?
3. What are appropriate dosing and administration guidelines for amphotericin B?
4. Should SB receive a colony-stimulating factor?

CASE 25

CC: RB is a 67-year-old male who presents to the adult cardiology clinic for evaluation of recent onset of fatigue, shortness of breath, and a pink discoloration in his urine.

History of Present Illness

The patient was diagnosed by his cardiologist with new-onset atrial fibrillation accompanied by mild shortness of breath and dizziness approximately two months ago. The ventricular response rate at that time was 110 beats/min. Procainamide and digoxin were initiated, and the patient chemically converted to normal sinus rhythm with complete resolution of symptoms two days later. Procainamide and digoxin were to be continued for three months to prevent recurrence of arrhythmia. Over the next four to six weeks, RB gradually began to experience increasing fatigue and difficulty catching his breath after only moderate amounts of physical activity. RB states that his current symptoms are different than those associated with atrial fibrillation. Five days ago, he returned to his cardiologist after noticing a pink discoloration in his urine. ECG performed at that time showed normal sinus rhythm, and RB was referred to this clinic for further evaluation and treatment.

Past Medical History
Recent-onset atrial fibrillation
Osteoarthritis (five-year history)
Seasonal allergic rhinitis

Allergies
NKDA
Nausea, abdominal distress with aspirin and most NSAIDs

Medication History
Procainamide (sustained-release tablets) 500 mg p.o. q6h (×
    2 months)
Digoxin 0.25 mg p.o. q.d. (× 2 months)
Naproxen 500 mg b.i.d. (taken with meals)
Antacids p.r.n. (magnesium/aluminum hydroxide suspension)
Pseudoephedrine 60 mg q4h p.r.n.

Physical Examination
GEN: Well-developed, well-nourished male appearing somewhat anxious about his current state of health
VS: BP 130/80, HR 75, RR 22, afebrile; Wt 82 kg, Ht 183 cm
HEENT: Pale conjunctiva, icteric sclera, rhinorrhea, swollen nasal mucous membranes
COR: Normal S1 and S2, no murmurs, rubs, or gallop
CHEST: Clear to auscultation and percussion
ABD: Soft, nontender, no masses, or organomegaly
GU: WNL
RECTAL: Guaiac-negative, enlarged prostate gland
EXT: Nail beds and palms of hands slightly pale, both knees swollen and mildly tender, limited range of motion in both knees and right hip
NEURO: Oriented × 3, cranial nerves grossly intact, reflexes within normal limits

Results of Laboratory Tests

Na 139 (139)	MCHC 350 (35)	Corrected 0.1 (10)
K 4.3 (4.3)	LDH 5.1 (300)	Haptoglobin 0.13 (13)
BUN 5.0 (14)	T Bili 41 (2.4)	Direct Coombs 2+
CR 99.5 (1.1)	D Bili 5 (0.3)	Procainamide 14.4 (3.4)
Hct 0.3 (30%)	Ind Bili 36 (2.1)	NAPA 31 (7.3)
Hgb 91 (9.1)	Retic 0.15 (15)	Digoxin 1.1 (0.9)
MCV 82 (82)		

Peripheral blood smear: normochromic, normocytic RBCs
ECG (12-lead): normal sinus rhythm
Urinalysis: hemoglobin present

PROBLEM LIST
1. Osteoarthritis
2. Seasonal allergic rhinitis ("hay fever")
3. Recent-onset atrial fibrillation (now sinus rhythm)
4. Hemolytic anemia

CASE 25 SOAP NOTES
Problem 4. Hemolytic Anemia
S: RB complains of fatigue, shortness of breath, and pink-colored urine. The physician has noted icteric (yellow) sclera, pale conjunctiva, and pale nail beds.
O: The patient's hemoglobin, hematocrit, and haptoglobin are decreased. Serum bilirubin and lactate dehydrogenase concentrations are elevated. Indirect (unconjugated) bilirubin is increased disproportionately relative to direct (conjugated) bilirubin. The reticulocyte count is markedly elevated.
A: RB states that his current symptoms are different than those he experienced while in atrial fibrillation, and the ECG indicates normal sinus rhythm. RB is exhibiting classic symptoms of anemia: fatigue and shortness of breath. Furthermore, decreased haptoglobin concentration along with elevated concentrations of total bilirubin, indirect bilirubin, and lactate dehydrogenase indicate red blood cell lysis. The increased levels of bilirubin account for the yellow discoloration of the patient's eyes (scleral icterus). Marked reticulocytosis and hemoglobinuria suggest that the hemolytic process is relatively severe. A strongly positive direct Coombs' test indicates an immune-mediated process. Because RB began experiencing his current symptoms shortly after he was initiated on a new medication, a drug-induced disorder should be considered. The procainamide initiated two months ago is the likely cause of this acute hemolytic anemia.
P: One should discontinue procainamide therapy. Most often, this leads to a gradual resolution of hemolytic anemia. Although moderately symptomatic, RB is not hemodynamically compromised, and other interventions, such as transfusion or pharmacologic treatment, will not likely be necessary. However, because of an accelerated rate of erythropoiesis and accompanying increased folate utilization, supplementation of 1 mg/day of folic acid should be provided. The patient's hematologic status (i.e., hemoglobin, hematocrit, and reticulocyte count) should be followed closely to ensure that stopping procainamide has reversed the hemolytic process and that no further treatment will be required.

Problem 3. Recent-onset Atrial Fibrillation
S: None.
O: RB is currently in normal sinus rhythm.
A: RB apparently converted to normal sinus rhythm secondary to the initiation of procainamide about two months ago. Two separate ECGs since that time indicate that he has remained in normal sinus rhythm. RB's ventricular rate is well-controlled with digoxin.
P: A type I antiarrhythmic agent, such as quinidine or procainamide, is frequently used in patients with new-onset atrial

fibrillation to restore and maintain normal sinus rhythm or to prevent relapse in patients converted to normal sinus rhythm by direct-current countershock. However, quinidine is generally preferred over procainamide for long-term use because of the high incidence of increased ANA titers and lupus erythematosus associated with the latter. Because RB's episode of atrial fibrillation two months ago was symptomatic and associated with a relatively rapid ventricular response, it may be prudent to continue digoxin and start prophylactic quinidine therapy for the remainder of the planned three-month period (i.e., one more month). An appropriate regimen for RB would be quinidine sulfate tablets 300 mg p.o. q6h. When this approach is chosen, the potential interaction between quinidine and digoxin must be addressed either by careful monitoring of digoxin plasma concentrations or by reducing the digoxin dose by 50% in anticipation of the interaction. The use of anticoagulants prior to converting patients to reduce the risk of thromboembolism is recommended if atrial fibrillation were to persist for more than a few days. In RB's case, normal rhythm was restored in two days; therefore, anticoagulation is not likely to be necessary.

Problem 1. Osteoarthritis

S: RB complains of mild pain and stiffness in both of his knees.
O: Limited range of motion in both knees and right hip were noted during physical examination.
A: The patient's subjective complaints of pain and stiffness along with range-of-motion deficits found on physical examination indicate moderately advanced osteoarthritis. Aspirin and ibuprofen have provided symptomatic relief but caused nausea and abdominal discomfort that RB found to be intolerable. The naproxen he is currently taking provides adequate pain relief while causing only minimal gastrointestinal distress.
P: RB should continue to take naproxen with meals. He should also be counseled that the quinidine may cause adverse gastrointestinal effects that are unrelated to NSAID therapy. Diarrhea, abdominal cramping, nausea, and vomiting occur commonly with quinidine and are believed to result primarily from local irritation of the gastric mucosa. If this were to occur, a sustained-release form of quinidine sulfate or quinidine gluconate may alleviate the gastric symptoms.

Problem 2. Seasonal Allergic Rhinitis ("Hay Fever")

S: Patient states he is always "stuffed up" this time of year.
O: Rhinorrhea and swollen nasal passages were noted during physical examination.
A: According to RB, he has been taking pseudoephedrine (60 mg) on a relatively regular schedule recently (q4-6h) due to seasonal allergies. This regimen has produced adequate symptom relief.
P: Pseudoephedrine is a sympathomimetic that may increase the irritability of the myocardium, especially when large doses are used or in patients who are inherently sensitive

to the myocardial effects of sympathomimetic agents. Because of RB's recent history of atrial fibrillation, he should be counseled to avoid oral decongestants, such as pseudoephedrine, or to use them sparingly at the lowest effective dose. Another potential alternative for RB may be the short-term use of a topically applied nasal decongestant, such as oxymetazoline.

QUESTIONS FOR CASE 25

1. Assuming procainamide had not induced hemolytic anemia in RB and was to be continued for three months, what maintenance dose of sustained-release procainamide tablets would have been required to achieve a steady-state procainamide plasma concentration of approximately 6 mg/liter?
2. By what mechanism is procainamide believed to initiate red blood cell hemolysis?
3. What is the incidence of procainamide-induced immunohemolytic anemia?
4. Why do serum levels of indirect bilirubin increase disproportionately higher than those of direct bilirubin during hemolytic anemia?
5. In RB's situation, discontinuing procainamide provided an acceptable resolution of the hemolytic process. What therapy is effective in treating clinically significant immunohemolytic anemias not amenable to discontinuing an offending agent or other means?

CASE 26

CC: AM is a 22 year-old female who presents to the ED with bloody diarrhea and complains of severe abdominal pain, arthritic pain in both knees, increased fatigue, and decreased appetite. Findings include T 99.8°F and pulse 94. AM states she is having a worsening of her ulcerative colitis.

History of Present Illness

AM was diagnosed 1½ months ago with ulcerative colitis by sigmoidoscopy. Extent of disease at that time was 22cm. Her symptoms at diagnosis included increased fatigue, moderate abdominal pain, and approximately six bloody stools/day. She was started on sulfasalazine 2gm/day and has been titrated up to 6gm/day due to persistence of symptoms. She began to experience increased headaches, intermittent nausea and vomiting, malaise, and anorexia. Over the last three weeks AM has had a weight loss of approximately 8 pounds. AM began menstruating four days prior to admission.

Past Medical History

Depression

Medication History

Lomotil p.r.n. for diarrhea (2 tabs p.o. q.i.d.)
Sulfasalazine 6gm/day
Fluoxetine 40mg p.o. q.d.

Allergies
PCN—rash

Social History
AM is a college student in her sophomore year and lives in a dormitory. She denies tobacco smoking, but has occasional alcohol binge drinking.

Review of Systems
AM has increased number bloody stools (nine/day) over last two weeks, not relieved by Lomotil. AM has noticed a decrease in appetite since she started taking fluoxetine for depression about 1½ years ago (with a 5-pound weight loss during this time).

Physical Examination
GEN:	Thin, pale female in moderate-to-severe distress
VS:	BP 120/84, HR 94, RR 18, T 99.8°F, Wt 43kg, Ht 156cm
HEENT:	WNL
COR:	Tachycardic
CHEST:	Lungs clear to auscultation and percussion
ABD:	Soft, lower abdomen tender to palpitation
GU:	WNL, menstruating
RECT:	Bloody, watery diarrhea
EXT:	Tenderness and warmth of both knees
NEURO:	WNL

Results of Laboratory Tests

Na 137 (137)	WBC 16 × 10^9 (16 × 10^3)	Alk Phos 3.0 (180)	Cr 68.63 (0.9)
K 3.3 (3.3)	Hct 0.28 (28)	AST 0.75 (45)	Glu 5.0 (90)
HCO$_3$ 24 (24)	Hgb 87 (8.7)	ALT 0.58 (35)	Ca 2.45 (9.8)
BUN 5.4 (16)	Plts 240 (240)	Uric Acid 120 (2.0)	Mg 1.0 (2.0)
TIBC 82.39 (460)	MCV 60 (60)	MCHC 240 (24)	S Ferr 11 (11)
Cl 96 (96)	T bili 13.68 (0.8)	Alb 41 (4.1)	ESR 60 (60)

Urinalysis, chest radiography, ECG: all WNL

Stool examination: numerous WBC, RBC

Stool culture: negative

Repeat sigmoidoscopy: edematous and friable mucosa, extent of disease 23cm

PROBLEM LIST
1. Ulcerative colitis
2. Iron deficiency anemia
3. Anorexia
4. Depression

CASE 26 SOAP NOTES
Problem 1. Ulcerative Colitis
S: AM complains of severe abdominal pain (tender to palpitation), arthritic pain in both knees (tender and warm), increased fatigue, and decreased appetite. She also complains of increased headaches, intermittent nausea and vomiting, malaise, and anorexia since her sulfasalazine dose has been increased.

O: AM's HR and T are elevated at 94 and 99.8°F, respectively. AM has increased bloody diarrhea, nine bloody stools/day (increased from 6/day) and weight loss of approximately eight pounds over the last three weeks. Stool examination shows numerous RBCs and WBCs; culture is negative. Sigmoidoscopy shows edematous and friable mucosa, with extent of disease to 23cm. Pertinent lab values indicate increased erythrocyte sedimentation rate, liver enzymes (AST, ALT, Alk Phos), and WBC, and low potassium.

A: AM is not responding to remission induction with sulfsalazine. AM has never received a trial of corticosteroids for remission induction. Sulfasalazine, which has been titrated up to its maximum dose, is not controlling her UC and is causing intolerable side effects. AM shows evidence of extraintestinal manifestations of UC: arthritis and elevated liver enzymes. Leukocytosis, fever, and increased sedimentation rate are manifestations of active inflammatory disease. AM's potassium is moderately low due to losses from severe diarrhea. It does not need to be replaced because she is not experiencing any symptoms of hypokalemia; however, it should be continually monitored.

P: AM needs to be hospitalized for parenteral corticosteroid administration to treat active UC. Corticosteroids are effective agents for the induction of remission of severe, acute UC exacerbations. Oral corticosteroids should not be used at this point due to their unreliable absorption and efficacy in patients with severe, acute UC. Methylprednisolone or prednisone are the most preferred agents because of their high antiinflammatory and low mineralocorticoid potencies. The initial dose and rate of taper need to be individualized, based on patient's signs and symptoms and extent of disease. Dosage ranges of 40–80 mg/day for methylprednisolone and 250–300 mg/day for hydrocortisone (in divided doses) are often used. Surgery may be indicated if AM were not to respond within 72 hours of starting high-dose steroids. The goal of surgery in UC is cure. AM should be switched to an oral corticosteroid once a satisfactory initial response is achieved (7–10 days). Prednisone is typically used and is dosed once daily in the morning. AM should be gradually tapered; the usual total course of corticosteroids is four to eight weeks. Due to extent of her disease, topically administered corticosteroids (enemas, foams, and suppositories) are not an option; they are effective for management of distal proctocolitis. Once AM is started on oral prednisone, an oral 5-ASA product should be started in order to maintain disease remission. Because she had intolerable side effects to sulfasalazine at 6gm/day, it would be reasonable to decrease the dose since the N/V, headache, malaise, and anorexia are dose-related (seen at doses > 4gm/day). Another option is to start her on olsalazine (500mg p.o. b.i.d.), which lacks the sulfapyridine moiety of sulfasalazine. Olsalazine 1 g provides amounts of 5-ASA comparable to 2.5 gm of sulfasalazine. The sulfapyridine moiety is believed to be responsible for the dose-related side effects. Because sulfapyridine is acetylated, AM may be a slow acetylator and, therefore, at greater risk for toxicity. AM should be cautioned that olsalazine may cause secretory diarrhea. This may be minimized by starting with a low dose of olsalazine and gradually increasing the dose.

Problem 2. Iron Deficiency Anemia
S: AM complains of fatigue and appears pale.

O: Pertinent lab values include decreased Hgb, Hct, MCV, MCHC, ferritin, and elevated TIBC.

A: The subjective complaints and laboratory values are consistent with iron deficiency anemia. Patients with UC are prone to develop iron deficiency anemia due to rectal blood loss. Her menses also may be contributing to anemia. Treatment objectives for iron deficiency anemia include (a) correcting the underlying causes of the iron deficiency, (b) administering supplemental iron to replenish iron stores, and (c) correcting the erythrocyte deficiency (normalization of Hgb and Hct). Because AM has severe diarrhea, adequate absorption of oral iron supplementation is unreliable. Therefore, parenteral iron should be administered.

P: The dose of parenteral iron to be administered is based on an approximation of total iron deficit using the following equation:

$$\text{Iron (mg)} = (\text{Pt's. wt. in lb.}) \times \left(\frac{100 - \text{Hgb} \times 100}{14.8} \right) \times 0.3$$

Utilizing the equation, AM requires 1170mg of parenteral iron-dextran. Iron-dextran may be administered undiluted IM or by slow IV injection. Because she is thin, AM does not have adequate muscle mass for IM administration and should be given intravenous iron-dextran. For a total dose IV infusion, AM should be pretreated with an antihistamine (diphenhydramine) 30 minutes before the iron dose to prophylaxis against potential hypersensitivity reaction to the drug. The total dose is diluted in 250–1000ml of 0.9% NaCl (preferably) or D5W. A test dose then needs to be administered (10–25mg) over 5–10 minutes. If no reaction to the test dose were to occur, the remainder of the dose may be administered over 2–6 hours (not to exceed 6mg/ minute). Alternatively, the dose may be split up into 100mg daily given by direct bolus injections (not to exceed 50mg/ min). Laboratory tests to monitor for response include Hct, Hgb, MCV, MCHC, TIBC, reticulocyte count, serum ferritin, and serum iron. Reticulocyte count generally increases within five days, peaks within 7–10 days, and returns to normal after 14 days.

Problem 3. Anorexia

S: AM complains of an acute decrease in appetite, increased fatigue, anorexia since her sulfasalazine dose was increased, and also a decrease in appetite since she began taking fluoxetine 1½ years ago.

O: Recent 8 lb. weight loss over 3 weeks, 5 lb. weight loss over 1½ years.

A: The reason for AM's acute decrease in appetite/anorexia and increased fatigue is most likely due to her increased dose of sulfasalazine (seen at doses of sulfasalazine greater than or equal to 4gm/day). These side effects correlate more specifically to serum concentrations of sulfapyridine of greater than 50 mcg/ml. The dose-related side effects tend to occur early in therapy. AM's anorexia and weight loss over the last 1½ years are due to the fluoxetine. Anorexia is a common side effect of fluoxetine, also dose-related, which occurs in up to 25% of patients.

P: As mentioned above, it is reasonable to either decrease the dose of sulfasalazine or try another agent, such as olsalazine. In terms of her therapy for depression, it would be reasonable to discontinue the fluoxetine and try another agent, such as a tricyclic antidepressant because she does not have any contraindications. A tricyclic antidepressant may be a good choice because one of its potential side effects is weight gain.

Problem 4. Depression

S: AM is not experiencing any depressive symptoms. Her increased fatigue is probably mostly due to her other problems.

O: None.

A: Elavil is an appropriate tricyclic antidepressant to begin therapy. It should be started at a dose of 25–50mg p.o. qHS or 25mg b.i.d. and titrated slowly, usually to about 150–200mg/day. It should be given at bedtime to avoid some of the sedative side effects and also so the peak serum levels occur at night. It takes approximately 7–10 days to reach steady state and up to eight weeks to manifest maximal response.

P: AM needs to be monitored to assess efficacy of therapy and also for potential side effects, such as dry mouth, sedation, orthostatic hypotension, constipation, tremor, tinnitus, photosensitivity, diaphoresis, and urinary retention. AM should be counseled on side effects and a health care provider should monitor AM's depression.

QUESTIONS FOR CASE 26

1. What are some potential side effects of glucocorticoid therapy?
2. What is the proposed mechanism of action of sulfasalazine?
3. Your M.D. has heard of the new drug Asacol. Is mesalamine (Asacol or Pentasa) use justified in this patient?
4. What is toxic megacolon?
5. Parenteral iron therapy has two types of reactions associated with its use. What are they?

CASE 27

CC: LP is a 23-year-old white female who presents to the local ED complaining of severe abdominal cramping, loose stools, and weakness.

Recent Medical History

LP reports a two-day history of mild abdominal cramping and four to five stools per day. She complains of decreased energy, generalized weakness, and anorexia over the past two weeks. She denies any nausea or vomiting. During this period, she lost eight pounds. This morning, abdominal cramping became more severe, and she noticed small tinges of bright blood in some of her stools. She called her local doctor, who referred her immediately to the ED.

Past Medical History

LP has a history significant for Crohn disease, which was diagnosed approximately one year ago. Her initial exacerbation lasted two months. Work-up of her disease showed involvement of the ileum. She was begun on oral sulfasalazine, but due to a lack of response was changed to prednisone 30 mg/day. Since then, she has been tapered to 10 mg of prednisone a day. She has a five-year history of menorrhagia, and occasional migraine headaches.

Allergies

None known

Physical Examination

GEN: Pale, thin, small-frame female; alert and oriented to place and time
VS: BP 128/60, HR 120, RR 28, Wt 48, Ht 162.5 cm, T 38°C
HEENT: Head without trauma, ears clear, PERRLA
NECK: WNL, no masses
COR: Tachycardic, no murmurs, no gallops
CHEST: Chest radiography clear, no rales, no rhonchi
ABD: Slightly distended, slight tenderness upper right quadrant, hyperactive bowel sounds
UR/GENT: WNL
EXT: Pale-appearing skin, nails brittle
NEURO: Reflexes + 3 throughout and symmetrical, motor intact
RECTAL: Guaiac-positive stool, fat-streaked

Medication History

Prednisone 10 mg q.d.
Ibuprofen 400 mg q.i.d. p.r.n. for headaches
Ranitidine 150 mg b.i.d.

Results of Laboratory Tests

Na 132 (132)	Hct 0.25 (25)	MCH 262 (26.2)	Mg 0.7 (1.4)
K 3.8 (3.8)	Hgb 81 (8.1)	MCHC 32.2 (32.2)	Sed Rate 70 (70)
Cl 100 (100)	Lkcs 13.3 × 10⁹ (13.3 × 10⁵)	Alb 35 (3.5)	S iron 12.5
HCO₃ 25 (25)	Plts 412 × 10⁹ (412 × 10⁵)	Glu 7.44 (134)	TIBC 85.9 (480)
BUN 1.4 (4)	RBC 3.09 × 10⁹ (3.09 × 10⁵)	Ca 2.1 (8.5)	S Ferr 5 (35)
CR 106 (1.2)	MCV 81.3 (81.3)	PO₄ 0.97 (3.0)	

Peripheral smear: microcytic, hypochromic RBCs

PROBLEM LIST

1. Crohn disease
2. Nutrition/malabsorption
3. Iron deficiency anemia

CASE 27 SOAP NOTES

Problem 3. Iron Deficiency Anemia

S: Pale-appearing, brittle nails, weakness.
O: Malabsorption disease with small bowel involvement, menorrhagia, decreased Hct, decreased MCV, decreased MCHC, and microcytic, hypochromic RBCs on peripheral blood smear, increased TIBC, and decreased plasma ferritin.

A: LP shows obvious signs and symptoms of iron deficiency anemia. Factors that are contributing to this include malabsorption due to Crohn disease, history of menorrhagia, increased need for iron because of age, and inhibition of iron absorption due to H₂-antagonists. LP may be at risk for folic acid and B₁₂ deficiency as well.
P: Because of LP's malabsorption problems, parenteral iron replacement therapy would be the route of choice initially. Her TPN solution would be the most appropriate vehicle for administering iron dextran. Low-dose iron therapy may be supplemented daily in LP's TPN and should be changed to an oral preparation when feasible.

Problem 2. Nutrition/Malabsorption

S: Weakness, weight loss, decreased energy, anorexia, diarrhea.
O: Decreased albumin, fatty stools.
A: LP is malnourished because of decreased oral intake and malabsorption from ileum involvement due to Crohn disease. She also has increased energy needs because of her increased catabolic state caused by Crohn disease.
P: Because of diarrhea, small bowel disease, malnutrition, and increased metabolic state, LP is at an increased risk of using her visceral protein stores. TPN at present would be the most beneficial therapy to meet her body's demands. TPN solution should contain dextrose, crystalline amino acids, electrolytes, vitamins, zinc, trace elements, and fat emulsion to meet her needs. Once she can tolerate an oral diet without difficulty, LP should be weaned from parenteral therapy. Renal function, volume status, electrolytes, and changing nutritional needs should be monitored regularly.

Problem 1. Crohn Disease

S: Abdominal cramping, loose stools.
O: Guaiac-positive, distended abdomen, tenderness upper right quadrant, sed rate increased, hyperactive bowel sounds, and T 38.0°C (100.4°F).
A: LP is having symptoms of Crohn disease. She has the typical features of diarrhea, abdominal pain, fever, and weight loss.
P: One should increase prednisone to a level to suppress her symptoms: begin with 30 mg prednisone per day. Once in LP is in remission, one should repeat efforts to reduce the dose. If unsuccessful, immunosuppressive therapy may be required to keep prednisone at a low dose. Monitor signs and symptoms of perforation of bowel, toxic megacolon infection, sepsis, and adverse effects of steroid use.

QUESTIONS FOR CASE 27

1. What is the importance of zinc supplementation in patients with Crohn disease?
2. Calculate the total iron dose in milligrams to replete iron stores.
3. Describe why you would administer a test dose of parenteral iron and how you would do it.

4. What are the common long- and short-term side effects of prednisone?
5. What drug interactions are possible with prednisone therapy?

CASE 28

CC: FP is a 78-year-old male admitted to the adult internal medicine service for evaluation of complaints of nausea, vomiting, and confusion consistent with digoxin toxicity.

History of Present Illness (given by grand-daughter)

Two days prior to admission, the patient reported nausea and vomiting unaccompanied by fever, chills, or cough. The morning of this admission, FP's granddaughter noted him to be confused, calling her by her grandmother's name. She promptly brought him to the ER for evaluation. FP was seen by his local medical doctor 10 days ago complaining of fatigue and was started on ferrous sulfate for presumed iron deficiency anemia. Verapamil was also prescribed at this time for hypertension uncontrolled by diuretic therapy. A digoxin level at that visit was 2.0 nmol/liter (1.6 µg/liter).

Past Medical History

Chronic atrial fibrillation
Hypertension
Rheumatoid arthritis
Anemia
Constipation

Allergies

Aspirin ("upset stomach")

Medication History

Digoxin 0.25 mg p.o. q.d.
Hydrochlorothiazide 50 mg p.o. q. AM
Verapamil 80 mg p.o. t.i.d. (× 10 days)
Ferrous sulfate 325 mg p.o. t.i.d. with meals
Ibuprofen 400 mg p.o. t.i.d. with meals
Docusate sodium 100 mg p.o. b.i.d.

Review of Systems (per granddaughter)

Joint pain and stiffness in the morning; tired and lethargic recently

Physical Examination

GEN: Thin, pale elderly man appearing somewhat confused
VS: BP 140/70, HR 40, RR 20, afebrile, Wt 64 kg, Ht 180 cm
HEENT: Pale mucous membranes; AV nicking and narrowing c/w chronic hypertension
COR: Normal S1 and S2; no murmurs
CHEST: No rales or rhonchi
ABD: Thin, no masses
GU: WNL
RECTAL: Enlarged prostate gland; guaiac-negative
EXT: No clubbing/cyanosis/edema; swelling of left knee and arthritic changes in metacarpal joints bilaterally
NEURO: Oriented × 1 (name only); CN II-XII difficult to assess, but grossly intact; reflexes WNL

Results of Laboratory Tests

Na 142 (142)	MCV 90.4 (90.4)	Digoxin 3.3 (2.6)
K 3.2 (3.2)	MCHC 339 (33.9)	Folate 45 (20)
BUN 10.4 (29)	MCH 30.7	B$_{12}$ 1005 (1362)
CR 124 (1.4)	Retic Count 0.01	Iron 2.7 (15)
Hct 0.328 (32.8)	Ca 2.2 (8.8)	TIBC 30 (168)
Hgb 113 (11.3)	Mg 0.86 (2.1)	Ferritin 330 (330)

Peripheral blood smear: normochromic, normocytic RBCs
Chest radiography: WNL
ECG: atrial fibrillation with slow ventricular response rate

PROBLEM LIST

1. Hypertension
2. Rheumatoid arthritis
3. Atrial fibrillation
4. Constipation
5. Anemia
6. Digoxin toxicity
7. Hypokalemia

QUESTIONS FOR CASE 28

1. Assuming all of the verapamil has been eliminated from his system, how long will it take for FP's digoxin concentration to decrease to the therapeutic range [i.e., to 2.6 nmol/liter (2.0 µg/liter)]?
2. By what mechanism does verapamil increase serum digoxin concentrations?
3. What diseases are associated with the anemia of chronic disease?
4. How can the anemia of chronic disease be differentiated from iron deficiency anemia?
5. Why doesn't iron therapy improve the anemia of chronic disease?

CASE 29

CC: AB is a 25-year-old black female with a history of sickle cell anemia admitted to the adult internal medicine service for management of dehydration and a painful crisis.

History of Present Illness

AB presented to the Hematology Clinic today complaining of diffuse pain affecting her abdomen, arms, and legs, which is typical of her previous painful crises. She has had malaise, fevers to 38.9°C, and diarrhea over the last three to four days. She has been unable to eat or drink much and reports recent contact with two children with the flu. She denies melena, BRBPR, cough, SOB, headache, or dysuria.

Past Medical History

Sickle cell anemia
Multiple admissions for painful crises
Narcotic dependence
Splenectomy
Pneumococcal pneumonia
Seizures (due to meperidine)

Family History

Mother, father, and 23-year-old brother have the sickle cell trait, and a 20-year-old brother has sickle cell anemia. Older sister died last year (at 27 years) of complications of sickle cell anemia.

Allergies

None known

Medication History

Hydromorphone 6–9 mg p.o. q4h p.r.n. (usually 24 mg/day)
Folic acid 1 mg p.o. q.d.

Review of Systems

Dizziness with standing since yesterday; continuous diffuse pain unrelieved by oral hydromorphone

Physical Examination

GEN: Black female appearing younger than stated age, in acute distress
VS: BP 100/60, HR 104, RR 18, T 38.0°C, Wt 46 kg, Ht 160 cm (usual weight 48 kg)
HEENT: Mildly icteric sclera, pupils equal and reactive, no sinus tenderness, pale and dry mucous membranes
COR: Nl S1 and S2; II/VI systolic ejection murmur
CHEST: Clear to auscultation and percussion
ABD: Hyperactive bowel sounds; + diffuse, nonlocalized tenderness; no hepatomegaly
GU: Deferred
RECTAL: Guaiac-negative
EXT: Dry skin; + clubbing; tenderness to palpation: legs ε arms; pale nail beds; no cyanosis or edema
NEURO: Alert and oriented × 3; CN II-XII intact; motor grossly intact

Results of Laboratory Tests

K 4.1 (4.1)	Hgb 81 (8.1)	MCH 30.2
BUN 5.0 (14)	Lkcs 13.6 × 10⁹ (13.6 × 10⁵)	Iron 16 (88)
CR 70 (0.8)	MCV 90.2 (90.2)	TIBC 68 (380)
Hct 0.243 (24.3)	MCHC 334 (33.4)	

Lkcs differential: Segs 48%, Bands 2%, Lymphs 45%, Monos 5%

Peripheral blood smear: widespread sickled cells and few schistocytes; normochromic, normocytic RBCs

Chest radiography: no infiltrates or effusions, enlarged cardiac shadow

ECG: normal sinus rhythm with rate of 100 beats/minute, left ventricular hypertrophy

PROBLEM LIST

1. Sickle cell anemia
2. Narcotic addiction
3. Painful sickle cell crisis
4. Viral gastroenteritis
5. Dehydration
6. Healthcare maintenance

CASE 29 SOAP NOTES
Problem 5. Dehydration

S: AB reports dizziness on standing.

O: Dry mucous membranes and skin, 2-kg weight loss, BP 100/60, HR 104.

A: AB's fever, diarrhea, and lack of oral intake resulted in dehydration. Fluid therapy must provide both replacement of prior losses as well as usual daily maintenance requirements. Fluid requirements for this patient may be calculated as follows:

Deficit = (kg body weight lost)(1000 ml/kg)
= (2 kg)(1000 ml/kg)
= 2000ml

Maintenance = (first 10-kg body weight)(100 ml/kg)
+ (second 10-kg body weight)(50 ml/kg)
+ (remaining kg body weight)(20 ml/kg)
= (10 kg)(100 ml/kg) + (10 kg)(50 ml/kg) + (28kg)(20 ml/kg)
= 1000 ml + 500 ml + 560 ml
= 2060 ml

In addition, maintenance fluid requirements are increased by 10% for every 1°C increase in temperature; because of her current fever, AB's maintenance requirements are increased to 2266 ml. Fluid and electrolyte losses from continued diarrhea must also be replaced. Therefore, the total amount of fluid (deficit + maintenance) to be administered the first day is 4266 ml plus the amount of any further gastrointestinal output. Intravenous repletion is indicated because of AB's present inability to ingest oral fluids.

P: One should give an intravenous bolus of 500 ml of 0.9% NaCl and then infuse 0.9% NaCl with 20 mEq/liter KCl intravenously at a rate of 200 ml/hr for 8 hr. Reduce the rate to 150 ml/hr for the next 16 hr. On the following day, infuse fluids at 100/hr to provide maintenance fluid requirements. Quantify losses due to diarrhea and replace ml for ml as needed. Encourage AB to drink, and reduce the intravenous infusion rate as oral intake increases and her temperature and gastrointestinal losses decrease. One should monitor fluid input, urine and stool output, weight, orthostatic BP, and heart rate daily. Monitor serum electrolytes (e.g., potassium) and replace as necessary. Also check skin turgor and moistness of skin and mucous membranes for improvement.

Problem 3. Painful Sickle Cell Crisis

S: AB complains of diffuse, continuous abdominal, arm, and leg pain refractory to oral hydromorphone and similar to her pain in previous sickle cell crises.

O: Peripheral blood smear reveals sickled cells and schistocytes. Icteric sclera are noted on physical examination.

A: Based on AB's recent history of contact with sick children, the painful crisis most likely resulted from an acute infection that led to temperature elevation and subsequent dehydration. Therapy should be supportive and aimed at reducing continued sickling (by improving oxygenation and hydration status) and further discomfort. AB complains that her present pain is unrelieved by oral hydromorphone. Pain medications, therefore, should be administered parenterally, as scheduled intermittent or continuous intravenous infusions, rather than as p.r.n. regimens, so that anxiety related to pain is minimized. Because AB takes hydromorphone chronically, she will be tolerant to the analgesic effects of usual doses of narcotic agents. A daily dose of morphine sulfate that exceeds the equivalent of hydromorphone taken as an outpatient should be calculated. Meperidine should be avoided because of AB's history of seizures with this agent.

P: One should replete fluids as listed above in Problem 5 and attempt to alleviate the underlying cause of the painful crisis. Give humidified oxygen 2 liters by nasal cannula. Initiate a continuous intravenous infusion of morphine sulfate at a rate of 2–6 mg/hr and titrate to pain relief. One should also closely monitor BP, respiratory rate, and level of sedation. Once pain is controlled, attempt to reduce AB's narcotic requirements over the next two to four days: change to intermittent IV doses of morphine sulfate q4-6h p.r.n., taper the narcotic dose down by 20–30% daily by initially reducing the dose—not the dosing interval, and convert to oral hydromorphone prior to discharge.

Problem 4. Viral Gastroenteritis

S: AB reports malaise, fevers to 38.9°C, and diarrhea over the past three to four days.

O: Lkcs 13.6, differential with 45% lymphocytes, hyperactive bowel sounds.

A: Elevated white blood cell count indicates an infection. The increased proportion of lymphocytes suggests a viral etiology and is consistent with AB's history of contact with sick children. Viral gastroenteritis is a self-limiting process and necessitates supportive therapy.

P: One should keep AB well-hydrated, replacing fluid losses due to diarrhea. Give an antipyretic (acetaminophen 650 mg p.o. q4-6h p.r.n.) for temperatures over 37.8°C, and monitor fluid input, urine and stool output, temperature, potassium level, and Lkcs count and differential.

Problem 1. Sickle Cell Anemia

S: None.

O: Physical examination findings include pale mucous membranes and nail beds, clubbing, icteric sclera, and a systolic ejection murmur. Peripheral blood smear reveals sickled cells and schistocytes. Left ventricular hypertrophy is noted on chest radiography and ECG. Hemoglobin and hematocrit levels are reduced, whereas iron and TIBC are WNL.

A: Elevated red cell production in patients with sickle cell anemia increases folic acid requirements. If these requirements were not met and folate deficiency were to result, an aplastic crisis may be induced. Although AB has clinical signs of anemia, red blood cell transfusion is not presently warranted because of the degree and chronicity of this problem.

P: One should continue treatment with folic acid 1 mg p.o. q.d, educate AB about the usual causes of painful crises, and encourage regular high oral fluid intake (3–5 liters/day) as an outpatient.

Problem 2. Narcotic Addiction

S: Medication history indicating chronic use of narcotics.

O: None.

A: AB appears to be taking oral narcotic analgesics continuously, which is not appropriate for this disease. Pain medications should be used only for acute, painful crises, not for prophylaxis, and should be tapered as pain subsides.

P: One should educate AB about the role of narcotic analgesics in sickle cell anemia and her probable addiction to these agents. Formulate a plan that AB will agree to and that incorporates close follow-up. Identify one primary care physician to coordinate all of AB's future therapy, including prescriptions for narcotic analgesics. One should gradually taper the oral hydromorphone as an outpatient and counsel her to use oral narcotics only after other pain relief measures (e.g., NSAIDS) have failed, and offer psychosocial counseling to enhance her ability to cope with her disease.

Problem 6. Healthcare Maintenance

S: None.

O: AB indicates a history of pneumococcal pneumonia.

A: AB's splenectomy puts her at risk for infections with *Streptococcus pneumoniae* and *Haemophilus influenzae*. Current recommendations include immunizing those over the age of two years with polyvalent pneumococcal vaccine. Infection prophylaxis with penicillin VK may also be advisable.

P: One should check AB's medical records and, if not previously immunized with the polyvalent pneumococcal vaccine, administer (0.5 ml s.c. or IM) as an outpatient after the present gastroenteritis has resolved. One should also initiate penicillin VK 250 mg p.o. q6h at that time.

CASE 30

CC: KL is a 62-year-old male who is brought to the hospital by his wife. KL is complaining of stomach pains, weakness, and dizziness.

History of Present Illness

KL has had stomach pain for the past few weeks. Lately he has noticed that his stools are loose and tarry. Today, he decided to come into the hospital after he started coughing up some material that looks like coffee grounds. He states that food relieves his stomach pain, but he has not been eating well due to his painful tongue. He has been self-medicating with antacids for a few weeks, but the pain only goes away for a short period of time. He has also been feeling depressed lately because he just received his second DUI in the past year. He has decided to try to quit drinking alcohol and is willing to do anything to stop so that his life can return to normal.

Past Medical History

None

Medication History

Ibuprofen 600–800mg q.i.d. p.r.n. for headaches
Maalox p.r.n. for stomach pain (~ one 8 ounce bottle per day)

Allergies

None known

Social history

Lives with his wife (his two grown children are still at home while going to college), and works at a business firm
Tobacco—1 ppd
Alcohol—approximately 5 martinis after work every day; lately he has a "pick-me-up" drink in the morning before work

Physical Examination

GEN: Pale, elderly-appearing male in moderate distress
VS: BP 110/65, HR 80, RR 12, T 37.5°C, Wt 75 kg (decrease of 5kg)
HEENT: PERRLA
COR: RRR
CHEST: Clear to auscultation and percussion
ABD: Soft, slightly tender, no hepatosplenomegaly
RECT: Guaiac-positive
EXT: Pale nail beds, bruising on upper arms and thighs
NEURO: Oriented to time, place, and person

Results of Laboratory Tests

Na 138	Hct 0.25 (25)	RBC 4.0 (4.0)
K 4.0 (4.0)	Hgb 100 (10)	Serum Vit B$_{12}$ 55 (80)
Cl 99 (99)	Plts 120 × 10^9 (120 × 10^3)	Serum folate 2 (1.2)
HCO$_3$ 22 (22)	WBC 3.8 (3.8)	Serum iron 4 (25)
BUN 3.6 (12)	MCV 60 (60)	
CR 80 (0.9)	MCH 22 (22)	

Endoscopy: 0.5 cm ulcer in the duodenum

PROBLEM LIST

1. Peptic ulcer disease
2. Anemia
3. Alcohol abuse

Use **SOAP** for the above problems.

CASE 30 SOAP NOTES
Problem 1. Peptic Ulcer Disease

S: KL complains of stomach pain, coughing up coffee ground-like material, and having loose, tarry stools.

O: Endoscopy is positive for duodenal ulcer.

A: KL has a duodenal ulcer. Contributing factors include alcohol abuse, smoking, and ulcerogenic medication, ibuprofen. KL has had stomach pain for several weeks. He has been coughing up coffee ground-like material and has had loose, tarry stools for a few days; these are signs of bleeding. KL needs to be admitted to the hospital to ensure that his blood loss is not chronic and to evaluate the severity of bleeding.

P: One should discontinue all oral medications and give IV fluids. For immediate IV treatment, H$_2$-receptor antagonists are the drugs of choice with ranitidine and famotidine having less potential for drug interactions than cimetidine. Antacids can be given concomitantly, as needed, for pain. Once KL is guaiac-negative, oral treatment should begin. KL should be treated for four to eight weeks with oral therapy. Five different classes of medications can be used: anticholinergics, antacids, sucralfate, H$_2$-receptor antagonists, and omeprazole. Anticholinergics are less effective than the other medications and have many side effects; therefore, they are not considered first-line agents. Antacids are also not preferred monotherapy due to the need for frequent dosing (6–8 doses/day). However, they are often given in conjunction with other medications on an as needed basis for pain. The mechanism of action of sucralfate is to coat the mucosa and promoting healing. Sucralfate is equally efficacious to H$_2$-receptor antagonists and omeprazole, but must be taken two to four times daily. H$_2$-receptor antagonists work by blocking secretion of acid. They are selective and reversible antagonists for the histamine receptor on the parietal cell, and can be given once daily. Omeprazole is a proton-pump inhibitor which can also be given once daily. It is as effective as H$_2$-receptors and sucralfate, but due to its cost and potency, it is reserved for failure of the other medications. For initial treatment, one should start ranitidine 50mg IV q8h until guaiac is negative. Initiate ranitidine 300mg po qHS for 4 to 8 weeks. Give antacids, such as Mylanta 30ml, as needed, for pain. One should encourage KL to stop smoking because smoking may delay ulcer healing, and alcohol should be discontinued as well because it can increase acid secretions and contribute to ulcer formation. KL also needs to discontinue ibuprofen because it is ulcerogenic; he should try acetaminophen for headaches. One should repeat endoscopy after 4 to 8 weeks to evaluate the extent of ulcer healing.

Problem 2. Anemia

S: KL complains of weakness, dizziness, and a painful tongue.

O: RBC, Hgb, Hct, serum folate, serum Vitamin B_{12}, serum iron, WBC, platelets, and MCV are low. Physical examination reveals guaiac-positive stools and multiple areas of bruising.

A: KL is suffering from several types of anemia. He has iron-deficiency anemia secondary to blood loss. He also has both folate deficiency anemia and Vitamin B_{12} deficiency anemia due to malnutrition and chronic alcohol use.

P: KL needs iron replacement for iron-deficiency anemia. The goal of iron therapy is to normalize the Hgb, Hct, and serum iron levels. When doses of elemental iron are sufficient, the reticulocyte count should start increasing within several days of starting therapy, peak by the end of ten days, and settle within the normal range after 14 days. Within three weeks there should be about a 2gm/dl increase in Hgb and a 6% increase in Hct. Iron therapy should continue for at least three months and preferably six months. Estimated folate body stores are approximately 5–10 mg; therefore, 1mg of folic acid given once daily for about two to three weeks should be enough to replace KL's depleted stores. Vitamin B_{12} deficiency is more insidious and requires lifelong treatment with cyanocobalamin injections to ensure adequate stores of this vitamin. One should give KL ferrous sulfate 325mg po t.i.d. with meals for six months, assess efficacy by observing an increase in the reticulocyte count, Hct, and Hgb in one month, and inform patient that the iron may produce many symptoms similar to those he has experienced with his ulcer, such as dark stools, stomach pain, and constipation. These effects should decrease after several days and can be alleviated by taking the iron with food. He should take folic acid 1mg po qd for three weeks. One should recheck folic acid levels in one month to make sure his stores have been repleted. Cyanocobalamin should be given 100 mcg IM qd for three weeks, then 100–200 mcg IM monthly for the rest of his life; lifelong treatment is required to maintain Vitamin B_{12}

stores. If he were to discontinue this therapy, the anemia may return within five years. Also, the neurologic damage he has experienced (tingling of feet, dizziness, and emotional instability) may not resolve completely.

Problem 3. Alcohol Abuse

S: None.

O: KL is drinking alcohol on a daily basis, including during working hours.

A: KL suffers from alcoholism. The etiology of alcoholism can be genetic, psychosocial, and/or biochemical. His folate and Vitamin B_{12} deficiency may be due to malnutrition from drinking alcohol instead of eating properly. KL would benefit from daily multivitamins and eating a regular diet. KL also needs counseling. Alcoholics Anonymous (AA) is one of the more successful support and counseling programs available. Disulfiram is potentially useful in alcoholic patients; it may be used as aversion therapy to prevent patients from ingesting alcohol, because of the reaction that ensues. A typical disulfiram reaction includes flushing, tachycardia, dyspnea, palpitations, and severe headache. These symptoms are usually followed by nausea and vomiting, thirst, sweating, dizziness, confusion, and require several hours of sleep for recovery. KL fits the criteria for those patients most likely to benefit from disulfiram: age > 40 years, highly motivated and willing to go through psychotherapy, socially stable, and has no contraindications to the medication.

P: The usual dose of disulfiram is 500mg/day for two weeks, then 250mg per day for about one month, or until KL feels he no longer needs the disulfiram as a deterrent. He should be warned to avoid all forms of alcohol, including alcohol in foods and OTC cough medicines. KL should wear a medical alert bracelet to warn medical practitioners that he is taking disulfiram. He also needs to be advised that a disulfiram reaction may occur up to 14 days after he takes his last disulfiram dose.

QUESTIONS FOR CASE 30

1. What is the best route of administration for thiamine to treat vitamin B_{12} deficiency?
2. Why are H_2-receptor antagonists administered at night?
3. Describe differences among the various salt formulations of iron.
4. Should this patient receive therapy for *H. pylori*?

ENDOCRINE AND METABOLIC DISEASES

CASE 31

CC: JG is a 45-year-old female with adult-onset diabetes mellitus (DM) who presents to the urgent care clinic with a three-day history of fever, chills, pleuritic chest pain, productive cough, and extreme fatigue.

Past Medical History

JG returned three days ago from a stressful five-day business trip to Mongolia. Since then, she has developed the symptoms described above. For one week, she has felt restless, anxious, and has been unable to sleep soundly. She complains that her frequent cough, tactile fever, and increased nocturia are not helping her to sleep either. She has noticed increased numbness in her toes and "burning" leg pain at night over the past two months.

Social History

Cigarettes—two packs per day for 15 years
Coffee—three cups per day, more on business trips
Compliant with ADA diet

Medication History

Pseudoephedrine 60mg po q.i.d. × 5 days
Glipizide 10mg po qd
Tylenol #3 po p.r.n. for leg pain (average 10 tablets per day for one month)

Allergy

NKDA

Physical Examination

Gen:	Tired, obese, agitated female in moderate respiratory distress
VS:	BP 140/90, RR 28, HR 125, T 39.5°C, Wt 70kg, Ht 5'4"
HEENT:	"Bags under the eyes," yellow purulent sputum for three days
COR:	Normal S_1S_2, no murmur, tachycardic
CHEST:	LLL dullness
ABD:	WNL
GU:	WNL
RECT:	Deferred
EXT:	Numbness to toes bilaterally
NEURO:	Decreased DTR lower extremities

Results of Laboratory Tests

Na 135 (135)	Hct 0.35 (35%)	Ca 2.2 (8.8)
K 4.5 (4.5)	Hgb 119 (11.9)	PO$_4$ 0.66 (2.0)
Cl 105 (105)	WBC 14 × 10^9 (14 × 10^3)	Mg 1.15 (2.8)
HCO$_3$ 25 (25)	Plts 2.1 × 10^9 (210 × 10^3)	Alb 37 (3.7)
BUN 7.1 (20)	MCV 90 (90)	Fast glu 12.2 (220)
Cr 126 (1.2)		HbA$_{1C}$ 12% (12%)

WBC differential: PMN 0.85 (85%), bands 0.12 (12%), lymphs 0.03 (3%)

Sputum: gram stain shows many pleomorphic gram (−) coccobacilli, few gram (+) cocci in pairs, chains and clusters, 30 neutrophils, < 10 epithelial cells per low-power field; culture pending

Blood: smear negative, culture × 2 pending

Urine: 1+ protein, (−) glucose, (−) ketone; culture pending

Chest radiography: LLL consolidation, no pleural effusion

Doppler: Negative

PROBLEM LIST

1. DM
2. Respiratory infection
3. Insomnia

CASE 31 SOAP NOTES

Problem 1. Diabetes Mellitus

S: Increased nocturia, toe numbness, "burning" leg pain, proteinuria, ADA diet.

O: Elevated HbA$_{1C}$ > 7% (7%), fasting glucose > 7.8 (140).

A: JG's elevated HbA$_{1C}$ is reflective of poorly controlled blood glucose for at least one to two months. She also has signs of vascular and kidney damage secondary to diabetes. Her glipizide dose can be increased to improve blood glucose control. Because her leg pain is refractory to narcotic-analgesic treatment, a trial of a tricyclic antidepressant may be warranted. Her increased nocturia may be the result of both her poorly controlled diabetes and her increased consumption of caffeine.

P: One should instruct JG to decrease coffee intake, increase glipizide to 10mg po qAM and 5mg po qPM, and monitor blood glucose at home twice a day. One should start amitriptyline 25–75 mg po qd for peripheral neuropathy.

Problem 2. Respiratory Infection

S: Fever, chills, pleuritic chest pain, and productive cough for three days.

O: Yellow purulent sputum with gram (–) coccobacilli, chest radiography, leukocytosis with left shift, tachycardia, increased respiratory rate, and chest exam.

A: JG has the classic signs and symptoms of community-acquired pneumonia, perhaps contracted from close contact and poor circulation in airplanes (or anywhere else). From the sputum gram-stain, the most likely pathogen is *Haemophilis influenza*. Other common pathogens include *Streptococcus pneumoniae* and *Moraxella catarrhalis*. Atypical pathogens are unlikely due to the rapid onset of symptoms, high fever, and consolidation seen on chest radiography. Oral antibiotics that cover *H. influenza* include trimethoprim/sulfamethoxazole (T/S), ampicillin or amoxicillin, amoxicillin/clavulanate, second- and third-generation cephalosporins (cefuroxime axetil and cefixime), and quinolones. Among these options, amoxicillin/clavulanate and quinolones should be reserved for documented β-lactamase-producing strains of *H. influenza* or patients who are unresponsive to T/S, ampicillin, or amoxicillin. Duration of therapy is 10–14 days.

P: One should start oral antibiotics for 10-14 days.

Problem 3. Insomnia

S: JG has not been sleeping well for one week.

O: None.

A: JG's transient insomnia (about one week) is probably caused by jet-lag, although her increased use of caffeine and over-the-counter (OTC) sympathomimetics also contribute to the problem. Smoking more than one pack per day is an independent cause of insomnia.

P: One should discontinue pseudoephedrine, and counsel JG to avoid use of OTC sympathomimetics. She should decrease tobacco and caffeine use. The tricyclic antidepressant given for peripheral neuropathy may also help in her insomnia. She should be counseled on relaxation techniques as well.

QUESTIONS FOR CASE 31

1. Name three of the most common chronic complications of DM and how they might manifest. What tests should be done to screen for these complications? Which are now evident in JG?
2. In light of JG's microproteinuria, what class of drugs can be used to prevent progression of diabetic nephropathy? What is the mechanism of action of this class of drugs?
3. Based on the mechanisms of action, is it reasonable to initiate metformin therapy in the presence of glipizide?
4. JG was given amoxicillin to treat her pneumonia. Two days later, the sputum culture results show growth of β-lactamase-producing *H. influenza* which is resistant to amoxicillin but sensitive to amoxicillin/clavulanate. What are the benefits of these β-lactam/β-lactamase inhibitor combinations?

CASE 32

CC: TT is a 40-year-old female who presents to the general medicine clinic complaining of polyuria, polydipsia, and chest pain.

History of Present Illness

TT has had a history of type I DM since the age of 30; insulin was started at diagnosis. Yesterday, she lost all her medications when her purse was stolen. Today, she complains of polyuria and polydipsia. She also had chest pain when she woke up this morning.

Past Medical History

TT has a long history of DM and hypertension. Five years ago, she developed pain and tingling sensation at her lower extremities requiring a tricyclic antidepressant for relief. She was diagnosed with hypercholesterolemia two years ago and was started on fluvastatin. She is currently followed by a dietitian once per week and she jogs every day for 30 minutes. Two weeks ago, she started to have chest discomfort that radiates to her left arm. She denies any history of peptic ulcer disease.

Medication History

Insulin regular 10U SQ qAM, 15U SQ qPM
Insulin NPH 20U SQ qAM, 30U SQ PM
Fluvastatin 20mg PO qHS
Benazepril 20mg PO qd
Nitroglycerin SL tablets p.r.n.
Amitriptyline 25mg PO qHS

Allergies

Penicillin (rash)

Social History

Tobacco—negative
Alcohol—one glass of wine per day at dinner

Family History

Mother died of myocardial infarction at age of 50
Father has diabetes and hypertension

Review of Systems

Noncontributory

Physical Examination

GEN: Obese, WDWN female in no apparent distress
VS: BP 165/100, HR 85, RR 14, T 37.5°C, Wt 100 kg, Ht 160cm
HEENT: PERRLA
COR: Normal S_1 and S_2
CHEST: Clear to auscultation and percussion
ABD: Soft, nontender, no hepatosplenomegaly
RECT: Guaiac-negative
EXT: No clubbing, cyanosis, or edema
NEURO: Oriented to time, place, and person; cranial nerves intact; decreased deep tendon reflexes

Results of Laboratory Tests

Na 140 (140)	Hct 0.40 (40)	ALT 0.33 (20)	TG 2.1 (186)
K 4.0 (4.0)	Hgb 130 (13)	AST 0.58 (35)	Ca 2.4 (9.6)
Cl 136 (136)	Lkes 10 × 10⁹ (10 × 10³)	Alk Phos 0.83 (50)	Po₄ 0.9 (2.8)
HCO₃ 25 (25)	Plts 170 × 10⁹ (170 × 10³)	Alb 55 (5.5)	Mg 0.98 (2.4)
BUN 7.1 (20)	MCV 85 (85)	T. bili 10.3 (0.6)	Uric Acid 333 (5.6)
Cr 132.6 (1,5)	LDL 4.1 (158)	LDH 1.34 (80)	Fasting Glu 13.32 (240)
		HDL 0.67 (26)	T. Chol. 6.2 (240)

Urinalysis: 2+ protein, 3+ glucose, no organisms seen, clear, pH 7.5, SG 1.020, and no RBC/leuk/casts

PROBLEM LIST

1. Type I diabetes mellitus
2. Isolated hypercholesterolemia
3. Hypertension
4. CAD
5. Peripheral neuropathy

Use **SOAP** for the above problems.

CASE 32 SOAP NOTES
Problem 1. Type I DM

S: TT complains of polydipsia and polyuria.

O: TT was diagnosed with type I DM 10 years ago. Her fasting blood glucose is elevated today. She also has 3+ glucose and 2+ protein in urine and elevated serum creatinine.

A: TT has type I DM. Her diabetes is not controlled today because she has not taken her insulin for longer than a day. She would be at risk for diabetic ketoacidosis (DKA) if she were not to resume therapy. She also has complications of diabetes, such as proteinuria, diabetic nephropathy, peripheral neuropathy, hypertension, and CAD. Strict glycemic control is necessary to prevent an acute episode of DKA, the progression of these long-term complications, and the development of other complications, such as retinopathy and stroke.

P: One should refill regular insulin and NPH insulin, encourage TT to start home blood glucose monitoring before meals and at bedtime, and inform her of the importance of euglycemia to prevent the long-term complications of diabetes. One should also educate her on the signs and symptoms of hyperglycemia (polydipsia, polyuria, polyphagia, fatigue) and hypoglycemia (blurred vision, sweating, hunger, and confusion). She should also have yearly eye examinations and should check her feet daily for signs of infection. She also needs to restrict her caloric intake to improve tissue responsiveness to insulin, avoid high-fat and high-cholesterol diet, and consume complex carbohydrates and high-fiber foods. Insulin, diet, and regular exercise are necessary to decrease the morbidity and mortality of diabetes.

Problem 2. Isolated Hypercholesterolemia

S: None.

O: She has elevated total cholesterol and elevated low-density lipoproteins.

A: TT suffers from isolated hypercholesterolemia. She has multiple cardiac risk factors for coronary heart disease: family history of premature CAD, DM, hypertension, low HDL, and high LDL. With her high LDL, dietary therapy and pharmacologic intervention are necessary to achieve a goal LDL of < 2.6 (100) and to prevent the progression of CAD. Bile acid sequestrants, such as cholestyramine and colestid, have a strong safety and efficacy profile and can achieve a 17–26% reduction in LDL. HMG-CoA reductase inhibitors, such as lovastatin, pravastatin, simvastatin, and fluvastatin, allow dose-dependent reduction of LDL ranging 20–40%. With the high LDL level of this patient, HMG-CoA reductase inhibitors are preferred to bile-acid sequestrants. Niacin should not be used because it can cause hyperglycemia and increase the insulin requirement of this patient. Gemfibrozil is usually reserved for patients with both hypercholesterolemia and hypertriglyceridemia. The relative potencies of different HMG-CoA reductase inhibitors are as follows:

Lovastatin	Pravastatin	Simvastatin	Fluvastatin	% LDL reduction
20mg	10mg	5mg	20mg	20%
40mg	20mg	10mg	40mg	30%
80mg	NA	40mg	NA	40%

NA = data not available

TT requires at least 30% reduction in LDL and fluvastatin 20mg is probably inadequate.

P: One should increase daily dose of fluvastatin to 40mg, and encourage patient to continue dietary therapy and lose weight by exercising regularly. Recheck lipid profile in four weeks and monitor adverse effects of fluvastatin, such as myositis, insomnia, headache, and gastrointestinal side effects (e.g., dyspepsia, diarrhea, nausea).

Problem 3. Hypertension

S: None.

O: Elevated BP 165/100.

A: TT's BP is most likely elevated today because she has been out of medication for two days. Proper control of her blood pressure is necessary to prevent end organ damage and to reduce the risk of stroke. Diuretics should not be used because they can increase serum cholesterol and triglycerides. Beta-blockers should be avoided because they may mask the signs and symptoms of hypoglycermia, prolong hypoglycemic episodes, and worsen glucose tolerance. Benazepril is a good choice for her because it has a neutral lipid profile and does not affect blood glucose. It has also been shown to be beneficial in the treatment of diabetic nephropathy and to improve proteinuria.

P: One should continue benazepril 20mg/day, and monitor BP over the next few clinic visits in order to assess her response to the current dose of benazepril. Monitor for adverse effects associated with benazepril, such as cough, angioedema, hyperkalemia, and hypotension. One should stress compliance with medications because hypertension is a silent disease; she should continue to take her medications even though she is asymptomatic.

Problem 4. CAD

S: TT complains of chest pain that radiates to her left arm.

O: None.

A: TT has multiple risk factors for CAD as mentioned in the problem above. Secondary prevention of hypercholesterolemia is necessary to prevent the progression of heart disease. TT is currently not on any medication for CAD. Usual treatment includes beta-blockers, nitrates, or calcium channel blockers. Beta-blockers should be avoided because they may mask the signs and symptoms of hypoglycemia. Both nitrates and calcium channel blockers may be used in TT. Nitrates are preferred at this point because most patients respond to nitrates; they also have a strong safety profile. One should start TT on scheduled nitrate therapy and short-acting nitrates for acute relief of chest pain.

P: One should start isosorbide dinitrate 10mg po three times daily. It should be taken three times daily, but not every eight hours, during the day. The dosing schedule should allow for a nitrate-free period at night to avoid nitrate tolerance. TT should also receive nitroglycerin sublingual tablets. She should be instructed to place one tablet under the tongue at the onset of chest pain. If chest pain were to persist, she may repeat an NTG tablet every five minutes, to a maximum of three tablets. If chest pain were not to be relieved after three nitroglycerin tablets, TT should call 911 or go to the ED. TT should return to the clinic in one month for follow-up.

Problem 5. Peripheral Neuropathy

S: TT has painful and tingling sensations in her lower extremities.

O: TT has decreased deep tendon reflexes.

A: Peripheral neuropathy is a long-term complication of DM. Tricyclic antidepressants are the drug of choice and patients usually respond to lower doses than doses used for the treatment of depression. TT's peripheral neuropathy has been controlled by amitriptyline for five years and she tolerates the medication well without side effects. She should continue current treatment.

P: One should refill amitriptyline 25mg tablets and review possible side effects of amitriptyline with TT, including dry mouth, blurred vision, urinary retention, and constipation.

QUESTIONS FOR CASE 32

1. What are the long-term complications of uncontrolled diabetes and how can these complications be avoided?
2. What type of antihypertensive medications should be avoided in TT based on her medical history?
3. What are TT's risk factors for CAD?
4. What are the treatment goals for hypercholesterolemia?
5. Should nonsteroidal antiinflammatory agents be used to treat TT's peripheral neuropathy?

CASE 33

CC: EM is a 65-year-old female who is brought into the ER by her husband because of an acute change in her mental status. Her husband states that she has become progressively more confused over the past 24–48 hrs, and is now only semiconscious. She had also been experiencing weakness, dizziness, diarrhea, and severe vomiting prior to the onset of her mental status changes. Her husband mentions that they had just returned from a vacation, during which EM ran out of the prednisone she has been taking for rheumatoid arthritis.

Past Medical History

EM has a five-year history of rheumatoid arthritis for which she has been taking prednisone for one year.

Medication History

Prednisone 10 mg p.o. q.d., discontinued one week ago
Conjugated estrogens 0.625 mg p.o. q.d.
Aspirin 325 mg, 2 tablets q.i.d. since prednisone ran out
Maalox Plus® 30 ml p.o. q.i.d. with aspirin

Physical Examination

GEN: Pale, semiconscious elderly female
VS: BP 100/52, P 112, RR 28, T 37.3°C, Wt 65 kg (72 kg one month ago)
HEENT: Moon facies, pale gums
CHEST: WNL
COR: Normal S_1, S_2; no S_3, S_4; rapid heart rate; mild mitral valve murmur suggestive of mitral valve prolapse
ABD: Obese; diffuse abdominal tenderness; normal bowel sounds
EXT: Thin, cool extremities; proximal muscle weakness; 1 – 2 + pulses throughout; pale nail beds
SKIN: Dry; + tenting; + striae on abdomen

Results of Laboratory Tests

Na 119 (119)	Hct .38 (38)	MCH 27 (27)	Glu 2.8 (50)
K 5.8 (5.8)	Hgb 110 (11)	ALT 0.37 (22)	Ca 5 (10)
Cl 92 (92)	Lkcs 6.5×10^9 (6.5×10^3)	LDH 1.43 (86)	Po_4 1.2 (3.8)
HCO_3 26 (26)	Plts 170×10^9 (170×10^3)	Alk Phos 1.3 (78)	Mg 0.9 (1.8)
BUN 17.8 (50)	MCV 80 (80)	Alb 30 (3.0)	Uric Acid 238 (4)
CR 150 (1.7)	MCHC 320 (32)	T Bili 14 (0.8)	

Stool: guaiac-positive
UA: SG 1.025
ECG: tachycardia, regular rhythm

PROBLEM LIST

1. Anemia
2. Addisonian crisis
3. Hypoglycemia
4. Dehydration/hyponatremia
5. Hyperkalemia

Problem 2. Addisonian Crisis

S: EM has been taking prednisone for one year for rheumatoid arthritis. She abruptly discontinued the prednisone when she ran out of it and was unable to obtain a refill.

O: EM is only semiconscious, and her vital signs include BP 100/52, HR 112, and RR 28. Serum potassium is elevated, and serum sodium and serum chloride are low. Hypoglycemia is present. The BUN-to-serum-creatinine ratio is > 20, signifying prerenal azotemia.

A: EM has HPA-axis suppression due to chronic administration of prednisone. The abrupt discontinuation of prednisone has resulted in acute adrenal insufficiency, with impending shock. Immediate treatment is required.

P: One should administer hydrocortisone sodium succinate or phosphate 100 mg IV immediately, and then continue with 100 mg IV q6h for the first 24 hrs. If EM's condition were stabilized within 24 hrs, the IV dose of hydrocortisone should be decreased to 50 mg IV q6h. This dose should be continued for one to two days, depending on her response. The IV hydrocortisone dose should be tapered rapidly (50% each day) and converted to an oral prednisone dose as soon as tolerated. During hydrocortisone treatment, one should monitor mental status, BP, serum electrolytes, signs and symptoms of hyperglycemia, signs and symptoms of infections, gastrointestinal distress, and stool guaiac.

Problem 3. Hypoglycemia

S: EM is semicomatose and has had severe vomiting and abdominal pain.

O: EM has experienced mental status changes, weakness, dizziness, and low serum glucose of 2.8 (50).

A: EM has developed hypoglycemia as a result of acute adrenal insufficiency. The serum glucose level may even be falsely high due to concurrent dehydration. EM needs immediate treatment to avoid coma and possible brain damage.

P: One should administer 50 ml of 50% dextrose immediately and follow with a dextrose 5% intravenous infusion as described in Problem 4. One should also monitor serum glucose and mental status.

Problem 4. Dehydration/Hyponatremia

S: EM has symptoms of weakness, dizziness, vomiting, and diarrhea.

O: BP is low; pulse and temperature are elevated. Pulses are thready, skin is dry and exhibits tenting, and extremities are cool. BUN-to-serum-creatinine ratio is > 20. Serum sodium level is low. Urine specific gravity is high.

A: EM has severe hyponatremia and hypotonic dehydration caused by adrenocorticoid deficiency, vomiting, diarrhea, and decreased fluid intake. She needs immediate treatment with intravenous fluids. One must calculate the serum osmolality as follows:

$$2 \, (119 + 5.8) + (50/18) = 254 \text{ mOsm/kg}$$

This is lower than normal serum osmolality; therefore, the serum is hypotonic. Calculate the fluid deficit as follows:

$$(140 - 119/140) \times (65 \text{ kg} \times 0.6 \text{ liter/kg}) = 5.4 \text{ liter}$$

Add to the daily fluid requirement as follows:

$$2.4 \text{ liter} + 5.4 \text{ liter} = 7.8 \text{ liter}$$

Calculate the sodium deficit as follows:

$$(140 - 119) \times (65 \text{ kg} \times 0.6 \text{ liter/kg}) = 819$$

Add to the daily sodium requirement as follows:

$$72 + 819 = 891 \text{ mEq}$$

P: One should administer 1000 ml of D5NS over 1 hr, and replace up to half of EM's sodium deficit over the first 24 hrs. If the sodium were replaced too rapidly, osmotic brain injury may occur. Increase serum sodium by 0.5–2.0 mEq/liter/hr. Administer a second 1000 ml D5NS at 125 ml/hr × 8 hr, then change to D5/0.45% NaCl at 125 ml/hr. One should monitor serum sodium at least q6h during the first 24 hrs, and adjust IV solutions based on laboratory test results. Monitor intake and output, other serum electrolytes, vital signs, and daily weight.

Problem 5. Hyperkalemia

S: EM complains of weakness.

O: Serum potassium of 5.8.

A: HPA-axis suppression has resulted from chronic prednisone treatment. Suppression of aldosterone without prednisone administration led to an increased serum potassium concentration. No cardiac conduction abnormalities are occurring; therefore, the only treatment required is adrenocorticosteroid administration as outlined in Problem 2.

P: One should administer corticosteroid as recommended in Problem 2, and monitor serum potassium level q6h over the next 24 hrs until the patient is stabilized.

Problem 1. Anemia

S: EM complains of weakness.

O: Hgb 110 (11), Hct 0.38 (38), HR 96, MCH 27 (27), MCV 80 (80), MCHC 320 (32), pale nail beds, and guaiac-positive stool.

A: Hgb and Hct are below normal yet falsely elevated due to dehydration. RBC indices are all low normal. EM has been taking aspirin for pain since she ran out of prednisone, which has probably caused gastric irritation and blood loss, although the values would not change this quickly. Prednisone is associated with peptic ulcer disease. EM should be evaluated to discover the cause of a positive stool guaiac when she is stable.

P: One should discontinue aspirin use and treat any gastric pain with antacids. Monitor Hgb, Hct, and stool for further blood loss.

QUESTIONS FOR CASE 33

1. Identify five physical findings in EM's admission examination that are markers of chronic steroid excess. List five other physical findings associated with chronic steroid use.

2. What monitoring parameters (at least three physical parameters and at least three laboratory parameters) should be followed to guide the tapering regimen of intravenous hydrocortisone in EM?
3. What, if any, ACTH-stimulation test had been performed on EM? Describe precisely how the tests are conducted and what results you would expect to see with EM.
4. If EM had developed acute gastrointestinal bleeding during her first day of hospitalization, what complications could this cause and how would it be treated?
5. When EM is discharged from the hospital, what patient education should she receive about steroid use?

CASE 34

CC: JK is a 30-year-old woman admitted to the Hospital Family Practice Ward for complaints of fever, palpitations, shortness of breath, insomnia, confusion, and progressive muscle weakness.

Past Medical History

JK was admitted nine months ago with "thyroid storm" secondary to Graves' disease and noncompliance with her antithyroid medications. Her Graves' disease was first diagnosed two years ago and was complicated by ophthalmopathy, pretibial myxedema, and pernicious anemia. At that time she was started on propylthiouracil (PTU) 200 mg p.o. q6h and vitamin B_{12} injections. Her symptoms improved initially, but she was lost to follow-up until her last admission. PTU was restarted after control of the thyroid storm. Her last known vitamin B_{12} injections were administered during her last hospitalization.

Social History

Alcohol binges, drinks two to four glasses of wine intermittently when anxious or depressed, nonsmoker

Family History

Graves' disease and ophthalmopathy

Medication History

Propylthiouracil 200 mg p.o. q6h
Vitamin B_{12} 100 µg IM q. month
Over-the-counter (OTC) Sudafed® 60 mg p.o. q6h p.r.n. for nasal congestion
Micnor-Q-D one tablet q.d. for contraception

Allergies

None known

Review of Systems

JK complains of generalized weakness, the "shakes," feelings of "burning up," palpitations, intermittent chest pain, shortness of breath, and "water in her legs." She is bothered by her forgetfulness and confusion, loss of her menstrual periods,

frequent, loose bowel movements, and an itchy rash all over her body. She states that it is difficult to take the medication and that the PTU tastes bitter and gives her diarrhea. She notes that her weight has increased 10 kg over the last few months and she has a ravenous appetite. She doesn't like the way her eyes have been looking lately and complains of protruding "big eyes," tearing, pain, double vision, and light sensitivity. She also notes increased numbness and tingling in both her legs and hands.

Physical Examination

GEN: 30-year-old tremulous, anxious, and restless female in apparent respiratory distress, intermittently stuporous
VS: BP 180/100, HR 130 ireg, T 39.0°C, RR 28
HEENT: Thin, fine hair with patches of baldness, bilateral proptosis R > L, (+) lid lag, (+) stare, (+) chemosis and conjunctivitis, (+) painful tongue, diffusely enlarged goiter five times normal size (approximately 100 g), (+) bruit in right thyroid lobe, (+) JVD
COR: Rapid, irregular rhythm, (+)S_3 (+) S_4; displaced PMI
CHEST: Bilateral rales and crackles
ABD: Soft, (−) masses, (+) abdominal tenderness, hepatomegaly, hyperdynamic bowel sounds
GU: WNL
RECT: Guaiac-negative
EXT: 2+ pitting edema bilaterally, (+) pretibial myxedema, hot flushed skin, (+) palmar erythema, and nail oncholysis
NEURO: Rapid DTRs with mild clonus, decreased pinprick and vibratory sensation in lower legs, weakness of large muscle groups, (+) coarse tremor

Results of Laboratory Tests

Na 130 (130)	CR 133 (1.5)	MCV 120 (120)	Alb 33 (3.3)
K 3.5 (3.5)	Hct 0.23 (23)	AST 2.5 (150)	T Bili 60 (3.5)
Cl 90 (90)	Hgb 80 (8)	ALT 2.42 (145)	Glu 19.7 (355)
HCO_3 26 (26)	Lkcs 14.3×10^9 (14.3×10^3)	LDH 4.67 (280)	PT 15
BUN 12.5 (35)	Plts 150×10^9 (150×10^3)	Alk Phos (5.8) (350)	

TSI 100%, TgAB 30%, Anti M 1:6400
TT_4 > 257 nmol/liter (> 20 µg/dl), TT_3 12.7 nmol/liter (830 ng/dl)
FT_4I > 20, TSH < 0.05 mU/liter (< 0.05 µU/ml)
Vitamin B_{12}, 59 pmol/liter (80 pg/ml)
Urinalysis: WNL, RAIU (one year ago) 93% uptake at 24 hr
Peripheral blood smear: macrocytic cells and abnormal platelet morphology
Chest radiography: cardiomegaly, pulmonary edema
ECG: HR 130–150, atrial fibrillation, (+) LVH

PROBLEM LIST

1. Atrial fibrillation
2. Congestive heart failure

3. Thyroid storm
4. Pernicious anemia
5. Graves' disease
6. Ophthalmopathy
7. Propylthiouracil toxicity
8. Hypokalemia

Problem 3. Thyroid Storm

S: JK complains of fever, agitation, restlessness, "burning up," shakiness, loose bowel movements, loss of menses, thinning of hair, palpitations, stomach and chest pains, insomnia, confusion, weakness, forgetfulness, and weight loss despite ravenous appetite.

O: Findings included T 39.0°C, R 28, glucose 19.7 mmol/liter (355 mg/dl), K 3.5 mmol/liter (meq/liter), T Bili 60 μmol/liter (3.5 mg/dl), PT 15, elevated TT_4, TT_3, FT_4I, and suppressed TSH. Positive physical findings were high fever, atrial fibrillation, congestive heart failure, tremor, goiter, stupor, confusion, pulmonary edema, hepatomegaly, and rapid deep tendon reflexes. Patient had a positive history of thyroid storm.

A: The fever and florid signs and symptoms of hyperthyroidism are consistent with thyroid storm. JK is taking birth control pills that do not contain estrogen and should not interfere with assessment of the thyroid function tests. JK is taking pseudoephedrine, which will interact with thyroxine and aggravate the symptoms of thyrotoxicosis. Immediate therapy of storm is required because of the high mortality rate. Despite some minor allergic reaction to PTU, PTU should still be the thioamide of choice over methimazole because it inhibits the peripheral conversion of T_4 to T_3 and increases control of the hyperthyroidism. Corticosteroids should be administered to reduce T_3 levels and to correct for unsuspected adrenal insufficiency. Additionally, steroids will control the allergic reaction to PTU. Because the beneficial effects of PTU will not be evident for at least two weeks, therapy with iodides or adrenergic antagonists should be instituted immediately to relieve the hyperthyroid symptoms. Iodides act rapidly, within two to three days, to block further thyroid hormone release. Theoretically, iodides should be given 1 hr after PTU administration to avoid blocking the effect of PTU and to avoid iodizing existing hormone stores, which will aggravate the storm. However, iodides interfere with the uptake of radioactive iodine ablative therapy for several weeks. β-Blockers should not be used because they could exacerbate asthma and possibly high-output congestive heart failure. Calcium-channel blockers, such as diltiazem, can be used to control the hyperthyroid symptoms and to reduce the heart rate and AV nodal conduction without adverse effects on asthma. The risk of aggravating CHF with calcium antagonists is minimal in patients with EF > 30%, which is likely in this patient without history of heart disease. Digitalization should control heart failure and ventricular rate (Problem 6). Thyroid storm is caused by her noncompliance with PTU; other precipitating factors, such as infection, should be eliminated.

P: One should eliminate and correct any underlying causes of thyroid storm. Institute supportive therapy with oxygen, sedation, antipyretics, and correction of electrolytes, as needed. One should give the following: KCl 10 meq IV q1h × 3 and repeat, as needed, to maintain K^+; hydrocortisone 100–200 mg IV q6–8h until stable and then taper; and PTU 200–300 mg q6h p.o. If she were unable to take p.o. PT, a rectal formulation could be administered. One hour after PTU administration, begin iodides, either Lugol's solution 10 gtt t.i.d. p.o. or ipodate 1 g p.o. q.d. or potassium iodide 1 g IV q.d. Give digoxin as described in Problem 2 to keep the HR < 100. Start diltiazem 90–120 mg p.o. t.i.d. for symptomatic relief of hyperthyroid symptoms to reduce the heart rate and titrate dose to symptoms. Monitor HR, BP, temperature, pulse, RR, and other symptoms of hyperthyroidism daily. Monitor TT_4, TT_3, TSH every three days initially until clinical resolution, then every four to six weeks. Patient education should include the following: (a) compliance with long-term thioamide therapy necessary to prevent recurrent hyperthyroidism and storm, (b) signs and symptoms of thyroid storm (i.e., fever, accentuated symptoms of hyperthyroidism), (c) use of diltiazem for first four to six weeks for symptomatic relief, then can taper or stop, and (d) avoid use of OTC sympathomimetics, which can aggravate signs and symptoms of hyperthyroidism. One should tell JK to consult the pharmacist for recommendations about use of OTC preparations.

Problem 2. Congestive Heart Failure

S: JK complains of shortness of breath, palpitations, intermittent chest pain, and "water in her legs."

O: HR 130–150 ireg, R 28, (+) S_3, displaced PMI, (+) JVD (+) rales and crackles, (+) hepatomegaly, (2+) pitting edema chest radiography, cardiomegaly, pulmonary edema, AST 2.50 μkat/liter (150 U/liter), ALT 2.42 μkat/liter (145 U/liter), T Bili 60 μmol/liter (3.5 mg/dl), LDH 4.67 μkat/liter (280 U/liter), PT 15, K 3.5 mmol/liter (3.5 mEq/liter), CR 133 μmol/liter (1.5 mg/dl), and ECG of LVH and atrial fibrillation

A: The signs and symptoms are consistent with congestive heart failure secondary to high-output failure from her thyrotoxicosis, atrial fibrillation, and pernicious anemia. Digitalization is necessary to decrease the heart rate and control the failure. Congestive heart failure secondary to thyrotoxicosis is relatively resistant to digoxin until normalization of thyroid function test results. Larger loading and maintenance doses of digoxin will be required because both the volume of distribution and the clearance are increased. Conversely, the low potassium concentration, impaired renal function, and potential digoxin-diltiazem interaction may increase the risk of digoxin toxicity. The dose of digoxin must be adjusted downward as the patient becomes euthyroid to avoid digoxin toxicity. Blood transfusions may improve heart failure, but packed red cells should be administered rather than whole blood, to prevent fluid overload and cardiovascular crisis.

P: One should control thyroid storm (Problem 3) and replace K^+ (Problem 8). Infuse packed red cells to bring Hgb up to 100 (10). Begin digoxin 0.25–.5 mg IV q6h for one day to keep the HR < 100, then 0.25 mg p.o./IV q.d., as needed, to keep HR < 100. Monitor signs and symptoms of CHF, digoxin levels, HR, K⁺, CR, and ECG q.d. until stable. Patient education should include the following: (a) signs and symptoms of digoxin toxicity, (b) signs and symptoms of congestive heart failure, (c) dietary restriction of salt and salty foods, and (d) compliance with follow-up visits as digoxin is tapered.

Problem 1. Atrial Fibrillation

S: JK complains of intermittent chest pain, palpitations, and symptoms of congestive heart failure. She is taking BCP.

O: HR 130 irregular, atrial fibrillation on ECG.

A: The signs and symptoms are consistent with new-onset atrial fibrillation secondary to congestive heart failure and thyrotoxicosis. Atrial fibrillation secondary to thyrotoxicosis carries a high risk of systemic embolism, and anticoagulation therapy should be strongly considered, especially in elderly patients. The nonestrogen-containing BCP carries a small risk of thromboembolism and should be discontinued when possible. In thyrotoxicosis, smaller doses of warfarin are required for anticoagulation because the turnover of the clotting factors is enhanced. Likewise, as euthyroidism ensues, the dose of warfarin should be increased to maintain adequate anticoagulation. However, JK is not a good candidate for anticoagulation because of heart failure, history of drinking, confusion, hepatomegaly, and poor compliance. JK is also somewhat anticoagulated from her heart failure and liver problems.

P: One should not begin anticoagulation now, but observe the patient for symptoms of systemic embolism. When warranted, begin heparin therapy IV. Patient education should include the following: (a) signs and symptoms of atrial fibrillation, (b) signs and symptoms of embolism, (c) avoid alcohol, and (d) alternative forms of birth control.

Problem 7. Propylthiouracil Toxicity

S: JK complains of bitter taste, itchy rash, diarrhea, fever, and poor compliance because of inability to tolerate medications. She denies arthralgias or joint pain.

O: JK has a fine, maculopapular, itchy rash over body and extremities, T is 39.0°C, and Lkcs and differential are not depressed.

A: The signs and symptoms are consistent with PTU toxicity. The elevated Lkcs, normal differential, and lack of arthralgias or joint pain are not consistent with agranulocytosis or serious systemic toxicities. The dose of PTU is appropriate for hyperthyroidism, but the thioamide of choice after control of the thyroid storm is methimazole because it can be dosed once daily, fewer tablets need to be administered, and it produces minimal taste (bitter) and gastrointestinal disturbances. Methimazole is 10 times more potent than PTU and is equally efficacious when administered in equipotent doses. Little cross-sensitivity between PTU and methimazole occurs with regard to rash.

P: One should discontinue PTU after resolution of thyroid storm, and begin methimazole 40 mg p.o. given in one daily dose or in divided doses if patient desires. Monitor resolution of rash, bitter taste, diarrhea, hyperthyroid symptoms, goiter reduction, and TFTs. TFTs should normalize four to six weeks after starting methimazole, then reduce the dose of methimazole by one-third every four to six weeks until a maintenance dose of 5–10 mg q.d. is reached. Patient education should include the following: (a) signs and symptoms of rash, hepatitis, or agranulocytosis; for sore throat, fever > 39.0°C for a few days, rash, or sores in the mouth, she should contact her physician or pharmacist immediately so that an Lkc with differential can be obtained, (b) signs and symptoms of hyperthyroidism, (c) compliance with regimen to ensure resolution of hyperthyroidism, and (d) delayed onset of resolution of hyperthyroidism.

Problem 4. Pernicious Anemia

S: JK complains of fatigue, muscle weakness, confusion, vertigo, tinnitus, diarrhea, palpitations, signs of congestive heart failure, and tingling and numbness in hands and both lower extremities.

O: JK has decreased Hct/Hgb, increased MCV, low B₁₂ level, negative guaiac test result, peripheral smear showing macrocytic cells and abnormal platelets, and history of PA treated nine months ago with B₁₂ injections. Physical examination showed decreased pinprick and vibratory sensation in lower legs, confusion, and painful tongue.

A: The signs and symptoms are consistent with pernicious anemia secondary to autoimmune Graves' disease. The goals of therapy are to reverse the hematologic manifestations, reverse or retard the central nervous complications, and replenish vitamin B₁₂ body stores. The IM or IV route should be used because oral bioavailability is poor and unreliable. JK receives an appropriate monthly dose of vitamin B₁₂ for maintenance therapy. However, because her last injection was nine months ago, repletion of body stores is required before initiation of maintenance therapy. Folate therapy should not be used alone to reverse macrocytosis because it does not prevent irreversible neurologic damage, although the anemia is improved. After receiving vitamin B₁₂, symptoms (e.g., painful tongue, affective disturbances, and megaloblastosis) reverse before neurologic problems. Increased erythropoiesis may produce severe hypokalemia and depletion of iron and folate stores.

P: One should check JK's folate level to eliminate the possibility of folate deficiency, and replace K⁺ deficiency as described above. Begin vitamin B₁₂ injections of 100 µg q.d. IV or IM × 1 week, then 100 µg q.o.d. for 7 doses when clinical improvement and a reticulocyte response occurs. After that, administer 100 µg/day every three to four days for another two to three weeks, and then maintenance therapy consists of 100–200 µg/month for life. Monitor Hgb, Hct, reticulocyte count, improvement of clinical manifestations, K⁺ concentration, and iron stores. Replace iron and K⁺, as necessary, to maintain normal levels. Patient education should include: (a) compliance with lifelong

B_{12} injections required to reverse anemia, (b) signs and symptoms of pernicious anemia, (c) signs and symptoms of hypokalemia, (d) avoid drugs (e.g., ASA, alcohol) that further aggravate platelet dysfunction, and (e) signs and symptoms of bleeding.

Problem 6. Ophthalmopathy

S: JK doesn't like the way her eyes look lately and complains of bulging "big eyes," tearing, pain, double vision, and light sensitivity.

O: History of Graves' disease diagnosed two years ago complicated by ophthalmopathy. Physical examination shows bilateral proptosis R > L, lid lag, stare, chemosis, and conjunctivitis.

A: Graves' disease is complicated by symptoms of progressive ophthalmopathy. Ophthalmopathy is not related to the activity of the thyroid gland but results from antigens and immunoglobulins from the thyroid gland directed against the eye and its muscles. The gland should be removed or ablated, and JK's thyroid status controlled to prevent further loss of vision. The ophthalmopathy may worsen after surgery or RAI therapy. The mild symptoms of eye irritation should be managed with lubricant eye drops, avoidance of dust and irritants, and protection from sunlight. If the eye were to become inflamed or irritated, corticosteroids could be given to reduce symptoms. Surgical correction may be needed later to correct double vision.

P: The patient's eyes should be protected from light. One should instruct the patient to stop smoking, and use artificial tears to decrease dryness. NSAIDs can be used to decrease inflammation. If no response were to occur, corticosteroids could be given (prednisone 60 mg q.d. until symptoms decreased then tapered to zero over three to four weeks). Patient education should include the following: (a) avoid bright lights, use sunglasses, (b) signs and symptoms of progressive ophthalmopathy (contact your physician), (c) signs and symptoms of steroid toxicity, and (d) ophthalmopathy not associated with thyroid status.

Problem 5. Graves' Disease

S: JK has symptoms of hyperthyroidism, ophthalmopathy, pretibial myxedema, and pernicious anemia.

O: Ophthalmopathy, goiter, pretibial myxedema, positive thyroid antibodies, (+) TSI, hyperthyroid indices, (+) family history, history for two years.

A: JK has signs and symptoms consistent with Graves' disease. After controlling the thyroid storm, the goal of thioamide therapy is to maintain euthyroidism until the disease goes into remission on its own. Remission of the Graves' disease is unlikely because she has had the disease for over two years, continues to have high levels of TSI, and her goiter has not regressed with thioamide therapy. Thioamides are appropriate initially to produce euthyroidism; however, JK should have definite therapy with either surgery or radioactive iodine because of the low likelihood of remission and the progression of ophthalmopathy. RAI may be preferable over surgery because it is quick, effective, and poses no risks to her cardiac status. Her noncompliance may be improved by changing to methimazole therapy prior to surgery or RAI.

P: One should consider RAI when hormone stores are normal to prevent recurrent storm, and change PTU to an equivalent dose of methimazole given once daily (100 mg PTU = 10 mg methimazole). Discontinue thioamides one to two weeks before RAI therapy. Because RAI may take one to three months to work, thioamides can be restarted one week after RAI therapy when necessary. One should monitor TFTs every four weeks. Patient education should include the following: (a) signs and symptoms of hyperthyroidism, (b) signs and symptoms of hypothyroidism, and (c) signs and symptoms of thioamide toxicity (Problem 6).

Problem 8. Hypokalemia

S: JK complains of weakness, fatigue, and frequent, loose bowel movements.

O: Findings include K 3.5 mmol/liter (3.5 mEq/liter), HCO_3 26 mmol/liter (26 mEq/liter), and Cl 90 mmol/liter (90 mEq/liter). Physical examination shows hyperdynamic bowel movements and ECG rapid AF. JK is positive for alcohol intake and CHF.

A: JK has hypokalemia secondary to diarrhea from hyperthyroidism, PTU, and hyperaldosterone state from heart failure. Because of her renal dysfunction, K^+ replacement must be done carefully. K^+ replacement will decrease her heart rate.

P: One should control hyperthyroidism, CHF, and hyperaldosteronism. Give KCl 10 mEq IV q.h. × 3. Repeat K^+ administration the next day, and replace as needed. Monitor resolution of diarrhea, CHF, and hyperthyroidism. Patient education should include the following: (a) signs and symptoms of hypokalemia, (b) K^+-rich dietary sources, and (c) signs and symptoms of hyperkalemia.

QUESTIONS FOR CASE 34

1. What is agranulocytosis? How is it monitored? What type of education should patients receive to prevent this toxicity?
2. Describe iodide-induced thyrotoxicosis.
3. If JK were to become pregnant, how should she be managed?
4. If surgery were required, explain what preparation and risks are to be expected?
5. What are the common adverse effects associated with the thioamides?
6. Describe the use of radioactive iodine in Graves' disease.

CASE 35

CC: KJ is a 29-year-old male with a history of type I DM, who reports to the diabetes clinic for adjustment of insulin doses. KJ uses two split and mixed injections of human NPH/REG and monitors blood glucose levels three to four times per day. KJ has ESRD and requires hemodialysis (HD) three times per week.

Past Medical History

Type I DM × 15 years
Graves' disease treated 10 years ago
Hypothyroidism secondary to thyroidectomy
ESRD treated with HD

Past Surgical History

Thyroidectomy 10 years ago

Medication History

Human insulin 20 units NPH/8 units regular q. AM, 12 units
    NPH/5 units regular before dinner (7 PM)
Levothyroxine 150 µg/day
B-complex vitamins q.d.
Vitamin C 500 mg b.i.d.
CaCO₃ 500 mg t.i.d.
1,25-dihydroxyvitamin D 0.25 µg/day
Folic acid 1 mg q.d.

Allergies

Allergy to beef/pork insulin (lipoatrophy)

Physical Examination

      GEN: Well-appearing male, 72 kg
       VS: BP 125/84, HR 84, RR 12, T 98.0°F
    HEENT: PERRLA, EOM intact
      COR: NSR
    CHEST: Without rales or rhonchi
      ABD: No organomegaly
      EXT: AV fistula—left arm
    NEURO: WNL

Results of Laboratory Tests

Na 138 (138)	Hct 0.43 (43)	Glu 7.5 (135)
K 3.9 (3.9)	Hgb 170 (17)	Ca 2.24 (9.0)
Cl 103 (103)	Lkc 5.7 × 10⁹ (5.7 × 10³)	Po₄ 1.38 (4.3)
HCO₃ 28 (28)	Plts 238 × 10⁹ (238 × 10³)	Mg 1.0 (2.0)
BUN 14 (39)	MCV 88 (88)	Glycosylated
CR 318 (3.6)	Alb 38 (3.8)	Hgb 10%

T_4 154 nmol/liter (12.0 µg/dl)
T_3 1.36 nmol/liter (89 ng/dl)
FTI 10.5
TSH < 0.4 µU/liter
UA: (−) glucose, (−) ketones, (−) albumin, SMBG
    (averages from last 2 months) fasting 6.4 (115),
    prelunch 6.7 (120), predinner 10.8 (195), bedtime
    6.6 (118)

PROBLEM LIST

1. Type I DM
2. Hypothyroidism
3. ESRD—treated with hemodialysis

Problem 1. Type I DM

S: KJ is without complaints of polydipsia, polyuria, or polyphagia.
O: KJ has a glycosylated hemoglobin of 10% and blood glucose
   levels as shown above. Urine is without glucose, protein,
   or ketones.
A: KJ is moderately well controlled on the current regimen.
   He appears to be compliant with insulin dosing and with
   blood glucose monitoring. SMGB reveals that the predinner blood glucose level is consistently elevated.
P: One should increase the morning NPH dose by 2 units,
   or have KJ decrease his caloric intake at lunch. Either of
   these measures should result in a decline in predinner
   blood glucose levels. Caution should be exercised with
   these changes because insulin requirements may decline
   when his thyroxine dose is decreased (Problem 2).

Problem 2. Hypothyroidism

S: KJ is without signs and symptoms of hypothyroidism or
   hyperthyroidism.
O: T_4 154 (12.0), T_3 1.36 (89), FTI 10.5, TSH < 0.4
A: KJ has a suppressed TSH level which indicates a mild hyperthyroid state.
P: One should decrease thyroxine dose by 25 µg to 125 µg/
   day, and monitor for signs and symptoms of hyper- and
   hypothyroidism. If he were to remain asymptomatic, one
   should repeat thyroid function tests in four to six weeks.
   If he were to have signs and/or symptoms of hyper- or
   hypothyroidism, one should repeat thyroid function panel
   at that time.

Problem 3. End-stage Renal Disease (Hemodialysis)

S: Patient is without complaints of renal failure and is being
   treated with hemodialysis.
O: Blood chemistries are WNL (with the exception of BUN
   and CR, which are unremarkable for a hemodialysis patient). CBC is WNL.
A: KJ appears to be tolerating chronic hemodialysis and is
   being well maintained on current medications. He is not
   on any medications that require adjustment for HD.
P: One should continue with current treatment plan: hemodialysis three times weekly, B-complex vitamins q.d., vitamin
   C 500 mg b.i.d., CaCO₃ 500 mg t.i.d., 1,25-dihydroxyvitamin
   D 0.25 µg/day, and folic acid 1 mg q.d.

QUESTIONS FOR CASE 35

1. This patient has a history of lipoatrophy. What is lipoatrophy, and what is its treatment?
2. How does thyroid function or thyroid replacement therapy
   affect insulin kinetics?
3. What is the appropriate method for mixing NPH and regular insulin?
4. Should this patient have a glucagon kit? Why?
5. How is glucagon administered?

CASE 36

CC: JN is a 55-year-old male who has returned to the general medicine clinic for a routine follow-up visit. His joint pain has been increasing lately and he has difficulty walking. He also complains of increasing abdominal discomfort when he takes some of his medications. He denies increased thirst or urination.

Past Medical History

JN has degenerative joint disease that has been treated with steroids for the last nine years. His pain was relatively well controlled until six months ago when increasing pain and morning stiffness required an increase in prednisone therapy from 10 mg q. AM to 15 mg q. AM. He was diagnosed with hyperthyroidism 20 years ago and treated with radioactive iodine, resulting in hypothyroidism requiring thyroid replacement therapy. He has had adult-onset DM for five years, which has only been moderately controlled with oral hypoglycemics. Three months ago, he was diagnosed with hypercholesterolemia and hypertriglyceridemia that was verified after repeated testing. He was started on niacin and diet therapy.

Medication History

Prednisone 15 mg p.o. q.AM
Levothyroxine 0.075 mg p.o. q.d.
Ibuprofen 400 mg p.o. q.i.d.
Glyburide 5 mg q.AM with breakfast
Niacin 500 mg p.o. t.i.d.

Allergies

Codeine—severe stomach distress
Ampicillin—rash

Physical Examination

GEN: Obese, cushingoid-appearing male in slight distress, mild swelling and tenderness in both knees
VS: BP 145/85, HR 87 regular, T 37.0°C, Wt 98 kg (ideal 85 kg)
ABD: Obese, soft, no masses
RECT: Guaiac-negative
EXT: Thin, wasted extremities, several ecchymoses, knees warm and tender to touch

Results of Laboratory Tests (fasting)

Na 138 (138)	BUN 6.4 (18)	AAST 0.4 (24)	ESR 47
K 3.9 (3.9)	CR 88.4 (1.0)	ALT 0.45 (27)	TFTs normal
Cl 108 (108)	Hct 0.42 (42)	Alk Phos 1.1 (68)	Total Chol 4.9 (190)
HCO₃ 19 (19)	Hgb 140 (14)	Glu 8.9 (160)	TG 2.54 (225)

Urinalysis: normal

PROBLEM LIST

1. Hypothyroidism × 20 years
2. Degenerative joint disease × 15 years
3. Chronic steroid toxicity
4. Type II DM × 5 years
5. Mixed hyperlipidemia × 3 months

Problem 4. Mixed Hyperlipidemia

S: Stomach distress when taking medication.
O: Total cholesterol 4.9 (190), fasting triglyceride 2.54 (225).
A: JN has two risk factors for CHD (diabetes and male sex) and, therefore, is "high risk." Cholesterol is under control and below target value of 5.2 (200). Triglyceride level is slightly elevated despite diet and drug therapy. Both diabetes and glucocorticoid therapy can aggravate hyperlipidemia. His diabetes is not well controlled, and the increase in prednisone dose six months ago could have precipitated hyperlipidemia and the subsequent diagnosis. His diabetes should be controlled before a diagnosis of hyperlipidemia is made and treatment initiated. Diet therapy was not unreasonable, but beginning niacin in JN was premature. In addition, triglycerides are not an independent risk factor for CHD, and the value of treating mild elevations is questionable. Niacin is most likely contributing to his stomach distress. Niacin can also aggravate diabetes. This drug was not a good choice for JN.
P: One should discontinue niacin therapy, but diet counseling for using NCEP step 1 diet can be continued. Do not initiate aggressive therapy for hyperlipidemia until the diabetes is under better control and it is clear that the prednisone dose cannot be lowered. Diet should be given a six-month trial before drug therapy is initiated.

Problem 5. Chronic Steroid Toxicity

S: Stomach upset.
O: Obese, cushingoid appearance, altered fat distribution with thin extremities, bruising on extremities, fasting glucose 160, fasting triglycerides 2.54 (225), and Lkcs 12.
A: Long-term side effects of treatment are unavoidable.
P: The patient should take prednisone with meals to avoid stomach distress. One should taper steroids; steroids are usually not required for DJD. NSAIDs are as effective as acetaminophen (Problem 2). After tolerating ibuprofen for DJD for four to six weeks, one should begin steroid taper to minimum effective dose. Reduce the dose in increments of 5 mg every other day (2.5 mg daily); therefore, the first dose of taper is 15 mg q.o.d., alternating with 10 mg q.o.d. (15 mg day 1, 10 mg day 2, 15 mg day 3, etc.). Dose should be reduced slowly and no more frequently than every two weeks to prevent addisonian crisis and flare of pain from withdrawal. Stop taper when pain flares, and increase prednisone dose to the previous step in the taper before pain returned. If a dose of prednisone of 5 mg q.d. (20 mg hydrocortisone equivalent) were achieved before pain returned, one should stop taper, switch to hydrocortisone 10 mg q.d., and maintain dose until AM cortisol level is normal, indicating the return of a pituitary-adrenal response. One should then discontinue steroids.

Problem 1. Hypothyroidism

S: None.

O: TFTs normal.

A: JN seems to be well-controlled on current dose of levothyroxine.

P: One should continue levothyroxine 0.075 mg daily.

Problem 2. Degenerative Joint Disease

S: Increasing pain and difficulty walking.

O: Knees warm and tender to touch; ESR 47.

A: Pain and inflammation are due to DJD and require drug therapy. One should avoid increasing prednisone unless absolutely required. JN should be maintained on a minimum effective dose to reduce long-term adverse effects of steroid therapy. Use optimal dose of NSAIDs; ibuprofen dose can be increased as high as 3200 mg daily.

P: One should increase ibuprofen to 600 mg q6h, and increase the dose in four to six weeks to 800 mg if pain and inflammation were still not relieved. Instruct JN to take medication with food to minimize stomach upset.

Problem 3. Diabetes

S: JN denies increased thirst or urination.

O: Fasting glucose 160 (8.9).

A: Glucose level is not well controlled. Prednisone may contribute to diabetes, and the recent dose increase may have worsened control. Addition of niacin therapy three months ago may have further aggravated JN's condition. Tight control may be difficult to achieve in JN because of prednisone therapy.

P: One should discontinue niacin for cholesterol as described above. If diabetes were still not controlled and prednisone therapy were stable, one could increase glyburide to 5 mg q.AM and 2.5 mg q.PM.

QUESTIONS FOR CASE 36

1. What are the chronic side effects of steroid therapy?
2. Is acetaminophen a therapeutic alternative for DJD?
3. Would sustained-release niacin have minimized JN's stomach upset?
4. What would be appropriate initial drug therapy for JN's hyperlipidemia if diet therapy were to fail and drug treatment were initiated?
5. What are some nondrug treatment options for DJD?

CASE 37

CC: RM is an obese 56-year-old male admitted to the hospital with complaints of extreme weakness of the arms and legs, headache, and increased thirst. He was examined in hypertension clinic one week ago, where BP was found to be elevated.

Past Medical History

This is RM's second hospitalization this year. During his previous admission eight months ago he was diagnosed as having tuberculosis and started on medications. RM also has a history of hypertension for the past 15 years. He has noticed a 12-kg weight gain over the past two months. He has a positive family history for DM.

Social History

History of alcohol abuse; tobacco (40 pack years)

Medication History

Isoniazid 300 mg p.o. q.d.
Rifampin 600 mg p.o. q.d.
Nifedipine XL 180 mg p.o. q.d.
Acetaminophen 650 mg p.o. p.r.n. for headache pain

Physical Examination

GEN: Obese male appearing very anxious
VS: BP 140/105, HR 84, RR 20, T 36.9°C, Wt 94 kg
HEENT: Rounded face, ruddy skin color, no hemorrhages or exudates
CHEST: Normal breath sounds
COR: Normal S1, S2, + S4
ABD: Protuberant abdomen, + striae, normal bowel sounds
EXT: Thin, wasted appearance; bilateral proximal muscle weakness of arms and legs; unhealed bruise on left lower leg; 2+ pitting edema of lower extremities
SKIN: Hyperpigmented

Results of Laboratory Tests

Na 140 (140)	Hct 0.36 (36)	ALT 0.55 (33)	Glu fasting 10.8 (195)
K 3.0 (3.0)	Hgb 120 (12)	LDH 1.8 (110)	Ca 4.6 (9.2)
Cl 100 (100)	Lkcs 8 × 10⁹ (8 × 10³)	Alk phos 1.7 (105)	Po₄ 1.3 (4.0)
HCO₃ 22 (22)	Plts 313 × 10⁹ (313 × 10³)	Alb 36 (3.6)	Mg 1.0 (2.0)
BUN 6.4 (18)	MCV 92 (92)	T bili 15.4 (0.9)	Uric acid 321 (5.4)
CR 106 (1.2)	AST 0.58 (35)		

Serum cortisol: 1048 nmol/liter (38 μg/dl)

Serum ACTH: 2.20 pmol/liter (10 pg/ml), UA 3+ glucose, no ketones, SG 1.022

Urine free cortisol: (24 h) 827 nmol/day (300 μg/24 hr)

ECG: WNL

PROBLEM LIST

1. Hypertension
2. History of tuberculosis
3. Cushing syndrome
4. Hyperglycemia
5. Hypokalemia

Problem 3. Cushing Syndrome

S: RM complains of proximal muscle weakness and weight gain.

O: Findings include truncal obesity; wasted extremities; anxiety; increased BP; hyperpigmented skin; abdominal striae; edema; increased serum sodium, glucose, and cortisol levels; decreased serum potassium concentration; elevated 24-hr urine free cortisol; and suppressed serum ACTH levels.

A: Signs and symptoms of chronic cortisol excess are present. The 24-hr urine free cortisol test is used as a screening test to verify hypercortisolism. The serum ACTH test is a localization test that, in this patient, suggests that the hypercortisolism is most likely secondary to an ACTH-independent cause, such as an adrenal tumor.

P: One should obtain CT scan of the adrenal glands to document an adrenal tumor. Treatment of an adrenal tumor is unilateral adrenalectomy of the affected gland. During the operative and immediate postoperative periods, it is important to administer corticosteroids until the remaining adrenal gland is fully functional. Therefore, one should administer hydrocortisone phosphate 100 mg (or equivalent) IV q8h beginning just before surgery is begun. Continue RM on this dose of IV hydrocortisone for at least 24–48 hrs. Taper the intravenous hydrocortisone by 50% each day for the next three days, convert to hydrocortisone 20 mg p.o. b.i.d. for one to two days, and then discontinue corticosteroid therapy. It may be necessary to continue corticosteroid treatment for a longer period, depending upon RM's response. Monitor for adrenocorticoid insufficiency: weakness, confusion, nausea, vomiting, hyperkalemia, hyponatremia, and hypoglycemia. One should also monitor BP, serum electrolytes, signs and symptoms of infection, gastrointestinal distress, stool guaiac tests, and the need for a higher steroid dose caused by increased drug metabolism by rifampin (hepatic microsomal oxidase enzyme induction).

Problem 4. Hyperglycemia

S: Increased thirst.

O: Serum glucose 10.8 (195), glucose in urine, and positive family history.

A: RM's hyperglycemia is secondary to hypercortisolism and a predisposition to type II DM. High serum levels of cortisol inhibit tissue responsiveness to insulin and stimulate hepatic gluconeogenesis. Nifedipine may also be contributing to hyperglycemia.

P: One should treat RM by administering regular insulin on a sliding scale based on serum glucose levels obtained q6h. It will probably be necessary to continue insulin postoperatively, until RM has stabilized and can be taken off of exogenous corticosteroids. The goal of insulin therapy is to keep the fasting serum glucose < 7.8 (140). Monitor serum glucose levels q6h, serum electrolyte levels, and signs and symptoms of hypoglycemia.

Problem 1. Hypertension

S: RM complains of a headache and attends hypertension clinic.

O: Elevated BP.

A: Increased BP is most likely due to sodium and water retention with hypercortisolism and increased fluid intake due to thirst. RM is on a high dose of nifedipine, which may be contributing to his leg edema.

P: One should institute a low-salt diet, administer p.o. furosemide 40 mg 1 dose, and then start furosemide 20 mg p.o. q.d. until postoperative steroids have been discontinued and RM has stabilized. Continue nifedipine XL 180 mg p.o. q.d., but hold the dose for systolic BP < 90 mm Hg. Once RM has stabilized off exogenous corticosteroids, decrease the nifedipine XL dose to < 120 mg q.d., and monitor intake and output, and serum electrolyte and calcium levels.

Problem 5. Hypokalemia

S: RM complains of weakness.

O: Serum potassium 3.0.

A: Hypokalemia is secondary to hypercortisolism which promotes potassium excretion. Insulin administration, as recommended in Problem 4, also exacerbates hypokalemia. Furosemide administration, as recommended in Problem 1, increases potassium loss in urine. Potassium replacement is recommended to prevent severe hypokalemia which may induce cardiac conduction abnormalities.

P: One should administer p.o. potassium 40 mEq one dose, and begin 20 mEq p.o. q.d. until postoperative steroids have been discontinued. One should also monitor serum potassium at least daily, ECG, and complaints of muscle aches.

Problem 2. History of Tuberculosis

S: RM is taking medications for tuberculosis.

O: Hospitalization eight months ago for tuberculosis.

A: Antituberculosis medications should be continued for at least nine months. Rifampin can interfere with the metabolism of corticosteroids by inducing hepatic elimination. Isoniazid and rifampin are associated with a high incidence of adverse hepatic effects.

P: One should continue rifampin and isoniazid, and monitor RM closely for signs and symptoms of adrenocorticoid deficiency due to increased hydrocortisone metabolism and use higher doses if this were to occur. Monitor for signs and symptoms of hepatitis and adrenocorticoid deficiency.

QUESTIONS FOR CASE 37

1. Identify three laboratory test abnormalities in RM's report that are associated with hypercortisolism. List five other laboratory tests that are also associated with hypercortisolism.
2. If the serum ACTH level evaluation were not conducted, what other testing procedures could be performed to diagnose hypercortisolism? Describe how these tests are conducted and how they can be used to determine the cause of hypercortisolism.
3. Describe the HPA-axis and the difference between ACTH-dependent and ACTH-independent hypercortisolism.
4. If RM were to begin to experience acute nausea and vomiting, confusion, hyperkalemia, hypoglycemia, and depression during his fourth postoperative day, what would be the most likely cause and how should this situation be managed?

5. If RM's surgery had to be delayed for a few months, what treatment could be given until then? Give specific drug recommendations including dosing regimen, adverse reactions, and drug interactions.

CASE 38

CC: EE is a 46-year-old commercial fisherman who is admitted for dehydration secondary to a combination of sun exposure and nausea and vomiting. He also complains of increased confusion and memory loss.

History of Present Illness

EE was diagnosed with primary hyperparathyroidism 10 years ago and refused surgery. At that time his serum calcium ranged 2.62–2.82 mmol/liter (10.5–11.3 mg/dl) and an intact PTH level ranged 60–70. He gave a history of passing two kidney stones but had no bone pain, constipation, numbness, tingling, cramps, muscle weakness, or other symptoms associated with hyperparathyroidism.

Past Medical History

He has hypertension, which was diagnosed four years ago, and is controlled with HCTZ 100 mg p.o. q.d. Hashimoto thyroiditis was diagnosed five years ago and he has been maintained on desiccated thyroid 3 g daily.

Social History

Cigarettes—two packs per day for 10 years
Alcohol—binges, especially when fishing
Cheese—daily intake

Family History

Postive for insulin-dependent diabetes, hypertension, gout, and CAD

Medication History

HCTZ 100 mg p.o. q.AM
Rolaids 1 p.o. q6h p.r.n. for abdominal pain
Multivitamins 1 p.o. q.d.
Senokot® 2 tablets q6h for last two weeks
OTC salt substitute p.r.n.
Desiccated thyroid 3 g p.o. q.d.

Allergies

None known

Review of Systems

EE complains of dizziness, fatigue, polyuria, polydipsia, nocturia, and feeling very thirsty despite increased liters of fluid and orange juice intake. Constipation has been particularly bothersome as he has had only one bowel movement every two weeks. Increased use of Senokot® tablets has been only slightly helpful. His joints have been aching more and interfering with his ability to fish. He is concerned that he has been forgetful, especially with taking his medications. However, he does recall intermittent palpitations soon after taking his thyroid tablets.

Physical Examination

GEN: Ill-appearing male in moderate distress
VS: BP 170/100, HR 100 (sitting), BP 130/60, HR 130 (standing), RR 22, T 37.0°C, Wt 60 kg
HEENT: PERRLA, (+) arteriolar narrowing, dry and pale mucous membranes and gums, (+) firm thyroid goiter 35 g
COR: Normal S_1, S_2, sinus tachycardia
CHEST: Clear to ausculation and percussion
ABD: Positive bowel sounds, lower quadrant tenderness
GU: WNL
RECT: Guaiac-negative, (+) impacted stool
EXT: (+) Bone tenderness, poor skin turgor
NEURO: 3 (+) deep tendon reflexes, (+) ataxia, unable to do "serial 7s"

Results of Laboratory Tests

Na 150 (150)	CR 221 (2.5)	MCV 100 (100)	Glu 20.3 (365)
K 6.8 (6.8)	Hct 0.43 (43)	AST 1.08 (65)	Ca 3.99 (16)
Cl 110 (110)	Hgb 160 (16)	ALT 0.92 (55)	PO₄ 0.58 (1.8)
HCO₃ 37 (37)	Lkcs 13 × 10⁹ (13 × 10³)	Alk Phos 3.3 (200)	Uric Acid 714 (12)
BUN 23.2 (65)	Plts 300 × 10⁹ (300 × 10³)	Alb 34 (3.4)	Chol 8.02 (310)

PTH 95 pg/ml, TT₄ 84 nmol/liter (6.5 μg/dl)
FT₄I 6.5, TSH 12 mU/liter (12 μU/ml)
Lkcs differential: no left shift
Urinalysis: 1.033, urine Na < 2 mmol/day (< 2 mEq/24 hr), urine K < 10 mmol/day (< 10 mEq/24 hr), 3+ glucose, (−) ketones, 0–2 rbc and Lkcs
Sonogram of neck: (+) parathyroid adenoma
ECG: Sinus rate 130, PR 0.22, QT 0.2, QRS 0.15, (+) wide T-waves

PROBLEM LIST

1. Hypertension
2. Hypovolemia/dehydration
3. Hyperparathyroidism
4. Acute hypercalcemia
5. Hypothyroidism
6. Hyperkalemia
7. Hyperglycemia
8. Constipation
9. Hyperuricemia

QUESTIONS FOR CASE 38

1. Discuss the use of plicamycin in the management of hypercalcemia secondary to primary hyperthyroidism.
2. Discuss the role of calcitonin in the management of hypercalcemia secondary to primary hyperparathyroidism.

3. Discuss when phosphates should be used in the acute and chronic management of hypercalcemia from primary hyperparathyroidism.
4. How should hypocalcemia be managed postparathyroidectomy?

CASE 39

CC: AH is a 57-year-old white male referred by a primary care physician to a diabetes clinic for evaluation of adverse drug reactions related to oral hypoglycemic agent therapy. The patient was diagnosed with noninsulin-dependent diabetes about two years ago. Despite numerous attempts with diet control, AH was unable to achieve satisfactory weight reduction and glycemic control with diet and exercise alone. His fasting blood glucose concentrations have been in the 9.4–10.0 mmol/liter (170–180 mg/dl) range over the last two months, with a glycosylated hemoglobin level of 11%. The patient complains of signs and symptoms (sweating, tremulousness, and hunger) of hypoglycemia on two occasions over the past week. AH has not required assistance for treatment of the hypoglycemia and has self-treated with orange juice. SMBG at these times revealed blood glucose levels of 3.0 mmol/liter (55 mg/dl) and 2.8 mmol/liter (51 mg/dl). AH also complains of dizziness and flushing last night after consumption of one glass of wine. The patient also complains of nocturia, polyuria, and fatigue.

Past Medical History
HTN × 10 years
Type II DM
Rheumatoid arthritis (mild)

Family History
Diabetes
HTN

Social History
Nonsmoker
Drinks wine on rare occasions

Medications History
HCTZ 50 mg q.d.
KCl 40 mEq q.AM
Prednisone 15 mg q.d. (× 10 months)
Chlorpropamide 250 mg q.d.

Physical Examination
GEN: Obese, pale-appearing male in NAD
VS: BP 154/94 (previous BP ranged from 150/92 to 160/96) HR 88 regular, RR 14, Wt 90 kg (up 3 kg), Ht 173 cm

HEENT: EOM intact, PERRLA, facial edema
COR: NSR
CHEST: Without rales, rhonchi
ABD: Normal, positive bowel sounds, no guarding, no organomegaly
EXT: No peripheral edema
NEURO: DTR intact, without signs of diabetic neuropathy

Results of Laboratory Tests

Na 140 (140)	CR one year ago 133 (1.5)	MCHC 310 (31)
K 4.5 (4.5)	Hct 0.32 (32)	Glu (Random) 10 (180)
Cl 98 (98)	Hgb 100 (10)	Chol 6.4 (250)
HCO$_3$ 21 (21)	Lkcs 6.8 × 10^9 (6.8 × 10^3)	TG 2.68 (238)
BUN 10 (28)	MCV 91 (91)	Hb$_{Alc}$ 11%
CR 221 (2.5)	MCH 24 (24)	

Folate 4.5 nmol/liter (2 µg/dl)
Fe 14.7 µmol/liter (82 µg/dl)
Vit B$_{12}$ 162 pmol/liter (220 ng/dl)
U/A: (–) glucose, (–) ketone, (1+) protein

PROBLEM LIST
1. DM
2. Rheumatoid arthritis
3. Anemia
4. Steroid use
5. Adverse drug reaction (oral hypoglycemic agent)

QUESTIONS FOR CASE 39
1. Why are β-antagonists not the drugs of choice for the hypertensive patient with diabetes?
2. What side effects are associated with chlorpropamide use?
3. Should patients who take oral hypoglycemic agents be instructed against alcohol consumption?
4. Should urine glucose testing be routinely practiced by AH?
5. What preventative measures may prevent the progression of renal failure in the patient with diabetes?

CASE 40

CC: PJ is a 42-year-old female who presents to thyroid clinic with complaints of increasing fatigue and muscle weakness that are interfering with her job and active lifestyle. She is also very concerned about a "lump" in her throat that interferes with her swallowing. She denies any choking or respiratory difficulties. Food does not get stuck in her throat.

Past Medical History
PJ has a one-year history of recurrent idiopathic thrombocytopenia purpura (ITP) that has been managed with chronic steroid therapy. ITP has caused bruising, chronic gastrointestinal bleeding, epistaxis, and menorrhagia. She was also diagnosed six months ago with iron deficiency anemia. Iron was prescribed, but she has not been compliant because the tablets upset her stomach and caused her to be constipated.

Family History

Her father was diagnosed with Graves' disease and her sister is taking thyroid for a "fat neck." Family history is positive for diabetes and heart disease.

Social History

Drinks two to three glasses of wine daily

Medication History

Prednisone 60 mg q.d.
FeSO$_4$ 325 mg t.i.d.
OTC ibuprofen 200 mg 2 tablets p.r.n. for menstrual cramps or ASA 325 mg q.i.d. p.r.n.
OTC Senokot® 1–2 tablets q.d. p.r.n. for constipation
Kelp tablets q.d. (bought in health food store) × one year
Lo-Ovral 1 tablet q.d. for contraception

Allergies

None known

Review of Systems

PJ complains of a "lump" in her throat, 10-kg weight gain over the last six months, decreased energy, "inability to think," and feeling "colder" than others. She also has more "painful and heavy periods" than is usual for her. Her skin has been dry and itchy, and her hair seems to be falling out. Constipation is bothersome as she only has one bowel movement per week. Her voice seems deeper, and she can no longer sing high notes. She complains of increased urinary frequency and hesitation. She claims she always has bleeding gums, some blood in her stools, and bruises on her arms and legs, but this is much better than it used to be.

Physical Examination

GEN: Lethargic, obese, cushingoid-appearing 47-year-old female in no apparent distress
VS: BP 160/95, HR 78, RR 10, T 37.8°C, Wt 60 kg
HEENT: Flaky, dry scalp; puffy, moon facies; periorbital edema; dry and pale mucous membranes and gums; epistaxis; conjunctival hemorrhages; diffusely enlarged goiter, approximately 55 g; right > left; no discrete nodules palpable
COR: Normal S$_1$, S$_2$, no S$_3$, S$_4$, or murmurs
CHEST: Clear to auscultation
ABD: Obese, soft, nontender; multiple striae, purpura, and petechiae
GU: WNL
RECT: Guaiac-positive but no bright red blood per rectum
EXT: (+) Thin, wasted lower extremities, (+) pretibial myxedema, (+) multiple purpura and petechiae on arms and legs, (+) dry scaly skin, (+) pale nail beds
NEURO: (+) Delayed DTRs, (+) proximal muscle weakness

Results of Laboratory Tests

Na 144 (144)	CR 88 (1.0)	MCV 78 (78)	TIBC 70 (390)
K 3.1 (3.1)	Hct 0.32 (32)	MCHC 260 (26)	T$_4$ 84 (6.5)
Cl 100 (100)	Hgb 120 (12)	Alb 32 (3.2)	FT$_4$I 4.5
HCO$_3$ 30 (30)	Lkcs 7.5 × 10^9 (7.5 × 10^3)	Glu 15.8 (285)	TSH 20 (20)
BUN 5.4 (15)	Plts 120 × 10^9 (120 × 10^3)	Chol 8.02 (310)	Thyroid antibodies (+)

Urinalysis: 10 RBC, 0–2 Lkcs, (+) blood (1+) glucose
ECG: NSR, PR 0.15 sec, (–) PVCs

PROBLEM LIST

1. Idiopathic thrombocytopenia purpura
2. Iron deficiency anemia
3. Steroid toxicity
4. Hyperglycemia
5. Hypokalemia
6. Hypothyroidism

CASE 41

CC: BK is a 23-year-old male with an 11-year history of type I DM. He was brought to the ER with a two-day history of nausea and vomiting, myalgias, polydipsia, and polyuria. BK states that he went to a party, drank excessive alcohol, and woke up two days PTA feeling "sick to his stomach." He has vomited six times since them. He denies HA, chest pain, cough, fever, URI symptoms, and abdominal pain. BK stated he last took his insulin one to two days PTA.

Past Medical History

Type I DM since age 12, several hospital admissions for diabetic keto acidosis (DKA); history of cardiac arrhythmias not requiring chronic therapy (occasional PVCs)

Family History
DM—negative

Social History

Works for father, mother died of suicide, social drinker, nonsmoker, negative IV drug abuse, poor understanding of his disease

Medication History
Human NPH 60 units q. AM

Physical Examination

GEN: Well-developed, well-nourished, pale, 23-year-old male in mild distress
VS: Breathing is deep and labored with fruity breath, BP 100/85 supine, HR 120, BP 99/60 sitting, HR 140, RR 34, T 37.0°C orally, Wt 65 kg (normal weight 72 kg)

HEENT: Dry tongue and mucous membranes
CHEST: Clear to A & P, no rales, no wheezing, no rhonchi
COR: Tachycardia, regular rate and rhythm
EXT: Poor skin turgor
NEURO: A & O × 3
ABD: + voluntary guarding 2° to nervousness + bowel sounds

Results of Laboratory Tests

Na 125 (125)	BUN 14.2 (40)	Lkcs 14 × 10⁹
K 7.7 (7.7)	CR 141 (1.6)	(14 × 10⁵)
Cl 96 (96)	Hct 0.457 (45.7)	Glu 57 (1033)
HCO₃ 14 (14)	Hgb 152 (15.2)	Po₄ 1.5 (4.8)

ABG pH 7.2
Urinalysis: trace protein, 4 + glucose, (+) ketone
Chest radiography: no acute infiltrate
ECG: WNL
BC × 2 pending
UC pending

PROBLEM LIST

1. Type I DM
2. Diabetic ketoacidosis
3. Rule out infection

CASE 42

CC: MG is a 63-year-old male who has come into clinic today for a follow-up visit after discovering an elevated cholesterol level during a health fair screening at a shopping mall one month ago.

Past Medical History

MG has been followed in the diabetes clinic for several years for type II DM that has been well controlled with attention to diet and oral hypoglycemic therapy. He was diagnosed with diabetes approximately five years ago, and he has been compliant with therapy. He is approximately 8–10 kg over his ideal body weight, but his weight has remained constant. He was diagnosed with hypothyroidism 20 years ago by his family physician. Last month, MG had a cholesterol determination performed as part of a health fair at a local shopping mall.

He was told that his cholesterol level was elevated and that he should notify his physician. He has no other complaints and denies increased urination or thirst and changes in energy or weight.

Social History

Retired for three years with a relatively sedentary lifestyle except for a passion for golf, which he plays three times weekly. Nonsmoker, he drinks two to three glasses of white wine with his evening meal.

Family History

Father died of presumed myocardial infarction at age 53. Brother recovered from acute myocardial infarction at age 44 and is otherwise healthy.

Medication History

Thyroid tablet 1½ grain daily
Glyburide 2.5 mg daily
Dipstick for urine glucose testing as needed

Allergies

None known

Physical Examination

GEN: Slightly overweight man in no apparent distress
VS: BP 150/88, HR 85 regular, RR 18, Wt 89 kg
HEENT: Normal
COR: Normal
ABD: Positive bowel sounds
EXT: Skin normal with good turgor
NEURO: Tendon reflexes normal

Results of Laboratory Tests (fasting)

Total cholesterol 5.95 (230)
HDL cholesterol 1.89 (73)
LDL cholesterol 3.89 (150)
Triglycerides 1.1 (97)
Thyroid function tests: normal
Glucose 7.5 (135)
U/A normal, glucose-negative

PROBLEM LIST

1. Hypothyroidism (× 20 years)
2. Type II DM (× five years)
3. Hyperlipidemia

RENAL DISEASES

CASE 43

CC: HJ is a 67-year-old male seen in clinic today for follow-up of chronic medical problems. His chief complaints are a 3-day history of frequent urination and urgency. He also complains of chronic fatigue, weakness, and occasional nausea/vomiting, which is unchanged from his last visit.

Past Medical History

Chronic renal insufficiency × two years secondary to analgesic abuse for chronic pain
Congestive heart failure (CHF) × five years
Hypertension (HTN) × 20 years

Medication History

Digoxin 0.25 mg p.o. q.d.
Lisinopril 30 mg p.o. q.d.
Triamterene/HCTZ 1 q.d.
Acetaminophen 650 mg p.o. q4–6h p.r.n. for pain

Allergies

None known

Physical Examination

GEN: Well-developed, well-nourished male in no acute distress
VS: BP 100/70, HR 60, RR 20, T 37.1°C, Wt 73 kg, Ht 173 cm
HEENT: Pale mucous membranes and skin
COR: Normal S1 and S2, early S3
CHEST: Few rales and dullness over bases of lungs
ABD: WNL
GU: No flank pain
RECT: WNL
EXT: Pale nail beds
NEURO: WNL

Results of Laboratory Tests

Na 130 (130)	Cr 309.4 (3.5)	MCV 85 fl	T bili 13.7 (0.8)
K 5.5 (5.5)	Hct .31 (31.1)	ALT 47 (28)	Ca 2.1 (8.4)
Cl 105 (105)	Hgb 104 (10.4)	Alk Phos 2.12 (127)	Po₄ 1.97 (6.1)
HCO₃ 22 (22)	Lkcs 5.4 × 10⁹ (5.4)	Alb 31 (3.1)	Mg 1.15 (2.8)
BUN 20 (56)	Plts 4.25 × 10⁹ (425)		

UA: Lkcs > 50 cells/hpf
Appearance: cloudy
Esterase: positive
Peripheral smear: normochromic, normocytic

Chest radiography: enlarged heart
ECG: prolonged P-R interval with occasional PVCs

PROBLEM LIST

1. HTN
2. Chronic CHF
3. Chronic renal insufficiency
4. Anemia
5. UTI

CASE 43 SOAP NOTES

Problem 3. Chronic Renal Insufficiency (CRI)

S: None.

O: BUN 20 mmol/liter (56), Cr 309.4 μmol/liter (3.5), Na 130 mmol/liter (130), K 5.5 mmol/liter (5.5), Po₄ 1.97 mmol/liter (6.1), and decreased Hgb and Hct.

A: HJ has CRI as evidenced by electrolyte changes and anemia. Cause of CRI from HJ's history is from continued analgesic use for chronic pain. A second possible cause for HJ's CRI is his long history of HTN. HJ is exhibiting a number of electrolyte disturbances secondary to CRI. At creatinine clearances (CrCl) < 0.4 ml/sec (25 ml/min), the kidney is unable to decrease sodium excretion to match sodium intake. Because HJ has a history of CHF and HTN, it is likely that he will require a low-sodium diet. However, this must be balanced with the kidney's inability to compensate for changes in sodium intake. In addition, HJ is taking an ACE-inhibitor and a diuretic, both of which act to increase sodium excretion that can contribute to hyponatremia. Hyperphosphotemia occurs frequently when CrCl < 0.4 ml/sec (25 ml/min). To prevent the development of renal osteodystrophy, it is necessary to control phosphate intake. Initially dietary restriction through reduction of high-phosphorus-containing foods (meat, milk, legumes, and carbonated beverages) can be attempted. Phosphate-binding antacids may be useful. Hyperkalemia is not usually found until CrCl < 0.08 ml/sec (5 ml/min). However, HJ is taking lisinopril and triamterene, both of which retain potassium in exchange for sodium. He may need to switch to a nonpotassium-sparing diuretic if two drugs were necessary to control HTN and chronic CHF symptoms.

P: One should discontinue triamterene/HCTZ, start aluminum hydroxide 500 mg p.o. three to four times daily, and counsel on dietary restriction of foods containing phosphate.

Problem 5. UTI

S: Frequent urination, urgency.

O: UA has Lkcs > 50 cells/hpf and is cloudy and esterase-positive.

A: HJ's symptoms are consistent with an uncomplicated UTI. He does not complain of flank pain, has no fever, chills, or other signs of systemic involvement. A possible cause of HJ's UTI is benign prostatic hypertrophy (BPH), which is common in males over 50 years of age. Approximately 3/4 of UTIs in males are due to gram-negative bacilli, which are most likely sensitive to trimethoprim/sulfamethoxazole.

P: One should start trimethoprim/sulfamethoxazole DS b.i.d. × 10–14 days. This dose is appropriate for a CrCl of 0.33 ml/sec (20 ml/min). A work-up for the etiology of HJ's UTI should be done as well as culture and sensitivity testing if symptoms were not to improve within two to three days.

Problem 2. Chronic CHF/Digoxin Toxicity

S: Nausea/vomiting, fatigue, and weakness.

O: Findings include few rales and dullness over bases of lungs, enlarged heart on chest radiography, and early S_2. Prolonged P-R interval occurred with occasional premature ventricular contractions (PVCs)

A: Although he exhibits many of the characteristics associated with CHF, HJ does not appear to be in any acute distress. Nausea/vomiting and ECG changes are consistent with digoxin toxicity. Expected parameters include the following:

1. Digoxin:

$$CrCl \ (ml/min/kg) = \frac{140 - Age}{Scr \ 72}$$

$CrCl = 0.29 \ ml/min/kg$
$Cl_{Dig} = 0.9 \ (CrCl) + 0.33$
$\quad = 0.59 \ ml/min/kg \ (73 \ kg)$
$\quad = 43.2 \ ml/min = 2.6 \ liter/hr$
$Vd = 3.8 + 3.1 \ (CrCl)$
$\quad = 4.7 \ liter/kg \ (73 \ kg) = 343 \ liter$
$Kel = Cl/Vd = 2.6/343 = 0.0076 \ hr^{-1}$
$T_{1/2} = 0.693/Kel = 3.8 \ days$

$$C_{ave} = \frac{SFD/\tau}{Cl}$$

$$C_{ave} = \frac{0.65 \ 250/24}{2.41} = 2.8 \ \mu g/liter$$

$\quad = 3.6 \ nmol/liter$

2. Both renal failure and CHF decrease the clearance of digoxin and are likely to prolong $t_{1/2}$ in HJ.

3. By halving the current maintenance dose, a steady-state level of approximately 1.8 nmol/liter (1.4 μg/liter) will be achieved. Based on expected parameters, assuming compliance, HJ's digoxin level is predicted to be 3.6 nmol/liter (2.8 μg/liter). Because HJ is not bradycardic, not exhibiting heart block, and not hypokalemic, digoxin antibodies are not indicated.

P: One should obtain serum digoxin level. If it were consistent with the predicted level, one should hold treatment for three to four days, which is approximately one half-life, and restart the dose at 0.125 mg p.o. q.d. to achieve a level of 1.8 nmol/liter (1.4 μg/liter). If symptoms of CHF were

to persist, one should consider adding furosemide at the next appointment.

Problem 4. Anemia

S: Fatigue, weakness, and pale nail beds.

O: Microcytic, hypochromic.

A: HJ's anemia most likely represents a reduced production of erythrocytes. Chronic blood loss secondary to uremia is a likely cause. HJ's anemia may be exacerbating his chronic CHF; therefore, occasional transfusions may be necessary to control anemia and CHF. If his anemia were to worsen, it may be necessary to start steroids and/or erythropoietin to stimulate erythropoiesis.

P: One should obtain transfusions p.r.n. and monitor CBC and signs and symptoms of anemia.

Problem 1. HTN

S: None.

O: BP 100/70.

A: BP appears well controlled on current regimen. Because lisinopril is primarily renally eliminated, it has potential for accumulating in renal failure. If diuretics were to be added to control HJ's CHF, it may be necessary to decrease the dose of lisinopril and/or switch to another, shorter-acting ACE-inhibitor to prevent the possibility of becoming hypotensive.

P: One should discontinue triamterene/HCTZ as described above, but continue with lisinopril treatment.

QUESTIONS FOR CASE 43

1. If the digoxin level were to come back as 2.7 nmol/liter (2.1 μg/liter), how would you explain it?

2. What would you do?

3. If HJ were septic and required an aminoglycoside for his UTI, what would be the dose of gentamicin? When should samples for gentamicin levels be drawn?

4. If HJ developed atrial fibrillation, what would be the dose of procainamide?

5. If HJ's atrial fibrillation were refractory to procainamide and quinidine were being considered, would the addition of quinidine affect any of the drugs HJ is currently receiving? How can this be managed?

CASE 44

CC: CL is a 37-year-old female who presents to the ED with nausea, chills, fever, palpitations, polyuria, polydipsia, and weakness.

History of Present Illness

CL has been treated for insulin-dependent diabetes mellitis (IDDM) for 21 years. She usually injects NPH insulin every morning and at bedtime. According to her husband, she has been sick with a bad cold for the past 10 days and she did not administer her bedtime insulin for the past three nights.

Two days ago, she started to experience polyuria and polydipsia. She also ran out of the strips that she uses with her One-Touch II machine to test her blood glucose once weekly.

Past Medical History

CL has a long history of noncompliance with insulin therapy. She experiences about one to two episodes of diabetic ketoacidosis per year. Her last episode was four months ago when she was hospitalized for three days and developed acute renal failure (BUN/creatinine: 20:1) secondary to dehydration. She missed her appointment at the diabetes clinic last month because she was feeling well and she did not need any insulin refills. She also has peripheral neuropathy and claims that amitriptyline helps to relieve the symptoms.

Medication History

Insulin NPH 40 U qPM and 20 U qAM
Captopril 25 mg PO t.i.d.
Ibuprofen 400 mg PO q4h (for the past three days)
Amitriptyline 150 mg PO qHS

Allergies

Penicillin: hives

Review of Systems

Noncontributory

Physical Examination

GEN: thin, ill appearing, lethargic female in acute distress
VS: BP 103/56 mm Hg, HR 125, RR 14, Wt 50 Kg, Ht 152 cm, T 39.5°C
HEENT: PERRLA
CHEST: clear to ascultation and percussion
ABD: soft and nontender
RECT: guaiac negative
EXT: dry mucous membranes, dry skin
Neuro: A&O ×3, cranial nerves intact

Results of Laboratory Tests

Na 149 (149)	BUN 12.5 (35)	Glu 37 (680)
K 5 (5)	Hct 0.47 (47)	Cr 212 (2.4)
Cl 105 (105)	Hgb 150 (15)	WBC 15,000
HCO₃ 6 (6)	Plts 150 × 10⁹ (15 × 10⁵)	

Urinalysis: 1+ Proteinuria, Glucose 2%, pH 5.1, Moderate ketones, SG 1.029, WBC (–), RBC (–), No bacteria or casts

PROBLEM LIST

1. Diabetic ketoacidosis
2. Diabetes
3. Acute renal failure

CASE 44 SOAP NOTES

Problem 1. Diabetic Ketoacidosis (DKA)

S: CL complains of nausea, chills, fever, polyuria, polydipsia,

and weakness.

O: SF has a history of diabetic ketoacidosis. She also has a high serum glucose concentration (750), dry mucous membranes, dry skin, urine PH 5.1, proteinuria, increased respiratory rate (20), low BP, serum HCO₃ 6, and increased HR.

A: Insulin requirements increase during the course of infection in patients with IDDM. In addition, poor compliance is one of the most common causes of DKA, particularly with recurrent episodes. After having polyuria and polydipsia for three days, CL is hypotensive and tachycardic, indicating fluid depletion. CL does not have mental status changes common during DKA. Patients with DKA are generally hypothermic, but CL has a fever as a result of her infection. Furthermore, CL has the classic laboratory findings of DKA (serum glucose: 750, elevated BUN, elevated Cr, low urine pH, ketonuria, and glycosuria). Patients, such as CL, with histories of noncompliance to insulin commonly omit their insulin doses during stressful situations, such as active infection, and predispose themselves to develop DKA.

P: *Hyperglycemia/dehydration:* A bolus dose of insulin (0.1–0.2 unit/kg) followed by a continous infusion of 0.1 unit/kg/hr should be administered concomitantly with normal saline at a rate of 0.5–1 liter/hr. Once the BP and pulse have been stabilized sodium chloride 0.45% may be substituted and once blood glucose begins to approach normal limits, D5 0.45% sodium chloride may be used.
Electrolyte imbalances—Na: Sodium is usually adequately replaced by sodium chloride. *K:* 10–20 meq/hr of potassium may be administered after CL demonstrates adequate urine output. Once the DKA is resolved, a key point in treatment plan for CL is education and counseling with an emphasizes on regular testing of blood glucose and insulin dosing.

Problem 2. Diabetes

S: CL experiences signs and symptoms of DKA and long-term complications of diabetes, including peripheral neuropathy.

O: CL has a history of IDDM for 21 years. Her serum glucose is 750 and she has proteinuria.

A: Patients like CL with IDDM have the tendency to develop DKA and require insulin to sustain life. Weight loss and ketoacidosis are common in poorly controlled IDDM patients. The Diabetes Control and Complications Trial (DCCT) supports the hypothesis that tight glycemic control improves long-term outcome in patients with IDDM. CL is currently experiencing peripheral neuropathy which is a long-term complication of diabetes.

P: IDDM is a chronic disease that requires ongoing care and education to prevent acute illnesses, such as DKA, and to reduce the severity of long-term complications. CL is on NPH insulin which is an intermediate-acting insulin. She should be advised to test her blood glucose frequently and to be able to identify her specific signs and symptoms of hypo- and hyperglycemia. In addition, a major part in CL's treatment plan is patient and family education.

Problem 3. History of Acute Renal Failure (ARF)

S: CL is experiencing dehydration.

O: CL's BUN (35) and Cr (2.4) are elevated.

A: CL developed acute renal failure during her past hospitalization secondary to dehydration. Currently, CL shows some signs and symptoms of dehydration such as dry mucous membranes, dry skin, hypotension, and tachycardia. Her dehydrated status could put her at risk of developing ARF. In addition, CL has other risk factors that predispose her to developing ARF. She is taking ibuprofen and captopril, both of which can induce renal dysfunction. Due to her poorly controlled IDDM, she may have diabetic nephropathy. All these risk factors can worsen her renal function. Because she already has high BUN and Cr levels, her renal function should be monitored closely. The maintenance of renal perfusion is also essential to prevent ARF. CL would most likely receive adequate volume replacement as she is being treated for DKA (which includes fluid replacement therapy).

P: CL's hemodynamic status should be monitored closely while she is receiving fluid replacement therapy. In addition, her BUN and Cr should be checked daily while she is in the hospital until they are normal and stable. Nephrotoxic agents, such as ibuprofen, should be avoided.

QUESTIONS FOR CASE 44

1. Why did CL develop diabetic ketoacidosis?
2. What are the therapeutic considerations when treating diabetic ketoacidosis?
3. What are some common long-term complications of diabetes?
4. Name four risk factors that put CL at high risk of developing acute renal failure.
5. How would you educate CL about the importance of testing her blood glucose at home?

CASE 45

CC: JW is a 37-year-old female admitted through the ED with increased nausea/vomiting and dizziness over the past two days, which she claims is worse after taking her procainamide. Patient states she takes two tablets every six hours.

Past Medical History

JW's history is significant for rheumatic heart disease (RHD) at age two. She was discharged two days ago status-post (S/P) redo mitral valve replacement (MVR) for prosthetic valve endocarditis (*Staphylococcus epidermidis*). JW had received a 2-week course of gentamicin/vancomycin therapy prior to discharge. During her last admission, JW developed perioperative atrial fibrillation and was subsequently started on procainamide. JW also has a history of partial complex seizures after a possible embolic event in 1988 and has been well controlled on phenytoin.

Social History

Tobacco—30 pack-year history
Alcohol—drinks occasionally

Medication History

Phenytoin 300 mg p.o. b.i.d. (increased on last admission from 300 mg HS)
Vancomycin 750 mg IV q12h (home IV therapy)
Procainamide SR 1 g p.o. q6h
Rifampin 300 mg p.o. b.i.d.
Warfarin 5 mg p.o. q.d.

Allergies

None known

Physical Examination

GEN: well-developed, well-nourished female in acute distress

VS: BP 120/74 (sitting), 128/70 (standing); HR 74 (sitting), 70 (standing); RR 20, T 36.9°C, Wt 64 kg (62 kg on last admission), Ht 168 cm

HEENT: nystagmus

COR: JV pulse 8 cm, quick S_1, normal S_2, 2/6 systolic ejection murmur, 2/6 early diastolic murmur

CHEST: clear to auscultation and percussion

ABD: WNL

GU: WNL

RECT: WNL

EXT: WNL

NEURO: ataxia
Abdominal sonography: no urinary obstruction

Results of Laboratory Tests

Na 132 (132)	Hct 0.31 (31.1)	ALT 28.5 (17)	Ca 2.2 (8.9)
K 3.7 (3.7)	Hgb 104 g/l (10.4)	Alk Phos 2.5 (154)	PO_4 1.4 (4.5)
Cl 98 (98)	Lkcs 6.7 × 10^9/l (6.7)	Alb 28 (2.8)	Mg 0.75 (1.8)
HCO_3 26 (26)	Plts 3.9 × 10^9/l (385)	T Bili 10.3 (0.6)	
BUN 8.8 (24)	MCV 68 fl (68)		
Cr 283 (3.2)			

Peripheral smear: macrocytic cells
Urine electrolytes: Cl 86 (86), Cr 539 g/liter (61 mg/dl), Na 74 (74), K 33 (33), osmolality 385 (mmol/kg)
Urine output: 1500 ml/24 hr
CrCl: 0.22 ml/sec (13 ml/min) (24-hr urine collection)
Antinuclear antibodies (ANA): < 40 (titer)
Sedimentation rate: 62 (mm/hr)
Phenytoin: 103.1 μmol/liter (26)
Procainamide: 113 μmol/liter (26.6)
N-Acetyl procainamide: 60.6 μmol/liter (16.8)
Chest radiography: mild increase in heart size, no signs of CHF
ECG: first-degree AV block

PROBLEM LIST
1. Anemia
2. S/P MVR for endocarditis
3. Atrial fibrillation/procainamide toxicity
4. Partial complex seizures/phenytoin toxicity
5. Acute renal failure

QUESTIONS FOR CASE 45
1. When should JW receive her next dose of vancomycin?
2. Would the addition of rifampin affect the dosing of any of the drugs JW is currently receiving?
3. How should this be managed?
4. If JW were to develop melenic stools during the course of treatment, what would be the possible causes?
5. How should this be managed?

CASE 46
CC: DH is a 27-year-old male who received a cadaveric renal transplant 14 days ago. He has an elevated serum creatinine level, decreased UO, and elevated BP.

Past Medical History
The patient has a history of congenital bladder neck obstruction and recurrent pyelonephritis. He underwent bilateral nephrectomy three years ago. Since that time, he has been on hemodialysis until his recent cadaveric renal transplant. He also has a history of hypertension.

Medication History
Cyclosporine 175 mg p.o. b.i.d.
Prednisone 15 mg p.o. b.i.d.
Azathioprine 50 mg p.o. q.d.
Clonidine 0.3 mg p.o. t.i.d.

Allergies
None known

Physical Examination
GEN: Male with cushingoid facies in no apparent distress
VS: T 38.2°C, HR 100, BP 160/110, RR 20, Wt 60 kg, Ht 168 cm
HEENT: Pupils equal, round, reactive to light and accommodation, extraocular muscles intact
COR: Prominent PMI, S1 + S2, II/VI soft systolic murmur, no gallop or rub
CHEST: Unremarkable, without rales, rhonchi, wheezes, or rubs
ABD: + BS, well-healed surgical scar, pain over graft
GU: Normal without mass or hernia
RECT: Guaiac-negative
EXT: Left-sided radial arteriovenous fistula, 1+ pitting edema LLE, good distal pulses, no calf tenderness

Results of Laboratory Tests

Na 140 (140)	Hct 0.24 (24%)	ALT .27 (16)	Glu 6.05 (10⁹)
K 5.0 (5.0)	Hgb 85 (8.5)	LDH 3.6 (215)	Ca 2.3 (9.1)
Cl 110 (110)	Lkcs 9.5 × 10⁹ (9.5 × 10³)	Alk Phos .83 (50)	Po₄ 0.87 (2.7)
HCO₃ 21 (21)	PLT 166 × 10⁹(166 × 10³)	Alb 40 (4.0)	Mg 1.2 (2.4)
BUN 11.1 (31)	MCV 90 (90)	T Bili 8.6 (0.5)	Uric acid 470 (7.9)
Cr 265 (3.0)	Ast 0.28 (17)		

Cyclosporine 94 μg/liter
Lkcs differential: Neutr 8.5 × 10^9/liter, Lymph 0.9, Mono 0.6, Eos 0.2, Baso 0.1
Urinalysis: Spgr 1.010, pH 6.5, 2+ prot, 2 + Hgb, 25–50 RBC, 3–10 Lkcs, occas renal tubule epithelial cells
Chest radiography: Clear
ECG: Normal

PROBLEM LIST
1. Hypertension
2. Cadaveric renal transplant
3. Rejection

CASE 46 SOAP NOTES
Problem 2. Cadaveric Renal Transplant
S: Tenderness, pain at site of transplanted kidney.
O: SCr 265 (3.0), decreased urine output.
A: Renal transplantation is an effective treatment for ESRD. This treatment reverses the undesirable effects of ESRD (e.g., uremia, anemia). Although very successful, cadaveric transplants have lower survival rates than living, related transplants. Reasons for loss of the transplanted kidney (graft) include rejection, infection, obstruction, and surgical failure. The major reason for graft loss is rejection; therefore, chronic treatment with immunosuppressives to prevent this is necessary. Close monitoring, particularly during the first six months after transplant, is needed to detect and treat rejection.
P: One should continue immunosuppressives, monitor for toxicities associated with these agents, and proceed with diagnostic evaluation to rule out rejection or other causes of decreased kidney function (obstruction, infection, cyclosporine toxicity).

Problem 1. Hypertension
S: No symptoms.
O: History of hypertension, BP now 160/110.
A: Hypertension is not uncommon in cadaveric kidney transplant recipients. DH has a previous history of hypertension secondary to renal disease. In addition, acute rejection, cyclosporine, and steroids may also contribute to hypertension. Because the dose of clonidine is maximized, one should consider use of another agent.
P: One should add nifedipine 10 mg p.o. t.i.d., and titrate the dosage regimen to BP, with the goal of maintaining systolic BP at 120–160 and diastolic 80–90.

Problem 3. Rejection
S: DH complains of tenderness on palpation over graft site.
O: Increased Scr from 203 (2.3) to 265 (3.0), decreased UO

from 100 ml/hr to 40 ml/hr, uncontrolled BP, temperature 38.2°C, weight gain from 57 kg to 60 kg, cyclosporine whole blood concentration 94 ng/ml, and 14 days post-transplant.

A: The patient appears to have acute rejection, based on the acute increase in serum creatinine level, graft tenderness, low-grade fever, and low cyclosporine concentration. To make the proper diagnosis, biopsy should be considered. High-dose steroids should be instituted. In addition, one should consider increasing the cyclosporine dose.

P: One should continue to monitor renal function (Scr and urine output) closely, obtain bleeding time to ensure it is within normal range prior to renal biopsy, and initiate high-dose methylprednisolone regimen of 500 mg IV q.d. for three days. Increase cyclosporine dose to 250 mg p.o. b.i.d.

QUESTIONS FOR CASE 46

1. High-dose steroids, such as methylprednisolone are considered first-line agents in treating acute rejection. However, some patients may not respond to this therapy. What alternatives are currently available for use in refractory rejection and what dosage regimens and duration are used for these agents?
2. If OKT3 were to be used in this patient, what precautions should be used?
3. Cyclosporine can also cause changes in renal function, resulting in nephrotoxicity. This must be differentiated from rejection. What signs and symptoms differentiate cyclosporine nephrotoxicity from acute rejection?
4. In this patient, cyclosporine concentrations are low. What could be the reason(s) for a low concentration?
5. Drug interactions are frequently reported with cyclosporine and include calcium-channel blockers. Nifedipine was chosen in this patient. Does this drug interact with cyclosporine? What about other calcium-channel blockers?

CASE 47

CC: HP is a 45-year-old female with a history of rapidly progressive glomerulonephritis (RPGN) and is in clinic for follow-up with complaints of sweating, irritability, and palpitations.

Past Medical History

HP has had RPGN for two years, which has been responsive to steroids; however, the steroids are currently being tapered because of side effects. HP also has had type II (adult-onset DM) for 10 years

Medication History

Hydrocortisone 20 mg qAM, 10 mg qPM
Cyclophosphamide 125 mg p.o. q.d.
Chlorpropamide 250 mg p.o. q.d. (recently changed from glipizide because of insurance reimbursement)

Allergies

None known

Physical Examination

GEN: Well-developed, well-nourished female in no acute distress
VS: BP 100/60, HR 92, RR 15, T 37.1°C, Wt 71 kg, Ht 163 cm
HEENT: Retinal edema, punctate hemorrhages
COR: WNL
CHEST: WNL
ABD: WNL
GU: WNL
RECT: WNL
EXT: WNL
NEURO: WNL

Results of Laboratory Tests

Na 128 (128)   Cr 345 (3.9)   MCV 85 (85)   Glu 2.7 (49)
K 4.7 (4.7)   Hct 0.36 (35.5)   ALT 0.7 (42)   Ca 2.3 (9.1)
Cl 102 (102)   Hgb 115 (11.5)   Alk Phos 2.1 ukat/l (127)   Po₄ 2.1 (6.6)
HCO₃ 20 (20)   Lkcs 3.3 × 10⁹/l (3.3 × 10³)   Alb 31 (3.1)   Mg 1.3 (3.1)
BUN 14 (38)   Plts 126 × 10⁹ (126 × 10³)   T bili 13.7 (0.8)

UA: Protein 3(+), RBC casts

PROBLEM LIST

1. Diabetes type II
2. Chronic renal failure (CRF)

CASE 48

CC: TR is a 67-year-old female who presents to the hospital with lethargy, confusion, nausea, and vomiting for the past three days.

History of Present Illness

TR notes she has chronic stomach problems. Recently she has been constipated and has had stomach pain. Less than one week ago she started some new medicines for these problems.

Past Medical History

TR has a long history of chronic renal failure secondary to a 15-year history of hypertension. She has sought attention for her stomach problems for the last 40 years and has been diagnosed with irritable bowel syndrome. She experiences intermittent diarrhea and constipation and has tried a variety of OTC medications.

Medication History

Calcium carbonate 1250 mg t.i.d.
Felodipine 5 mg po q.d.
Erythropoietin 4000 U SQ three times weekly for eight weeks
MOM 60 cc/day for one week
Mylanta II 30 cc po 5/day for one week

Allergies
None known

Social History
Tobacco—negative
Alcohol—negative

Physical Examination
GEN: Thin, elderly female in moderate distress
VS: BP 100/ 55, HR 110, RR 22, T 37.0°C, Wt 50 kg, Ht 165 cm
HEENT: WNL
COR: Normal S_1 and S_2, no murmurs
CHEST: Clear to auscultation
ABD: Intermittent crampy lower abdominal pain, decreased bowel sounds
GU: WNL
RECT: Guaiac-negative
EXT: No edema
NEURO: Oriented to person; disappearance of patellar reflex, diminished tendon reflexes

Results of Laboratory Tests

Na 142 (142)	Hct 0.26 (26)	AST 0.47 (28)	Glu 8.32 (150)
K 4.6 (4.6)	Hbg 85 (8.5)	ALT 0.53 (32)	Ca 2.0 (8.0)
Cl 107 (107)	Lkcs 6.0×10^9 (6.0×10^3)	LDH 1.2 (70)	PO_4 3.0 (9.2)
HCO_3 19 (19)	Plts 120×10^9 (120×10^3)	Alk Phos 1.17 (70)	Mg 3.4 (6.8)
BUN 21.4 (60)	MCV 75 (75)	Alb 35 (3.5)	Uric Acid 535 (9)
CR 247 (2.8)	MCH 28	T Bili 17.1 (1.0)	
	Iron 6.3 (35)	B_{12} 295 (400)	
	TIBC 86 (480)	Folate 34 (15)	
	Ferritin 10 (10)		

ECG: no acute changes

PROBLEM LIST
1. Hypermagnesemia
2. Chronic renal failure
3. Iron deficiency anemia
4. Irritable bowel syndrome
5. Hypertension

Problem 1. Hypermagnesemia
S: TR complains of nausea, vomiting, lethargy, and confusion.
O: Mg level is elevated 3.4 (6.8); TR is hypotensive and is exhibiting decreased deep tendon reflexes.
A: TR's renal failure together with her recent increased intake of magnesium-containing laxatives and excessive use of magnesium-containing antacids have brought her magnesium to a dangerously high level. TR is symptomatic and thus needs immediate attention. She is at risk for seizures, respiratory paralysis, and heart block. If TR were to have normal renal function, we could more confidently rely on renal excretion; however, because her renal function is severely impaired, symptomatic resolution will be slower. In the absence of cardiac symptoms and respiratory depression, calcium injections need not be given.
P: TR should be gently hydrated with 0.45% sodium chloride and intravenous furosemide to attempt to accelerate renal magnesium clearance. All magnesium-containing products

should be discontinued as should her felodipine because she is hypotensive. Symptoms and serum magnesium should be monitored over the next 24 hours. If symptoms were to worsen or if TR were to fail to diurese with hydration and furosemide, hemodialysis may be necessary.

Problem 2. Chronic Renal Failure
S: Lethargy.
O: Increased SCr 247 (2.8), increased BUN 21.4 (60), increased Mg 3.4 (6.8), decreased Ca 2.0 (8.0), increased Po_4 3.0 (9.2), decreased HCO_3 19, increased uric acid 535 (9), and decreased platelets 120×10^9 (120×10^3).
A: TR has developed chronic renal failure (CRF) secondary to hypertension. Her CRF has likely progressed over the years such that her CL_{cr} is currently only 15 ml/min:

$$CL_{cr} = (140 - 67)(50)/72(2.8) \times 0.85 = 15.3 \text{ ml/min}$$

CRF leads to a multitude of problems with treatment measures usually focused on correcting electrolyte and acid-base abnormalities, anemia, and hypertension. TR's low HCO_3 is consistent with metabolic acidosis seen in CRF due to decreased acid excretion. Until the acidosis is severe, treatment is not necessary. TR's hyperphosphatemia, however, should be managed to prevent cardiac and neurologic problems, in addition to preventing problems associated with calcium-phosphate precipitation and hypocalcemia. Despite calcium supplementation, TR's calcium remains low. Because the calcium-phosphate product (Ca × P) is > 70 (5.63), TR is at risk for soft-tissue calcification; therefore, one needs to reduce serum Po_4 levels before further supplementing calcium. Aluminum-containing antacids given with meals are used to complex dietary phosphate. Dietary phosphate restriction in TR should also be encouraged. Because TR's renal failure predisposes her to chronic aluminum toxicity, she should be closely monitored. Once her Po_4 has come down and the calcium-phosphate product is reduced to below 70 (5.63), calcium supplementation can be continued or vitamin D can be tried to further correct the serum calcium. If these methods were to fail, hemodialysis may be necessary. TR's platelet count is low but not yet low enough to require treatment. TR's uric acid is elevated but TR remains asymptomatic and has no history of gout; therefore, elevated uric acid does not require treatment.
P: TR's calcium should be temporarily stopped and she should start aluminum hydroxide (e.g., 600 mg AlOH/5 ml; give 15 ml with meals and qHS). TR should be instructed to restrict dietary phosphate (high in meat, milk, legumes, and carbonated drinks). Unfortunately, TR is already complaining of constipation which the Al may worsen. A stool softener may be helpful. TR needs to be instructed to avoid all magnesium-containing OTC drugs and K-containing salt substitutes. Special attention should be paid to reducing doses of drugs that are eliminated renally.

Problem 3. Iron deficiency anemia
S: Increased fatigue.

O: Decreased ferritin, iron, MCV, MCH, and increased TIBC.

A: TR, like most patients with chronic renal disease, developed anemia of chronic disease and has been treated with erythropoietin for eight weeks. However, her Hct and Hgb are still low even though the erythropoietin has been prescribed at appropriate starting doses. The laboratory results now show that TR has iron deficiency anemia in addition to anemia of chronic disease. Her anemia is not normochromic and normocytic as is the anemia of chronic diseases but is consistent with the microcytic, hypochromic anemia associated with iron deficiency. Iron deficiency is likely the reason why TR's Hgb and Hct are still below goal levels after eight weeks of treatment with erythropoietin. Iron indices should be monitored closely with patients on erythropoietin because Hgb synthesis stimulated by erythropoietin is dependent on sufficient Fe stores; TR has not be on supplemental iron therapy and needs to be. TR is elderly and a poor nutritional intake may also contribute to iron deficiency anemia. Blood loss also needs to be ruled out as an etiology. Oral iron can cause abdominal cramps, constipation, or diarrhea which are already a problem for this patient; however, oral iron should be tried before starting parenteral iron due to higher cost, more difficult administration, and the adverse reaction profile of parenteral iron.

P: One should start FeSO$_4$ 325 mg po t.i.d. for six months. A reduction in dose may be possible after six months but iron supplementation will likely be needed as long as erythropoietin is given. TR needs to be instructed to take her AlOH at least one hour before or two hours after the iron to prevent decreased iron absorption. If GI side effects were a problem, the dose may be initiated at 325 mg q.d. and increased incrementally over several days until the full dose can be tolerated. Although absorption of iron is better on an empty stomach, most patients do not tolerate iron without food; thus, TR should be instructed to take iron with food if necessary. TR's Hgb and Hct should be monitored with some expected increase within four to six weeks.

Problem 4. Irritable Bowel Syndrome

S: Constipation, abdominal pain.

O: History of the syndrome.

A: TR is experiencing altered bowel habits and abdominal pain. This has been a chronic problem for her, and she has been given the diagnosis of irritable bowel syndrome. Irritable bowel syndrome is fairly benign, yet it is important that other diagnoses have been ruled out. No evidence appears to suggest that any therapy is effective in treating the underlying problem. Rather, a symptomatic approach is taken . Antacids provide no relief. TR particularly needs to watch magnesium intake and needs some guidance in choosing appropriate therapy.

P: While TR is experiencing constipation and abdominal pain, fiber supplementation may be tried with wheat bran or psyllium. If this were unsuccessful, TR may try an antispasmodic, such as belladona 5–10 drops po t.i.d before meals or dicyclomine 10–20 mg t.i.d.—q.i.d. For periods when TR is experiencing diarrhea, an antidiarrheal, such as loperamide, should be tried.

Problem 5. Hypertension

S: None.

O: History of hypertension.

A: TR's current hypotension is likely due to hypermagnesemia. TR has had a history of hypertension. In addition, her CRF may contribute to hypertension due to renin excess and increased sodium retention. TR also is taking erythropoietin which may further exacerbate hypertension.

P: One should discontinue TR's felodipine until the hypotension resolves, and continue to monitor BP and, when necessary, restart felodipine. (See question 2)

QUESTIONS FOR CASE 48

1. If TR could not tolerate oral iron supplementation, how should parenteral iron therapy be dosed and administered?

2. Two weeks later, TR's BP is 170/100. The team asks for your recommendation on treating her hypertension. What would you say?

3. TR begins to complain of headaches and the intern asks you if it is okay to start TR on aspirin. What would you recommend?

4. What would you say to an intern who asks you if Vitron C (125 mg Vitamin C + 66 mg iron) is a better choice than iron sulfate for TR?

5. What are the dangers of chronic aluminum ingestion in patients with chronic renal failure?

GASTROINTESTINAL DISEASES

CASE 49

CC: AJ is a 35-year-old female who comes to clinic today complaining of abdominal pain for the last three weeks, which awakens her at night and is relieved by food and antacids.

Past Medical History

AJ was diagnosed two months ago with Graves' disease. At that time, she had symptoms of hyperthyroidism, including tachycardia, that has been treated with propranolol. AJ has had chronic renal dysfunction for many years because of polycystic kidney disease. AJ has had irritable bowel syndrome (IBS) since high school, with intermittent complaints of diarrhea and constipation. Her diarrhea has increased over the last two months but is still mild. Laboratory results are consistent with iron deficiency anemia, but she has not received treatment.

Medication History

Propylthiouracil 200 mg p.o. q6h for two months
Magnesium hydroxide 300 mg/5 ml, aluminum hydroxide 600 mg/5 ml 15 ml p.o. p.r.n.
Propranolol 20 mg p.o. q.i.d.

Allergies

None known

Social History

Cigarettes—1/2 pack per day
Alcohol—drinks two to three glasses of wine per day with dinner
Coffee—two to six cups of coffee per day

Physical Examination

GEN: Well-developed, thin female in mild distress
VS: BP 140/88, HR 84, RR 18, T 37.0°C, Wt 55 kg, Ht 165 cm
HEENT: Small, symmetric goiter, much smaller than two months ago
COR: NL S1 and S2; no murmurs, rubs, or gallops
CHEST: WNL
ABD: Intermittent, crampy, lower abdominal pain relieved by passage of flatus, point tenderness between the xiphoid and umbilicus
GU: WNL
RECTAL: Guaiac-positive
EXT: Pruritic pretibial myxedema
NEURO: WNL

Results of Laboratory Tests

Na 128 (128)	Hgb 100 (10)	Alk Phos 1.1 (65)	Uric Acid 535 (9)
K 4.8 (4.8)	Lkcs 5×10^9 (5000)	Alb 35 (3.5)	TT_4 100 (7.8)
Cl 102 (102)	Plt 120×10^9 (120×10^3)	T bili 15.4 (0.9)	RT_3U 0.3 (30%)
HCO_3 20 (20)	MCV 68 (68)	Glu 4.7 (84)	FT_4I 34 (2.6)
BUN 28.6 (80)	AST 0.42 (25)	Ca 2.1 (8.6)	TSH 5 (5)
Cr 283 (3.2)	ALT 0.45 (27)	Po_4 1.6 (4.8)	Fe 9.8 (55)
Hct 0.29 (29%)	LDH 1.1 (65)	Mg 1.35 (2.7)	

Lkcs differential: WNL
Urinalysis: Hematuria, proteinuria
Chest radiography: WNL
ECG: WNL
Endoscopy: Two small duodenal ulcers
Peripheral blood smear: Microcytic anemia

PROBLEM LIST

1. Chronic renal dysfunction
2. Irritable bowel syndrome (IBS)
3. Graves' disease
4. Iron deficiency anemia
5. Peptic ulcer disease (PUD)

CASE 49 SOAP NOTES

Problem 3. Graves' Disease

S: AJ has a small, symmetric goiter that has reduced in size over the last two months. She also has a pruritic pretibial myxedema. Her eye examination yielded normal results.

O: AJ's TT_4, RT_3U, FT_4I, TSH, BP, and HR are in the normal range.

A: The thioamides (PTU) are preferred in young adults with Graves' disease. Thyrotoxicosis of Graves' disease is self-limiting. PTU controls symptoms until spontaneous remission occurs. PTU does not carry the added risk of hypothyroidism associated with RAI and surgery. Conversely, induction doses require that the patients take a large number of tablets at frequent intervals because of tablet size and a short half-life; therefore, patient compliance may be an issue. Adverse reactions of PTU (rashes, agranulocytosis, GI symptoms, and hepatitis) and long treatment duration must also be considered. AJ has pretibial myxedema, which occurs in patients with past or present Graves' disease. Half the cases occur during the active stage, and the remainder develop after treatment. This is a self-limited disorder. She does have pruritus, which can be treated topically. AJ has been treated for two months with a high dose of PTU and now has a normal TSH with no objective symptoms. Therefore, her dose can be reduced to 50–100 mg p.o. q.d. for maintenance for six months to two years. AJ is no longer tachycardic because of the Graves' disease. It may be possible to taper off the propranolol.

P: One should taper AJ's PTU on a monthly basis to 50–100 mg p.o. q.d. with continued monitoring for exacerbation of Graves' disease. Decrease propranolol dose to 20 mg p.o. t.i.d. and continue the taper until discontinuation if possible, while monitoring HR and BP. Start topical hydrocortisone cream 1% and apply q.i.d. p.r.n. for pruritus.

Problem 1. Chronic Renal Dysfunction

S: None.

O: AJ has increased creatinine, BUN uric acid, and magnesium levels. She also has low sodium and bicarbonate levels, low platelet count, and high-normal phosphate and potassium levels. Urinalysis demonstrates hematuria and proteinuria.

A: Polycystic renal disease is a genetic disorder that is marked by multiple spherical cysts in both kidneys, which are believed to compress the nephrons and cause local obstruction. Although AJ has an elevated uric acid level, patients with renal-failure-induced hyperuricemia rarely develop gout unless they have a history of gout. In addition, little evidence suggests that hyperuricemia in these patients leads to further deterioration of renal function. For these reasons, treatment of AJ's hyperuricemia is not necessary. AJ has low sodium and bicarbonate levels, which could be normalized with oral sodium bicarbonate administration. Her platelet count is not low enough to require treatment.

$$Cr_{cl} = \frac{(140 - 35)55}{72(3.2)} \times (0.85) = 21 \text{ ml/min } (0.35 \text{ ml/sec})$$

P: Other than renal transplant, which is not indicated at present, no treatment will cure this problem. The treatment approach should be directed at avoiding situations that worsen the patient's kidney function, such as nonsteroidal antiinflammatory agents, urinary infections, nephrotoxic drugs, and hypertension. Due to AJ's decreased renal function currently, it is important to adjust doses of drugs that are eliminated renally. To replace sodium and bicarbonate, give NaHCO$_3$ 650 mg p.o. t.i.d., with titration based on response. AJ is hypermagnesemic because of the magnesium-containing antacid and her renal dysfunction. The magnesium-containing antacid should be discontinued.

Problem 2. Irritable Bowel Syndrome (IBS)

S: AJ has complained of worsening but still mild diarrhea. She has intermittent, crampy, lower abdominal pain relieved by passage of flatus. She also complains of intermittent constipation.

O: AJ's sodium level is low, and potassium and magnesium concentrations are high.

A: IBS is a chronic and relatively benign syndrome and, therefore, AJ's treatment should be conservative. IBS nearly always lacks objective gastrointestinal findings other than intermittent diarrhea/constipation. The diarrhea tends to be associated with stress. AJ's diarrhea has worsened over the last two months, which may be related to the PTU therapy. This may resolve with the decrease in PTU dose (Problem 1). She also has been taking a magnesium-containing antacid that can cause diarrhea. Because of the high placebo effect in the treatment of this syndrome, it has been difficult to assess the efficacy of various treatments. High-fiber diets appear to be beneficial in some patients. Bran and bulk laxatives may or may not be effective. In addition, although not well documented, relaxation techniques or biofeedback may be of use. Although AJ's diarrhea has worsened over the last two months, it is still considered to be mild, and aggressive treatment cannot be justified. The final assessment of this should be based on how many stools she is actually having per day and whether she is having any weight loss or orthostatic hypotension. AJ has had IBS for almost 20 years without major distress.

P: AJ should be monitored for number of stools per day, serum electrolyte levels, and body weight. One should decrease AJ's PTU dose as described in Problem 1, discontinue the magnesium antacid, and consider instituting a high-fiber diet and biofeedback.

Problem 4. Iron Deficiency Anemia

S: None.

O: AJ has a decreased Hct, Hgb, MCV, and serum iron levels. Her peripheral blood smear shows microcytic anemia. Her stool is guaiac-positive.

A: Active PUD and menstruation are contributing to AJ's anemia. Ferrous sulfate is preferred over ferrous gluconate because the cost of the sulfate is much lower and the gluconate offers no additional benefit. To replace iron stores and reverse the anemia, 200 mg of elemental iron per day for six months is necessary. This converts to FeSO$_4$ 325 mg p.o. t.i.d. for six months. Iron therapy can cause either diarrhea or constipation, either of which may be a problem for this patient. The black stools caused by the oral iron must be distinguished from blood in the stool (black, tarry stool). PUD is a relative contraindication for oral iron replacement. Parenteral iron therapy is usually reserved for extreme situations in which patients cannot take orally administered iron. This reservation is due to cost and an adverse reaction profile with parenteral iron.

P: AJ should be started on FeSO$_4$ 325 mg p.o. t.i.d. for six months. She should be instructed to take it on an empty stomach, avoid antacids, and keep it out of the reach of children. She should also be educated about iron's adverse reaction (dark stools, constipation, and diarrhea). Stressing the importance of compliance for the full six months is also important. Her reticulocyte count should increase in one week and Hgb/Hct values in about four to six weeks.

Problem 5. Peptic Ulcer Disease

S: AJ complains of abdominal pain for the last three weeks, which awakens her at night and is relieved by food or antacids. She has point tenderness between the xiphoid and umbilicus.

O: Endoscopy revealed two small duodenal ulcers. AJ has guaiac-positive stools, and low Hct and Hgb values.

A: AJ has active PUD, which is contributing to anemia. The antacid she has been taking to relieve the pain is contributing to her diarrhea and hypermagnesemia. Her smoking, drinking and coffee consumption potentiate her ulcers. In addition, continuation of smoking delays ulcer healing. Cimetidine decreases the clearance of propranolol. This interaction can be managed with adjustment in the propranolol dose (which will be tapered anyway) or by avoidance of the interaction. Antacids decrease the absorption of $FeSO_4$ and should be avoided or at least given one hour before or two hours after the iron. Magnesium-containing antacids are a problem for AJ because of the diarrhea and renal dysfunction. Sucralfate and aluminum-containing antacids are a potential problem for AJ because of their constipating effect. Histamine antagonists are primarily renally eliminated. For that reason, the dosage should be reduced in this patient [$Cr_{Cl} = 0.35$ ml/sec (21 ml/min.)].

P: One should start ranitidine 150 mg p.o. qHS for treatment of AJ's PUD and discontinue the oral antacids. AJ should be counseled about avoiding foods that are irritating: discontinuing smoking, drinking ethanol, and coffee; and avoiding nonsteroidal antiinflammatory agents (aspirin and ibuprofen).

QUESTIONS FOR CASE 49

1. If AJ were to become pregnant, what would be done for her Graves' disease therapy?
2. If AJ's renal function were to decline and she would require dialysis, how would this affect her drug therapy?
3. What if AJ were still anemic after six months of ferrous sulfate therapy?
4. If AJ's PUD were not to heal after six weeks of ranitidine, should sucralfate be added?
5. Should AJ receive prophylaxis for her PUD after completion of treatment?

CASE 50

CC: GK is a 32-year-old male admitted to the hospital with severe recurrent Crohn disease of the terminal ileum and colon, uncontrolled with oral steroid therapy. Current symptoms include severe abdominal pain, crampy diarrhea, and a recent 10-lb weight loss. Because he did not respond to a 72-hr course of intravenous steroid therapy, resection of the terminal ileum was performed. Postoperatively, he complains of nausea and vomiting, possibly secondary to narcotic medication for pain control.

Past Medical History

GK was first diagnosed with Crohn disease at age 18. At the age of 23, recurrence of the disease within the colon and terminal ileum and a mucosa appearing patchy and cobblestoned confirmed the diagnosis. Since then, GK has had numerous relapses despite continual sulfasalazine and oral steroid therapy. Several years ago, he developed arthritis in both knees. NSAIDs have been effective in controlling the arthritic pain that flares in concert with exacerbations of his intestinal disease. One year ago, he developed a gastric ulcer that was believed to be NSAID-induced. The gastric ulcer was successfully healed with famotidine.

Past Surgical History

GK underwent a small bowel resection three years ago. Following surgery, he relapsed and was treated with a course of azathioprine (1.5 mg/kg). After eight weeks of therapy, the azathioprine was discontinued because of leukopenia.

Medication History (prior to admission)

Prednisone 30 mg qAM and 20 mg qPM for three years
Sulfasalazine 1 g q.i.d. for three years
Ibuprofen 600 mg q4-6h p.r.n. for arthritic and muscle pain; past two weeks has taken an average of 2400 mg/day of ibuprofen
Oxycodone/aspirin 1–2 tablets p.o. q4-6h p.r.n. for abdominal pain; began taking 4 tablets/day about two weeks ago

Allergies

None known

Review of Systems

GK complained of severe abdominal pain and cramping, watery diarrhea (> 10 bowel movements/day), which has become increasingly worse over the last two weeks. As a result of long-term steroid administration, he has developed a cushingoid appearance, suffers from general myopathy, and recently fractured his tibia. Three days of intravenous steroid therapy (methylprednisolone 20 mg q6h) was unsuccessful, and emergency bowel resection was performed. GK is nauseated and vomited postoperatively.

Physical Examination

GEN: Ill-appearing thin male, febrile, and in acute distress
VS: BP 145/85, HR 95, T 38.0°C, RR 14, Wt 61.4 kg, Ht 173 cm (68 inches)
HEENT: WNL
CHEST: WNL
ABD: Abdominal tenderness and guarding
RECT: Guaiac-positive
EXT: Reduced reflexes, swollen knees, mild lower extremity edema, dry skin, ecchymosis

Results of Laboratory Tests

Na 135 (135)	Hct 0.37 (37%)	AST 0.65 (39)	Glu 10 (180)
K 3.5 (3.5)	Hgb 130 (13)	ALT 0.53 (32)	Ca 2.3 (9.2)
Cl 98 (98)	Lkcs 1.4×10^9 (1.4×10^3)	LDH 3.2 (190)	Po$_4$ 1.4 (4.3)
HCO$_3$ 22 (22)	Plts 260×10^9 (260×10^3)	Alk Phos 1.5 (90)	Mg 1.2 (2.4)
BUN 11.4 (32)		Alb 23 (2.3)	Uric Acid 357 (6)
CR 115 (1.3)		T Bili 13.7 (0.8)	

PROBLEM LIST

1. Crohn disease
2. Arthritis
3. Steroid stress management
4. Stress ulcer prophylaxis/history of PUD
5. Nausea and vomiting
6. Nutritional support

Problem 1. Crohn Disease

S: GK complains of severe abdominal pain, crampy diarrhea, and a recent 10-lb weight loss.

O: GK has Crohn disease with confirmed terminal ileum and colonic involvement, one prior resection of the small intestine, and low-grade fever. Physical examination showed abdominal tenderness and guarding, guaiac-positive stool, and watery diarrhea (> 10 bowel movements/day).

A: Surgical intervention is not curative in Crohn disease. Indications for surgery include failed medical therapy, perforation, toxic dilation, strictures, and obstruction.

P: GK has refractory Crohn disease and failed high-dose intravenous steroid therapy; surgery is warranted. Based on GK's previous clinical course, medical management following convalescence will be necessary. Prior to this present exacerbation, GK was treated with sulfasalazine and oral steroids. Although drug-free remission appears to be unattainable for GK, his past drug regimen helped to control the symptoms of the disease. Therefore, once clinical stabilization has been achieved, sulfasalazine should be reintroduced at 1–2 g/day in divided doses with meals. GK will probably require a minimum daily sulfasalazine dose of 4 g/day to obtain a clinical response. Therefore, sulfasalazine should be titrated upward by 500 mg every two to three days, if tolerated, until a dosage of 4 g/day is achieved. Steroid therapy must also be continued. The daily dose required will depend upon the disease progression and the steroid replacement need.

Problem 3. Steroid Stress Management

S: None.

O: Long-term steroid therapy, cushingoid appearance, tibia fracture secondary to osteoporosis, general myopathy, ecchymosis, glucose 10 mmol/liter (180 mg/dl), and BP 145/85.

A: Chronic steroid therapy results in adrenal suppression. The degree and duration of adrenal suppression depends upon the exogenous steroid administered, its dose, and the duration of steroid therapy. Chronic exogenous steroid therapy followed by increased physical and/or psychologic stress may result in increased exogenous steroid requirements. This increased requirement results from the suppression of corticotropin release from the pituitary and the inability to provide necessary steroid levels. Adrenal insufficiency may persist for up to 12 months in patients who have received large dosages of steroids for prolonged periods.

P: GK is receiving intravenous methylprednisolone (MP) 20 mg q6h for treatment of possible residual colonic disease and to provide exogenous corticosteroid replacement therapy. He should be maintained on this steroid regimen until he is clinically stable. Following clinical improvement, a taper of the intravenous steroid regimen may be initiated, followed by the conversion from intravenous methylprednisolone to oral prednisone. An example of a steroid-tapering regimen is MP 20 mg q6h for three days; MP 15 mg q6h for two days; MP 10 mg q6h for two days; followed by the conversion of the MP 10 mg × 6 hr (40 mg/day) to the equivalent oral prednisone dose of 50 mg/day. An appropriate initial oral dosage regimen is prednisone 30 mg qAM and 20 mg qPM. The rapidity of the steroid dose reduction and the conversion from intravenous administration to oral steroid therapy depend upon the occurrence of disease relapse, the development of remission, and his ability to take oral medication. GK should be monitored for disease exacerbation and signs and symptoms of adrenal insufficiency, which include a flulike syndrome, orthostatic hypotension, decreased serum glucose concentrations, and altered electrolyte levels.

Problem 4. Stress Ulcer Prophylaxis

S: None.

O: GK has had long-term steroid therapy, undergone major surgery, and has a history of possible NSAID-induced PUD.

A: GK is at risk for developing stress-related mucosal bleeding because of major surgery and poor nutrition. He is also at risk for upper GI bleeding because of a history of PUD and long-term steroid therapy. Concurrent intravenous H2-receptor antagonist (H2RA) therapy admixed with his total parenteral nutrition (TPN) solution may provide more consistent H_2RA blood levels and better pH control.

P: GK is currently receiving central TPN and intermittent infusions of ranitidine 50 mg q8h. One should admix ranitidine with TPN and administer it by continuous intravenous infusion at a rate of 6.25 mg/hr. Monitor gastric pH q6h. If pH were < 4 and his renal function were to remain stable, one should increase the ranitidine to 8.5 mg/hr or administer antacids (Mylanta®) 30 ml to maintain the pH > 4. Monitor nasogastric aspirate for signs of overt bleeding. As an outpatient, GK controlled his abdominal pain with oxycodone and aspirin. If GK were to continue p.r.n. oxycodone combination therapy, the prescription should be changed to Percocet®, which contains acetaminophen. Aspirin should be avoided because of his history of PUD.

Problem 5. Nausea and Vomiting

S: Nausea and vomiting postoperatively.

O: Current pain medication.

A: Postoperative pain management is required in GK. Morphine is a common narcotic used in pain management, but morphine has emetic properties. The addition of an antiemetic agent to GK's drug therapy is appropriate.

P: GK does not have any contraindications to phenothiazines. Therefore, prochlorperazine 5-10 mg IM/IV q6h p.r.n. for nausea and vomiting is an appropriate antiemetic choice and regimen. Oral administration at present is not appropriate because of his nausea and vomiting and the possibility of compromising drug absorption. Once the acute episodes of nausea and vomiting have subsided, prochlorperazine may be administered orally. One should monitor GK for a decrease in nausea and vomiting, dystonic reactions, sedation, and/or BP changes.

Problem 6. Nutritional Support

S: Severe Crohn disease symptoms.

O: IBW 68.4 kg (150 lbs), actual weight 61.4 kg (135 lbs), recent 10-lb weight loss, Alb 23 g/liter (2.3 g/dl); previous short-bowel resection.

A: Several pathophysiologic mechanisms result in nutritional problems in Crohn disease patients. Inflammation of the small intestine may decrease absorption of nutrients, induce digestive enzyme deficiencies, and cause protein-losing enteropathies and iron deficiency. Small-bowel bacterial overgrowth and resection results in cobalamin malabsorption and an imbalance in the bile salt intestinal recycling pattern. Anorexia and self-imposed dietary restrictions add to an overall poor nutritional status. These mechanisms of malnutrition may result in diarrhea, steatorrhea, microcytic or megaloblastic anemia, hypoproteinemia, edema, demineralization of the bone and acid-base disturbances. The maintenance of adequate nutrition is often difficult in severe Crohn disease, especially following small bowel resection. Replacement therapy of vitamins D and K, calcium, folic acid, and iron is usually warranted. Administration of vitamin B_{12} is indicated after resection of the terminal ileum. Supplemental enteral and TPN regimens are alternatives in maintaining adequate nutritional requirements.

P: To permit bowel rest after surgery, to establish fluid balance, and to provide adequate nutrition, GK receives 2 liters of TPN centrally at a rate of 80 ml/hr, consisting of amino acids 4.25%/liter providing 85 g of protein/day, and dextrose 25%/liter providing 500 g of carbohydrates/day and approximately 1700 kcal/day. Each liter of TPN solution contains Ca 5 mEq, Mg 5 mEq, K 40 mEq, Na 35 mEq, acetate 50 mEq, Cl 35 mEq, and Po_4 12 mM. Multivitamins with B_{12} and trace elements are added to the first liter each morning, and vitamin K is added weekly. GK also receives 500 ml of 10% fat emulsion at a rate of 20 ml/hr twice a week to prevent fatty acid deficiency and provide an additional 1000 kcal/week. Triglyceride and cholesterol levels should be obtained the morning after the administration of fat emulsion. Daily monitoring parameters include serum electrolyte levels, liver function tests, and serum and urine glucose, BUN, and creatinine levels. Daily weight should be monitored, and an average weight should be calculated on a weekly basis to monitor weight gain. A 2 lb/week dry weight gain is the desired goal, and his caloric intake should be adjusted to attain and maintain this goal.

Problem 2. Arthritis

S: Arthritic pain in knees bilaterally.

O: Physical examination showed reduced reflexes and stiff, swollen knees; increased ibuprofen use was also noted.

A: Extraintestinal manifestations of IBD occur in approximately 10–20% of patients and usually follow the clinical activity of intestinal disease. Systemic involvement commonly includes arthritis and arthralgias, skin manifestations, and ocular lesions. Arthritis and arthralgias are the most frequent manifestations of both Crohn disease and ulcerative colitis. Arthritis is usually bilateral and occurs most commonly in large peripheral joints and joints of the lower extremities.

P: GK's arthritic pain is likely to subside after surgery. The severity of the extraintestinal manifestation usually correlates with the severity of the intestinal disease. Current medication includes IV morphine for pain control and corticosteroids for adrenal insufficiency during this crisis period. This medication regimen should also control GK's arthritic pain.

QUESTIONS FOR CASE 50

1. In the past, GK was treated with azathioprine 1.5 mg/kg for eight weeks. What are the indications for immunosuppressive therapy?
2. Cyclosporine (CsA) is an investigational agent in the treatment of Crohn disease. What role does CsA play in Crohn disease?
3. If Crohn disease were confined to the ileum, would sulfasalazine be appropriate drug therapy?
4. What is toxic megacolon? Are antimotility drugs or narcotics contraindicated in GK because of Crohn disease?
5. If GK's Crohn disease were also to include perianal involvement, would metronidazole be appropriate drug therapy?
6. On rounds, one of the interns asks if GK's methylprednisolone should be changed to ACTH. Would this be an appropriate therapeutic intervention?
7. Have NSAIDs been associated with inducing exacerbations of Crohn disease?

CASE 51

CC: DH is a 55-year-old male who presents to the walk-in clinic with complaints of fatigue, weakness, and abdominal discomfort.

Past Medical History

Chronic renal failure on hemodialysis
Hypertension
Parkinson disease
Benign prostatic hypertrophy (BPH)

Family History

History of hypertension (mother)

Medication History

Verapamil SR 240 mg p.o. qAM for one month
Clonidine 0.2 mg p.o. b.i.d. (dose for one month)

Benztropine 2 mg p.o. qHS
Aluminum hydroxide suspension 2 tbsp p.o. t.i.d.
Allopurinol 100 mg p.o. q.d.
Sodium bicarbonate 650 mg p.o. t.i.d.
Calcitriol 0.5 μg p.o. q.d.
Epsom salt p.o. p.r.n. for constipation

Allergies

None known

Review of Systems

DH states he has experienced straining upon passing stools for three weeks. He describes his stools as hard and difficult to pass. He usually has one bowel movement every other day. He recently admits to passing stool only two times per week. He states that he has visited the local pharmacy for laxatives on several occasions, with little relief. DH states that the dose of his antihypertensive medication has been recently increased. DH states that his antihypertensive medication has recently changed.

Physical Examination

GEN: Pale 55-year-old male appearing listless, with c/o gastrointestinal discomfort
VS: BP 130/82, HR 60, T 37.6°C, RR 22, Wt 71 kg, Ht 177.8 cm
HEENT: Dry mucous membranes
COR: WNL
CHEST: Clear to auscultation
ABD: Nontender; decreased bowel sounds
GU: WNL
RECT: Guaiac-negative
EXT: No edema
NEURO: Resting hand tremor

Results of Laboratory Tests

Na 142 (142)   Hct 0.24 (24)   AST 0.47 (28)   Glu 6.0 (10^9)
K 4.5 (4.5)   Hgb 83 (8.3)   ALT 0.53 (32)   Ca 2.32 (9.3)
Cl 103 (10^3) Lkcs 4.5 × 10^9 (4.5 × 10^3) LDH 1.2 (70)   Po$_4$ 122 (3.8)
HCO$_3$ 24 (24) Plts 180 × 10^9 (180 × 10^3) Alk Phos 0.95 (57) Mg 1.2 (2.4)
BUN 17.1 (48) MCV 75 (75)   Alb 45 (4.5)   Uric Acid 297 (5.0)
CR 274 (3.1)   MCH 24 (24)   T Bili 2.6 (0.15)   Fe 7 (40)
               MCHC 300 (30)   TIBC 81 (450)
               Retic 0.0005 (0.5)   Ferritin 9.0 (9.0)
                                                             Folate 11 (5)
                                                             B$_{12}$ 443 (600)

PROBLEM LIST

1. Chronic renal failure
2. Hypertension
3. Iron deficiency anemia
4. Constipation
5. Parkinson disease

Problem 3. Iron Deficiency Anemia

S: c/o fatigue and weakness; pale, listless-appearing male on physical examination.
O: Hgb 83 (8.3), Hct 0.24 (24), MCV 75 (75), MCH 24 (24), MCHC 300 (30), Retic 0.0005 (0.5), Plts 180 × 10^9 (180 × 10^3) Fe 7 (40), TIBC 81 (450), ferritin 9.0 (9.0), folate 11 (5), and history of chronic renal failure.
A: The subjective complaints of DH and the laboratory results are consistent with iron deficiency anemia. Patients on hemodialysis are prone to iron deficiency due to blood loss with dialyzer use. Folate and B$_{12}$ levels are normal, which rules out mixed anemia. DH has a transferrin saturation ratio (Fex 100/TIBC) of 8.9%. Anemia often results in patients with chronic renal failure due to a decrease in the kidneys' ability to produce erythropoietin. Recombinant human erythropoietin (EPO) therapy is necessary for the treatment of anemia of CRF. However, patients with low baseline iron profiles prior to erythropoietin therapy should be supplemented with oral or parenteral iron to support the demands placed on body stores. If iron deficiency were to occur, supplemental iron would be necessary to replenish iron stores. Oral iron may be inappropriate in this patient with acute, chronic constipation. Parenteral iron may be administered upon assessment of total iron deficit.

$$\text{Total iron (mg)} = (0.66)\,(71\text{ kg})\left[100 - \frac{(100)(8.3)}{14.8}\right]$$

$$= 2058\text{ mg}$$

Volume of iron dextran injection

2058 mg × 1 ml/50 mg elemental iron

$$= 41\text{ ml iron dextran}$$

P: DH does not have contraindications to IM injection use. One should initiate therapy with a 25-mg test dose. Wait one hour before remainder of initial dose is administered to monitor for anaphylactic reactions. The Z-track technique of injection should be recommended to avoid staining the skin. Daily injections of < 250 mg (generally 100 mg is associated with fewer adverse effects) may be administered safely until the total calculated dose has been given. Erythropoietin should be initiated at a dose of 50–100 units/kg of dry body weight SQ three times a week. Monitor Hct for improvement (30–33%) or increases by four points in any two-week period, then reduce the dose by 25 units/kg. Supplemental iron therapy may be necessary with continued use of erythropoietin when serum ferritin is < 100 ng/ml or the transferrin saturation is < 20%. It may be administered IV as a postdialysis dose. Laboratory tests to monitor should include Hgb, reticulocyte counts, serum ferritin, serum iron, and TIBC levels. If symptoms of anemia were to persist despite correction of iron deficiency, a trial of androgens may be prudent because the patient has chronic renal failure. Baseline LFTs should be WNL. Monitoring of LFTs would be necessary due to the risk of hepatotoxicity and hepatocellular carcinoma with androgens. D/C androgens after six months. Recombinant human erythropoietin therapy is also a good alternative in treating the underlying cause of anemia.

Problem 4. Constipation

S: c/o abdominal discomfort, experiencing straining for

three weeks, stools hard and difficult to pass, decrease in frequency of bowel movements, and no relief of constipation with OTC laxatives.

O: On physical examination, abdomen is nontender with decreased bowel sounds: guaiac-negative, Lkcs normal, and patient afebrile.

A: Based on DH's history, changes in his bowel habits have several contributing factors. Parkinson disease may cause chronic constipation. His acute constipation could be due to a recent change in antihypertensive therapy to verapamil in addition to the anticholinergic side effects of benztropine. Aluminum hydroxide suspension also causes constipation. Because DH has Parkinson disease, chronic therapy for constipation is necessary in addition to acute therapy. DH should avoid p.r.n. use of Epsom salt (magnesium sulfate) because of the risk of hypermagnesemia in chronic renal failure.

P: One should evaluate medications that have contributed to DH's constipation (Problems 1, 2, and 5). Nonpharmacologic treatment of constipation should be emphasized to DH, which includes increased fluid and fiber intake and exercise. DH does not appear to have any contraindications for laxative use. For acute relief of constipation, a glycerin suppository would be appropriate. For chronic relief, a daily regimen of bulk-forming laxatives is safe and effective. One should recommend psyllium one teaspoon in 8 oz. of liquid p.o. t.i.d. DH should be instructed to follow each dose with an additional glass of liquid. DH should monitor the frequency and consistency of stools until he returns to his "normal" pattern of defecation.

Problem 1. Chronic Renal Failure (CRF)

S: None.

O: BUN 17.1 (48), CR 274 (3.1); history of chronic renal failure and dialysis dependent.

A: DH has a family history of chronic renal failure, which suggests hereditary renal disease. His laboratory data (BUN and CR) support the history. His estimated Clcr is 0.45 ml/sec (27 ml/min). Presently, the complications (metabolic and electrolyte imbalances) associated with CRF are controlled on the current regimen. DH should be instructed to avoid magnesium-containing products (Epsom salts) for constipation because his Mg level is presently high-normal. No treatment is necessary for this problem. Aluminum phosphate binder, which may be contributing to DH's constipation, may place him at risk of aluminum toxicity.

P: Routine monitoring of renal function and electrolyte levels is prudent during clinic visits. One should recommend alternative phosphate binder—calcium acetate 2 tabs (0.66 g) p.o. t.i.d.—because it has fewer gastrointestinal side effects. Monitor $PO_4 < 1.6$ (5.0). Continue current medications for control of electrolytes; due to DH's decreased renal function, verapamil SR should be used with caution because the drug and its active metabolite may accumulate in some patients. DH's heart rate is 60 beats/minute which may suggest that this is occurring.

Problem 2. Hypertension

S: None.

O: History of hypertension; no edema in extremities.

A: Hypertension is currently controlled (130/82), but a recent change in medication to verapamil has caused acute constipation. Changes in other factors contributing to constipation in addition to treatment may obviate the need to alter current antihypertensive therapy.

P: One should discontinue verapamil and replace it with an α-1-blocker (prazosin, terazocin, or doxazocin). Start prazocin at 1 mg/day. These types of agents are appropriate because the patient has a history of BPH and no adjustments in dose are required with decreased renal function. One should caution DH to take the initial dose at bedtime or observe him for up to three hours because of the possibility for first-dose syncope. Monitor BP and HR within one to two weeks to determine whether his dose needs to be increased.

Problem 5. Parkinson Disease

S: None.

O: Resting hand tremor.

A: DH is experiencing some resting hand tremor while taking benztropine. Anticholinergics generally improve tremor. However, DH's constipation and BPH may be complicated by benztropine-induced anticholinergic side effects.

P: One should taper benztropine, and start selegiline 5 mg p.o. with breakfast and after lunch. Counsel DH not to take selegiline in the evening.

QUESTIONS FOR CASE 51

1. After two weeks of using psyllium, DH occasionally experienced constipation. He began taking bisacodyl 10-mg tablets p.o. qHS for 1½ weeks and subsequently noticed very loose stools. How should DH be advised on the use of this laxative?

2. Develop a treatment plan for DH if he were to become fecally impacted. Include drug(s), dose(s), route(s), schedule(s), and duration. List three items of patient information that should be provided about the nonpharmacologic treatment of constipation.

3. Recommend androgen therapy for DH in an effort to increase erythropoiesis. Include drug(s), dose(s), route(s), schedule(s), and duration. Discuss the monitoring parameters necessary while DH is on this agent. List eight side effects commonly reported of androgens in chronic renal failure patients. Which agent has the highest anabolic:androgenic ratio? Why is this ratio significant in the selection of these agents?

4. DH's anemia did not respond to androgen therapy after six months. Baseline LFTs began to elevate slightly while on therapy. Recommend a starting dose of erythropoietin for this patient. What dosage adjustments should be recommended during therapy? What monitoring parameters are necessary while on therapy?

5. DH ran out of allopurinol and requested a refill. The doctor prescribed allopurinol 300 mg p.o. q.d. Why is this an inappropriate dose for DH?

CASE 52

CC: GG is a 65-year-old male who presents to clinic today with complaints that his ulcer has been acting up for the last month. His major complaints are nausea, diarrhea, and abdominal pain.

Past Medical History

GG was diagnosed 12 years ago with a duodenal ulcer that has been treated and has resolved on 6 different occasions over the years.

GG has had Crohn disease for several years and is currently receiving prednisone.

GG claims to have "rheumatism" for which he has been taking aspirin for the last month.

GG has benign prostatic hypertrophy and developed prostatitis for which he was started on ciprofloxacin 3 days ago.

Medication History

Prednisone 20 mg p.o. q.d. × 1 month
Aspirin 650 mg p.o. q4h p.r.n. leg pain × 1 month
Ciprofloxacin 500 mg p.o. b.i.d.
Allergies
Sulfa—rash
Social History
GG drinks 6 cups of coffee per day.
Physical Examination
    GEN: Well-developed, well-nourished male
      VS: BP 148/90, HR 90, RR 16, T 37, Wt 75 kg (down 5 kg from last month), Ht 178 cm
  HEENT: WNL
    COR: NL S_1 and S_2; no murmurs, rubs, or gallops
  CHEST: WNL
    ABD: Abdominal pain that wakes him up at night
     GU: Urinary retention
 RECTAL: Guaiac-positive, moderately enlarged prostate
    EXT: One plus pitting edema × 1 month, sore legs since he started a daily walking program (rheumatism)
  NEURO: WNL

Results of Laboratory Tests

Na 138 (138)	Hct 0.32 (32%)	AST 0.42 (25)	Glu 6.1 (110)
K 4.0 (4.0)	Hgb 100 (10)	ALT 0.45 (27)	Ca 2.2 (9)
Cl 102 (102)	Lkcs 10 × 10⁹ (10000)	LDH 1.1 (65)	PO₄ 0.87 (2.7)
HCO³ 24 (24)	Plt 160 × 10⁹ (160 × 10³)	Alk Phos 1.1 (65)	Mg 0.85 (1.7)
BUN 5.4 (15)	MCV 150 (150)	Alb 40 (4.0)	Uric Acid 557 (9)
Cr 88.4 (1.0)		T bili 15.4 (0.9)	

Lkcs differential: left shift
Urinalysis: hematuria
Chest x-ray: WNL
ECG: WNL

Endoscopy/colonoscopy: 1 cm duodenal ulcer; skip lesions in the distal ileum and right colon c/w mild Crohn disease

PROBLEM LIST

1. Peptic ulcer disease
2. Crohn disease
3. "Rheumatism"
4. Prostatitis
5. Anemia

QUESTIONS FOR CASE 52

1. GG fails cimetidine, sucralfate, and antacids for his ulcer treatment. He receives omeprazole and his ulcer heals. What should be done for ulcer prophylaxis?
2. If GG's rheumatism turns out to be rheumatoid arthritis, should he receive misoprostol along with his nonsteroidal antiinflammatory therapy?
3. After GG's Crohn disease goes into remission, can his prednisone be discontinued?
4. While tapering GG's prednisone, it is found that every time the dose is below 15 mg, his Crohn disease flares. Would azathioprine be useful in this patient?
5. GG is found to have a low folate level and macrocytic anemia. How should he be treated?

CASE 53

CC: DD is a 35-year-old woman who has an appointment with her gastroenterologist because of recurrent ulcerative colitis (UC). For the past month she has been feeling increasingly fatigued. Two weeks ago, she began to experience an increase in the frequency of her bowel movements, rectal bleeding, and abdominal cramping that is usually relieved upon defecation. The number of bloody bowel movements has increased to 6–7/day.

Past Medical History

Proctosigmoiditis was first diagnosed 3 years ago. DD was treated initially with sulfasalazine. The dose was titrated to 4 g/day, at which time she began to experience severe headaches, increased fatigue, malaise, upset stomach with nausea, and an itchy rash. At that time the sulfasalazine was discontinued. Hydrocortisone enemas were begun, and remission of her UC was achieved in 1 month.

Social History

An increase in work-related stress, alcohol consumption, late night working hours, and poor nutrition has occurred during this past month.

Medication History

PAST MEDICATION
Hydrocortisone enema 100 mg/60 ml q. h.s. for 1 month
Sulfasalazine 2–4 g/day for 6 weeks

CURRENT MEDICATION
Multivitamin with minerals q. AM
Calcium carbonate 1250 mg q. AM
Loperamide p.r.n. diarrhea (Rx—With onset of diarrhea take
4 mg followed by 2 mg q4-6h until diarrhea resolves.)

Allergies
Sulfasalazine

Review of Systems

DD was first diagnosed with UC 3 years ago. Following a 6-week upward titration of sulfasalazine to 4 g/day, she began to experience headaches, upset stomach with nausea, fatigue, and an itching rash that covered her upper torso and arms. The sulfasalazine was discontinued, and successful remission was achieved within 1 month with hydrocortisone enemas. She has remained in remission with only mild gastrointestinal discomfort until this present episode.

Physical Examination
GEN: Thin female in mild-to-moderate distress
VS: BP 128/80, HR 85, T 37.5, Wt 45.5 kg, Ht 157 cm (62 inches)
HEENT: WNL
CHEST: WNL
ABD: Mild tenderness, hyperactive bowel sounds
RECT: Bloody, watery diarrhea

Results of Laboratory Tests

Na 135 (135)	Hct 0.32 (32)	AST 0.45 (27)	Glu 3.9 (70)
K 3.9 (3.9)	Hgb 102 (10.2)	ALT 0.5 (30)	Ca 2.2 (8.9)
Cl 95 (95)	Lkcs 1.2×10^9 (1.2×10^3)	LDH 2.0 (120)	PO_4 1.4 (4.2)
HCO_3 27 (27)	Plts 270×10^9 (270×10^3)	Alk Phos 1.6 (95)	Mg 1.3 (2.5)
BUN 8.9 (25)		Alb 30 (3)	Uric Acid 297 (5)
CR 97 (1.1)		T. Prot 59 (5.9)	

Sigmoidoscopy Report—Mucosal surface irregular and granular in appearance; mucosa is friable with spontaneous bleeding.

PROBLEM LIST
1. Ulcerative colitis (proctosigmoiditis)
2. Sulfa intolerance
3. Nutritional support

QUESTIONS FOR CASE 53
1. Are corticosteroids absorbed systemically when administered rectally?
2. If DD requires maintenance therapy, what drug and dosage regimen would you recommend?
3. Is DD at a greater risk than the general population for developing colon cancer?

4. DD read an article in the *Wall Street Journal* on the use of fish oil in the treatment of ulcerative colitis (UC). What is the proposed mechanism of action of fish oils in the investigational treatment of UC?
5. What steroid-related adverse effects might DD develop if long-term corticosteroid therapy became necessary?
6. Are sulfasalazine and corticosteroids contraindicated in pregnancy?

CASE 54
CC: KT is a 39-year-old American male who has traveled to Guatemala. On day 5 of the trip, KT presents to the hospital with abdominal cramps, diarrhea, vomiting, fatigue, polydipsia, and blurred vision. He denies having proper oral intake × 2 days. He admits to "sipping on ice cubes to keep fluid down."

Past Medical History

KT developed type II diabetes mellitus 4 years ago, which was initially diet-controlled. He has been controlled on tolbutamide × 1 year. Six weeks ago, KT was hospitalized with his first episode of deep venous thrombosis (DVT). He was diagnosed with hyperlipidemia 1 year ago [(total cholesterol = 5.25 mmol/liter (203 mg/dl), LDL = 170 mg/dl]. KT was initiated on AHA diet, since he had several risk factors for coronary artery disease (CAD). He admits to a diet rich in fresh leafy green vegetables, fruit, fish, and chicken.

Social History
Smokes one pack of cigarettes/day

Family History
History of angina (father)

Medication History
Warfarin 5 mg p.o. q.d. (× 5 weeks)
Tolbutamide 500 mg p.o. t.i.d.
Simvastatin 20 mg po q evening

Allergies
No known drug allergies

Review of Systems
KT admits to having five to six loose stools/day × 2 days

Physical Examination
GEN: Obese male complaining of abdominal discomfort, diarrhea, and vomiting; decreased skin turgor
VS: BP 116/72, HR 100 (lying); 100/66, 110 (sitting); T 37.9; RR 18, Wt 84 kg (usual wt 88 kg); HT 175.3 cm

HEENT: Dry mucous membranes
COR: Tachycardia
CHEST: WNL
ABD: Soft, hyperactive bowel sounds; pain on palpation
GU: WNL
RECT: Stool guaiac-negative
EXTR: (–) edema; (–) pain
NEURO: WNL

Results of Laboratory Tests

Na 132 (132)	Hct 0.45 (45)	AST 0.50 (30)	Glu 16.8 (303)
K 2.7 (2.7)	Hgb 150 (150)	ALT 0.40 (24)	Ca 2.3 (9.2)
Cl 100 (100)	Lkcs 7.1 × 10^9 (7.1 × 10^3)	LDH 0.82 (50)	PO$_4$ 0.80 (2.5)
HCO$_3$ 20 (20)	Plts 350 × 10^9 (350 × 10^3)	Alk Phos 0.80 (48)	Mg 0.90 (1.8)
BUN 13.2 (37)	MCV 90 (90)	Alb 42 (4.2)	Uric Acid 178.4 (3.0)
CR 114 (1.3)		T Bili 3.6 (0.21)	

PT (control) 12.0

PT 16.2

INR 2.3

Total plasma cholesterol: 4.1 mmol/liter (160 mg/dl)

Fasting plasma triglyceride: 1.58 mmol/liter (140 mg/dl)

High density lipoprotein cholesterol 29 mg/dl (0.75mmol/liter)

Low density lipoprotein cholesterol 125 mg/dl (3.3mmol/liter)

Stool culture: Pending

PROBLEM LIST

1. Type II diabetes mellitus
2. Deep venous thrombosis
3. Hypercholesterolemia
4. Traveler's diarrhea (TD)
5. Dehydration/hypovolemia

QUESTIONS FOR CASE 54

1. What organism is most commonly identified as the cause of traveler's diarrhea (TD)?
2. After 6 days, KTs symptoms have not resolved, and he reported to the hospital with complaints of fever and chills. KT was noted to be guaiac-positive, and stool cultures returned positive for enterotoxigenic *E. coli*. Is antibiotic therapy appropriate at this time? What treatment would you recommend? Include drug(s), dose(s), route(s), schedule(s), and duration.
3. The doctor prescribed trimethoprim/sulfamethoxazole (TMP/SMX) 160 mg/800 mg p.o. b.i.d. for 5 days for treatment of TD. What possible drug interaction(s) may occur with this agent, considering KT's medication history?
4. What alternative rehydration solution may be extemporaneously prepared by KT for use in TD?

5. After adequate fluid replacement and discontinuance of the insulin sliding scale, KT's fasting blood glucose level was 9.4 mmol/liter (170 mg/dl) and his preprandial glucose level was 10.0 mmol/liter (181 mg/dl). What may be an appropriate dosage adjustment for KT's tolbutamide regimen?

CASE 55

CC: RU is a 42-year-old female who presents to clinic today complaining of heartburn, morning hoarseness, and laryngitis for which she has been taking Gaviscon-2, which has not helped.

Past Medical History

RU has had moderate gastroesophageal reflux for years, but it has worsened over the last week.

RU has had hypertension for 5 years and is currently being treated with verapamil and propranolol.

RU was diagnosed 3 weeks ago with deep vein thrombosis for which she receives warfarin.

RU has problems with motion sickness. She has been traveling a great deal over the last month. One week ago she started using scopolamine patches to try to reduce the nausea.

Medication History

Aluminum hydroxide 160 mg and magnesium trisilicate 40 mg with alginic acid (Gaviscon-2) 1 tab p.o. q2h p.r.n. heartburn

Verapamil 80 mg p.o. t.i.d.

Propranolol 40 mg p.o. q.i.d.

Warfarin 10 mg p.o. q.d.

Scopolamine patch 1 topically q. 3 days × 1 week

Allergies

None known

Social History

RU smokes 1 pack per day × 20 years and drinks 3–4 glasses of wine daily.

Physical Examination

GEN: Well-developed, obese female in moderate pain
VS: BP 130/85, HR 80, RR 16, T 37, Wt 90 kg, Ht 157 cm
HEENT: Dysphagia
COR: NL S$_1$ and S$_2$; no murmurs, rubs, or gallops
CHEST: WNL
AD: Nontender, no masses
GU: Deferred
RECTAL: Guaiac-positive
EXT: Few small healing bruises, right calf larger than left
NEURO: WNL

Results of Laboratory Tests

Na 140 (140)	Hct 0.35 (35%)	AST 0.42 (25)	Glu 4.4 (80)
K 3.8 (3.8)	Hgb 130 (13)	ALT 0.45 (27)	Ca 2.2 (9)
Cl 102 (102)	Lkcs 5 × 10⁹ (5000 mm⁻³)	LDH 1.1 (65)	PO₄ 0.87 (2.7)
HCO³ 24 (24)	Plt 160 × 10⁹ (160 × 10³)	Alk Phos 1.1 (65)	Mg 0.85 (1.7)
BUN 5.4 (15)	MCV 68 (68)	Alb 40 (4.0)	Uric Acid 557 (9)
Cr 88.4 (1.0)		T bili 15.4 (0.9)	

Lkcs differential: WNL
Urinalysis: WNL
Chest x-ray: WNL
ECG: WNL
Endoscopy: Moderate esophagitis, friable mucosa

PROBLEM LIST

1. Gastroesophageal reflux disease
2. Hypertension
3. Deep vein thrombosis
4. Motion sickness

CASE 56

CC: BD is a 34-year-old female who is admitted to the hospital today after calling her physician complaining of dizziness, abdominal cramping, and profuse diarrhea. She reports having eaten a normal diet at home for the past 8 days, since her return from a vacation.

History of Present Illness

Twenty-two days prior to admission, BD suffered a puncture wound on the left heel while wading in a river during a vacation trip to the Rocky Mountains. Although the wound was cleansed and bandaged, medical attention was not sought until 3 days later (in another city on the vacation route), when the left heel could no longer bear weight and had become tender to touch, swollen, and erythematous. She was admitted to the local hospital for treatment of osteomyelitis. Cultures taken during surgical debridement showed mixed flora, including *Pseudomonas aeruginosa* and *Staphylococcus aureus*. Antimicrobial therapy was initiated with tobramycin, ticarcillin, and nafcillin. This therapy was changed to ceftazidime (1 g q12h IV) and vancomycin (750 mg IV q 24 h) on day 8, when laboratory results indicated that her serum creatinine level rose from a baseline level of 88 μmol/liter (1 mg/dl) to 176 μmol/liter (2 mg/dl) on the 7th day, and 212 μmol/liter (2.4 mg/dl) on the 8th day. The wound was responding appropriately to therapy. BD was discharged on day 12 to fly home to have therapy continued by her personal physician with the assistance of a home-healthcare agency for a 28-day course.

The patient was seen in her physician's office on day 13 for examination and review of therapy. The heel wound was responding well, with minimal tenderness and no erythema. Pertinent laboratory results at this time were: Cr 150 μmol/liter (1.7 mg/dl), vancomycin peak level of 18 μmol/liter (26.1 mg/liter), and a trough level of 3.6 μmol/liter (5.2 mg/liter). Roentgenograms of left and right heels showed no evidence of osteomyelitis in the left heel.

Past Medical History

BD has a history of peptic ulcer disease treated with cimetidine 1 year ago. She also has a history of generalized tonic-clonic seizures secondary to a motor vehicle accident 4 years ago.

Medication History

Ceftazidime 1 g every 12 hr IV
Vancomycin 750 mg q 24 hr IV
Maalox TC, 12 ozper week × 2 weeks for "upset stomach"
Carbamazepine 400 mg b.i.d.

Allergies

None known

Physical Examination

GEN: Well-developed, well-nourished, pale, mildly anxious female
VS: BP 130/85 (lying), 120/65 (standing), HR 95 (lying), 115 (standing); T 40.0, RR 20, WT 52 kg (usual Wt 55 kg); Ht 64″ (163 cm).
HEENT: No lymphadenopathy, sticky mucous membranes
COR: Sinus tachycardia
CHEST: WNL
ABD: Diffuse tenderness in lower abdomen, no rebound, no quadrant pain; hyperactive bowel sounds
GU: Deferred
RECT: Guaiac-positive
EXT: Wound on left heel nontender, nonswollen; healing well, cool extremities, borderline decreased skin turgor
NEURO: WNL

Results of Laboratory Tests

Na 131 (131)	Hct 0.35 (35%)	AST WNL	Glu 5 (90)
K 2.9 (2.9)	Hgb 120 (12)	ALT WNL	Ca 2.1 (8.4)
Cl 95 (95)	Lkcs 22 × 10⁹ (22,000)	LDH WNL	PO₄ 1.1 (3.4)
HCO₃ 22 (22)	Plts 250 × 10⁹ (250,000)	Alk Phos WNL	Mg 0.7 (1.4)
BUN 13.2 (37)		Alb 29 (2.9)	
Cr 150 (1.7)			

Carbamazepine 30 mol/liter (7 mg/liter)
Urinalysis: WNL
Cultures and sensitivity: Stool positive for *Clostridium difficile* toxin
Sigmoidoscopy: Whitish-yellow raised plaques on the mucosal surface consistent with pseudomembranous colitis.

PROBLEM LIST (on day 22)

1. Seizures
2. Peptic ulcer disease
3. Osteomyelitis
4. Diarrhea
5. Hypovolemia
6. Hyponatremic dehydration
7. Electrolyte abnormalities

HEPATIC AND PANCREATIC DISORDERS

CASE 57

CC: SR is a 41-year-old male with type II (adult-onset insulin-dependent) diabetes mellitus (DM), a known alcohol abuser who is brought semicomatose to the ER by paramedics. His wife reports that he had an episode of hematemesis about 36 hrs prior to admission and has remained asleep and poorly responsive. SR appears to be acutely ill, showing a yellowish tinge to the skin, pale nail beds, and clammy skin.

Past Medical History

SR has had type II DM for eight years and has been stable on NPH insulin, 30 u/day. He is an admitted alcohol abuser but denies other substance abuse. He has had alcohol-withdrawal seizures, but has been in good general health, with no known liver problems. He is reported to have been without alcohol for two months. Shortly after stopping the alcohol he had several seizures and on his own began taking previously prescribed valproic acid. The last dose of valproic acid was approximately 48 hrs ago.

Medication History

NPH insulin (human) 30 u s.c. q.d.
Valproic acid (dose not known)
Aspirin 650–1300 mg p.r.n.

Physical Examination

GEN: Thin male, semicomatose, responding only to noxious stimuli, looks much older than stated age

VS: BP 110/60, HR 92, T 38.0°C, RR 16, Wt 59 kg, Ht 177.5 cm

HEENT: Semicomatose, pupils unequal, dried blood around mouth and in throat

ABD: Slightly rotund, SR responds to RUQ pressure, liver enlarged

EXT: Reflexes equal but exaggerated, poor skin turgor, dry skin

Results of Laboratory Tests

Na 142 (142)	Hct 0.18 (18.2)	AST 1.5 (90)	Glu 27.7 (499)
K 4.6 (4.6)	Hgb 63 (6.3)	ALT 1.2 (72)	Ca 1.97 (2.9)
Cl 109 (109)	RBC 1.77×10^{12} (1.77×10^6)	LDH 3.8 (229)	PO_4 1.36 (4.2)
HCO_3 11 (10.8)	Lkcs 18×10^9 (18×10^3)	Alk Phos .71 (43)	PT 33.1
BUN 12.8 (36)	Plts 94×10^9 (94×10^3)	Alb 26 (2.6)	PTT 90
CR 186 (2.1)	MCH 35 (35)	T Bili 70.1 (4.1)	Ammonia 106

Lkcs differential: 0.37 segs, 0.29 stabs, 0.19 lymph, 0.3 mono, 0.7 eosin

Toxicology screen: negative for 27 drugs, including cocaine
Alcohol screen: < 10 µg/dl
Valproic acid: 305 µmol/liter (44 µg/ml)
Blood, urine, CSF cultures pending
Hepatitis screen: HBsAg (–), HBsAb (+), anti-HCV (+), anti-HCV IgM (–), HAV (–), anti-HAV (+)

PROBLEM LIST

1. Type II DM
2. Alcohol abuse with withdrawal seizures
3. Acute drug-induced hepatitis
4. Hepatic encephalopathy
5. Upper GI bleeding
6. Severe anemia
7. Jaundice
8. Elevated Lkcs
9. Thrombocytopenia

Problem 3. Acute Drug-induced Hepatitis

S: Reports of nausea/vomiting, lethargy, semicomatose state.

O: Mild jaundice, T bili 70.1 (4.1), elevated AST and ALT, hepatomegaly, viral hepatitis screen conclusive for past exposure with immunity, negative exposure to hepatotoxins.

A: Valproic-acid-induced acute hepatitis (steatonecrosis) is diagnosed. SR is an admitted alcohol abuser but had no reports of liver problems until after this round of valproic acid. Antigen-antibody profile indicates immunity to the three major types of viral hepatitis. Valproic acid (like alcohol) causes hepatocyte necrosis by indirectly increasing the synthesis of fatty acids in the liver. The extra fatty acids are taken up by the hepatocyte, which swells and bursts. An inflammatory response follows. No specific diagnostic test exists to detect drug-induced hepatitis. The determination is made primarily by ruling out other possibilities. The clinical and laboratory profiles are similar to those with viral hepatitis and cirrhosis: elevated AST, ALT, bilirubin levels, and jaundice. In severe situations where portal hypertension develops, serum albumin levels are low, PT is prolonged, and gastrointestinal bleeding is likely. This represents a poor prognostic sign.

P: One should discontinue valproic acid, and begin methylprednisolone 40–60 mg IV q8h, phytonadione 10 mg s.q. q.d. for three days, folic acid 1 mg IV q.d. for three days, thiamine 100 mg IV q.d. for three days, gradual rehydration, and nutrition with TPN containing 0.8–1 g protein/kg/day and 2000–3000 cal/day. Begin TPN after the blood glucose level is down to 16 mmol/liter (288). Monitor liver function tests, bilirubin level, PT, PTT, icterus, and clinical symptoms for recovery. Treat other consequential problems (see below).

Problem 4. Hepatic Encephalopathy

S: Poorly responsive, semicomatose patient.

O: Elevated ammonia level is likely contributor to clouding of sensorium in hepatitis.

A: Encephalopathy is secondary to the inability of the liver to convert blood ammonia to urea for excretion by the kidney. Serum ammonia accumulates, interfering with normal metabolic pathways in brain. A reduction in ammonia production in the GI tract is the best approach.

P: One should place an n/g tube for medication administration, and begin lactulose 30 g via n/g tube q.i.d. Monitor for diarrhea and clearing of sensorium.

Problem 1. Type II DM

S: None.

O: Blood glucose is 27.7 (499). Wife reports no insulin given in the preceding 36 hrs, but can't recall when the last dose was given.

A: Previously-controlled diabetes is now out of control because of sporadic insulin dosing and liver damage. One should regain control with intravenous insulin and reestablish insulin needs.

P: One should give 20 u regular insulin s.c., followed by 10 u regular insulin every hour until the blood glucose level is down to 14 (252), then give regular insulin by sliding scale. Reevaluate insulin needs for maintenance when acute illness resolves.

Problem 5. Upper GI Bleeding

S: Wife reports that the patient vomited bright red blood.

O: Crusted blood is noted around the mouth; coffee-ground-looking material recovered via suction. Prothrombin time and partial thromboplastin time are prolonged and platelet count is decreased, making bleeding likely.

A: This problem is secondary to Problem 1. Acute necrosis and swelling in the liver has led to portal hypertension and gorging of capillaries in the GI tract. Aspirin probably contributed to the situation.

P: One should suction and lavage to remove old blood. One should also administer appropriate vitamins, hydration, and treatment for hepatitis (Problem 1).

Problem 6. Severe Anemia

S: No complaints.

O: Hgb, Hct, RBC, and other red blood cell indices are well below normal.

A: Although no conclusive information is given by the wife, SR has probably been bleeding into the GI tract for some time. Guaiac stool test was not performed.

P: One should transfuse with whole blood to replace serum protein, platelets, and RBC. Monitor red blood cell indices

for return toward normal and repeat transfusion, if needed.

Problem 7. Jaundice

S: No complaints.

O: Icterus is noted in the sclera. Bilirubin is elevated.

A: This problem is secondary to Problem 1. The ability of the liver to conjugate bilirubin is impaired. Increased red blood cell destruction may be leading to larger amounts of bilirubin in the serum.

P: See Problem 3. Monitor scleral icterus and bilirubin levels.

Problem 2. Alcohol Abuse with Withdrawal Seizures

S: No complaints.

O: By history; no alcohol currently in blood.

A: Alcoholism is a chronic problem. The withdrawal seizures are not documented by medical records.

P: When acute problems resolve, SR should be admitted into a rehabilitation program. One should impress upon him the seriousness of his condition. If seizures were to return, one should consult a neurologist for thorough evaluation and therapy. Avoid valproic acid.

Problem 8. Elevated Lkcs

S: No complaints.

O: WBC is 18. Differential pattern does not point to viral or bacterial infection. Blood, urine, and CSF cultures are pending.

A: Elevated Lkcs is probably not due to infection but to the stress of acute illness and massive inflammatory process in the liver. However, because SR is alcoholic, appropriate antibiotic coverage is needed until cultures are returned. Broad-spectrum gram-negative coverage, including *Pseudomonas,* with minimal hepatic/renal toxicity is desired.

P: One should begin ceftazidime 1 g IV q12h [creatinine clearance calculated from the serum creatinine is 0.85 ml/sec (50.7 ml/min.)]. Continue antibiotic until cultures return; change or discontinue antibiotic as cultures indicate. Monitor for adverse affects.

Problem 9. Thrombocytopenia

S: No complaints.

O: Platelet count is critically low.

A: Thrombocytopenia is noted to be an adverse effect of valproic acid, occurring in 6–40% of those receiving the drug. Aspirin is an inhibitor of platelet aggregation, but it is not believed to cause massive thrombocytopenia as is seen here.

P: One should recheck platelet count after transfusion with whole blood (Problem 5). If platelet count were below 200, one should give 1–2 units of platelets. Continue to monitor platelet count.

QUESTIONS FOR CASE 57

1. Can this patient be fed orally?
2. Are there any particular considerations for deciding the specific TPN formulation or oral diet?

3. The patient had a slightly rounded abdomen, which could have been ascites. If ascites were present, what treatment should be recommended?
4. Given SR's alcoholism and severe anemia, what other laboratory test results were probably abnormal? What, if any, maintenance therapy would you recommend?
5. How could SR's compliance with insulin therapy be assessed?

CASE 58

CC: LF is a 54-year-old female brought to the ambulatory care clinic by her husband who states she did not sleep well overnight and has been "shaking, sweating, and acting paranoid" all morning long. He says she quit drinking alcohol "cold turkey" yesterday. LF's husband brought her into clinic because he was "afraid she would start seizing." In the clinic waiting room, LF became increasingly agitated.

Past Medical History

LF was first diagnosed with alcoholic liver disease six months ago after an emergent hospital admission for bleeding esophageal varices. At that time, LF was experiencing hematemesis and melena. The hemorrhage stopped without intervention while LF was stabilized in the intensive care unit. Fiberoptic esophagoscopy provided positive evidence of esophageal varices. LF was also started on spironolactone to treat mild ascites. Since her hospital discharge, LF has been considering discontinuing her alcohol intake.

Social History

LF's husband states she does not smoke cigarettes or use recreational drugs. She has a 32-year history of drinking alcohol, up to a bottle of wine per day, until she quit yesterday.

PROBLEM LIST

1. Alcohol withdrawal
2. Esophageal varices
3. Ascites

Medication History

Spironolactone 50 mg po qd
Conjugated estrogen 0.625 mg po qd
Medroxyprogesterone 10 mg po qd

Allergies

Sulfa—rash

Physical Examination

GEN: tremulous, diaphoretic obese female in moderate distress
VS: BP 150/98, HR 96, RR 24, T 38, Wt 84 kg, Dry Wt 81 kg, Ht 173 cm

HEENT: PERRLA, EOMI, anicteric, + facial flushing
COR: tachycardic, no S3 or S4, no murmurs
CHEST: lungs clear to auscultation and percussion
ABD: increased girth, + hepatomegaly, + fluid wave, + shifting dullness
RECT: guaiac negative
EXT: 1 + edema
NEURO: WNL, no asterixis

Results of Laboratory Tests

Na 140 (140)	Hct 0.36 (36)	AST 1.95 (117)	Glu 6.1 (110)
K 3.9 (3.9)	Hgb 110 (11)	ALT 1.47 (88)	Ca 9.3 (9.3)
Cl 104 (104)	WBC 7.1 × 10⁹ (7100)	TBili 22 (1.3)	Po₄ 1.2 (3.7)
HCO₃ 27 (27)	Plts 140 × 10⁹ (140 × 10⁹)	Alk Phos 2.47 (148)	Mg 0.9 (1.8)
BUN 3.6 (10)	MCV 96 (96)	Alb 39 (3.9)	PT 14.7
Cr 80 (0.9)			INR 1.5
			PTT 29.9

WBC differential: WNL
Urinalysis: WNL
Chest radiography: WNL
ECG: WNL

Problem 1. Alcohol Withdrawal

S: LF reports difficulty sleeping, paranoia, and agitation. She presents with tremors, diaphoresis, and facial flushing.

O: Increased BP, HR, RR, and temperature.

A: LF is experiencing signs and symptoms consistent with acute alcohol abstinence (withdrawal) syndrome. LF's physical examination has confirmed her condition is not caused by other sequelae of chronic alcohol use, such as glucose or electrolyte imbalance. The goal of alcohol detoxification is to remove alcohol from her system while minimizing withdrawal symptoms from the CNS-depressant effects. Presently, her symptoms are mild-to-moderate; however, more severe and even life-threatening withdrawal reactions may occur. The use of benzodiazepines, which are long-acting sedative-hypnotics compared to alcohol, may minimize the adverse withdrawal effects. While other sedative-hypnotics are effective, benzodiazepines are longer-acting, safer, do not produce gastritis, have antiseizure activity, and are available in convenient dosage forms. It may be possible for LF's withdrawal syndrome to be managed as an outpatient, with adequate social support. LF could receive appropriate doses of benzodiazepines, return to clinic daily for evaluation of vital signs, and have her husband bring her to the ER if her withdrawal syndrome were to progress. To maintain abstinence, LF will likely benefit from participating in Alcoholics Anonymous.

P: Patients going through alcohol withdrawal often require high doses of benzodiazepines to control their withdrawal symptoms. One should start Diazepam 10 mg orally q4–6h on the first day. Initially, the benzodiazepine dose should be titrated to the desired effect (alleviation of most of the withdrawal symptoms), and then the drug should be gradually tapered. The dose should be decreased by about 20% daily, rather than increasing the dosing interval. The dosing regimen should be reevaluated every few hours the first day, and then at least daily until the drug is discontinued. In addition to drug treatment, refer LF and her husband to Alcoholics Anonymous.

Problem 2. Esophageal Varices

S: LF has a history of bleeding esophageal varices.

O: None.

A: LF has a positive history of bleeding esophageal varices; therefore, she is at high risk for another bleeding episode. Any episode of bleeding esophageal varices is life-threatening. Esophageal varices are likely secondary to portal hypertension from alcoholic cirrhosis. LF may benefit from secondary intervention with β-adrenergic blockers, which decrease portal venous pressure and theoretically decrease the risk of gastrointestinal bleeds. LF does not have any condition for which β-adrenergic blockers may be contraindicated, such as asthma or DM. The dose should be titrated to reduce the resting pulse by 25%.

P: One should start propranolol 20 mg orally twice daily, and increase the dose until LF's resting pulse is reduced by 25%. Monitor LF for bradycardia, weakness, lethargy, gastrointestinal disturbances, and lipid levels.

Problem 3. Ascites

S: None.

O: Weight three kilograms greater than dry weight, presence of increased abdominal girth, shifting dullness, fluid wave, and peripheral edema.

A: LF has ascites secondary to portal hypertension caused by alcoholic liver cirrhosis. Therapeutic intervention prevents progressive increase in ascites and potential complications, such as abdominal and back pain, gastroesophageal reflux, and shortness of breath secondary to impaired diaphragm movement. Treatment to reduce ascites should be gradual to allow for adequate fluid remobilization from the ascitic compartment to the intravascular compartment, otherwise renal failure may result. Therapy includes bed rest, salt restriction, fluid restriction if the patient were hyponatremic, and diuretics. The goal of treatment is to remove 500–1000 ml of fluid per day. Spironolactone is the diuretic of choice because it is slow-acting, potassium-sparing, and more specifically, it is an aldosterone antagonist (many patients with ascites exhibit hyperaldosteronism). The dose may be increased by 50 mg every three to five days, as needed, to reach treatment goals. Spironolactone may be given once daily to treat ascites. LF has been taking spironolactone for six months (since her hospitalization) without resolution of her ascites; therefore, her dose should be increased. If her ascites were not to resolve after spironolactone has been titrated to maximal doses of about 400 mg per day, she may benefit from the addition of a loop diuretic to her regimen.

P: One should increase spironolactone to 100 mg orally per day and monitor LF's weight, serum electrolytes, abdominal girth, shifting dullness, fluid wave, peripheral edema, and renal function. One should also monitor for adverse effects of Spironolactone, such as hypotension and gynecomastia. Educate LF about a salt-restricted diet and increased bed rest.

QUESTIONS FOR CASE 58

1. What type of vitamin supplementation should LF receive with her history of chronic alcohol use?
2. LF is at risk for what type of anemia?
3. Should LF receive prophylaxis for alcohol withdrawal seizures?
4. Is LF at risk for peritonitis?
5. Should LF receive gastrointestinal ulcer prophylaxis?
6. When is paracentesis appropriate treatment for LF's ascites?

CASE 59

CC: BB is a 26-year-old female who has been on outpatient hemodialysis for the past four years. Both kidneys were severely injured in an automobile accident. She has tolerated dialysis well, with the exception of several episodes of anemia during the first year of treatment. She is otherwise healthy. After this dialysis she was noted to be pale, very weak, nauseated and slightly febrile (T 38°C). She was admitted for a short hospitalization to evaluate her symptoms.

Past Medical History

BB's medical history was unremarkable until six years ago when an automobile accident resulted in severe internal injuries to her kidneys. Although BB recovered from the accident, over the next three years, kidney function deteriorated. Outpatient renal dialysis became necessary four years ago. BB is compliant with treatment and claims compliance with medications. She had received all childhood immunizations prior to the accident. She was given a tetanus booster at the time of the accident. She had a moderately severe dermal reaction, which her mother attributed to the tetanus shot. She has continuously refused the hepatitis vaccine. She has had only one blood transfusion. She admits to SOB, dyspnea on exertion, weakness, and lethargy, all of which she believes are transient and stress-related. She denies substance and alcohol abuse. One of her roommates was recently diagnosed hepatitis-B-positive. They have shared razors, eating and drinking utensils, and clothes.

Medication History

Multivitamin, 1 daily
Calcium carbonate 1250 mg p.o. t.i.d.

Allergies

Dermal inflammatory response six years ago, attributed to tetanus injections. No other known allergies.

Physical Examination

GEN: Well-developed, slightly underweight, pale female, unable to stand without assistance; complains of nausea and abdominal cramping

VS: BP 100/58, HR 10³, T 38.2°C, RR 24, Wt 50 kg, HT 160 cm

HEENT: Pale mucous membranes, no other assessment made

COR: Mild sinus tachycardia

CHEST: Slight dry cough

ABD: Unremarkable

GU: No assessment

RECT: Deferred

EXT: Pale

Results of Laboratory Tests

(Blood was drawn before dialysis)

Na 138 (138)	RBC 1.6	AST .5 (30)	Glu 7 (126)
K 3.6 (3.6)	Hct .14 (14.6)	Alk Phos 2.8 (173)	Ca 2.4 (9.5)
Cl 100 (100)	Hgb 46 (4.6)	LDH 4.4 (265)	Po₄ 1.2 (3.6)
HCO₃ 21 (21)	Lkcs 15.3 × 109 (15.4 × 10³)	Alb 22 (2.2)	
BUN 12.8 (36)	Plts 260 × 109 (260 × 10³)	T. Bili 6.8 (.4)	
Cr 504 (5.7)	MCV 85 (85)		

Lkcs differential: PMN 46, Lymph 50, Mono 3
RBC morphology: Fragmented RBC, microcytosis, anisocytosis

PROBLEM LIST

1. Renal failure
2. Severe anemia
3. Hepatitis B exposure

QUESTIONS FOR CASE 59

1. What are the mode of transmission and incubation period of hepatitis B? Why is BB in a high-risk group?
2. Why is hepatitis B immune globulin given?
3. How can it be confirmed that BB is protected against hepatitis B?
4. Why is epoetin used to treat anemia in renal failure patients?

CASE 60

CC: JG is a 59-year-old male who comes to the ER complaining of abdominal pain, nausea, and vomiting. He admits that he went on an alcohol binge two days ago because of problems at work. He awoke this morning with the above complaints that have continued throughout the day. He also complains of feeling thirsty and having to urinate frequently throughout the day.

Past Medical History

JG has a 10-year history of insulin-dependent diabetes due to chronic pancreatitis. He has a long history of polysubstance abuse including alcohol and IV drug abuse (cocaine). JG complains of years of chronic diarrhea and abdominal pain that worsen with meals. He reports a loss in weight of approximately 20 pounds over the past six months.

Social History

Cigarettes—smokes 1 pack daily.
Alcohol—1-2 quarts of beer daily and occasional binges with scotch

Medication History

NPH insulin 15 units s.c. 8 AM and 6 PM
Regular insulin 5 units s.c. 8 AM and 6 PM
Viokase 2 caps p.o. t.i.d. ac
Pancrease 2 caps p.o. t.i.d. ac
Cimetidine 400 mg p.o. b.i.d.

Allergies

None known

Physical Examination

GEN: Disheveled, thin-appearing male

VS: BP 110/50–75, HR 88-regular, T 37.0°C, RR 20, Ht 182 cm, Wt 80 kg, Usual Wt 88 kg (six months ago)

HEENT: Nystagmus, sclera anicteric, poor dentition

COR: RRR

CHEST: Clear to auscultation and percussion

ABD: Midepigastric pain, (–) BS

RECT: Guaiac-negative, ileus by rectal examination

EXT: R AKA, ulcerations of L leg, foot and L elbow

NEURO: Uncooperative

Results of Laboratory Tests

Na 133 (133)	CR 251 (3.3)	AST 0.57 (34)	Ca 1.62 (6.5)
K 3.4 (3.4)	Hct 0.36 (36)	ALT 0.58 (35)	Po₄ 1.13 (3.5)
Cl 104 (104)	Hgb 108 (10.8)	Alk Phos 3.67 (220)	Mg 0.86 (2.1)
HCO₃ 29 (29)	Lkcs 8.9 × 109 (8.9 × 10³)	Alb 19 (1.9)	Trig 3.23 (286)
BUN 7.14 (20)	MCV 91 (91)	T Bili 25.65 (1.5)	Amylase 6.17 (370)
		Glu 15 (270)	

PROBLEM LIST

1. Chronic pancreatitis
2. Alcoholism with cirrhosis
3. Peptic ulcer disease
4. Insulin-dependent DM
5. Malnutrition
6. Acute pancreatitis

QUESTIONS FOR CASE 60

1. JG's serum calcium level is below normal. What ionized (free) level does his calcium level represent? Is the ionized level normal or abnormal?
2. JG has some chronic renal insufficiency. What electrolyte abnormalities would you anticipate JG to experience due to his renal insufficiency in conjunction with electrolytes he may receive in his maintenance fluids and TPN?

3. Days after admission, JG has a serum potassium level of 6.5 mmol/liter (mEq/liter) with peaked T waves on ECG. What treatment would you recommend for his condition?

4. JG may be at risk for vitamin deficiencies because of his history of alcoholism. Which vitamin deficiency may be the cause of his nystagmus? How would you prevent worsening of the syndrome that this vitamin deficiency can cause?

5. Following discharge, JG still complains of diarrhea and foul-smelling, oily stools. His abdominal pain continues to worsen with food. How would you adjust JG's therapy for chronic pancreatitis to lessen his symptoms?

6. JG is brought to the ER months later by a friend and is diagnosed with hepatic encephalopathy caused by worsening liver failure from cirrhosis. Serum ammonia level is 70.46 μmol/liter (120 μg/dl). What drug and nondrug interventions would you institute to immediately treat his condition?

CASE 61

CC: SB is a 38-year-old lawyer who is admitted to the hospital after vomiting bright red blood. For the past two weeks he has complained of increasing nausea, abdominal pain, and bloody stools. The last two days he has become increasingly lethargic and disoriented and complains of being light-headed.

Past Medical History

SB has a long history of alcohol abuse since age 15. He is a successful lawyer in a large corporate firm. His alcohol use consists of nightly beer or wine with heavy binges on the weekends. Despite heavy use, he has had no apparent complications until now. Past medical history includes a gastric ulcer which was treated two years ago empirically with ranitidine and intermittent bouts of gastritis since then. He broke his ankle playing basketball six months ago and still complains of pain, despite using large quantities of Tylenol 3 and OTC Tylenol.

Social History

Alcohol—heavy use in the past
Tobacco—1/2 ppd × 15 years

Allergies

NKDA

Medication History

Acetaminophen with codeine p.r.n. up to 10 tablets per day
Acetaminophen 500 mg caps up to 6 caps per day
Ranitidine 150 mg po qHS

Review of Systems

SB is confused as to time and place, distressed over vomiting blood, and complains mostly of abdominal pain.

Physical Examination

GEN: Confused, middle-aged man looking older than stated age

VS: BP 100/60 supine; BP 90/40 sitting, HR 90 supine; HR 110 sitting, RR 20 T 37.0°C, Wt 70 kg, Ht 172.7 cm

HEENT: PEERLA, icteric sclera, mouth covered with blood, foul breath with possible fetor hepaticus

COR: Regular rate and rhythm, no gallops, no rubs

CHEST: lungs clear A&P

ABD: Enlarged abdomen, liver enlarged and palpable 6 cm at the costal margin, mild pain to percussion

GU: Normal

RECT: Nonbleeding hemorrhoids, hemocult (+) for blood

EXT: Mild swelling in both ankles, appears jaundiced

NEURO: Asterixis in both hands, AxOx2

Results of Laboratory Tests

Na 143 (143)	Hct .25 (25)	LDH 3 (180)	Ca 2.24 (9.0)
K 4.2 (4.2)	Hgb 90 (9)	Alk Phos 1.7 (100)	Po$_4$ 1.4 (4.3)
Cl 100 (100)	WBC 12 × 10^9 (12 × 10^3)	Glu 6.6 (120)	Alb 30 (3.0)
HCO$_3$ 23 (23)	Plts 120 × 10^9 (12 × 10^3)	ALT 4 (240)	T bili 87 (5.1)
BUN 2.9 (8)	MCV 91 (91)		Mg 1.03 (2.1)
Cr 71 (.8)	AST 5 (300)		Uric acid 357 (6)

Prothrombin time: 16 sec/control 11 sec
WBC differential: wnl
Urinalysis: wnl
Chest radiography: heart and lungs normal
ECG: WNL
Endoscopy: shows actively bleeding esophageal varices

PROBLEM LIST

1. Massive GI bleed (variceal bleeding)
2. Coagulopathy
3. Altered mental status
4. Alcoholic liver disease

CASE 61 SOAP NOTES
Problem 1. Variceal bleeding

S: SB complains of nausea and light-headedness.

O: SB vomited large quantities of bright red blood at home and once since admission. Hemocult test is positive. Active bleeding is noted on endoscopy. Hct 0.25 (25) and Hgb 90 (9) were found on admision. Orthostatic BP was obtained.

A: SB has active bleeding esophageal varices with probable volume depletion, hypotension, and decreased Hct. The treatment of choice for bleeding varices is sclerotherapy to stop the bleeding. Vasopressin usually is not given immediately due to the risk of side effects. However, SB has no known CAD and may benefit from vasopressin therapy if sclerotherapy were not available, or to reduce the bleeding in order to better visualize the varices before sclerotherapy. H2-receptor antagonists should be started at treatment doses to prevent reflux into the esophagus. Antacids may also be administered. Iced saline lavage may be used to slow bleeding. After bleeding has stopped, sucralfate suspension and β-blocker therapy should be started to protect the variceal bleeding sites and to lower portal venous pressure, respectively, and lower the risk for rebleeding.

P: One should inject each bleeding variceal site with sclerosing agent, the choice of which may depend on the institution. Monitor for recurrent episodes of bleeding, volume and color of future vomitus, and further decreases in Hgb and Hct. Ranitidine should be started at 50 mg IV q8h. Monitoring should include gastric pH measurements and guaiac testing. β-Blocker therapy should not be initiated until SB's BP and fluid status are stabilized.

Problem 2. Coagulopathy

S: None.

O: Prothrombin time 16 sec/control 11 sec, Hct 0.25 (25), bleeding esophageal varices, and positive hemocult test.

A: Prothrombin time is most likely prolonged secondary to decreased liver production of vitamin-K-dependent coagulation factors (II, VII, IX, X). The prolonged prothrombin time is also contributing to SB's active bleeding from variceal sites. SB also has anemia due to blood loss and probably suffers from anemia secondary to nutritional deficiency from poor intake of both folate and iron (common to patients with alcoholic liver disease). Whole blood transfusions should be administered to achieve Hct 0.3 (30). Vitamin K should be administered to correct any defiency in clotting factors.

P: One should administer whole blood transfusions to keep Hct 0.3 (30). Vitamin K, 10 mg per day, should be given for three days or until protime is normalized.

Problem 3. Altered Mental Status

S: Patient is confused, demented, and not oriented to place.

O: Asterixis, serum ammonia level not determined; serum glucose 6.6 (120), bicarbonate 23 (23), possible fetor hepaticus.

A: The cause of encephalopathy in this patient is most likely due to underlying disease (alcoholic hepatitis resulting in cirrhosis) and increased protein in the GI tract from GI bleeding. Serum glucose and bicarbonate levels are normal. A serum ammonia level should be obtained to confirm the diagnosis of hepatic encephalopathy. The use of CNS depressants should be minimized and dietary protein intake should be restricted. Therapy involves decreasing serum ammonia levels. Lactulose is the drug of choice; neomycin is an alternative for patients who do not tolerate or obtain benefit from lactulose.

P: One should minimize the use of drugs with CNS depressant activity, and restrict daily protein intake to 30 g/day. Start lactulose 30 g p.o. t.i.d. via N/G tube. Titrate dose until improved mental status or two to three loose stools/day are obtained. Continue to monitor for asterixis. If neomycin were indicated, one should give 1 g q.i.d. via N/G tube.

Problem 4. Alcoholic Liver Disease

S: Patient is confused and disoriented.

O: SB has elevated AST, ALT, T bili, decreased serum albumin, and is suffering from bleeding esophageal varices, hepatic encephalopathy, and coagulopathy. On examination, the patient is noted to be jaundiced with an enlarged liver.

A: SB likely has permanent damage to his liver (cirrhosis). The cause is his long-standing alcohol abuse and his recent large intake of acetaminophen. Cirrhosis is an irreversible process and the goal is to prevent any further damage to the liver and treat the patient symptomatically. The primary treatment is to encourage the patient to abstain from alcohol. Vitamin replacement is also essential for patients with recent alcohol intake. The patient should also avoid future contact with other hepatotoxins, specifically eliminating the use of acetaminophen intake. The patient should be cautioned not to use NSAIDS or aspirin for pain relief because they may aggravate GI bleeding.

P: One should give thiamine 100 mg p.o. q.d., folate 1 mg p.o. q.d., MVI 1 p.o. q.d. Discontinue acetaminophen use and encourage the patient to abstain from alcohol and educate him that stopping alcohol is the only way to stop the progression of his disease. One should consider checking B12 level as well. Continue to monitor LFT's, folate, B12, albumin, and signs and symptoms of bleeding, bruising, and mental status changes.

QUESTIONS FOR CASE 61

1. What are the mechanisms of action of neomycin and lactulose in the treatment of hepatic encephalopathy?
2. How should vasopressin be given to patients with bleeding esophageal varices? What are the limitations to the drug?
3. What is the ideal form of vitamin K and rate of administration for SB?
4. Can lactulose and neomycin be used together?

RHEUMATIC DISEASES

CASE 62

CC: VB is a woman, age 72, who arrives at the general medicine clinic complaining of nausea, right upper quadrant abdominal pain, and aching pain in the left knee.

History of Present Illness

VB takes acetaminophen and PRN ibuprofen for her degenerative joint disease. These analgesics give her intermittent relief. Recently, her pain level has increased, and 6 weeks ago, her orthopaedic surgeon prescribed Darvocet-N-100 for 7 days. The orthopaedic surgeon asked VB to return for reevaluation of her pain after finishing the course of Darvocet, but VB did not return. Instead, she cajoled her internist and her dentist son-in-law into providing additional prescriptions of Darvocet-N-100, and also obtained a prescription from an outpatient "Emergi-Center" one weekend. She resumed her weekly bowling and ballroom dancing sessions, which she had not participated in for more than a year. She takes extra doses of Darvocet after these activities. In the past week, she has noted a new onset of joint swelling.

Past Medical History

VB has a 20-year history of degenerative joint disease (DJD). She experiences morning stiffness and aching pain after completing daily chores. Last year she underwent replacement of her right knee. Although she admits her right knee feels better, her convalescence following the surgery was lengthy and difficult. Her orthopaedic surgeon has suggested that she consider having her left knee replaced, but she is very reluctant to undergo another uncomfortable and temporarily disabling procedure. VB's husband passed away approximately 3 years ago. She has had difficulty falling asleep since that time. Initially, triazolam was prescribed, which "sometimes helps." For the last 6 weeks, her knee pain has been keeping her awake, which has resulted in her becoming irritable and "snapping" at family members often.

Social History

She lives alone and stubbornly refuses offers from her children and grandchildren to provide assistance for household chores. She performs weight bearing tasks (e.g., mowing the lawn, moving furniture to vacuum) around the house regularly and hosts tea for neighborhood women daily. Drinks 2 glasses of sherry nightly to "help her fall asleep."

Medication History

Acetaminophen, 325 mg PO Q6H PRN pain × 15 years
Ibuprofen, 200 mg PO Q6H PRN pain, occasionally × 2 years
Darvocet-N-100 (acetaminophen 650 mg/propoxyphene 100 mg); 1 tab PO Q4H PRN pain (per physician's order) and 2 tabs PO PRN for severe pain (self-initiated); typically takes 6 to 8 tablets daily × 6 weeks
Triazolam, 0.0625 to 0.125 mg PO QHS PRN for sleep × 3 years (takes occasionally)

Allergies

Aspirin causes a macular rash

Physical Examination

GEN: thin, pale elderly woman in moderate distress
VS: BP 140/80; HR 85; RR 20; T 37.0°C; Ht 150 cm
HEENT: PEERLA
COR: nl
ABD: RUQ tenderness; mild guarding
EXT: limited range of motion of left knee; mild swelling
NEURO: oriented × 3
X-RAY: joint-space narrowing consistent with osteoarthritis, left knee

Results of Laboratory Tests

Na 140 (140)	Hct 0.36 (36)	AST 6 (360)	Glu 140 (140)
K 3.9 (3.9)	Hgb 120 (12)	ALT 4.7 (180)	Ca 2.2 (8.9)
Cl 103 (103)	WBC 8.5 × 10⁹	Alk phos 3 (200)	PO₄ 1.19 (3.7)
HCO₃ 27 (27)	Plts 180 × 10⁹	Alb 33 (3.3)	Mg 1.0 (2.0)
BUN 10.4 (29)	MCV 91 (91)	T bili 17.1 (1.0)	PT/PTT 11.2/28.7
Cr 115 (1.3)	MCHC 32 (32)		

PROBLEM LIST

1. Degenerative joint disease
2. Elevated liver function tests
3. Chronic insomnia

CASE 62 SOAP NOTES
Problem 1. Degenerative Joint Disease

S: VB complains of joint stiffness and swelling and aching knee pain which keeps her awake.

O: X-ray films reveal joint-space narrowing consistent with osteoarthritis in the left knee.

A: VB's DJD is worsening. Her pain is likely a result of her frequent heavy weight bearing activities. Treatment of DJD is directed toward alleviating pain. Acetaminophen is an appropriate agent for management of DJD; however, VB has been receiving 3.9 to 5.6 g daily, receives minimal relief and is experiencing acetaminophen toxicity. Propoxyphene has limited efficacy in relieving pain and may increase the incidence of central nervous system (CNS) side effects, especially in elderly patients. Nonsteroidal antiinflammatory drugs (NSAIDs) may be considered if there is evidence of swelling, warmth, or inflammation. VB has new evidence of inflammation, so antiinflammatory activity may provide her with additional relief. Although VB experiences a rash when taking aspirin, she appears to tolerate ibuprofen. If VB had a history of a more serious allergic reaction to aspirin (e.g., bronchospasm, anaphylaxis), the potential for cross-reactivity would have to be considered and NSAIDs should be avoided. Opiates do not have a role as regular therapy for DJD and should be used for short periods only. VB has recently exhibited a propensity to procure prescriptions from multiple providers and to abuse Darvocet-N-100. She needs to be taught about the role of different types of pharmacologic and nonpharmacologic therapies and to develop reasonable expectations of their effectiveness.

P: Discontinue Darvocet-N-100. Start ibuprofen scheduled at 600 mg PO Q6H, rather than "as needed." Teach VB the necessity of balancing exercise and rest and of recognizing the need to decrease activity when she has pain. Formal physical therapy may be useful.

Problem 2. Elevated Liver Function Test Levels

S: VB complains of right upper quadrant abdominal pain and nausea.

O: Mild guarding; elevated levels of AST, ALT, and alkaline phosphatase.

A: VB is experiencing hepatoxicity from chronic acetaminophen use. The dose of acetaminophen should be limited to 2.6 g daily in cases of prolonged use. Her occasional alcohol use and age may make her more susceptible to toxicity from acetaminophen. Generally, liver function abnormalities from chronic acetaminophen use resolve when the dose is decreased or the drug is discontinued. Acetylcysteine is not indicated for chronic toxicity.

P: Discontinue Darvocet-N-100 and monitor liver function tests.

Problem 3. Chronic Insomnia

S: VB reports difficulty falling asleep and sleeping poorly.

O: None.

A: VB has chronic insomnia, which may be caused by pain, the stress of coping with her DJD, and stress from the death of her husband. She drinks tea in the afternoon, which may interfere with her ability to fall asleep. Her nightly sherry (contains alcohol) may also disrupt sleep, since alcohol has a short duration of action. Upon withdrawal, her sleep may be fitful. VB needs to change lifestyle habits that may be interfering with her ability to fall asleep. VB's triazolam dose is appropriate for a patient of her age; however, VB likely has a tolerance to triazolam. Hypnotic agents, including the benzodiazepines, barbiturates, nonbarbiturate nonbenzodiazepines, and antihistamines, are indicated for short-term (1 to 2 weeks) relief of acute insomnia. There is little data supporting efficacy and safety of hypnotics for longer than 1 to 2 months. If temporary relief is necessary, diphenhydramine may be considered, but is associated with anticholinergic side effects that may be troublesome to elderly patients. Chloral hydrate may have less abuse potential than the barbiturates or benzodiazepines, but patients may become tolerant to chloral hydrate almost as rapidly as they do to barbiturates. Barbiturates have a narrow margin of safety, moderately high abuse potential, and potential drug interactions caused by liver enzyme induction.

P: Review proper sleep hygiene with VB: Set a regular time to go to bed and to wake up; make the sleep environment comfortable and secure; omit alcohol and caffeine in the late afternoon and evening; develop a sleep habit and use the bedroom only for sleep or sexual activity; carefully time meals and exercise; learn relaxation techniques; and consider psychotherapy.

Discontinue triazolam; taper by half the dose for 3 nights, then half the dose again for the next 3 nights, then stop. While VB is adjusting to new sleep habits, consider chloral hydrate, 500 mg PO QHs for 1 week.

CASE 62 QUESTIONS

1. Are glucocorticoids a good therapy option for treatment of this patient's DJD?
2. What nonpharmacologic therapies may be recommended for VB's DJD?
3. What are the causes of VB's chronic insomnia?
4. VB's dentist son-in-law suggests that she try flurazepam, 30mg PO QHS, for her insomnia, since triazolam does not seem to work. Do you agree or disagree with this recommendation?

CASE 63

CC: JM is a woman, age 34, with a 3-year history of rheumatoid arthritis who presents to the clinic with a 3-week history of increased pain, swelling, and stiffness in fingers and wrists. She has also experienced increased fever, malaise, and back tenderness over the past 2 weeks.

Past Medical History

Three years ago, just following delivery of her second child, JM began to notice mild bilateral swelling and tenderness of the small joints of her hands and feet. Workup also revealed about 1 hour of morning stiffness. Ibuprofen, 300 mg QID, was started, but was increased to 400 mg QID 6 months ago due to increased disease activity. Her current regimen also includes daily range-of-motion exercises and as needed rest periods. One year before this visit, her rheumatoid factor was 1:640 and periarticular osteopenia and soft tissue swelling were noticed on x-ray studies of hands. Over the past month, she has missed numerous days of work because of her arthritis and is on the verge of being fired because of her lack of productivity. Three weeks ago her dose of ibuprofen was increased to 800 mg QID, with little relief. She has not previously received corticosteroids or secondline agents.

Social History

The patient is an active mother of two children who continues to work because of financial need. Husband is very supportive.

She denies smoking and recreational drug use, with the exception of occasional alcohol socially.

Past Surgical History

No major surgeries.

Medication History

Ibuprofen, 800 mg QID
Multiple vitamins, 1 QD

Review of Systems

As noted in previous medical history and chief complaint
Fatigues easily
Itchy rash on chest for 1 week
Denies other problems (e.g., visual, GI, urinary, neurologic)

Physical Examination

GEN:	Well-developed, well-nourished woman in some discomfort.
VS:	BP 125/76, HR 64, RR 16, T 38.3°C, weight 63 kg, height 163 cm
HEENT:	PERRLA, EOMI
DERM:	Macular, papular rash on chest
COR:	RRR
CHEST:	Normal breath sounds throughout
ABD:	CVA tenderness; otherwise soft, nontender; no organomegaly
GU:	Deferred
RECT:	Guaiac-negative stools
EXT:	Considerable swelling and tenderness of the second, third, and fourth MCPs and PIPs and the wrists of both hands. Mild synovitis in MTPs.
NEURO:	DTRs and cranial nerves intact

Results of Laboratory Tests

Na 140	Hct 0.30 (30)	ALT 14	Ca 2.3 (9.2)
K 4.9	Hgb 103 (10.3)	LDH 255	PO_4 1.1 (3.4)
Cl 104	WBC 6.9	Alk Phos 1.1 (66)	Mg 1.1 (2.2)
CO_2 24	Plts 490	Alb 38 (3.8)	Urate 0.25 (4.1)
BUN 11.4 (32)	MCV 92	T Bili 3 (0.2)	
SCr 150 (1.7)	AST 25	Glu 5.6 (100)	

WBC differential: 76% Segs, 1% Bands, 17% Lymphs, 6% Eosin

Urinalysis: pH 6.5, Spec Grav 1.026, Epith cells 1-2/hpf, 2+ Eosin

Chest x-ray: not performed

EKG: not performed

ESR: 65 mm/hr

PROBLEM LIST

1. Rheumatoid arthritis in flare.
2. Renal insufficiency, interstitial nephritis.
3. Anemia, mild.

CASE 63 SOAP NOTES

Problem 1. Rheumatoid Arthritis

S: Fatigue and increased pain, swelling, and stiffness in fingers and wrists over previous 3 weeks despite an increased dose of ibuprofen. Patient is in jeopardy of losing her job.

O: Considerable swelling and tenderness of the second, third, and fourth MCPs and PIPs and the wrists of both hands. Mild synovitis in MTPs. ESR 65 mm/hr, platelet count 490 (increased with an increase in arthritis), Hct 0.30 (30), Hgb 103 (10.3), MCV 92 (anemia of chronic disease)

A: Flare of rheumatoid arthritis despite high doses of ibuprofen. The patient probably has progressive, destructive joint disease, judging from the nature of her disease activity. Patient has not previously received glucocorticoids or second-line agents, but now needs immediate relief as well as aggressive long-term therapy.

P: Obtain x-ray films of hands and feet. Change NSAID from ibuprofen to sulindac, 150 mg BID, because of loss of effectiveness of ibuprofen and the development of renal insufficiency and interstitial nephritis while on ibuprofen (see below).

Start prednisone 10 mg QAM to rapidly relieve the arthritis flare and improve the patient's function at work and home. In 2 weeks, attempt to decrease this dose to 7.5 mg QAM. This is not an ideal long-term choice of therapy because of the potential development of chronic adverse effects (e.g., osteoporosis).

Start methotrexate, 7.5 mg PO weekly in one dose. Monitor WBC and differential, Hct, Hgb, platelets, LFTs, skin, mucous membranes, GI tolerance, breathing, and joint inflammation every 2 weeks for 2 months, then less often. Consider adding folic acid 4 days per week.

Encourage the patient to increase rest periods and calcium intake, and diminish any use of alcohol. The patient should be educated regarding the immediate benefits and delayed adverse effects of prednisone and the delayed benefits and adverse effects of methotrexate. Many of these adverse effects can be seen by the patient, but certain serious adverse effects can be detected only through physical examination and laboratory studies.

Problem 2: Renal Insufficiency and Interstitial Nephritis

S: No history of renal disease before the increase in ibuprofen dose to 800 mg QID. No other drug allergies. No other risk factors for NSAID-induced, prostaglandin-mediated renal dysfunction (i.e., the patient is not elderly; there is no underlying cardiovascular, renal, or hepatic disease).

O: SCr 176 (2.0), BUN 12.5 (35), increased eosinophils in blood and urine, rash, CVA tenderness, increased temperature

A: Mild, hopefully fully reversible renal insufficiency caused by allergic reaction to ibuprofen and possibly a result of the increase in ibuprofen dose. However, patient still needs an NSAID to alleviate the activity of her arthritis.

P: Discontinue ibuprofen and add sulindac, 150 mg BID. Check serum creatinine, BUN, WBC and differential, CVA tenderness, rash, temperature, blood pressure, and heart rate in 2 weeks.

Problem 3: Anemia of Chronic Disease (Mild)

S: Fatigue

O: Hct 0.3 (30), Hgb 103 (10.3), MCV 92, guaiac-negative on rectal exam

A: Mild anemia of chronic disease as evidenced by low Hct and Hgb level, normal RBC indices, and presence of active rheumatoid arthritis

P: Treat the rheumatoid arthritis. If it worsens, consider workup for iron-deficiency anemia.

CASE 63 QUESTIONS

1. What are the major differences in adverse effects among the NSAIDs, particularly as they relate to this patient?
2. Which of the following would be most prudent in this patient?
   (a) Intraarticular corticosteroid injection
   (b) Intravenous high-dose pulse corticosteroid
   (c) Oral low-dose daily corticosteroid
3. What are the likely reasons for discontinuation of methotrexate or other second-line agents (e.g., antimalarial, injectable or oral gold salt, penicillamine, sulfasalazine, azathioprine, or cyclophosphamide) in this patient?
4. The patient experiences an initial response to methotrexate, but 1.5 years later her arthritis begins to worsen with increased pain and swelling. Is it necessary to discontinue the methotrexate?

CASE 64

CC: MJ is a woman, age 56, who presents to clinic today with multiple complaints, including lower abdominal cramping and constipation with intermittent watery diarrhea, usually in the morning. She has no energy and lately has noticed increasing fatigue and lethargy, malaise, and worsening pain in her hands, wrists, and feet.

Past Medical History

MJ received a diagnosis of irritable bowel syndrome 4 years ago when she complained of chronic constipation characterized by small, hard, mucus-covered stools and morning diarrhea. Sigmoidoscopy, barium enema, and stool examination revealed no pathology. A trial of propantheline, 15 mg TID, was unsuccessful, and low doses of diazepam caused intolerable sedation. Since these medication trials, the patient has just "coped" with her alternating bowel function. MJ has had osteoarthritis (OA) of both knees and the left hip for 20 years, which she attributes to the traumatic birth of her last child. She complains of moderate stiffness in the morning (of 10 minutes duration) and significant pain and stiffness after riding 4 hours in a car to visit her daughter in a nearby city. MJ denies any joint swelling or redness. In 1988, MJ received a diagnosis of premature ventricular contractions after complaining of her "heart jumping out of her chest," but she has been without symptoms on procainamide therapy for the last 2 years.

Social History

MJ drinks about 8 to 10 cups of coffee per day and has a 40 pack-year history of cigarette smoking.

Medication History

Procainamide SR, 500 mg PO TID
Aspirin, 650 mg PO QID
Milk of magnesia, 2 tablespoonfuls "as needed" for dyspepsia

Allergies

None known

Physical Examination

GEN: Slightly anxious, mildly obese woman, age 56, complaining of abdominal cramping, irregular bowel function, increasing fatigue, and multiple arthralgias

VS: BP 130/80, HR 120, RR 18, T 382, Wt 63 kg, Ht 165 cm

HEENT: Dry tongue and mucous membranes

COR: Tachycardia at 120 bpm

ABD: Right upper quadrant soft, tender, painful

RECTAL: Guaiac-negative, small, hardened stool present

EXT: Mild tenderness noted on both hands, wrists, and feet, decreased range of motion (ROM) of left knee, left hip, and wrists bilaterally; poor skin turgor

Results of Laboratory Tests

Na 146 (146)	CR 97.2 (1.1)	ALT 0.43 (26)	ANA (+)
K 4.8 (4.8)	Hct 0.457 (45.7)	ESR 80 (80)	LE (+)
Cl 105 (105)	Hgb 152 (15.2)	T4 112 (8.7)	RF (−)
HCO$_3$ 27 (27)	Lkcs 1.0 × 10^9 (1.0 × 10^3)	TSH 0.45 (0.45)	VDRL (+)
BUN 14.6 (41)	AST 0.25 (15)		

Procainamide concentration: 25.5 μmol/L (6 mg/L)
Sigmoidoscopy: WNL
Stool: negative for ova and parasites
X-ray films of knees: bilateral joint-space narrowing consistent with OA

PROBLEM LIST

1. Irritable bowel syndrome
2. Osteoarthritis
3. Procainamide-induced lupus-like syndrome
4. History of premature ventricular contractions (PVCs)

CASE 64 SOAP NOTES

Problem 1. Irritable Bowel Syndrome

S: MJ complains of lower abdominal cramping, right upper

quadrant pain, alternating constipation and diarrhea, morning diarrhea, and increasing fatigue and lethargy.

O: Stools are negative-guaiac and negative for ova and parasites; sigmoidoscopy WNL; small hardened stool on rectal examination

A: MJ has signs and symptoms characteristic of irritable bowel syndrome exacerbation. The irregular bowel function without identifiable pathology is consistent with this diagnosis. She also appears dehydrated as indicated by tachycardia (heart rate, 120 bpm); BUN/SCr ratio more than 20:1; high-normal level of serum electrolytes; high-normal hematocrit and hemoglobin level; dry tongue and mucous membranes; and poor skin turgor. Dehydration may be contributing to the pathogenesis of chronic constipation, even though most of MJ's symptoms are likely a result of an exacerbation of irritable bowel syndrome.

P: Emphasize the importance of adequate daily fluid intake. Encourage at least six 8-ounce glasses of water per day. This may help relieve some of her chronic constipation. Reassure her that irritable bowel syndrome will not progress to inflammatory bowel disease or colon cancer. Tell her that irritable bowel syndrome is a chronic condition characterized by remissions and exacerbations but symptoms can be controlled, even during periods of disease exacerbation. The constipation may be reduced by increasing dietary fiber, e.g., bran or psyllium, one to two teaspoonfuls two to four times daily. Each dose should be administered with at least one 8-ounce glass of water or juice and followed with another glass. The potential for impaction without adequate fluid intake with these agents should be stressed. Discontinuing the magnesium-containing antacid with reevaluation of "dyspepsia" may reduce the diarrhea. Otherwise, antidiarrheal agents, such as loperamide, for troublesome diarrhea may be helpful.

Problem 2. Osteoarthritis

S: MJ complains of moderate morning stiffness of short duration and significant pain and stiffness after long periods of inactivity.

O: Bilateral x-ray films of her knees show narrowed joint spaces consistent with OA; ESR 80 mm/hr (80 mm/hr); RF-negative; no palpable warmth or inflammation in joints

A: Although MJ has an elevated ESR, examination results of her affected joints is consistent with noninflammatory OA, which can be successfully managed with a combination of simple analgesia and physiotherapy. MJ's elevated ESR may be attributed to other causes (see problem 3). She currently takes two aspirin tablets four times daily and complains of dyspepsia. Considering MJ's present disease status, there appears to be no need for the antiinflammatory action of aspirin or the NSAIDs. Aspirin may exacerbate MJ's gastrointestinal complaints and should therefore be discontinued.

P: Discontinue ASA, 650 mg QID. Explain to the patient that the current status of her disease does not warrant treatment with aspirin or other antiinflammatory agents, although it may require more aggressive therapy in the future. Recommend acetaminophen 650 mg PO Q4-6H for her pain. Ex-

plain the principles of joint protection. Weight reduction (ideal body weight is 56.5 kg for MJ), strengthening of periarticular musculature by means of moderate exercise such as walking, and avoidance of heavy weight bearing activities will reduce the symptoms of OA and protect damaged joints from further injury. Mild ROM exercises during prolonged periods of inactivity will alleviate associated joint stiffness. MJ should monitor her pain as a response to therapy.

Problem 3. Procainamide-induced Lupus-like Syndrome

S: MJ complains of a recent onset of increasing fatigue and lethargy, malaise, and multiple arthralgias.

O: Mild tenderness noted on both hands, wrists, and feet; LE (+), ANA (+), ESR 80 mm/hr (80 mm/hr), VDRL (+), T 382

A: The patient has signs and symptoms consistent with drug-induced lupus-like syndrome. Symptoms will resolve if the offending agent is discontinued, but they may be treated with mild analgesia if necessary in the interim. A multitude of reports have indicated a strong and consistent association between procainamide and a lupus-like syndrome. Since procainamide is the most likely causative agent in MJ's therapeutic regimen, it would be prudent to discontinue its use. The clinical manifestations of procainamide-induced lupus-like syndromes resolve within days to a few weeks following drug withdrawal. Laboratory manifestations are much slower to resolve; LE cells may remain for up to 10 months, ANA positivity may take up to 2 years to resolve.

P: Discontinue procainomide SR. Assure MJ that this syndrome is a process without the renal and CNS complications of idiopathic systemic lupus erythematosus.

Problem 4. History of PVCs

S: MJ has no symptoms associated with PVCs.

O: HR 120 bpm

A: Reassure MJ that PVCs are not life-threatening and not all cases need to be treated with medication, especially the lower-grade PVCs (MJ's PVCs were graded 2 on a scale of 5). Tell her that PVCs may be precipitated by caffeine and stress, so she should try to minimize these influences.

P: Discontinue procainamide SR as mentioned above. In patients complaining only of palpitations, the benefits of PVC suppression must be weighed against the risk and cost of therapy. MJ had palpitations in 1988, but she is otherwise relatively free of significant systemic disease. Therefore, drug therapy is not necessarily indicated. The development of signs and symptoms consistent with procainamide-induced lupus-like syndrome further precludes the use of this particular agent in MJ.

CASE 64 QUESTIONS

1. What is the cause of osteoarthritis (OA)? Is it possible that trauma during the birth of her child could have caused MJ's OA?
2. MJ returns to your clinic 2 years later with complaints of painful knees. Her knees are swollen and tender with de-

creased range of motion bilaterally. She states that the acetaminophen is no longer effective. What would you recommend?

3. What are the clinical and laboratory manifestations of drug-induced lupus-like syndrome?

4. What drugs are commonly associated with drug-induced lupus-like syndrome?

5. If MJ had had a positive rheumatoid factor test result, would it have been appropriate to diagnose rheumatoid arthritis?

CASE 65

CC: AT is a white woman, age 62, complaining of fatigue, arthralgias of both hips and knees and the small joints of both hands, and a red scaly rash on her upper torso, extremities, and face. She says that sunlight aggravates the rash and that she has had all of these problems for approximately 2 months but is most disturbed by the itching rash. She says the rash has made her very depressed, and she has trouble sleeping at night and concentrating at work during the day.

Past Medical History

AT has a history of: allergies to penicillin drugs (but has not received them in the past 5 years); osteoarthritis for 10 years; depression for 4 years; severe gastroesophageal reflux disease (GERD) that often interferes with her job; and hypertension for 7 years.

Medication History

Fluoxetine 20 mg QAM
Naproxen sodium 550 mg BID
Omeprazole 40 mg QAM
Hydralazine 50 mg BID
Diltiazem 30 mg QID
AT is a very compliant patient.

Social History

Tobacco: Negative

Ethanol: Used to consume large amounts 7 to 8 years ago around the time of her husband's death, but has not had a drink in 7 years.

Physical Examination

GEN: Obese female who appears anxious about her condition

VS: BP 130/74, HR 76, RR 20, T 36.7, Wt 78.6 kg (84.6 kg 3 months ago), Ht 153 cm

HEENT: Patient has circular, erythematous, scaly plaques on cheeks of face, upper torso, and upper extremities

COR: Normal S_1 and S_2, no murmurs or gallops

CHEST: Clear to auscultation and percussion

ABD: Soft, nontender; no masses upon palpitation

GU: NL

EXT: Rash as described under HEENT. Limited ROM of both knees and hips; pain upon movement of hands (small joints), but no noticeable swelling.

NEURO: Oriented × 3 (time, place, person)

Results of Laboratory Tests (Today)

Na 138 (138)	Hct .396 (39.6)	AST 0.33 (20)	Glu 5.66 (102)
K 4.1 (4.1)	Hgb 130 (13.0)	ALT 0.233 (14)	Ca 2.34 (9.4)
Cl 99 (99)	Lkcs 4.1×10^9 (4.1×10^3)	LDH 1.47 (88)	PO_4 1.36 (4.2)
HCO_3 23 (23)	MCV 93 (93)	Alk Phos 1.07 (64)	Mg 1.0 (2.0)
BUN 6 (17)		Alb 42 (4.2)	ANA (+), 1:1280
CR 70.7 (.8)		T Bili 11.97 (0.7)	

Urine: protein (−)

Skin scrapings: KOH (−)

PROBLEM LIST

1. Arthralgias and arthritis
2. Hypertension
3. Depression
4. GERD
5. Rash

CASE 65 SOAP NOTES
Problem 5. Rash

S: AT complains of round, itching lesions on her face, chest, and arms for the last 2 months. She says that she was given clotrimazole cream by her physician when the rash first appeared, but the cream did not work. The rash appeared 10 months after starting fluoxetine therapy. Her fluoxetine was stopped for 3 weeks, because it can induce rashes; she became very depressed and the rash did not heal. She says she tried different antidepressants (i.e., amitriptyline, nortriptyline, trazodone), and they all made her sleepy so she would prefer to be placed back on fluoxetine. AT also admits she is taking hydralazine from a prescription she has had with another physician. She admits to taking hydralazine 50 mg BID for the last 3 years.

O: KOH: negative (45 days ago), ANA: positive (1:1280)

A: AT probably has drug-induced lupus. However, 2 months ago her physician did not know of her hydralazine prescription and felt the rash looked like a fungal rash (tinea corporis). Upon scraping the lesion, the KOH test to confirm the fungal infection had negative results. Clotrimazole did not resolve the rash. The rash was then thought to be caused by fluoxetine (side effect incidence is 5% for rash), so antidepressant therapy was terminated for 3 weeks. Since the rash did not begin to resolve, the patient was placed back on fluoxetine. Recently, AT was discovered to be taking hydralazine 50 mg BID for her hypertension. Since AT also had arthralgias, drug-induced lupus (DIL) must be considered. The fluorescent antinuclear antibody (ANA) test result was highly positive (1:1280) today, which is consistent with DIL.

P: AT should have her hydralazine therapy stopped immediately and have her blood pressure monitored. AT was instructed to wear long-sleeved shirts when outside to minimize exposure to sunlight, which irritates the rash. She should also to be instructed to wear sunscreen on areas of the rash (e.g., face, extremities) that could be exposed to sunlight. Hydroxychloroquine therapy will be started at 200 mg BID, but she should have an ophthalmologic examination before initiation of hydroxychloroquine therapy to make sure she has no retinal abnormalities before therapy. The patient should be monitored over the next several weeks for resolution of rash, fatigue, and arthralgias. Ophthalmologic examinations should be performed every 3 to 6 months if the patient is expected to remain on chronic therapy.

Initial doses of hydroxychloroquine are 400 mg/day. AT should be told to split the dose (200 mg BID) to minimize GI upset (especially with her GI history). If necessary, hydroxychloroquine can be taken with food to further reduce the chances of GI upset. After 2 weeks of 400 mg/day, AT should be placed on a maintenance regimen of 200 mg QAM until the rash resolves. If resolution is not seen after several weeks of therapy, glucocorticoid (prednisone) therapy should be instituted. AT was also told that, at the beginning of therapy, hydroxychloroquine can often cause headaches, which respond to acetaminophen therapy.

Problem 1. Arthralgias and Osteoarthritis

S: AT complains of increasing pain similar to her arthritis in both hips and knees and in the small joints of her hands, which she says is unusual for her. She says she has used naproxen sodium in the past for her arthritis with relief, but it often upsets her stomach and makes her reflux worse. AT admits she has never tried acetaminophen for her osteoarthritis.

O: Pain in both knees and hips with some limited ROM. Pain in her small finger joints on both hands.

A: AT has arthralgias, possibly caused by DIL. Although she has had some success with naproxen, when taking it she experiences worsening of her GERD. AT may benefit from acetaminophen therapy until the DIL has resolved. Hydroxychloroquine should also help AT with the resolution of her DIL arthralgias.

P: AT is instructed to initiate acetaminophen at a dose of one to two 325 mg tablets every 4 to 6 hours (not to exceed 4 g (10 to 11 tablets) per day). If acetaminophen does resolve the arthritic pain, AT should use naproxen sodium, 550 mg BID with food as needed for the arthritic pain. Liver function test results are currently normal, but they should be checked every 6 months if AT receives chronic high-dose therapy with acetaminophen.

Problem 3. Depression

S: AT says she feels depressed because she cannot go out in public with her rash. She says she can't stop scratching because of all the itching from the lesions. She is a widow, has no local family support mechanisms, and relies on social activities to keep her active and motivated. AT admits to re-

ceiving behavioral counseling for depression surrounding her husband's death. She also received several antidepressant medications (i.e., amitriptyline, trazodone, and nortriptyline) all of which made her feel sedated during the day. AT feels that fluoxetine has helped more than any other antidepressant in relieving her depression. Recently, AT says she has not been able to become involved socially, has difficulty sleeping at night, has lost her appetite, and has difficulty concentrating on her job. She admits that she is depressed despite being compliant with her fluoxetine therapy. She said the doctor stopped her fluoxetine therapy for 3 weeks because he thought it might be the source of her rash, but her depression became worse and the rash did not resolve with discontinuation of the fluoxetine.

O: Weight is 78.6 kg (decrease of 6 kg in 3 months). Patient has depressed affect.

A: AT has a history of a depressive disorder successfully treated by increasing her social activities and by the use of fluoxetine. The drug-induced rash makes AT so uncomfortable that she can't engage in social activities. She feels that her constant itching affects her ability to do her job, which entails working with the public. She has also shown weight loss and a decrease in appetite.

P: AT should be referred to a clinical psychologist or psychiatrist to receive behavioral therapy to provide her with social support and teach her ways to modify her outlook toward her situation. AT should also have the dose of her fluoxetine increased to 40 mg/day, divided into two doses with 20 mg given with breakfast and 20 mg with lunch. Doses of fluoxetine of more than 20 mg/day should be split because fluoxetine can cause abdominal cramping and pain. AT was reinstructed that fluoxetine should not be taken in the evening hours (unlike other antidepressants) because it produces a stimulatory effect that may keep patients awake at night. The fluoxetine therapy should be maintained for approximately 6 months and then be tapered to 20 mg QAM if her psychologist or psychiatrist feels she is stable enough to warrant tapering. After 4 to 6 months of fluoxetine, 20 mg QAM, attempts should be made to discontinue therapy.

Problem 4. GERD

S: AT had no complaints of reactivation of her GERD upon this clinic visit. AT says her GERD has often flared when she used naproxen sodium or aspirin and on the one occasion when she used prednisone. She remarks that she has received ranitidine 300 mg QHS, metoclopramide 10 mg QID, and nizatidine 300 mg QHS in the past for her reflux disease, with only marginal relief. She was then placed on omeprazole 20 mg QAM, which helped some, but the combination of omeprazole 40 mg QAM and diltiazem 30 mg QID. has markedly improved her symptoms of reflux.

O: Nothing done on this visit.

A: AT's GERD is currently under control, but AT has a history of reactivation of GERD symptoms when using NSAIDs or prednisone.

P: Observe AT while she is receiving hydroxychloroquine and higher-dose fluoxetine (20 mg BID) therapy to determine if GERD is reactivated. If it is reactivated, AT should increase the dose of her omeprazole or diltiazem and use antacids as needed for pain relief. If her GERD symptoms do not respond to these measures, refer AT to her gastroenterologist for further evaluation. The long-term safety of omeprazole has not been established.

Problem 2. Hypertension

S: AT has no complaints consistent with hypertension.

O: BP 130/74, HR 76

A: AT's blood pressure is currently under control with hydralazine, 50 mg BID, and diltiazem, 30 mg QID.

P: Discontinue hydralazine because of DIL and monitor AT's blood pressure. If her blood pressure exceeds 160/95, suggest increasing the diltiazem dose to 180 mg/day. This can be done using diltiazem 60 mg TID or diltiazem SR 90 mg BID.

CASE 65 QUESTIONS

1. What are the most common clinical presentations in drug-induced lupus (DIL)?
2. What laboratory values help confirm a diagnosis of idiopathic systemic lupus erythematosus (SLE) or DIL?
3. What are the major differences between DIL and idiopathic SLE?
4. Why do many patients with SLE often suffer from depression, and what considerations are involved in selecting an antidepressant medication?
5. Which two drugs are most commonly associated with DIL? Describe the theory explaining why certain patients experience DIL, the relationship between dose and DIL for each drug, and the percentage of patients who have a positive ANA titer and then go on to have symptomatic DIL.

CASE 66

CC: CJ is an obese woman, age 70, with a 10-year history of rheumatoid arthritis who presents to clinic for routine follow-up. She complains of fatigue, diarrhea, dry mouth, morning stiffness, and swelling and stiffness of her hands, elbows, and knees.

Past Medical History

CJ has had rheumatoid arthritis for 10 years. Previous trials of aspirin, ibuprofen, and naproxen at maximum doses have not provided optimal effects. Injectable gold salts resulted in some permanent decrease in disease, but she did not want to continue on injections, so therapy was stopped 3 years ago. Since then, penicillamine has caused a rash and hydroxychloroquine has caused intolerable GI distress. She has been receiving auranofin for 3 months, which was increased in dose from 6 mg/day to 9 mg/day two weeks ago, and piroxicam, 20 mg/day for the past 8 months. She has been experiencing 3 to 4 bowel movements daily for the past week, which is a change from her baseline of one every other day.

Other medical history reveals that CJ was admitted with a diagnosis of deep vein thrombosis (DVT) 2 months ago. For the past 5 years, she has complained of gastroesophageal reflux, with nightly discomfort. She also has had hypothyroidism for 12 years.

Social History

CJ is widowed, lives with her sister, drinks one to two glasses of wine almost every day, and smokes 1 pack of cigarettes per day, as she has for the past 50 years.

Past Surgical History

No major surgeries.

Medication History

Auranofin 9 mg QD
Piroxicam 10 mg QD
Warfarin 5 mg QD
l-Thyroxine 0.1 mg QD

Review of Systems

As described in previous medical history

Physical Examination

GEN: Obese elderly woman appearing pale and tired.
VS: BP 110/70, HR 84, RR 16, T 37.0°C, Wt 80 kg, Ht 150 cm
HEENT: PERRLA, EOMI
COR: RRR
CHEST: Normal breath sounds throughout
ABD: Obese, soft; without guarding or pain
GU: Deferred
RECT: Guaiac-positive
EXT: Swelling and tenderness in joints of the hands and elbows, with tenderness in the knees.
NEURO: No abnormalities in deep tendon reflexes (DTRs) or cranial nerves

Results of Laboratory Tests

Na 142	Hct 0.27 (27)	ALT 12	Ca 2.2 (8.9)
K 4.1	Hgb 90 (9.0)	LDH 188	PO_4 0.9 (2.8)
Cl 104	WBC 8.2	Alk Phos 1.5 (87)	Mg 1.0 (2.0)
CO_2 23	Plts 440	Alb 35 (3.5)	Urate 0.2 (3.5)
BUN 8.9 (25)	MCV 84	T Bili 15 (0.9)	SCr 115 (1.3)
AST 21	Glu 6.2 (111)		

WBC differential: 72% Segs, 26% Lymphs, 1% Monos, 1% Eosin

Fe 4.5 (25), TIBC 51 (286), Ferritin 205 ng/mL

Urinalysis: pH 7.2, Spec grav 1.031, RBCs 0-2/hpf, dip negative

Chest x-ray films: not performed

ECG: not performed

PROBLEM LIST

1. Diarrhea of recent onset
2. Anemia

3. Rheumatoid arthritis, active
4. History of DVT on chronic anticoagulation
5. Hypothyroidism
6. GERD
7. Obesity
8. Chronic cigarette use

CASE 66 SOAP NOTES
Problem 1: Diarrhea of Recent Onset
S: Fatigue; and three to four bowel movements daily, which started after auranofin dose was increased

O: Na 141, Cl 104, BUN 8.9 (25), SCr 115 (1.3), BUN:SCr ratio (19:1)

A: Diarrhea, resulting in minor dehydration, is caused by the increased dose of auranofin, which is commonly associated with diarrhea, particularly in higher doses. Diarrhea is much less commonly associated with injectable gold salt therapy.

P: Discontinue auranofin for 1 week; if diarrhea resolves, restart auranofin at a dosage of 6 mg/day. Encourage consumption of fluids. Explain to the patient the implications of diarrhea caused by auranofin therapy.

Problem 2: Anemia
S: Fatigue

O: Hct 0.27 (27), Hgb 90 (9.0), MCV 84 (84), guaiac-positive stool, PT 15 sec, Fe 4.5 (25), TIBC 51 (286), Ferritin 205

A: Low blood counts and iron deficiency with normal TIBC and slightly elevated ferritin levels indicate iron deficiency anemia in patients with active arthritis. The anemia is secondary to GI bleeding probably caused by piroxicam therapy or, less commonly, by auranofin-induced gastroenteritis.

P: Discontinue piroxicam therapy. Discontinue auranofin therapy temporarily (as noted above).Begin cimetidine therapy at 300 mg QID and FeSO₄ at 325 mg TID. Obtain GI series to determine whether peptic ulcer is present. Help patient learn to recognize the signs and symptoms of GI bleeding and ulceration, to realize that these disorders may be asymptomatic, and to understand the implications of such disorders.

Problem 3. Rheumatoid Arthritis, Active
S: Fatigue as well as swelling and stiffness of hands, elbows, and knees despite therapy with piroxicam and auranofin; dry mouth

O: Swelling and tenderness in joints of hands and elbows, with tenderness in the knees; platelet count 440, ferritin (205)

A: Arthritis symptoms show active arthritis; elevated platelet count and increased level of ferritin are signs of ongoing inflammation. There is continued activity of rheumatoid arthritis and the possibility of development of an associated condition, despite apparently adequate NSAID therapy and 3 months of auranofin therapy. It is still relatively early in the course of auranofin therapy, and the patient has a history of failure of therapy with other second-line agents.

P: Restart auranofin therapy after diarrhea has resolved. Dis-

continue piroxicam therapy. Evaluate patient for Sjögren's syndrome, and discuss Sjögren's syndrome with patient. Explain the possible flare in arthritis that may occur when drug therapy is temporarily discontinued.

Problem 4. History of Deep Vein Thrombosis while on Chronic Anticoagulation Therapy
S: No bruising or overt bleeding; no signs or symptoms of deep vein thrombosis (DVT) or pulmonary embolism (PE)

O: Hct 0.27 (27), Hgb 90 (9.0), MCV 84, guaiac-positive stool, PT 15 sec

A: Anticoagulation seems appropriate and is not a major reason for GI bleeding. Although the initial plan was for 12 weeks of therapy, 6 weeks may prove adequate in selected patients.

P: Discuss with physician whether to continue warfarin therapy.

If patient is to continue warfarin therapy, keep at the current dose, but monitor PT closely because of the addition, and subsequent discontinuation, of cimetidine therapy. Instruct patient about the importance of warfarin therapy and the signs and symptoms of GI bleeding, DVT, and PE.

CASE 66 QUESTIONS
1. The patient is not experiencing GI pain or discomfort consistent with an ulcer. Is this common with NSAID-induced ulcers?
2. Should piroxicam be continued given the diagnosis of GI bleeding and possible peptic ulcer disease?
3. Should this patient receive therapy to prevent GI bleeding or ulceration in the future if another NSAID is started?

CASE 67
CC: PS is a woman, age 40, who presents to the hospital with fever, fatigue, joint tenderness and swelling, and chest pain with mild dyspnea. She also complains of a dry mouth.

History of Present Illness
PS has had a low-grade fever for 48 hours with increasing fatigue and joint tenderness and swelling. In the past 10 hours she has been experiencing pleuritic chest pain with some dyspnea.

Past Medical History
PS has a 3-year history of systemic lupus erythematosus (SLE), first recognized when she noticed a rash appearing over her cheeks and the bridge of her nose. Since her diagnosis, she has felt weak and had a weight loss of 15 pounds. PS has experienced multiple problems resulting from SLE with periods of remissions and exacerbations. Her SLE flares have consisted of joint pain, fatigue, worsening facial rash, increasing serum creatinine levels with proteinuria, fever, and pleu-

risy. Since her diagnosis and subsequent flares, PS has been discouraged, sad, and withdrawn from family and friends. She began amitriptyline therapy approximately 1 year ago; the dose was increased to 100 mg approximately 4 months ago. She is often unable to sleep at night and has been feeling weak and tired.

Social History:

Occupation: Elementary school teacher
Tobacco use: negative
Alcohol use: Negative

Medication History

Sulindac, 200 mg PO Q12H
Sunscreen, apply to skin QID or as needed
Hydroxychloroquine, 200 mg PO QD
Amitriptyline, 100 mg PO QHS

Allergies

None known

Physical Examination

GEN: Pale, thin woman with complaints of chest pain and mild shortness of breath
VS: BP 150/90, HR 60, RR 20, T 38.2, Wt 56 kg, Ht 5'2"
HEENT: Butterfly-shaped erythema covering the cheeks and bridge of nose
COR: Normal S_1 and S_2
CHEST: Clear to auscultation and percussion
ABD: Soft, nontender, no distention
GU: WNL
RECT: Guaiac-negative
EXT: Joint swelling and tenderness at ankles, knees, and wrists; warm to touch
NEURO: Oriented to time, place, and person

Results of Laboratory Tests

Na 135 (135)	Hct .33 (33)	Alt .58 (35)	Ca 1.996 (8.0)
K 5.0 (5.0)	Hgb 120 (12.0)	LDH 1.7 (101)	PO₄ 1.94 (6.0)
Cl 98 (98)	WBC 3.0 (3000)	Alk Phos 1.08 (65)	Mg 1.20 (2.4)
HCO₃ 22 (22)	Plts 60,000 (60,000)	Alb 32 (3.2)	Uric Acid 446.1 (7.5)
BUN 12 (35)	MCV 76 (76)	T Bili 13.7 (0.8)	ESR 50 (50)
Cr 221 (2.5)	AST .47 (28)	Glu 5.55 (100)	

Urinalysis: 3+ proteinuria, granular casts, WBC 1+, RBC 2+, Nitrates (–), Estrase (–)
CXR: NL
ANA titer: 1:480 with a rim fluorescent pattern
Positive LE cell test
Positive anti-DNA antibodies
Positive anti-Sm
Serum complement (C3,C4) decreased

PROBLEM LIST

1. SLE flare
2. Chronic renal failure (lupus nephritis)
3. Depression
4. Drug-induced problem

CASE 67 SOAP NOTES

Problem 1. Systemic Lupus Erythematosus (SLE) Flare

S: PS complains of fatigue, joint swelling, and some chest pain with mild dyspnea.

O: PS has a history of SLE and presents with a fever, joint swelling with warmth to the touch, and a malar rash. Laboratory values consistent with lupus include low platelets; positive ANA with a titer of 1:480, described by a rim fluorescent pattern; a positive LE cell test; positive anti-DNA antibodies; positive anti-Sm antibodies; ESR of 50; and decreased serum complement.

A: PS is experiencing an active flare of SLE. Clinical manifestations include joint involvement with swollen and tender joints. Also typical in SLE patients is a malar rash (classic red butterfly rash over bridge of nose and cheeks). PS also is experiencing pleurisy and mild dyspnea which brought her into the hospital. Other symptoms of SLE that she has include fatigue, weight loss, renal insufficiency, and depression. Laboratory findings consistent with SLE are also part of her diagnosis.

P: Corticosteriod therapy is indicated for PS's symptomatic SLE flares, especially flares that include major organs, such as the kidney (glomerulonephritis) and lung (pneumonitis). PS's other symptoms of SLE are currently managed appropriately. Patients presenting with lupus-induced malar rash, fever, and joint pain may be treated with NSAIDs and an antimalarial agent. Sunscreens should be applied to avoid rashes on sun-sensitive skin. PS should be started on a dose of prednisone, 25 mg/day, in addition to her current therapy of sulindac and hydroxychloroquine. Corticosteroids are the mainstay of therapy for SLE in reducing signs and symptoms during acute episodes of the disease. Slow tapering of corticosteroids is required to avoid a disease flare. Nonpharmacologic therapy should also be included. Proper diet and resting habits should be followed. Minimum exposure to direct sunlight and proper exercise may help relieve and prevent complications and symptoms.

Problem 2: Chronic Renal Failure (Lupus Nephritis)

S: None

O: Her serum creatinine and BUN are 221 (2.5 mg/dL) and 14 (40), respectively; her calculated creatinine clearance is 26.4 mL/min. Urinalysis indicates high levels of 3+ proteinuria and urinary casts. PS also has electrolyte abnormalities including a high normal potassium level at 5.0, low serum calcium level of 1.996 (8.0), elevated phosphate level at 1.94 (6.0), and slightly elevated uric acid level at 446.1 (7.5). PS is hypertensive (blood pressure of 150/90).

A: PS has a history of SLE, and most SLE patients can eventually expect to have some degree of renal insufficiency as a result of their disease. PS's renal failure may improve with treating the SLE. However, if PS's renal function does not improve following SLE therapy, treatment for renal dysfunction should be initiated. Monitoring of electrolyte abnormalities, blood pressure, urine output, and BUN and creatinine levels will indicate when therapy should be considered. Prednisone, immunosuppressive agents, and possibly plasmapheresis may be tried. If worsening renal failure persists, dialysis or transplantation may be required.

P: Corticosteroids are the mainstay of therapy for lupus nephritis secondary to SLE. Patients with mild nephritis but no proteinuria do not require therapy. Patients with proteinuria, hematuria, and a calculated creatinine clearance of less than 50 mL/min are often given prednisone at 0.5 to 1.0 mg/kg/day, which results in improvement at 2 to 4 weeks. If no improvement in renal function is seen, increasing the dose to 1.5 mg/kg/day may be useful, or bolus doses of 1 gm/day of intravenous methylprednisolone for 3 days may be effective. Patients who fail to respond to large doses of corticosteroids may be given immunosuppressive therapy to reverse worsening renal function. Azathioprine, cyclophosphamide, and chlorambucil have been beneficial when used in clinical trials. PS should be started on a dose of 0.5 mg/kg/day (approximately 25 to 30 mg) of prednisone (similar to the previous dose given for SLE symptoms) and should continue therapy until renal function improves. If no improvement is noted, doses may be increased or immunosuppessive therapy may be added (allowing for a reduction of prednisone dose when used in combination). Other considerations include electrolyte abnormalities and monitoring of blood pressure. Calcium supplements may be recommended if PS has low serum calcium; aluminum hydroxide may be given to lower phosphate levels; allopurinol may be started if high uric acid levels lead to gout attacks or stones; blood pressure should be monitored to ensure no further progression of worsening renal function secondary to hypertension. Long-term therapy for chronic renal failure may require dialysis or kidney transplant as renal function worsens to end-stage renal disease (ESRD).

Problem 3: Depression

S: PS appears discouraged and sad and has withdrawn from family and friends. She feels tired and weak and is unable to sleep at night.

O: Weight loss of 15 pounds (could also result from SLE)

A: SLE patients may experience many emotional reactions with the progression of disease. Psychological problems may also be the result of the disease. PS may have anxiety and depression resulting from dealing with her disease state. Corticosteroid therapy has also been linked to depression or mild euphoria in patients. However, less than 2% of patients have experienced these effects with low doses. PS is currently taking amitriptyline, 100 mg PO QD. Amitriptyline is a good choice for PS, since it has a sedative effect and she is experiencing insomnia. Amitriptyline may help PS sleep better and feel less fatigue. The dose may be increased gradually to 300 mg/day, if the desired effects are not achieved over time. PS is not responding to the current dose; her dose should be increased. Note that PS is experiencing dry mouth, which may be caused by the

anticholinergic effects of amitriptyline.

P: Increase amitriptyline dose to 150 mg PO QHS. If she does not feel better in 2 to 4 weeks, her dose may be increased by 50 mg/week to a maximum of 300 mg QD. Alternative therapy, such as other tricyclics or selective serotinon-reuptake inhibitors, may be initiated if PS does not respond to the maximum dose of amitriptyline. Psychological (nonpharmacologic) support is appropriate for PS. Support groups for SLE patients may be helpful. Therapy should continue as considered appropriate by her psychiatrist or her primary physician.

Problem 4: Drug-induced Problem

S: PS complains of dry mouth.

O: None

A: Dry mouth may be caused by amitriptyline. Tricyclic antidepressants have been associated with many anticholinergic side effects including dry mouth, urinary retention, constipation, and others.

P: PS's dry mouth is not unbearable. As she continues her therapy with antidepressants, the anticholinergic side effects should resolve with time. Artificial saliva, hard candy, or sips of water may also be recommended to help alleviate dry mouth. Other antidepressant medications without anticholinergic side effects may be used if PS feels her symptoms have not improved or resolved.

CASE 67 QUESTIONS

1. Name two drugs that have been associated with drug-induced lupus-like syndrome. What is the typical clinical presentation of patients with drug-induced lupus-like syndrome?
2. Which antibody test is specific for SLE?
3. For which potential toxicity should PS be regularly monitored during antimalarial therapy?
4. How would hyperkalemia be managed in PS?
5. What methods may be used to treat hyperkalemia caused by renal failure in symptomatic patients?

CASE 68

CC: BN is a Scandinavian woman, age 62, who is hospitalized for acute pain in the low back and left hip region after falling from a standing position.

Past Medical History

Osteoporosis was suspected in BN 2 years ago after a minor fall resulted in right hip pain. X-ray revealed a fracture of the (R) femoral neck. Calcium supplementation was started. A diagnosis of rheumatoid arthritis (RA) was given 15 years ago; numerous trials of NSAIDs failed, and BN has been "steroid-dependent" for 8 years. There is a history of recurrent peptic ulcer disease (PUD) managed with antacids and cimetidine. Gastroscopy, 1 year PTA, revealed duodenal ulcer and gastric erosions consistent with NSAID therapy. Chronic active hepatitis B was detected 3 months PTA. Menopause occurred at approximately age 55.

Family History
Breast cancer in mother and one sister.

Medication History
Acetaminophen, two 500 mg tabs QID PRN for arthritis pain

ASA, two 325 mg tabs 5 × daily (discontinued because of GI upset)

Ibuprofen, 800 mg TID (discontinued because of GI upset)

Naproxen, 375 mg BID (discontinued because of guaiac-positive stool)

Piroxicam, 20 mg/day (discontinued because of GI upset)

Indomethacin, sustained-release, 75 mg/day (discontinued because of dizziness and confusion)

Cimetidine, 400 mg BID for several years (compliance related to GI symptoms)

Prednisone, up to 40 mg/day; 10 mg BID for last 6 months (makes her "feel better")

Tums, 1 BID

Vitamin D and fluoride, doses unknown (friend's recommendation)

Unknown antacid, used PRN

Allergies
None known

Physical Examination
GEN: White woman of Scandinavian descent with truncal obesity, appearing tired
VS: VSS
HEENT: Pale mucous membranes; moon facies
COR: RRR
CHEST: Clear to auscultation and percussion
ABD: Right upper quadrant (RUQ) pain; liver nonpalpable; striae
GU: Atrophy of urogenital area
RECT: WNL; guaiac-negative
EXT: Ecchymoses on both arms; MCP and PIP tender and swollen bilaterally
NEURO: MS WNL; proximal muscle weakness in both legs

Results of Laboratory Tests

Na 139 (139)	Hct 0.35 (35)	AST 8.00 (480)	Glu 7.8 (140)
K 3.2 (3.2)	Hgb 122 (12.2)	ALT 8.66 (520)	Ca 2.10 (8.4)
Cl 101 (101)	Lkcs 14.1 × 10⁹ (14.1 × 10³)	LDH 6.00 (360)	PO₄ 1.61 (5.0)
HCO₃ 25 (25)	Plts 240 × 10⁹ (240 × 10³)	Alk Phos 1.0 (60)	Mg 0.74 (1.8)
BUN 5.4 (15)	MCV 76 (76)	Alb 31 (3.1)	Uric Acid 178 (3.0)
Cr 71 (0.8)		T Bili 8.6 (0.5)	PT 11.6

Lkc differential: PMN 72, Lymph 15, Mono 9, Eos 0, Baso 1, Bands 3

ECG: NSR

X-ray Films: L2-L4 anterior wedge compression fractures; simple fracture of (L) femoral neck; decreased opacity suggestive of osteoporosis.

Muscle biopsy of vastus lateralis: selective atrophy of type II muscle fibers

PROBLEM LIST
1. Rheumatoid arthritis
2. PUD
3. Postmenopausal osteoporosis
4. Chronic active hepatitis B

CASE 68 QUESTIONS
1. BN is started on meperidine, 50 mg IM Q3H, for low back pain. After receiving two doses, BN is reported to be disoriented, confused, and mildly sedated with slow, shallow respirations. What is the likely explanation for this response? What recommendation will you make to avoid this type of reaction?
2. List four factors (drug and nondrug) that have contributed to the development of osteoporosis in BN and explain their pathophysiologic effects.
3. Why should the vitamin D and fluoride be discontinued?
4. What different therapeutic approaches have been used for glucocorticoid-induced osteoporosis? Should this therapy be considered in your initial recommendations for BN?
5. How will BN's prednisone therapy affect the management of chronic active hepatitis B? What recommendation will you offer?

CASE 69
CC: JN is a former professional football player, age 53, who presents with complaints of bilateral knee pain associated with motion. The pain has been present for many years but has recently become severe enough to limit ambulation. JN finds stair climbing and walking uphill particularly difficult. The pain is characterized as a dull ache in both knees, exacerbated with activity and improved with rest. The left knee occasionally "locks" and requires gradual passive movement to "unlock.". Stiffness is present after long periods of inactivity and in the morning, but it abates with movement and never lasts more than 10 to 15 minutes. When questioned, JN also notes occasional lower back pain, hip pain, and hand stiffness, but he did not spontaneously report these symptoms.

Past Medical History
JN has had osteoarthritis (OA) for 20 years and had a right arthroscopic meniscectomy 10 years ago without complications. JN has a 5-year history of type II (non-insulin-dependent) diabetes mellitus (DM). He originally presented with polyuria and polydipsia and is now taking an oral hypoglycemic after failure of diet alone. He admits to noncompliance with drug therapy, reporting that it makes him feel sick. JN has mild renal insufficiency secondary to diabetic nephropathy, with a baseline serum creatinine level of 159.1 µmol/L

(1.8 mg/dL) and blood urea nitrogen level of 12.14 μmol/L (34 mg/dL). Hypercholesterolemia was noted on JN's last medical visit, during which a total cholesterol level of 9.28 mmol/L (359 mg/dL) was measured. No medications have been prescribed for this problem. JN has a 20-year history of morbid obesity, beginning 3 years after the end of his professional football career. He also has mild cirrhosis secondary to alcohol use.

Social History

JN admits to a history of alcohol abuse for 20 years, but he now consumes only two to four cans of beer a day.

Medication History

Chlorpropamide, 500 mg/day orally
Acetaminophen, 650 mg PO Q4H "as needed" for pain (uses about two doses per day)

Allergies

ASA causes bronchospasm.

Physical Examination

GEN: A 53-year-old man with bilateral knee pain associated with ambulation
VS: BP 170/90, HR 90, RR 20, Wt 126 kg, Ht 185.4 cm
HEENT: Normocephalic/atraumatic; PERRLA, EOMI, sclera-anicteric, mucous membranes moist and pink
COR: Normal
CHEST: Clear to auscultation and percussion bilaterally
BACK: Midline spine, no tenderness
ABD: Obese, soft, nontender without organomegaly, normoactive bowel sounds
RECT: Guaiac-negative
EXT: No cyanosis, clubbing or edema; 25° varus deformity of knees bilaterally. Mild joint swelling with effusion, no erythema or warmth. No appreciable crepitus, decreased range of motion (ROM) bilaterally. Heberden's nodes on fingers 2 to 5 bilaterally with 15° ulnar deviation at the DIP joint

Results of Laboratory Tests

Na 140 (140)	CR 150.3 (1.7)	AST 2.02 (121)	Chol 9.05 (350)
K 4.1 (4.1)	Hct 0.42 (42%)	ALT 1.9 (114)	TG 1.58 (140)
Cl 102 (102)	Hgb 140 (14)	T Bili 25.7 (1.5)	ESR 41 (41)
HCO₃ 26 (26)	Lkcs 5.9 × 10⁹ (5.9 × 10³)	D Bili 6.84 (0.4)	HgbA₁c 14 (14)
BUN 12.5 (35)	Plts 323 × 10⁹ (323 × 10³)	Glu 10.05 (181)	

X-ray: AP knees. Notable for subchondral sclerosis, with joint-space narrowing medially more than laterally, and osteophyte formation medially more than laterally, bilaterally on tibias.

PROBLEM LIST

1. Osteoarthritis for 20 years
2. Obesity
3. Mild alcoholic cirrhosis
4. Type II diabetes mellitus for 5 years
5. Renal insufficiency
6. Type IIb hypercholesterolemia

CASE 70

CC: EK is a woman, age 75, who is admitted to the hospital with a 2-week history of pain, redness, swelling, and ulceration of her right foot with drainage.

History of Present Illness

EK states that, approximately 3 months ago, she had cellulitis of her right foot that was treated with ciprofloxacin for 3 weeks. Following this episode, she states that she did not notice anything wrong with her foot until approximately 2 weeks ago when she began experiencing pain, swelling, and redness in her foot, with a mild discharge that has increased over the past 2 weeks.

Past Medical History

EK has a 25-year history of insulin-dependent diabetes mellitus that has been poorly controlled in the past as a result of noncompliance and has resulted in peripheral neuropathy in her feet and worsening retinopathy. She also reports numerous cases of cellulitis and ulcerations of her feet. Over the past year, EK has had worsening stiffness with decreasing range of motion in her hands and wrists for which she has tried four different NSAIDs (i.e., ibuprofen, indomethacin, diflunisal, naproxen sodium). She complains of abdominal pain, especially when she eats, with occasional nausea and vomiting for the last 4 months.

Social History

Cigarette smoking: 2 pack/day for 15 years
Alcohol use: denies

Medication History

Insulin NPH, 15 units QAM and 25 units QPM
Insulin regular, 15 units QAM and 10 units QPM
Naproxen sodium, 500 mg PO TID
Magnesium and aluminum hydroxide: 2 tablets PO QID for abdominal pain for 4 months
Ciprofloxacin, 750 mg PO BID for 3 weeks (approximately 3 months ago)
Multivitamin with minerals, 1 tablet PO QD
Diazepam, 10 mg PO HS

Allergies

Penicillin causes a maculopapular, nonurticarial rash.
Physical Examination
GEN: Elderly thin woman in mild distress
VS: BP 142/82, HR 90, RR 20, T 37°C, Ht 160 cm, Wt 75 kg

HEENT: PERRLA
   COR: RRR; S_1,S_2, no S_3, S_4
CHEST: Clear to auscultation
   ABD: Mildly tender without guarding
    GU: Unremarkable
  RECT: Heme +
   EXT: Red, erythematous right foot, especially 1st and 2nd digit, foul-smelling; synovitis of PIP joints of both hands, right more than left, with swan neck deformity of both hands, right more than left
NEURO: No reflexes in either foot; no grip strength in either hand

Results of Laboratory Tests:

Na 140 (140)	Hct .331 (33%)	Alk Phos 1.3 (80)
K 4.4 (4.2)	Hgb 110 (11)	Glu 12.2 (220)
Cl 100 (100)	WBC 6500/mm³	Stool: Guaiac-positive
HCO_3 18 (18)	Plts 235 × 10⁹/L (235 × 10³/mm³)	ESR 55 (55)
BUN 5.4(15)	AST 0.4 (25)	
Cr 159 (1.9)	ALT 0.5 (31)	

Blood culture: Negative
Wound culture (prelimary results): num PMN's, num Gm-bacilli, num gram-positive aerobic cocci, few gram-negative anaerobes
X-ray film of foot: Unremarkable
Bone scan: positive for osteomyelitis

PROBLEM LIST
1. Osteomyelitis
2. Rheumatoid arthritis
3. Peptic ulcer disease

CASE 70 SOAP NOTES
Problem 1: Osteomyelitis
S: EK has a 2 week history of pain, redness, swelling, and ulceration of her right foot, with drainage. This is occurring after treatment of cellulitis of the same area 3 months ago.
O: On physical examination, EK was found to have a red, erythematous right foot, especially surrounding her 1st and 2nd digit, with a foul smell. WBC count is 6500/mm³; temperature is 37°; blood cultures are negative; wound cultures are pending, preliminary results reveal numerous polymorphonucleocytes, gram-negative bacilli, gram-positive aerobic cocci, and few gram-negative anaerobes. ESR is 55. X-ray film of foot is negative; bone scan of foot is positive for osteomyelitis.
A: This patient's history, in conjunction with her laboratory test results, is consistent with the diagnosis of osteomyelitis. The past medical history of cellulitis in the same affected area, poorly controlled diabetes mellitus, and chronic cellulitis with ulcerations of her feet also contribute to the diagnosis. Radiographic changes may not be seen for up to 4 weeks after infection; white blood cell counts may be normal in 40 to 75% of patients; and the ESR often is elevated. Blood cultures may be positive only in 50% of cases. While waiting for the final results of the wound culture and sensitivities to return, empiric antibiotic therapy should be initiated on the basis of this patient's history and preliminary wound culture results. As would be expected from a patient with osteomyelitis and with chronic,

poorly controlled diabetes, Gram's stain shows a mixed aerobic and anaerobic pattern. The gram-positive aerobic cocci are most likely *Staphylococci* species (i.e., *S.aureus*) or *Streptococcus* species; the gram-negative bacilli most likely are Enterobacteriaceae (i.e., *Pseudomonas, Proteus*) and the gram-negative anaerobes are most likely *Bacteroides fragilis*. In order to cover all of these pathogens, more than one antibiotic will probably be necessary. The patient's allergy to penicillin and her poor renal function (creatinine clearance, 30 mL/min) potentially limits the options. Clindamycin, 900mg IV Q8H (no renal dose adjustment is needed since clindamycin is cleared hepatically), would provide adequate coverage for this patient's presumed *Staphylococci*, *Streptococcus*, and *B. fragilis* infections. Coverage of the Enterobacteraceae infection is not as simple. Choices are limited; an antipseudomonal penicillin or cephalosporin may not be suitable for this patient because of her allergy. Cross-reactivity (IgE-mediated) between the cephalosporins and penicillins has been reported in the literature to have an incidence of 5 to 15%. An aminoglycoside, e.g., gentamicin or tobramycin, would be an alternative; however, in this elderly patient with decreased renal function and in whom long-term therapy may be required, the risks may outweigh the benefits. Since this patient's reaction to penicillin presents as a rash (maculopapular) and not as an immediate urticarial reaction (i.e., a non-IgE-mediated reaction), initiating ceftazidime, 1 to 2 gm IV Q12H (renal dose adjustment) and monitoring closely for signs of an allergic reaction (e.g., rash, difficulty breathing or swallowing) is appropriate. If this reaction was a true IgE-mediated reaction, aztreonam would be an appropriate alternative. The optimal duration of therapy for this patient is not well defined. Current recommendations for an acute case of osteomyelitis include at least 4 to 6 weeks of antibiotic therapy (i.e., 2 to 3 weeks of parenteral therapy, followed by oral therapy to complete the regimen)
P: Initiate clindamycin, 900 mg IV Q8H, and ceftazidime, 1 to 2 gm IV Q12H. Monitor the patient for difficulty breathing or swallowing and for a rash. Diphenhydramine and epinephrine should be kept at bedside in case an anaphylactoid-like reaction occur. Therapy may need to be tailored when the final culture and sensitivities results from the wound return. Parenteral therapy should be continued for 2 to 3 weeks or until clinical resolution of symptoms occurs, then begin oral therapy to complete a total of 4 to 6 weeks of therapy.

Problem 2: Peptic Ulcer Disease
S: EK complains of abdominal pain, especially when she eats, with occasional nausea and vomiting for the last 4 months. EK also reports using a magnesium and aluminum hydroxide preparation on a daily basis for 4 months (2 tablets PO QID).
O: Mildly tender abdomen without guarding. Heme +; stool guaiac +. Hgb 110 (11); Hct .331 (33%)
A: This patient's complaints, laboratory results, and history of 15 years of smoking and 1 year of NSAID use are suggestive of a gastric ulcer. Diabetic gastroenteropathy is also

in the differential diagnosis; however, the presentation in conjunction with guaiac-positive stools and a heme-positive rectal examination are more suggestive of a peptic ulcer. Smoking and NSAID use impair the gastric mucosal barrier's ability to protect the stomach and increases the risk for ulceration. Therapeutic options that exist for this patient include antacids, sucralfate, and H2-receptor antagonists. Antacids have failed to relieve this patient's abdominal pain in the past and therefore other alternatives should be pursued. Sucralfate is an effective agent for the management of duodenal ulcers; however, in this patient, the presentation is more consistent with a gastric ulcer. Sucralfate's QID dosing schedule may also not be suitable for this noncompliant patient. H2 blockers have been shown to be safe and effective agents for the treatment of gastric and duodenal ulcers. In this patient, any H2 receptor antagonist would be of benefit; however, cimetidine will decrease the hepatic metabolism of diazepam, thereby potentially increasing its effects. Ranitidine, 300 mg PO QHS, would be a good choice because of its beneficial schedule, adequate efficacy, and minimal drug interactions. The duration of therapy should be 4 to 8 weeks, after which the patient should be evaluated for improvements in subjective complaints and subsequent stool guaiac and heme tests should be scheduled.

P: Initiate ranitidine, 300 mg PO QHS, and reevaluate the patient in 4 to 8 weeks. Assess the patient's subjective complaints of abdominal pain and repeat stool guaiac and heme tests in 4 to 8 weeks.

Problem 3: Rheumatoid Arthritis

S: EK complains of worsening stiffness and decreasing range of motion in her hands and wrists over the last year, which has not been relieved by trials of three different NSAIDs.

O: ESR 55; synovitis of PIP joints with swan-neck deformity in both hands, right more than left; no grip strength in either hand

A: This patient has failed to have an adequate response to NSAIDs (four agents over the past year) and is therefore a candidate for more aggressive therapy with a slow-acting antirheumatic drug (SAARD). These agents include gold salts, hydroxychloroquine, methotrexate, sulfasalazine, penicillamine, azathioprine, and cyclophosphamide. There is a delay of 2 to 6 months between initiation of therapy and onset of action for these agents. Azathioprine and cyclophosphamide are reserved for patients who fail to respond to other SAARDs. Of the remaining agents, gold salts, hydroxychloroquine, and methotrexate are considered to be first-line SAARDs for the management of rheumatoid arthritis. Any of these agents may be used in combination with NSAIDs; however, the patient's renal dysfunction and diabetes should be taken into consideration. Methotrexate, hydroxychloroquine, and injectable gold are all excreted by the kidneys, whereas oral gold is primarily excreted by the intestines. Methotrexate toxicity may occur in patients with altered renal function as a result of decreased clearance and would therefore be of limited use in this patient. The risk of retinopathy with hydroxychl-

oroquine may limit its use, because differentiating drug toxicity from advancing diabetic retinopathy may be difficult. Oral gold therapy may be an alternative and has fewer side effects than the injectable form; however, oral gold is also considered to be less effective than injectable gold. Injectable gold would provide a reasonable selection for this patient, but careful monitoring is advised because of this patient's renal dysfunction and gold's renal clearance. Adverse effects of injectable gold therapy include mucocutaneous reactions, dermatitis, urticaria, stomatitis, alopecia, and chrysiasis, and these effects most often occur after 2 to 3 months of therapy. Therapy should be discontinued if a pruritic dermatitis develops to avoid development of a susequent exfoliative dermatitis. Hematologic side effects, such as leukopenia and thrombocytopenia, should also be watched for carefully during therapy. An initial test dose of 10 mg of gold salts is given intramuscularly (IM) in the gluteal muscle and is followed by doses of 25 to 50 mg weekly. In this patient, the lower dose of 25 mg should be used because of the renal dysfuntion. Weekly doses should be continued until a cumulative dose of 1 gm is reached, toxicity occurs, or a benefit is derived.

P: Initiate injectable gold therapy. An initial test dose of 10 mg IM should be followed by 25 mg IM weekly. Monitor the patient's CBC with platelets throughout therapy and watch for dermatologic reactions. Administer until a total cumulative dose of 1 gm is reached, toxicity occurs, or benefit is derived. Continue naproxen sodium at current schedule.

CASE 70 QUESTIONS

1. The final cultures from EK's wound results return and are as follows:

Numerous *Staph aureus* Sensitive to Penicillin;Clindamycin;TMP/SMX	Numerous *P aeuroginosa* Sensitive to Ciprofloxacin;Ceftazidime	Few *B.fragilis* Sensitive to Metronidazole;Clindamycin;Imipenem

The physician on your team is surprised that this isolate grew out *P.aeruginosa* (especially an isolate that is sensitive to ciprofloxacin) since she was treated with ciprofloxacin in the past. The team asks you to look into this. Upon questioning the patient, she tells you that in the past she did not take all of her medications but is positive that she has not missed one dose of her antibiotics. What other explanation may there be for the continued sensitivity of isolates to ciprofloxacin?

2. Why was ciprofloxacin a bad choice to treat this patient's infection initially?

3. After 2 weeks of parenteral therapy, EK's wound has improved significantly and is no longer painful,swollen and red. What oral antibiotic(s) would you recommend to complete therapy?

4. The physician on your team prescribes sucralfate instead of ranitidine. What additional information should you tell the patient?

5. If this patient's rheumatoid arthritis had been treated with only ibuprofen and naproxen sodium, would it still be reasonable to initial gold therapy?

CASE 71

CC: NA is a woman, age 26, with a 6-year history of systemic lupus rythematosus (SLE) who presents at the kidney dialysis center with complaints of hip pain and increasing weakness and fatigue. She also has experienced an increase in seizure frequency over the past several weeks.

Past Medical History

NA has experienced a progressive course of SLE, with development of chronic renal failure secondary to proliferative glomerulonephritis, which was detected a year ago. She has undergone hemodialysis three times weekly for the past 6 months. Two years ago, NA experienced several separate episodes of tonic-clonic seizures, presumably caused by SLE since no other metabolic or neurologic cause could be found. She was started on phenytoin, 300 mg PO QHS., which decreased the frequency of her seizures to two per week and produced a serum concentration of 31.2 μmol/L (8 μg/mL) after 6 weeks of drug therapy. The dose was increased to 400 mg PO QHS, with a resulting serum concentration of 59.5 μmol/L (15 μg/mL) after 2 months. NA is homebound by SLE photosensitivity and has minimal physical activity except for dialysis sessions. She eats only two meals daily.

Medication History

Phenytoin, 400 mg QHS
Naproxen, 500 mg TID (with adequate symptom control most of time)
Aluminum carbonate, 4 caps QID with meals and HS

Allergies

None known

Physical Examination

      GEN: NAD; patient complains of hip pain
       VS: VSS, Ht 168 cm, Wt 57 kg
    HEENT: Sclera clear, neck supple, malar rash
      COR: R R
    CHEST: Clear to auscultation and percussion
      ABD: Soft, nontender; positive bowel sounds
       GU: WNL
     RECT: WNL
      EXT: Tender, swollen hands, wrists, and knees
    NEURO: Decreased alertness; memory intact but slow; diplopia; lateral nystagmus bilaterally; bilateral proximal muscle weakness in both lower extremities; moderate ataxia

Results of Laboratory Tests

Na 137 (137)	Hct 0.25 (25.2)	ALT 0.4 (24)	Ca 2.0 (8.0)
K 5.5 (5.5)	Hgb 89 (8.9)	LDH 2.56 (154)	PO₄ 1.78 (5.5)
Cl 108 (108)	Lkcs 5.7 × 10⁹ (5.7 × 10³)	Alk Phos 1.1 (67)	Mg 1.4 (2.8)
HCO₃ 21 (21)	Plts 80 × 10⁹ (80 × 10³)	Alb 17 (1.7)	Uric Acid 392 (6.6)
BUN 27.8 (78)	MCV 82 (82)	T Bili 3.4 (0.2)	ESR 89 (89)
Cr 442 (5)	AST 0.4 (24)	Glu 4.7 (84)	Aluminum 8,598 (232)

LE test (+), ANA titer 1:200
Lkc differential: PMN 58, Band 3, Eos 2, Lymph 30,
Mono 7
Urinalysis: 3+ protein, no casts, no bacteria
X-ray films: (L) inner aspect of femoral neck characterized by Looser's transformation zones; pelvis with ground-glass appearance; no articular destruction

PROBLEM LIST

1. SLE
2. Seizures secondary to SLE
3. Chronic renal failure secondary to SLE
4. Osteomalacia secondary to dialysis and phenytoin

CASE 72

CC: TF is a woman, age 60, who presents with new-onset back pain of 2 days duration, joint pain, and stomach pain.

History of Present Illness

TF has a 10-year history of rheumatoid arthritis, for which she takes prednisone. She previously tried NSAIDs without adequate pain relief. TF also describes stomach pain with occasional coffee-ground emesis. Antacids have not relieved her pain.

Past Medical History

TF has a history of peptic ulcer disease and chronic alcoholism. She denies drinking any alcohol presently; however, she is known to occasionally "sneak" a few drinks. Her rheumatoid arthritis has been stable for the past 10 years. She had a hip fracture after a fall in the bathtub. She has been postmenopausal for 4 years.

Social History

Alcohol: (+) 4 to 6 drinks per day in the past
Tobacco: (+) 22 pack-year history

Medication History

Prednisone, 5 mg PO QD
Ranitidine, 150 mg PO QHS
Diazepam, 5 mg PO QHS PRN for sleep

Allergies

None known

Physical Examination

      GEN: Thin, elderly-appearing woman in no acute distress
       VS: BP 140/80, HR 70, RR 14, T 373, Wt 55 kg, Ht 5'3"
    HEENT: WNL
      COR: Normal S₁ and S₂
    CHEST: Clear to auscultation and percussion
      ABD: Soft, nontender; liver palpable; hepatomegaly
       GU: WNL
     RECT: Guaiac-positive
      EXT: No cyanosis, clubbing, or edema
    NEURO: Oriented to time, place, and person

Results of Laboratory Tests

Na 138 (138)	CL 98 (98)	BUN 3.6 (10)
Hct .25 (25)	WBC 3	MCV 105 (105)
ALT .58 (35)	Alk Phos 2.0 (120)	T Bili 18 (1.0)
Ca 2.2 (8.8)	Mg 1 (2)	Vit B$_{12}$ 177.1 (240)
K 4.2 (4.2)	HCO$_3$ 22 (22)	Cr 106 (1.2)
Hgb 100 (10)	Plts 100	Ast .58 (35)
LDH 1.7 (101)	Alb 25 (2.5)	Glu 5.55 (100)
PO$_4$ 1.07 (3.3)	Folate 9.064 (4)	

PROBLEM LIST

1. Osteoporosis
2. Peptic ulcer disease
3. Chronic alcoholism

CASE 72 SOAP NOTES

Problem 1 : Osteoporosis

S: TF complains of back pain.

O: None

A: TF has many risk factors for osteoporosis, and treatment is required. TF is a postmenopausal woman and has a history of hip fracture. She has a history of alcohol abuse, which may contribute to osteoporosis. TF has had long-term, low-dose corticosteroid therapy, which has been known to induce osteoporosis.

P: TF should be treated for osteoporosis because she has numerous risk factors. She should be started on calcium supplements, since many elderly patients do not obtain sufficient calcium in their diets. The National Osteoporosis Foundation recommends a total calcium intake of 1500 mg/day for postmenopausal women who are not on estrogen replacement and 1,000 mg/day for postmenopausal women on estrogen replacement therapy. Depending on TF's dietary calcium intake, up to 200 mg of elemental calcium may be taken with each meal. Calcium supplements are available in a number of preparations providing elemental calcium in amounts from 200 mg to 600 mg per tablet. Calcium supplements are beneficial; however, the diet is probably the best source of calcium. Vitamin D deficiency has been associated with increasing age. Often vitamin D is given in conjunction with calcium. Approximately 400 to 800 units of vitamin D per day should be added to TF's regimen. Estrogen replacement therapy should also be initiated for TF. Estrogen replacement therapy has been shown to prevent bone loss and reduce fracture risks. Estrogen is useful for the relief of postmenopausal symptoms. Beneficial effects of estrogen are usually seen in women who continue to take estrogen after therapy is initiated early after the start of menopause. TF can be started on estrogen 0.625 mg plus 2.5 mg medroxyprogesterone acetate given daily. This therapy is appropriate for women who are 3 to 5 years past menopause. Nonpharmacologic measures are also important in osteoporosis therapy. Physical activity, specifically weight bearing exercise such as walking, and some modest weight training should be incorporated into TF's daily routine. Lifestyle changes, including reducing alcohol consumption, may also reduce the risk of osteoporosis.

Problem 2: Peptic Ulcer Disease

S: TF complains of stomach pain with hematemesis.

O: TF has a history of peptic ulcer disease, has guaiac-positive stools, and has a low hematocrit of 25.

A: TF has a history of peptic ulcer disease and is currently taking ranitidine, 150 mg PO QHS (maintenance dose). She is also known to be an alcoholic and a smoker. Since her hematocrit is low and there is evidence of bleeding, TF should be treated. Her symptoms could a result of many factors, including prednisone therapy, infection with the gram-negative bacilli *Helicobacter pylori*, alcohol consumption, or smoking.

P: TF should be treated and then given prophylactic therapy for further peptic ulcers. Start ranitidine, 150 mg PO BID for 6 to 8 weeks, then return to a maintenance dose of 150 mg PO QHS. Discontinue alcohol and cigarettes. Because TF has not responded to maintenance therapy with ranitidine, *H. pylori* infection may be implicated and treatment of this pathogen should be considered. Start bismuth subsalicylate (Peptol Bismol), tetracycline, and metronidazole. The use of antibacterial drugs for 2 weeks in addition to a histamine$_2$ receptor antagonist decreases the incidence of recurrence of active peptic ulcers.

Problem 3: Chronic Alcoholism

S: TF is a thin-appearing woman.

O: TF has an increased MCV of 105, a low serum folate level of 9.064, a low WBC count of 3.0, and a platelet count of 100. She also has a palpable liver, and on physical examination hepatomegaly was noted.

A: Folate deficiency is a common sign of malnutrition in chronic alcoholics. TF's anemia should be treated, especially since she has active peptic ulcer disease.

P: TF should be counseled on the benefit of discontinuing alcohol consumption; a support group such as Alcoholics Anonymous may be helpful. Her nutritional status may improve after she has stopped drinking. TF should be started on a daily multivitamin and 1 mg daily of folic acid to improve her nutritional status and reduce anemia. She should also receive thiamine, 100 mg daily, to prevent Wernicke's encephalopathy. Folate, hemoglobin, hematocrit, and vitamin B$_{12}$ levels should be monitored.

CASE 72 QUESTIONS

1. What alternative regimens could have been used to eradicate *H. pylori* in TF?
2. What are the therapy options for treatment of active peptic ulcer disease?
3. What risk factors should be considered when deciding on a diagnosis of osteoporosis?
4. Describe any contraindications to estrogen replacement therapy in women.

RESPIRATORY DISEASES

CASE 73

CC: BJ is a woman, age 54, who comes to the emergency room with a 2-day history of shortness of breath, dyspnea, inability to speak without difficulty, and flu-like symptoms (nausea, vomiting, and fatigue). She also complains of palpitations, insomnia, and irritability of recent onset (1 week).

Past Medical History

BJ has a history of chronic steroid-dependent asthma. Over the past year, BJ has been admitted to the hospital twice for acute exacerbations of her asthma, which have required intubation. Two days before coming to the ER, BJ abruptly stopped her prednisone because "it was making me sick." Since then she has increased her use of inhalers because of increasing shortness of breath. Now, she complains that her inhalers "just aren't working any more." Three weeks before admission a diagnosis of gastroesophageal reflux disease (GERD) was made, and BJ was started on cimetidine. She states this has worked well for her. BJ also has a history of asymptomatic atrial fibrillation. BJ takes indomethacin three times daily for degenerative joint disease (DJD), which she has had for "years," and DJD has not been a problem. Although BJ is compliant with her medications, she has difficulty using her inhalers.

Medication History

Theophylline, 400 mg PO BID (clinic visit 2 month PTA: 94.4 μmol/L(17 mg/L)
Cimetidine, 400 mg PO BID (started 1 week ago)
Indomethacin, 50 mg PO TID
Prednisone, 20 mg PO QD (stopped 3 days ago)
Metoproterenol inhaler, 2 puffs PRN
Cromolyn inhaler, 1 puff PRN
Beclomethasone, 2 puffs PRN
Erythromycin, 500 mg PO QD

Allergies

None known

Physical Examination

GEN: Cushingoid appearance; in obvious respiratory distress
VS: BP 100/60 (sitting), BP 90/50 (standing), RR 27, HR 130, T 37.5, Wt 65 kg

HEENT: Moon facies, hirsutism
COR: No murmurs, n1 S1, S2
CHEST: Decreased breath sounds bilaterally, inspiratory/expiratory wheezing and rhonchi
ABD: Truncal obesity
GU: Unremarkable
EXT: Pale skin with tenting, bruising
NEURO: Oriented × 2, alert but confused

Results of Laboratory Tests

Na 125 (125)	BUN 10.7 (30)	Lkcs 9.0×10^9 (9.0×10^3)	T Bili 5.1 (0.3)
K 5.9 (5.9)	SCr 212 (2.4)	Plts 250×10^9 (250×10^3)	Ca 2.4 (9.8)
Cl 94 (94)	Hct 0.41 (41)	AST 0.3 (22)	PO_4 1.45 (4.5)
HCO_3 33 (33)	Hgb 140 (14)	Alb 41 (4.1)	Mg 0.78 (1.9)

Pulmonary function tests: FEV_1/FCV: 55% (before β_2-agonist dose); FEV_1/FCV: 70% (after β_2-agonist dose)

ECG: Atrial fibrillation and occasional premature ventricular contractions

PROBLEM LIST

1. Degenerative joint disease (DJD)
2. Atrial fibrillation
3. Steroid-dependent asthma with acute exacerbation
4. Gastroesophageal reflux disease (GERD) for 3 weeks
5. Theophylline toxicity
6. Cushingoid signs and symptoms and adrenal insufficiency

CASE 73 SOAP NOTES
Problem 3. Steroid-dependent Asthma with Acute Exacerbation

S: BJ complains of increasing shortness of breath, dyspnea, and difficulty speaking.

O: On physical examination, patient has decreased breath sounds bilaterally, inspiratory and expiratory wheezing, and rhonchi. The FEV_1/FCV ratio and $PaCO_2$, PO_2, and SaO_2 levels are decreased and consistent with an acute asthma exacerbation. Heart rate and respiratory rate are increased.

A: BJ is experiencing an acute asthma exacerbation, which is probably secondary to her abrupt discontinuance of prednisone. The results of pulmonary function tests before and after β_2-agonist therapy show significant airway responsiveness. Therefore, a nebulized treatment of a β-agonist is indicated for BJ. Excessive use of β_2-agonist therapy should be avoided in BJ because systemic absorption of β_2-agonists is known to occur at high doses, and the side-effect profile of these agents includes tachycardia and arrhythmias. BJ has a history of atrial fibrillation, which could be exacerbated by excessive β_2-agonist use. If BJ does not respond to nebulized treatment or if the PCO_2 level increases at a rate of 5 to 10 mm Hg per hour, respiratory failure is likely. BJ should be monitored closely for diaphragmatic fatigue and significant changes in arterial blood gas levels during her therapy.

Patients with steroid-dependent asthma who require more than two hospitalizations per year with subsequent intubation often require slow tapering of steroids to prevent disease exacerbation. They may also require long-term, low-dose steroids to control their disease. The role of steroids in other patient populations is unclear, but recent studies have supported the role of inflammation as a cause of bronchial airway constriction. BJ has steroid-dependent asthma, so steroids should be initiated to alleviate the symptoms of steroid withdrawal (see problem 6) as well as to reverse the inflammatory response associated with asthma. The choice between oral and intravenous (IV) administration is controversial. Onset of the antiinflammatory action of steroids is delayed by several hours, and therefore steroids should be administered as soon as possible by either route. The ability of a patient to take oral medications and other medical problems precluding the use of oral steroids should be considered when choosing the route of administration. Many patients can tolerate a rapid taper of steroids, but patients who are steroid-dependent usually require long slow tapers. After IV therapy, BJ should be switched to oral medications as soon as possible, and the dose should be slowly titrated to control her symptoms. Once BJ's inhaler regimen is reevaluated and she is taught the proper use of her inhalers, the need for chronic systemic prednisone can be reevaluated, because she has obvious physical signs of steroid excess.

BJ has been using her inhalers on an "as needed" basis. She should be instructed to use her steroid inhaler on a scheduled basis for optimal results. Maximal treatment with an inhaled steroid and β_2-agonists should precede the use of cromolyn. Since recent evidence supports the theory that inflammation plays a major role in development of bronchial constriction, high-dose inhaled steroids have been used for the treatment of asthma. BJ should be instructed to increase the dose of her steroid inhaler and use it on a scheduled basis. Inhaled steroids may decrease the need for systemic prednisone, alleviating some of the symptoms of steroid excess that BJ is experiencing; however, at high doses inhaled steroids may also have increased systemic absorption, so monitoring of steroid excess is still required. Inhaled steroids should be reinstituted when BJ has recovered from her acute exacerbation, because inhaled steroids can irritate bronchial airways, resulting in additional complications.

New recommendations state that β_2-agonists should be used on a PRN basis. BJ should be instructed to use her metoproterenol inhaler PRN. Tolerance to β_2-agonists has been reported, especially with repeated excessive use. BJ should be instructed to return to the emergency room if she has increasing shortness of breath despite appropriate use of the β_2-agonist inhaler. Although tolerance appears to be a result of receptor down-regulation, large doses of steroids reverse this effect rapidly.

P: Begin nebulized albuterol, 5 to 10 mg in 0.3 mL normal saline, followed by 2 to 5 mg in 0.3 mL normal saline every 20 minutes until symptoms improve. Monitor arterial blood gases, chest examination, respiration rate, and breathing patterns to assess the efficacy of treatment. Begin methylprednisolone, 125 mg IV every 8 hours until it is appropriate to start oral medications, then start prednisone, 20 mg PO QID with a slow taper (start with a decrease of 5 mg every 3 days and titrate to symptoms). Instruct BJ on the proper use of inhalers when acute symptoms have resolved: metoproterenol, 2 puffs QID PRN; beclomethasone, 4 puffs QID. Discontinue cromolyn and monitor her response as an outpatient.

Problem 5. Theophylline Toxicity

S: BJ complains of insomnia, irritability, and palpitations.

O: BJ has a theophylline level of 138.7 μmol/L (25 mg/L). Her ECG shows atrial fibrillation that was stable before admission.

A: The role of theophylline in the treatment of asthma is also controversial; its use is indicated mainly in patients unresponsive to standard therapy. BJ has steroid-dependent asthma and may benefit from theophylline. However, after a trial of scheduled inhaled medications, theophylline may not provide additional benefit, and its use in BJ should be reevaluated. The theophylline level taken in the emergency room was 138.7 μmol/L (25 mg/L), which is above the therapeutic range of 55.5 to 111 μmol/L (10 to 20 mg/L). Symptoms of theophylline toxicity include headache, nausea, insomnia, irritability, vomiting, diarrhea, hyperactivity, arrhythmias, and seizures. BJ is currently experiencing the signs and symptoms of theophylline toxicity. The onset of symptoms, together with the therapeutic theophylline level before the initiation of cimetidine, supports the hypothesis of a drug interaction. Cimetidine is an enzyme inhibitor that can significantly inhibit the metabolism of theophylline (decreases clearance by 20 to 30%). The effect of this inhibition is immediate, because the drug competes with P-450 enzymes. This is different from enzyme-inducers, which require time to synthesize new proteins before an interaction is seen. When cimetidine is initiated in a patient stabilized on theophylline, the daily dose should be reduced by 50% empirically, with follow-up monitoring of levels; or a different H_2-antagonist, such as ranitidine, which does not interact with theophylline, may be used. Erythromycin is also an enzyme inhibitor that interacts with theophylline. However, erythromycin is probably not contributing to the increase of theophylline concentration, because BJ has been stabilized on the current dose of theophylline while concurrently receiving erythromycin.

P: Based on BJ's calculated pharmacokinetic parameters, her theophylline half-life is 16.5 hours. Therefore, her next theophylline dose should be held, and the dose decreased to 200 mg PO BID ($Cp_{desired}/Cp_{ss}$ = X/Dose).

Problem 6. Cushingoid Signs and Symptoms and Adrenal Insufficiency

S: Nausea, vomiting, and fatigue (flu-like symptoms) are symptoms of adrenal insufficiency, which BJ is currently experiencing. She also states that she stopped her prednisone because it was "making her feel sick."

O: Several objective symptoms of adrenal insufficiency appear in BJ's laboratory test and physical examination results (i.e., hypotension, hyponatremia, hyperkalemia, and changes in mental status). BJ has also been experiencing emesis after steroid withdrawal and subsequently has objective symptoms of hypochloremic metabolic alkalosis and dehydration caused by excessive loss of HCl from the GI tract. Symptoms include pale skin, tenting, orthostatic hypotension, increased SCr level, a BUN/SCr ratio indicating prerenal azotemia, and increased bicarbonate concentration with increased pH and hypochloremia.

After long-term steroid treatment, BJ has several symptoms of steroid excess; moon facies, hirsutism, truncal obesity, and bruising are classic findings on physical examination. Some laboratory abnormalities, such as hypokalemia and glucose intolerance, are not apparent in BJ because she has adrenal insufficiency.

A: The baseline production of endogenous hydrocortisone is approximately 30 mg daily. Hydrocortisone production is regulated by several feedback systems, both positive and negative. When exogenous steroids in excess of 30 mg hydrocortisone are given for prolonged durations, the pituitary-adrenal axis shuts down by negative feedback, and the body stops producing endogenous hydrocortisone. This phenomenon develops over time and depends on variables such as patient response, dose of steroid, and duration of therapy. In turn, the pituitary-adrenal axis requires time to recuperate from exogenous steroid intake, so steroids are normally tapered to prevent symptoms of adrenal insufficiency. Fortunately, adrenal insufficiency secondary to steroid withdrawal is reversible with early detection and exogenous steroid replacement. BJ has been treated with prednisone, 20 mg daily for a prolonged period of time. This is approximately equivalent to 80 mg of hydrocortisone, which is in excess of normal endogenous production. Subsequently, BJ experienced adrenal insufficiency when she abruptly discontinued her prednisone. Treatment with methylprednisolone or hydrocortisone with isotonic fluids will reverse the electrolyte abnormalities and metabolic alkalosis. Since BJ's symptoms are severe and can progress to cardiovascular failure, intravenous steroids should be initiated.

Since BJ was receiving exogenous steroids in excess of normal endogenous production for long periods of time, she has physical signs of steroid excess. Many of these result from tissue redistribution and collagenous changes. As long as BJ is receiving high-dose steroids, she will continue to experience these symptoms. Many of the symptoms can be alleviated if the steroid dose is decreased or (if possible) discontinued. Once restarted on prednisone, BJ should be tapered to the lowest dose possible without aggravating symptoms of her disease.

P: A methylprednisolone regimen for the treatment of asthma should be sufficient to treat BJ's adrenal insufficiency. An isotonic solution of 0.9% normal saline without potassium should be instituted and titrated to blood pressure and urine output. Electrolytes, BUN, SCr, and other pertinent levels should be monitored closely. The metabolic/respiratory alkalosis will resolve with the administration of chloride (0.9% normal saline) and the resolution of the acute asthma exacerbation.

BJ should be switched to oral medications as soon as possible. Prednisone, 20 mg QID PO, is appropriate. A taper should begin at decreases of 5 mg every 3 days and be titrated to control BJ's asthma. As the prednisone dose reaches the physiologic hydrocortisone range (7.5 mg prednisone is equivalent to 30 mg hydrocortisone), the dose should be tapered more slowly, with special emphasis on monitoring for symptoms of adrenal insufficiency. BJ should be taught about compliance and the signs and symptoms of disease exacerbation and adrenal insufficiency.

Problem 4. Gastroesophageal Reflux Disease

S: BJ is not experiencing any symptoms of GERD and describes improvement with the addition of cimetidine.

O: None

A: Cimetidine has been FDA-approved for the treatment of GERD. Currently, BJ's calculated creatinine clearance is 0.4 mL/sec (24.0 mL/min). Since cimetidine is partially cleared by the kidney, decreased renal function can cause accumulation. BJ's renal dysfunction will probably resolve when she is treated for dehydration; therefore, dosing adjustment is not required at this time.

P: Continue cimetidine. Tell BJ about other nondrug methods that improve GERD, e.g., small, frequent meals; decreased coffee intake; not eating just before bedtime. Monitor renal function; if improvement does not occur, decrease the cimetidine dose.

Problem 2. Atrial Fibrillation

S: BJ is experiencing palpitations, but before admission she was asymptomatic.

O: ECG consistent with atrial fibrillation; occasional PVCs

A: BJ is probably experiencing an exacerbation of her atrial fibrillation as a result of theophylline toxicity and dehydration. With resolution of these problems, the arrhythmia should resolve. If BJ becomes symptomatic, digoxin or another rate-controlling antiarrhythmic agent may be instituted.

P: Monitor ECG, heart rate, theophylline level, resolution of dehydration, and subjective symptoms (palpitations).

Problem 1. Degenerative Joint Disease

S: BJ is currently asymptomatic.

O: None

A: DJD is not always an inflammatory disease, so pain associated with it can usually be controlled with acetaminophen PRN. The need for scheduled indomethacin should be reevaluated. Indomethacin is a nonsteroidal antiinflammatory drug (NSAID), and the potential for renal toxicity with it is significant, especially in older patients. Also, NSAIDs can disrupt the mucous layer that protects the stomach, which can lead to gastritis and possible ulcer formation. Prednisone has similar effects, and the use of both agents in combination warrants evaluation. Since BJ has been asymptomatic for a long time, a trial of acetaminophen or a less potent NSAID, such as sulindac, may be appropriate.

P: Discontinue indomethacin. Begin acetaminophen, one or two 325 mg tablets every 6 hours as needed for pain.

CASE 73 QUESTIONS

1. Calculate BJ's pharmacokinetic parameters for theophylline (i.e., clearance, half-life, volume of distribution, and elimination rate constant).
2. Using the above parameters, calculate an appropriate aminophylline dose to be given intravenously.
3. Should prophylactic antibiotics be used in asthma patients? Give recommendations about BJ's erythromycin.
4. Would an inhaled anticholinergic provide additional benefit for BJ?
5. Instruct BJ on the proper use of her inhalers.

CASE 74

CC: SB is a man, age 65, who presents to the general medicine clinic with a 1 week history of nausea, agitation, and tremors and an increased number of anginal attacks associated with palpitations.

History of Present Illness

SB underwent treatment for smoking cessation and had his last cigarette 2 months ago. SB was treated for an acute gouty attack with colchicine 1 week ago.

Past Medical History

Past medical history includes angina for 5 years; SB was previously stable on isosorbide dinitrate. Lately he reports chest pain with exertion. SB has a 10-year history of hypertension controlled with hydrochlorothiazide, and a 3-year history of chronic obstructive pulmonary disease (COPD), which has been stabilized with theophylline and albuterol inhaler PRN.

Social History

Tobacco: 1 pack/day for 30 years (discontinued 2 months ago)
Alcohol: occasional use

Family History

Mother had COPD; father had coronary artery disease and gout

Medication History

Hydrochlorothiazide, 50 mg PO QD
KCl, 20 mEq PO QD
Isosorbide dinitrate, 30 mg po TID
Theophylline SR, 300 mg PO BID
Albuterol inhaler, 2 puffs q4h PRN
Nitroglycerin, .4 mg sublingual (SL) PRN chest pain
Enteric-coated aspirin, 325 mg PO QD

Allergies

NKDA

Physical Examination

GEN: Well-developed man in mild distress
VS: BP 155/95, HR 100, RR 16, T 37.5, Wt. 70 kg, Ht. 177.8 cm
HEENT: Mild AV nicking
COR: S_1, S_2, no S_3, sinus tachycardia
CHEST: Barrel chest, increased accessory muscle use
ABD: Soft, nontender
GU: WNL
RECT: Heme-negative
EXT: MTP of left toe is erythematous, tender, warm to touch (1 week ago), now WNL
NEURO: A × O × 3

Results of Laboratory Tests

Na 139 (139)	Hct .40 (40)
ALT .38 (23)	Ca 2.02 (8.1)
K 4.6 (4.6)	Hgb 135 (13.5)
LDH 1.42 (85)	PO_4 1.03 (3.2)
Cl 96 (96)	WBC 9.5×10^9 (9.5×10^3)
Alk Phos .92 (55)	HCO_3 27 (27)
Plts 253×10^9 (253×10^3)	Alb 43 (4.3)
BUN 6.78 (19)	MCV 90 (90)
T Bili 17 (1)	Mg .95 (1.9)
Cr 106 (1.2)	AST .467 (28)
Glu 6.1 (110)	Uric acid 582 (9.8)

WBC differential: WNL
Theophylline: 21
Urinalysis: WNL
FEV/FVC=35%
Chest X-ray: clear
FEV_1: 700 mL
ECG: Sinus tachycardia, occasional PVC's
FEV_1: after bronchodilator, 900 mL

PROBLEM LIST

1. Chronic obstructive pulmonary disease
2. Hypertension

3. Angina
4. Hyperuricemia

CASE 74 SOAP NOTES

Problem 1. COPD

S: SB complains of nausea, agitation, tremors, and palpitations.

O: FEV/FVC is 35%; FEV_1 is 700 mL before bronchodilator and 900 mL after bronchodilator; theophylline level is 21 mg/L

A: SB's COPD has been controlled on his present medications. SB was previously stable on the present theophylline dose. He is now experiencing signs of theophylline toxicity and possibly of overuse of albuterol. SB quit smoking 2 months ago, and this change likely led to an increase in theophylline level and toxicity. Consideration must also be given to whether theophylline is the best choice in this patient; it has limited value in the treatment of COPD. Anticholinergic agents, such as ipratropium, may have more benefit because they reverse the cholinergic component of bronchoconstriction. Excessive β-agonist use may exacerbate his angina. If ipratropium does not control symptoms, a trial of a steroid inhaler may be warranted. Patients with COPD are at greater risk for upper respiratory infections and are candidates for the pneumococcal and *Haemophilus influenzae* vaccine.

P: Discontinue theophylline and albuterol. Start ipratropium, 1 puff QID. Administer pneumococcal and *H. influenzae* vaccine. Encourage continued abstinence from cigarettes.

Problem 2. Hypertension

S: SB is currently asymptomatic

O: BP 155/95; previously controlled on hydrochlorothiazide; mild AV nicking on examination

A: SB's BP was previously well-controlled on hydrochlorothiazide (HCTZ). The current high reading is most likely a result of theophylline toxicity. SB has evidence of end-organ damage (mild AV nicking). HCTZ may contribute to SB's hyperuricemia and switching to another agent is indicated. Using a β-blocker or calcium channel blocker will also treat SB's angina. β-blockers should be used with caution in SB, as they may aggravate COPD by blocking $β_2$ receptors, causing bronchoconstriction.

P: Discontinue HCTZ and start diltiazem CD, 120 mg PO QD. May titrate up to 380 mg PO QD as needed to control BP.

Problem 3. Angina

S: SB complains of relatively new-onset chest pain on exertion and recent anginal pain accompanied by palpitations.

O: None

A: SB is currently taking isosorbide dinitrate (ISDN), 30 mg PO TID, which results in moderate control of anginal symptoms. SB still complains of chest pain on exertion. Options to further control anginal symptoms are to increase the ISDN dose or add another agent. Diltiazem, while also controlling blood pressure, will decrease myocardial oxygen demand, thereby treating his angina as well. Diltiazem can be titrated as high as needed to provide optimal control of angina, provided SB's blood pressure does not drop too low.

P: Continue ISDN, 30 mg PO TID, and start diltiazem as stated above in treatment of hypertension.

Problem 4. Hyperuricemia and Gout

S: SB is currently asymptomatic; suffered first gouty attack 1 week ago.

O: Uric acid 9.8, (+) family history

A: SB suffered his first gouty attack 1 week ago. Reducing his uric acid level to normal levels (i.e., < 6.0) may help prevent further gouty attacks and potential complications. Hydrochlorothiazide is known to increase uric acid levels and may have contributed to the recent attack. SB also occasionally drinks alcohol (EtOH), which can precipitate acute gouty attacks. Discontinuing HCTZ may lower uric acid levels. SB should be encouraged to limit or discontinue EtOH intake. Low-dose aspirin is also known to increase uric acid levels. However, SB has active coronary artery disease (CAD), and the benefits of decreased mortality from aspirin therapy likely outweighs the risk of another gouty attack. Since SB has had only one gouty attack, uricosuric agents are not yet indicated.

P: Discontinue HCTZ and alcohol intake. Recheck uric acid level in 3 months.

CASE 74 QUESTIONS

1. How should SB properly use his nitroglycerin (NTG)?
2. Are all calcium channel blockers equally efficacious in treating angina?
3. If SB's uric acid level does not normalize with the discontinuation of HCTZ, what could be done to further treat SB for hyperuricemia?

CASE 75

CC: JU is a man, age 59, who presents with a 2-week history of dyspnea, wheezing, headache, insomnia, and irritability. He also complains of generalized weakness over the past month.

Past Medical History

JU has a 20-year history of asthma that is fairly well controlled with metaproterenol and triamcinolone inhalers. He was doing well until 2 months ago, when he started to have increased wheezing and shortness of breath, at the start of the allergy season. Subsequently, he was started on theophylline to control his symptoms. Now, he presents to the clinic requesting refills for his inhalers and claiming that he is not experiencing any benefit from increased use of his inhalers. He also has hypertension, for which he takes propranolol. In addition, he has had a 1-year history of mild ulcerative colitis that is well controlled on mesalamine enema.

Social History

Occasional wine with dinner; 10-year smoking history (quit 20 years ago)

Medication History

Metaproterenol MDI, 2 puffs QID
Triamcinolone MDI, 2 puffs QID (lost inhaler 2 weeks ago)
Theophylline (sustained-release), 400 mg PO BID
Mesalamine, 4 g pr QHS
Diphenhydramine, 50 mg PO Q8H (started 2 months ago)
Propranolol, 40 mg PO BID (started last month)
Acetaminophen, 325 mg PO PRN for headache (1 to 2 tabs daily for the past 2 weeks)

Allergies

Penicillin

Physical Examination

GEN:	59-year-old man in moderate respiratory distress
VS:	BP 145/92, RR 22, HR 56, T 37, Wt 75 kg
HEENT:	WNL
COR:	Sinus rhythm
CHEST:	Wheezes on inspiration and expiration
ABD:	No pain, no guarding
GU:	WNL
RECT:	Guaiac-positive, negative BRBPR
EXT:	Pale, dry skin
NEURO:	Unremarkable

Results of Laboratory Tests

Na 137 (137)	Hct 0.3 (30)	AST 0.53 (32)	Glu 6.1 (110)
K 3.9 (3.9)	Hgb 110 (11)	ALT 0.35 (21)	TIBC 88 (460)
Cl 101 (101)	Lkcs 8×10^9 (8×10^3)	Alb 39 (3.9)	Ferritin 10 (10)
HCO$_3$ 28 (28)	Plts 175×10^9 (175×10^3)	T Bili 3.4 (0.2)	
BUN 7.1 (20)	MCV 75 (75)		
CR 88.4 (1.0)	MCH 24 (24)		

Theophylline 55 (10) (1 month ago)

PROBLEM LIST

1. Asthma/hay fever
2. Hypertension
3. Ulcerative colitis
4. Anemia
5. Theophylline toxicity

CASE 75 QUESTIONS

1. Would JU benefit from anticholinergic inhalers? If so, give dose, route, and frequency.
2. What are the advantages and disadvantages of using salmeterol in treating asthma in JU?
3. Further evaluation indicates that JU does not use his inhalers appropriately. Should he receive a spacing device?
4. Describe the role of antihistamines in respiratory diseases.
5. JU does not like using enemas. What alternative route of administration is available to control his ulcerative colitis?

CASE 76

CC: YM is a woman, age 30, who presents to the clinic with a mild cough, slight fever, DOE, occasional wheezes, and decreased appetite. She also states that she has not been feeling herself lately. She has been sleeping a lot and doesn't seem to enjoy her usual activities. She has been experiencing crying spells approximately 3 to 4 times a week for the past month.

History of Present Illness

YM has a history of multiple pulmonary bacterial infections with pathogens including: *Haemophilus influenzae, Pseudomonas aeruginosa,* and *Staphylococcus aureus.* YM was seen in the emergency room 2 days before this clinic visit and cultures were taken. She was empirically started on Septra DS twice daily. It has not helped her symptoms much.

Past Medical History

YM was diagnosed with cystic fibrosis at 5 years of age. She has had multiple hospitalizations for pulmonary infections and is seen regularly for nutritional support. She has had chronic renal failure for approximately 2 years.

Medication History

Septra DS, 1 tablet PO BID
Pancrease MT4, 3 capsules PO TID with each meal
Albuterol MDI, 2 puffs QID PRN for shortness of breath
Hydrochlorothiazide, 25 mg PO QD
Vitamin A, 5000 U PO QD
Vitamin E, 400 U PO QD
Vitamin D, 800 U PO QD

Allergies

None known

Physical Examination

GEN:	Disheveled, depressed-looking woman in no acute distress.
VS:	BP 136/82, HR 70, RR 12, T 38.7, Wt 55 kg, Ht 165cm
HEENT:	PERRLA
COR:	Normal S$_1$ and S$_2$
ABD:	Soft, nontender, no hepatosplenomegaly
NEURO:	Oriented to time, place, and person
CHEST:	Mild rales at base
EXT:	Slight bruising on upper thighs

Results of Laboratory Tests (from emergency room data)

Na 140 (140)	WBC 12 (12)	INR 1.4 (1.4)
K 4.0 (4.0)	Vit A 0.28 (8)	Cl 100 (100)
Vit E 14 (0.6)	Culture (sputum): *Pseudomonas aeruginosa*	Culture (blood): (−)
HCO$_3$ 24 (24)	AST 0.58 (35)	Cr 178 (2.0)
BUN 8.5 (24)	ALT 4.6 (21)	

Chest X-ray film: bronchovascular markings
O_2 sats = 97%

PROBLEM LIST
1. Pseudomonas infection
2. Cystic fibrosis
3. Depression
4. Chronic renal failure

CASE 76 SOAP NOTES
Problem 1. *Pseudomonas* Infection
S: Dyspnea on exertion and cough

O: History of recurrent pulmonary infections; rales, slight fever, and increased WBC count. Sputum is culture positive for *Pseudomonas aeruginosa*. Blood culture is negative.

A: YM has a mild upper respiratory tract infection that is not susceptible to her current antibiotic, Septra. Her O_2 saturation test results are normal, and her blood culture is negative. However, the culture of her sputum is positive for *Pseudomonas aeruginosa*. This organism commonly colonizes patients with cystic fibrosis for most of their lives, and appropriate management of these organisms is important in order to prevent resistance from occurring. The rationale behind treatment of pulmonary infections in cystic fibrosis patients is not to eradicate the organism, but to treat the infection. There are several different treatment options. Antibiotics can be given by three different routes: intravenous, inhalation, or oral. The intravenous antibiotics are used in severe cases or in patients who have strains of *Pseudomonas* resistant to quinolones. Parenteral antibiotics with antipseudomonal activity include tobramycin, amikacin, mezclocillin, ticarcillin, piperacillin, ceftazidime, imipenem, ciprofloxacin, and aztreonam. Tobramycin may also be administered by inhalation; this route of administration is still controversial. For treatment of an active infection, it should not be prescribed as monotherapy, but is usually given in combination with intravenous antipseudomonal antibiotics. The only oral antibiotics with antipseudomonal activity are the quinolones and oral carbenicillin. To appropriately dose antibiotics in patients with cystic fibrosis, several things must be considered. These patients often have mucus plugs in many organs of their body. To treat pulmonary infections, enough antibiotic must be given to penetrate the mucus in the lung. Also, cystic fibrosis patients have a higher clearance of some antibiotics. Because of these factors, antibiotic doses in patients with cystic fibrosis should be as aggressive as possible to ensure adequate serum levels and to reduce the likelihood of resistance developing.

Since YM's illness appears to be mild, she can treated with oral antibiotics and close monitoring.

P: Discontinue Septra. Start ciprofloxacin 750mg PO TID for 14 days. Counsel YM on proper use of ciprofloxacin. She must complete the full regimen even if she feels better before completing therapy. She should not take the ciprofloxacin concomitantly with antacids, iron, or dairy products, as divalent cations (Fe++, Mg++, Ca++) may che-

late with ciprofloxacin, reducing absorption. If her symptoms worsen or do not seem to improve in the next few days, she should return to the clinic.

Problem 2. Cystic Fibrosis
S: Patient history of cystic fibrosis; history of recurrent respiratory infections.

O: History of cystic fibrosis; chest X-ray results are positive for bronchovascular markings, which are consistent with cystic fibrosis.

A: Cystic fibrosis patients have a missing conductance protein that regulates mucus secretions from exocrine glands. The absence of this protein causes an increase in production and decrease in dilution of mucus from all exocrine glands. Anywhere exocrine glands exist, thick mucus is secreted. There are three organ systems affected by these secretions, although others may become involved. These three areas are the GI tract, where maldigestion of fat-soluble vitamins occurs; the lungs, where chronic infections occur; and the skin, where sweat is produced that contains increased sodium chloride concentrations. YM has normal levels of both vitamin A and vitamin E. Her INR level is slightly elevated and she has mild bruising, which is indicative of either poor absorption of vitamin K (a fat-soluble vitamin) or liver dysfunction. Other than the elevated INR, she does not have other symptoms or risk factors for liver dysfunction. Therefore, it is likely that YM is not absorbing vitamin K very well. She should be given oral vitamin K to supplement her deficiency. YM is currently taking pancreatic enzymes to help her digestion and she appears to be stable on her current dose. She does not complain of diarrhea, fatty stools, or constipation. Her respiratory status was addressed in the previous problem. However, as her disease progresses, she may need medication to help the air flow through her lungs. At this time she only uses an albuterol MDI as needed.

P: In addition to her other fat-soluble vitamin supplements, she should start phytonadione (Vitamin K), 5 mg PO QOD. She should monitor herself for other signs of bleeding, such as spontaneous nosebleeds, bleeding gums, hematuria, or black stools. She should see her primary practitioner if she develops abdominal pain. Her INR level should be checked on a regular basis until it is normalized to determine if the phytonadione dosing is appropriate. The serum levels of the other fat-soluble vitamins are within normal limits.

Problem 3. Chronic Renal Insufficiency
S: None

O: Elevated BUN and serum creatinine levels. History of chronic renal insufficiency.

A: YM has mild renal failure. Her creatinine clearance can be estimated with the equation created by Cockcroft and Gault:

$$ClCr = \frac{140 - \text{age})(\text{weight [kg]})}{(72)(SCr)} \times 0.85 \text{ (females)}$$

Chronic renal insufficiency progresses differently in each patient. Most patients function without acute complications until their creatinine clearance rate is less than 25 mL/min. Below this clearance rate, many patients are managed well with medication alone until their creatinine clearance rate is less than 10 mL/min. Some long-term complications (both acute and chronic) can include hypertension, metabolic acidosis, hypermagnesemia, hyperkalemia or hypokalemia, anemia, hyperuricemia, impaired cardiac function, and uremia. YM currently has mild hypertension that is controlled by hydrochlorothiazide, a thiazide diuretic. Hypertension appears to be the only development that may be attributed to her chronic renal insufficiency. As her chronic renal insufficiency progresses and her creatinine clearance rate approaches less than 25 mL/min, it may be necessary to change to a loop diuretic. The thiazides become less effective as creatinine clearance rate decreases.

P: Monitor electrolyte levels, blood pressure, BUN level, serum creatinine level, hematocrit, and hemoglobin level on a regular basis. YM needs to be advised to follow a low-sodium diet. She should avoid salt substitutes because of the high potassium content, which could lead to hyperkalemia in a patient with chronic renal insufficiency. Currently, her chronic renal insufficiency is stable.

Problem 4. Depression

S: YM has not been feeling herself lately. She has had a loss of appetite, frequent crying spells, and anhedonia over the past month.

O: None

A: YM has signs that suggest she may be going through an episode of major depression. She is no longer interested in activities previously enjoyed; her accustomed level of hygiene is decreased; and she has crying spells for no apparent reason. Before starting therapy, a differential diagnosis should be done to rule out illnesses or medications that are associated with depressive symptoms. YM does not have any of the illnesses and does not take any of the medications that may induce depressive symptoms. However, she does have a chronic illness (cystic fibrosis), which may contribute to her depression. YM will probably receive a diagnosis of major depression. To treat affective disorders, most practitioners agree that a combination of psychotherapy and medication gives the best outcome. There are many antidepressants that can be prescribed for YM. The classes include tricyclic antidepressants, monoamine oxidase inhibitors (MAOIs), selective serotonin reuptake inhibitors (SSRIs), and other second-generation antidepressants, such as trazodone and bupropion. The choice of agent depends on the side effect profile and YM's specific type of depression. The MAOIs are primarily used in atypical depression, phobias, and in cases refractory to other therapy. Dietary restrictions accompany MAOI therapy because a hypertensive crisis may follow ingestion of foods that contain tyramine. It would be easier for YM to start on a different class of medications because of this potentially dangerous side effect. Tricyclic antidepressants are often used as initial agents for depression. They have primarily anticholinergic side effects that can be bothersome, but not life-threatening. Tricyclic antidepressant doses are started low and titrated every 2 to 3 weeks depending on the tolerance of side effects. Trazodone and bupropion are second-generation agents that do not have the anticholinergic side effects of tricyclic antidepressants. However, bupropion has a low threshold for seizures and trazodone is very sedating. The SSRIs are widely used because of their lack of unpleasant side effects and efficacy in treating depression. However, these agents have only become available in the past few years, therefore, long-term side effects are still to be determined. None of the antidepressants take effect immediately, and patients should be aware that several weeks may go by before they notice an effect on their mood.

P: Psychiatric consultation is essential to a diagnosis of the extent and type of depression. Tricyclic antidepressants or SSRIs can be used in YM. She should be seen in several weeks to document progress. She should be informed that antidepressants do not work instantaneously, and that psychotherapy is needed for maximal results.

CASE 76 QUESTIONS

1. Would the dexamethasone suppression test (DST) be appropriate in assessing YM's depression?
2. Should ciprofloxacin be used for prophylaxis in cystic fibrosis?
3. Why does chronic renal failure result in both hyperkalemia and hypokalemia?
4. Is monitoring serum drug levels of tricyclic antidepressants worthwhile?
5. Is theophylline effective in cystic fibrosis patients?

CASE 77

CC: MM is a man, age 64, who presents to the emergency department with shortness of breath, wheezing, and coughing. These symptoms were associated with a flu-like illness and have resulted in chest tightness and palpitation that keeps him awake at night.

Past Medical History

MM has a 15-year history of chronic steroid-dependent asthma. He was doing well until 5 days ago, when he started having increased shortness of breath and cough. Even though he admits to being compliant with his medications, he has been out of his prednisone for 10 days. He also has hypertension, which was diagnosed 6 years ago, and is treated with hydrochlorothiazide. He was last seen in the emergency room 1 week ago for high blood pressure. His blood pressure was 165/102, and nadolol was added to his regimen. His other significant illness is congestive heart failure, for which he receives digoxin.

Medication History

Metaproterenol MDI, 1 to 2 puffs PRN

Prednisone, 20 mg PO BID

Theophylline (sustained-release), 300 mg PO QD

Digoxin, 0.125 mg PO QD

Hydrochlorothiazide, 50 mg PO QAM

Nadolol, 80 mg PO QAM

Alka-Seltzer, PRN for GI upset

Allergies

None known

Social History

Occasional ethanol

Physical Examination

GEN: Confused and pale elderly man in acute respiratory distress, complaining of chest pain and palpitations.

VS: BP 145/94, HR 140, RR 26, T 37.0, Wt 65, Ht 178 cm

HEENT: PERRLA

COR: Jugular venous distention

CHEST: Inspiratory and expiratory wheezing, rales, and rhonchi

ABD: Hepatojugular reflux, hepatomegaly

RECT: Guaiac-negative

NEURO: Oriented × 1, confused

EXT: 2+ pedal edema

Results of Laboratory Tests

Na 134 (134)	Hct 0.35 (35)	AST 0.33 (20)	Ca 2.3 (9.4)
K 3.1 (3.1)	Hgb 90 (9.0)	ALT 0.42 (25)	Mg 1.1 (2.2)
Cl 95 (95)	Lkcs 8 × 10⁹ (8 × 10³)	Alb 38 (3.8)	B₁₂ 66 (90)
HCO₃ 20 (20)	Plts 280 × 10⁹ (280 × 10³)	T Bili 15 (0.9)	Digoxin 0.9 (0.7)
BUN 12 (35)	MCV 105 (105)		Theophylline 39 (7)
CR 213 (2.8)	Retic 0.0003 (0.3)		

ABG pH 7.4, PO_2 52, PCO_2 50

ECG: rhythm irregular/irregular, no real P waves (atrial fibrillation)

Pulmonary function tests: prebronchodilator FEV_1: 1.5 L; postbronchodilator FEV_2: 2 L

PROBLEM LIST

1. Asthma exacerbation/steroid-dependent asthma
2. Congestive heart failure
3. Hypertension
4. Atrial fibrillation
5. Hypokalemia

CASE 78

CC: RP is a woman, age 52, who was seen in the emergency department last night after experiencing an acute asthma attack. She complained of severe wheezing and shortness of breath and was unable to speak more than a few words without taking a breath. She reported wheezing and coughing "much more than usual," but attributes this to the rainy weather. Initial peak flow was 75/min, and a second reading, taken an hour after beginning treatment with aerosolized albuterol and oxygen, was 102/min. FEV_1 on admission was 1.8 L, FVC was 3.0 L, and FEV_1/FVC was 60%.

History of Present Illness

RP has been experiencing frequent asthma attacks for the past 2 months. Ten weeks ago, RP was in a serious motor vehicle accident (MVA), in which she sustained a concussion as well as a broken left leg and many contusions. Two weeks after the accident, RP's husband came home after work and found RP lying on the kitchen floor. She was "awake, but confused" according to her husband, and she had "wet herself." RP's MD, after learning that RP had no previous history of seizures, presumed that RP had suffered a posttraumatic seizure, and she was placed on anticonvulsant therapy with phenytoin. She has not experienced any seizure activity since the initiation of therapy.

Past Medical History

RP has a history of periodic asthma attacks since her early 20s. She has used an albuterol inhaler and has taken theophylline "for years." Three years ago, after a 6-year period of uncontrolled hypertension (average blood pressure, 165/98), RP began to experience increased SOB, DOE, and ankle swelling. Her work-up revealed an ejection fraction (EF) of 52%, cardiac dilatation, and a normal sinus rhythm, and she was diagnosed with mild congestive heart failure (CHF). She was placed on a sodium-restricted diet and HCTZ. Last year she began to exhibit signs of worsening CHF, with increasing peripheral edema and DOE, and she was placed on enalapril. Her symptoms have been well controlled for the past year.

Medication History

Theophylline SR, 300 mg BID

Albuterol MDI, PRN

Phenytoin, 300 mg QHS

HCTZ, 50 mg BID

Enalapril, 5 mg BID

Social History

Tobacco use: None

Alcohol use: None

Caffeine use: 4 cups of coffee and 4 diet colas per day

Family History

Father died at age 59 of kidney failure secondary to hypertension.

Mother died at age 62 of congestive heart failure

Physical Examination

GEN: pale, well-developed, anxious-appearing woman.

VS: Emergency department admission: BP 171/94, HR 122, RR 31, T 38.5, Wt 6 1kg, Ht 161cm; current: BP 142/79, HR 80, RR 18, T 38.3

HEENT: PEERLA, oral cavity without lesions, TM without signs of inflammation; no nystagmus noted, positive for AV nicking

COR: RRR, normal S_1 and S_2

CHEST: bilateral expiratory wheezes

ABD: nontender, nondistended, no masses

RECT: guaiac-negative

EXT: 1+ ankle edema on right, no bruising, normal pulses

NEURO: oriented to person, time, and place; cranial nerves intact

Results of Laboratory Tests

Na 134 (134)	Hct 0.37 (37)	LDH 2.5 (150)	Glu 6.1 (110)
K 4.9 (4.9)	Hgb 8.1 (13)	Alk Phos 1.32 (79)	Ca 2.23 (8.9)
Cl 100 (100)	WBC 5.2×10^9 (5.2)	Alb 38 (3.8)	PO_4 0.872 (2.7)
HCO_3 30 (30)	Plts 201 (201)	T Bili 3.4 (0.2)	
Mg 0.65 (1.3)	BUN 7.5 (21)	AST 0.45 (27)	PT 12 sec.
CR 106.1 (1.2)	ALT 0.4 (24)		

Theophylline level: 6.2 mcg/mL

Phenytoin level: 17 mcg/mL

Chest X-ray results: blunting of the right and left costophrenic angles

ECG: voltage changes consistent with left ventricular hypertrophy (LVH)

PROBLEM LIST

1. Asthma
2. Seizure disorder
3. CHF

CASE 78 SOAP NOTES

Problem 1: Asthma

S: RP complains of severe wheezing, SOB, and coughing, and was unable to speak full sentences without pausing to catch her breath.

O: On admission, RP had elevated HR, RR, and BP, and decreased FEV_1, FVC, and peak flow. RP also has a positive history for periodic asthma attacks, and her theophylline level is below therapeutic range at 6.2 (therapeutic range is 10 to 20).

A: RP experienced an acute asthma attack last night but also admits to worsening respiratory function, which correlates with the start of her antiseizure regimen with phenytoin approximately 2 months ago. Phenytoin enhances the metabolism of theophylline by inducing the cytochrome P-450 enzyme system, leading to a reduction in the steady-state theophylline concentration, and putting RP at risk for acute asthma attacks. The role of theophylline in the treatment of asthma is very controversial; it is used primarily in patients who are unresponsive to the standard therapies of inhaled β_2-agonists and inhaled steroids. Considering that RP will have to continue her phenytoin for seizure control, that she suffers only periodic asthma attacks, that she has a history of hypertension, and especially that she has never had an adequate trial of inhaled β_2-agonists, RP should be taken off theophylline and should be initiated on a trial of inhaled selective β_2-agonists (such as albuterol, pirbuterol, or terbutaline). The β_2-agonists act as sympathomimetic bronchodilators and should be administered only on a PRN basis (with the exception of salmeterol) in order to decrease the incidence of adverse effects and the development of tolerance. This patient should also be given a spacer device to assist her with proper administration of the inhaled medicine. Inhalation technique should be taught and monitored.

P: Albuterol should be administered, 1 to 2 puffs Q4-6H PRN and before exercise. RP should be monitored for inhalation technique, asthma exacerbation, FEV_1, FVC, peak flow, BP, and HR. Dose-related reflex tachycardia occurs from both peripheral vasodilation and from direct cardiac stimulation. Systemic side effects, such as tremor, palpitations, and nausea, are commonly seen with systemic administration of these agents, but are much less common with administration by inhalation. RP should be directed to contact her health care provider if, at any time, she experiences increasing SOB despite proper use of her inhaled β_2-agonist.

Problem 2: Seizure Disorder

S: None.

O: RP was found down and in a presumed postictal state after head trauma. She has not experienced any seizure activity since starting phenytoin, and her serum phenytoin level of 17 mcg/mL is within the therapeutic window.

A: Serum drug concentration is a less important monitoring parameter than the frequency of seizure activity; however, in patients such as RP who have infrequent seizures, maintenance of steady-state drug levels within the therapeutic range can help decrease the risk of seizure recurrence. RP has a phenytoin level within the therapeutic range and has not experienced seizure activity since the initiation of therapy. Also, she has not experienced any adverse effects from the phenytoin. For RP, the goal of therapy is to prevent seizure recurrence, maintain adequate therapeutic drug concentration between 10 and 20 mcg/mL, and to avoid unnecessary toxicity.

P: Continue RP on antiseizure medication for now. Her condition has been well-controlled and, as long as it continues to be controlled without experiencing significant toxicity, she should be maintained on phenytoin for 1 to 2 years free from seizures. CBC count, LFTs, and phenytoin level should be monitored periodically. RP should report any feelings of sedation, mental status changes, or blurred vision, as this may indicate that her drug level should be adjusted. While on therapy, RP should be seen by a dentist on a regular basis in order to manage gingival hyperplasia. All of RP's health care practitioners should be informed that RP is taking phenytoin, as this drug is associated with numerous drug interactions.

Problem 3: Congestive Heart Failure (CHF)

S: At the time of diagnosis, RP complained of DOE, SOB , and ankle swelling.

O: The patient was diagnosed with CHF 3 years ago according to symptoms, an ejection fraction of 52%, and evidence of cardiac dilitation. Today, only the ECG shows cardiac dilatation, and RP has mild, 1+ ankle edema.

A: RP's primary risk factor for CHF was uncontrolled hypertension. At the time of diagnosis, RP had uncontrolled hypertension with an average BP of 165/98. Also, RP has a strong family history of hypertension: both her mother and father died of complications of hypertension. Uncontrolled hypertension places increased afterload on the left ventricle. The goal of therapy in CHF is to provide symptomatic control and to improve the patient's quality of life. These goals are being met with RP's current therapy. A sodium-restricted diet results in decreased blood volume and prevents abnormal sodium retention by the kidney. Thiazide diuretics enhance renal excretion of sodium and water, thereby decreasing vascular volume. Decreased vascular volume relieves ventricular and pulmonary congestion and decreases peripheral edema (ankle swelling). Thiazide, rather than loop, diuretics are indicated in mild to moderate CHF, because they are less likely to cause volume depletion. Angiotensin-converting enzyme (ACE) inhibitors are very useful in the treatment of CHF because they decrease PCWP and SVR while increasing the cardiac index. The combination of these effects results in decreased preload as well as afterload.

P: No change in therapy is indicated at this time. Since RP is symptomatically controlled, the plan is to continue RP on diuretic therpy, to prescribe an ACE inhibitor, and to encourage her to continue to follow a sodium-restricted diet (2 g sodium per day). The adverse effects of ACE inhibitors include hypotension and hyperkalemia. The patient should be monitored for signs and symptoms of volume depletion, hypotension, hypokalemia, hyperuricemia, and hyperglycemia, as well as signs and symptoms consistent with worsening CHF. The use of NSAIDs, which cause sodium and water retention, should be avoided. The patient should be instructed to use acetaminophen for pain.

CASE 78 QUESTIONS

1. How long should RP continue to take her antiseizure medication?
2. What is the mechanism of action of phenytoin?
3. Should RP also be started on an inhaled steroid to help control her asthma?
4. Why is RP *not* taking digoxin for her CHF?
5. Seven months from now, RP returns to your clinic with signs of worsening CHF. How should she be managed?

CARDIOVASCULAR DISORDERS

CASE 79
CC: GH is a man, age 57, who presents to the anticoagulation clinic with complaints of frequent nosebleeds (three in the last week), easy bruising, palpitations, weakness, swelling in the feet and lower legs, abdominal discomfort, and a lack of appetite. In addition, GH complains that he has a cold.

History of Present Illness
GH has a history of atrial fibrillation, but has been in normal sinus rhythm for 3 years while receiving procainamide. GH has a history of alcoholism and has been alcohol-free for 3 years, but admits he has been drinking heavily for the last month. One month ago, GH was given a prescription for cimetidine to treat nocturnal heartburn and esophagitis and was instructed to stop taking antacids.

Social History
Tobacco use: 15 pack-years; quit 10 years ago
Alcohol use: binge drinking for the last month

Past Surgical History
Noncontributory

Medication History
Warfarin, 6 mg QD
Digoxin, 0.375 mg QD
Procainamide SR, 500 mg QID
Cimetidine, 300 mg QID
Pseudoephedrine SR, 120 mg BID
Mylanta, 15 mL TID (discontinued 1 month ago)

Allergies
No known drug allergies

Physical Examination
GEN: Well developed, well nourished (WDWN) man in distress
VS: HR 105, irregularly irregular; BP 175/96, RR 25; Wt 96 kg, Ht 174cm
HEENT: WNL
COR: Slight atrial enlargement
CHEST: WNL
ABD: (+) bowel sounds
EXT: Bruising on arms and knees; 1+ ankle edema
NEURO: A & O × 3
ECG: Atrial fibrillation

Results of Laboratory Tests
Na 143 (143)   Hct 0.43 (43)
K 4.8 (4.8)   Hgb 140 (14.0)
Cl 98 (98)   BUN 4.3 (12)
Cr 79 (0.9)   Procainamide 6 ug/mL
PT Control 11.7   PT 33
INR 4.7   Digoxin 2.0 ng/mL

PROBLEM LIST
1. Congestive heart failure
2. Atrial fibrillation
3. Gastroesophageal reflux disorder
4. Warfarin toxicity

CASE 79: SOAP NOTES
Problem 2. Atrial Fibrillation
S: GH complains of palpitations and weakness.
O: GH has an irregularly irregular heart rate of 105 bpm, atrial enlargement, and electrocardiographic evidence supporting the diagnosis of atrial fibrillation.
A: GH currently has atrial fibrillation (AF), which is normally controlled with procainamide. GH needs to discontinue alcohol consumption and pseudoephedrine, because they are the likely cause of his AF. In addition, his congestive heart failure (CHF) and elevated blood pressure may be contributing to AF. Since he is hemodynamically stable, his AF should be treated with medication rather than electric cardioversion. He is currently anticoagulated, so conversion to normal sinus rhythm may be attempted without concern about emboli. GH's digoxin, used to treat his CHF, is currently controlling his ventricular rate. Since the current dose of procainamide has been effective at controlling GH's AF in the past, discontinuing the use of alcohol and pseudoephedrine should be the first-line treatment. If this fails to resolve the AF, then the dose of procainamide SR may be increased to 750 mg QID.
P: Treatment should include discontinuing the alcohol and pseudoephedrine. If this fails to resolve GH's AF after 1 week, then the dose of procainamide SR should be increased to 750 mg PO QID. For anticoagulant dosing, see problem 4. The goals of therapy are to convert his heart rate to normal sinus rhythm and to reverse all signs and symptoms of AF. Furthermore, GH should be monitored for drug side effects. Procainamide has been shown to cause a systemic lupus erythematosus syndrome, GI side effects, and rash.

Problem 4. Warfarin Toxicity
S: GH has symptoms of bruising on the arms and knees and has had three nosebleeds in the last week.

110

O: GH has a PT 2.8 times more than control and an INR of 4.7.

A: GH is experiencing a mild case of warfarin toxicity that is likely caused by the cimetidine-warfarin drug interaction. Cimetidine inhibits the metabolism of warfarin, thus enhancing its anticoagulant effects. Furthermore, alcohol is thought to enhance the clearance of vitamin K-dependent clotting factors, which leads to an increased anticoagulant effect. GH has symptoms of bleeding and bruising and needs treatment. Since the PT is 2.8 times more than control, further warfarin doses should be temporarily held.

P: Treatment of GH's warfarin toxicity may be accomplished by holding warfarin for 2 days, then restarting at 5 mg PO QD followed by a reassessment of PT/INR the following week. Goals of therapy are to keep the PT between 1.5 and 2 times more than control and the INR between 2 and 3 and to prevent any further episodes of bleeding. Upon discharge, GH should be told to eat a steady diet, avoid aspirin and NSAIDs, and report signs of bleeding to the clinic.

Problem 1. Congestive Heart Failure

S: GH has symptoms of swelling in the lower legs and feet, abdominal discomfort, lack of appetite, and weakness.

O: GH has 1+ ankle edema and an elevated respiratory rate (25/min).

A: GH's signs and symptoms suggest that he is suffering from right-sided heart failure, which may be exacerbated by his atrial fibrillation, elevated blood pressure, weight, and acute viral infection. Treatment is necessary to prevent progressive left-sided heart failure, but because his symptoms are not life-threatening, he may be treated on an outpatient basis. A diuretic, such as furosemide, should be added to reduce GH's pedal edema. Now that GH is no longer taking antacids, the digoxin may have a greater bioavailability and serum concentration.

P: Continue digoxin, 0.375 mg PO QD, and add furosemide, 20 mg PO QD. Goals of treatment are to prevent worsening of CHF and to improve GH's quality of life. Monitoring parameters should include resolution of GH's presenting signs and symptoms, digoxin level, and signs of drug side effects. Monitoring of electrolyte levels is especially important when combining furosemide with digoxin, because electrolyte abnormalities may precipitate potentially fatal arrhythmias.

Problem 3. Gastroesophageal Reflux Disease

S: GH is currently not complaining of any symptoms of gastroesophageal reflux disease (GERD).

O: GH has esophagitis.

A: GH is currently without GERD symptoms, but he needs continued treatment for 12 to 16 weeks for his esophagitis. GH should avoid alcohol and lose weight, because these factors are known to exacerbate GERD. Mixing cimetidine and warfarin therapy together is no longer contraindicated, because the warfarin dose has been adjusted, taking cimetidine into consideration. The patient should be instructed to return to the anticoagulation clinic if any changes are made in his cimetidine regimen.

P: Continue cimetidine, 300 mg PO QID. Goals of therapy are to treat esophagitis and to prevent symptoms of heartburn. GH should be instructed to avoid alcohol, lose weight, decrease fat in his diet, and avoid food and liquid at bedtime.

CASE 79 QUESTIONS

1. What commonly prescribed medications are known to enhance the effect of warfarin?
2. What commonly prescribed medications are known to decrease the effect of warfarin?
3. What are the target INR values in a patient with atrial fibrillation? Mechanical prosthetic heart valves? Treatment of venous thrombosis?
4. What drugs are known to increase the severity of GERD?
5. List several compensatory mechanisms in response to heart failure.

CASE 80

CC: ED is a woman, age 72, who presents to the emergency department with a 2-day history of increasing shortness of breath, swollen legs, malaise, weakness, and a rash on her face. ED states that she stopped taking her newer medications (i.e., hydralazine and lisinopril) when she noticed a rash on her face 2 days ago. ED also states that she has gained weight over the past few days.

Past Medical History

ED has severe congestive heart failure (CHF) (ejection fraction, 6%; NYHA class IV), which requires her to sleep sitting up. She also has a history of sustained ventricular tachycardia (V-tach), controlled with amiodarone and a pacemaker. In addition, ED has a history of coronary artery disease (CAD) and angina for many years; has a history of hypertension; and has had four myocardial infarctions (MI).

Past Surgical History

ED has had three coronary artery bypass grafts (CABG).

Medication History

Amiodarone, 300 mg PO QD
Digoxin, 0.125 mg PO every 3 days
Furosemide, 80 mg PO QAM and 40 mg PO QPM
Maxzide, 1/2 tab PO QAM
Lisinopril, 5 mg PO QD
Nitroglycerin, 0.4 mg sublingual PRN for chest pain
Hydralazine, 50 mg PO TID for 7 months

Allergies
None known

Physical Examination
GEN: Well-developed, well nourished woman with no-
ticeable SOB
VS: BP 170/94, HR 84, RR 26, T 37.8, Wt 64 kg, Ht
157 cm
HEENT: WNL
COR: +S$_3$, displaced PMI
CHEST: Bibasilar rales
ABD: WNL
GU: Deferred
RECT: Deferred
EXT: 2+ edema bilat LE
NEURO: Alert, O × 4

Results of Laboratory Tests

Na 136 (136)	Hct 0.35 (35)	AST 0.50 (30)	Glu 6.1 (110)
K 4.0 (4.0)	Hgb 130 (13)	ALT 0.50 (30)	Ca 2.2 (8.8)
Cl 98 (98)	Lkcs 8.2 × 10^9 (8.2 × 10^3)	LDH 1.7 (100)	PO$_4$ 0.92 (3.0)
HCO$_3$ 26 (26)	Plts 200 × 10^9 (200 × 10^3)	Alk Phos 1.5 (90)	Mg 1.2 (2.5)
BUN 7.5 (21)	MCV 80 (80)	Alb 40 (4.0)	Uric Acid 190 (3.2)
CR 123 (1.4)		T Bili 3.4 (0.2)	

Dig   1.3   (0.9)
ANA   +
ESR   100 (100)
Lkc differential: WNL
Urinalysis: 2 + protein
Chest x-ray films: Enlarged cardiac silhouette, Ker-
ley's B lines
ECG: Pacer rhythm 84, wide complex

PROBLEM LIST
1. Hypertension
2. Chronic renal insufficiency
3. Angina
4. H/O sustained ventricular tachycardia
5. H/O four myocardial infarctions
6. CHF exacerbation
7. Rash

CASE 80 SOAP NOTES
Problem 6. CHF Exacerbation
S: Swollen legs, SOB, orthopnea, weight gain
O: Left ventricular ejection fraction (LVEF) 6%, rales, peripheral edema, enlarged cardiac silhouette and Kerley's B
lines on chest x-ray, displaced PMI, + S$_3$, h/o multiple MIs,
proteinuria
A: ED is experiencing an exacerbation of her CHF secondary
to stopping lisinopril and hydralazine. ED's other medications include digoxin and furosemide. ED has both right-
sided (ankle swelling, peripheral edema) and left-sided
(orthopnea, pulmonary edema) heart failure and is classified as NYHA class IV because of her symptoms at rest and
other evidence of advanced failure (e.g.,sleeping sitting

up, LVH, +S$_3$, LVEF 6%). ED should be treated for her
acute symptoms.
P: ED should receive intravenous furosemide now to remove
some of the excess fluid. Furosemide IV is preferred, because it may have more vasodilatory properties than the
oral formulation. Furosemide should be given in 20 mg
increments Q2H PRN until there is a response. Ideally,
the amount of fluid lost per day should be no more than
1 L. The hydralazine should be discontinued secondary
to drug-induced systemic lupus erythmatosus (SLE). ED
should be continued on digoxin, which is beneficial in
patients with a + S$_3$ heart sound and those considered to
have severe heart failure.

Problem 7. Rash
S: Rash on face
O: Increased ESR, + ANA, increased SCr, proteinuria, low-
grade fever
A: ED appears to have SLE, most likely hydralazine-induced.
Hydralazine causes a relatively high frequency of SLE (up
to 19%). It usually occurs after at least 2 years of treatment,
but has been reported as early as 1 month after starting
therapy. Risk factors for the development of hydralazine-
induced SLE include advanced age, female sex, Caucasian
race, slow-acetylator status, daily doses of more than 100
mg, and prolonged exposure. ED may be predisposed to
SLE, since she is an elderly white female taking more than
100 mg of hydralazine per day.
P: ED's hydralazine should be discontinued at this time. Since
ED was relatively well controlled on her previous regimen,
the first option should be to maximize the doses of her
lisinopril and furosemide before adding another medication. ED's current dose of lisinopril may be increased to
10 mg/day now and to a maximum of 40 mg/day; her
furosemide may be increased to 120 mg QAM and 40 mg
QPM at this time, up to a recommended maximum daily
dose of 480 mg. If her CHF is uncontrolled after optimizing
her previous regimen, alternative medications that may
be considered include minoxidil, prazosin, nitrates, and
calcium-channel blockers.

Problem 1. Hypertension
S: None
O: BP 170/94
A: ED's blood pressure is higher than the desired range of
120 to 140 mm Hg systolic and 80 to 90 mm Hg diastolic,
but no acute treatment is needed. ED's current therapy
should be adequate to control her hypertension if she is
compliant with her medications.
P: By increasing the doses of lisinopril and furosemide to
better control ED's CHF, her blood pressure should also
decrease. If the blood pressure remains elevated despite
increasing the doses of the antihypertensive medications,
a nitrate could be added to the regimen. For example,
isosorbide dinitrate, 10 mg PO TID, titrated to 40 mg PO
TID as needed for blood pressure control. Thrice daily
dosing is recommended over QID to allow for a 12-hour

nitrate-free period to avoid tachyphylaxis. The goal blood pressure may be lower than normal to aid in slowing the progression of heart failure.

Problem 2. Chronic Renal Insufficiency

S: None

O: BUN 7.5 (21), Cr 123 (1.4), estimated creatinine clearance 36 mL/min (0.6 mL/sec), 2 + proteinuria

A: ED's decreased renal function is most likely caused by her CHF, but the hydralazine-induced SLE may also be contributing.

P: No interventions are needed at this time, but caution should be used with renally cleared medications, and doses should be adjusted to allow for ED's decreased renal function.

Problem 3. Angina

S: None

O: History of angina, CAD, multiple MIs, CABGs

A: ED's angina appears to be controlled at this time.

P: Continue PRN sublingual (SL) nitroglycerin (NTG). ED should be instructed to keep her NTG tablets in the original container and store them at room temperature away from moisture. Unused tablets should be discarded 6 months after the bottle is opened. Instructions for use: One tablet should be dissolved under the tongue at the first sign of an angina attack. A lack of burning sensation does not indicate a lack of potency. The dose may be repeated at 5-minute intervals for a total of three doses in 15 minutes. If at this time the pain is not controlled, ED should go directly to the nearest emergency department.

Problem 4. Sustained Ventricular Tachycardia

S: None

O: History of V-tach, multiple MIs, pacemaker

A: ED is currently on amiodarone, which has prevented any recurrences in her V-tach. Amiodarone is considered an ideal antiarrhythmic for patients with CHF because it does not cause left ventricular dysfunction. In addition, some researchers have shown amiodarone to have a beneficial effect in patients with CHF, possibly by decreasing myocardial oxygen consumption.

P: No therapy change is necessary. Monitor for adverse effects to amiodarone, including photosensitivity, pulmonary toxicity, increased LFTs, and abnormal TFTs.

CASE 80 QUESTIONS

1. Calculate the expected digoxin levels from population parameters. What factors could be affecting ED's digoxin level?
2. Would you expect ED to have a normal serum potassium level while taking furosemide without potassium supplements? Explain.
3. When would metolazone be indicated in ED?

4. If ED's SLE does not clear, would steroids be helpful?
5. If ED's heart failure became worse, what would be the next step?

CASE 81

CC: SB is a man, age 62, who presents to the emergency department with lightheadedness, palpitations, and shortness of breath, which have lasted for 2 days.

History of Present Illness

SB is an active senior who walks 2 miles daily and rides an exercise bicycle three times a week. He states he has previously felt palpitations, but they were associated with exercise and usually went away with rest. Two days ago, while washing the dishes he began feeling short of breath and felt that his heart was "racing." He hoped that the palpitations would go away as they usually did, but when they continued, he came to the hospital.

Past Medical History

SB has a history of hypertension for 20 years, hyperlipidemia for 5 years, chronic renal failure for 2 years, and rheumatic heart disease (mitral valve) as a child. SB reports adhering to a step 1 diet for the last 2 years.

Review of Systems

Noncontributory

Medication History

Enalapril, 10 mg PO BID
Furosemide, 20 mg PO QD
Gemfibrozil, 600 mg PO QD

Allergies

NKDA

Physical Examination

GEN: Well developed male in moderate distress
VS: BP 110/65 (usually 145/85), HR 146, RR 22, T 37.2, Wt 80 kg, Ht 177.8 cm
HEENT: PEERLA, (–) JVD, mild AV nicking
CHEST: Clear to auscultation
COR: Rate irregular irregular, no murmurs or gallops.
ABD: Soft, nontender, active bowel sounds.
GU: Deferred
RECT: WNL
EXT: No edema, normal pulses throughout
NEURO: A × O × 3

Results of Laboratory Tests

Na 136 (136)   Hct 0.26 (26%)   Alk Phos 1.08 (65)   Glu 6.1 (120)
K 4.5 (4.5)   Hgb 95 (9.5)   AST .58 (35)   Ca 1.62 (6.5)
Cl 97 (97)   MCV 90 (90)   ALT .5 (30) PO_4 2.03 (6.3)
CO_2 22 (22)   WBC 8×10^9 (8×10^3)   Mg 1.05 (2.1)   Uric acid 440 (7.4)
BUN 21 (60)   Plts 175×10^9 (175×10^3)   Alb 51 (5.1)   LDL 4.4 (170)
Cr 309.4 (3.5)   Triglycerides 2.03 (180)   Cholesterol 6.2 (240)
HDL .88 (34)

WBC differential: WNL

Prothrombin time: 13.0 sec/ 12.5 sec control

Urinalysis: no RBC, no WBC, (+) protein, (+) hyaline casts

Chest X-ray: clear

ECG: atrial fibrillation, no P waves, variable R-R interval, normal QRS

Echocardiogram: enlarged atria, mild left ventricular hypertrophy, no thrombi seen

PROBLEM LIST

1. Atrial fibrillation
2. Hypertension
3. Hyperlipidemia
4. Chronic renal failure

CASE 81 SOAP NOTES

Problem 1. Atrial Fibrillation

S: Patient complains of dizziness, SOB, palpitations

O: BP 110/65, HR 146, pulse irregular irregularly, ECG: atrial fibrillation

A: The cause of SB's atrial fibrillation (AF) is most likely his history of childhood rheumatic heart disease. However, atrial fibrillation may occur in patients with hypertension as well. On echocardiogram, the atria are enlarged and mild hypertrophy of the left ventricle is noted. These changes are long-term results of hypertension. Rarely is atrial fibrillation a cause of mortality, but it can be a significant cause of morbidity. The detrimental effects of AF are hemodynamic compromise and thromboembolic events. Both can be prevented by returning the heart to normal sinus rhythm. Direct current (DC) cardioversion is the most effective method to convert AF to normal sinus rhythm (NSR) with an 85 to 90% success rate. Chemical conversion with antiarrhythmics has a lower success rate, especially after AF has been present for longer than 24 hours. SB is at risk for a thromboembolic event at the time of cardioversion, even though no thrombi were seen on the echocardiogram. The risk for emboli is significant when the duration of AF is 2 days or more, because atrial function may not return for up to 2 weeks even after normal sinus rhythm is restored. The current standard of practice is to anticoagulate for 3 weeks before cardioversion and for 4 weeks thereafter in patients at risk for clot formation. In the interim, because SB is symptomatic, the ventricular rate must be controlled to maintain adequate cardiac output. Digoxin, β-blockers, and calcium-channel blockers are all useful in controlling the ventricular rate by slowing conduction through the AV node. Digoxin is not the best choice in SB because of the potential for toxicity if renal function continues to deteriorate. Furthermore,

digoxin is not effective in controlling AF during exercise, and SB has reported palpitations during exercise. β-blockers could be used but there is the potential for decreased exercise tolerance. Calcium-channel blockers have been reported to have no effect or improve exercise tolerance in patients with AF. Calcium-channel blockers may also be used to control hypertension, potentially allowing the removal of other antihypertensives from the regimen SB is currently following.

P: Start either verapamil or diltiazem IV to control ventricular rate. Initiate anticoagulation with warfarin. Plan direct current cardioversion in 3 weeks.

Problem 2. Hypertension

S: None

O: History of hypertension for 20 years, mild AV nicking, renal insufficiency, mild LVH, (+) proteinuria.

A: SB's hypertension was reasonably controlled (BP 145/85) before his AF developed. A calcium-channel blocker will be initiated to control the ventricular rate. Potentially the choice of a calcium channel blocker can be used to control hypertension as well, eliminating the need for enalapril. However, SB may benefit from enalapril because of his proteinuria. A β-blocker could also be used to treat both disease states, but is not a good a choice in SB because of his hyperlipidemia and the potential for β-blockers to increase serum triglyceride levels. Control of blood pressure in SB is imperative, because end-organ damage is present, and the risk of coronary artery disease should be decreased. Once a dose of verapamil or diltiazem is established to control the ventricular rate, the enalapril may be reduced if necessary. Furosemide should be continued to prevent fluid retention and maintain urine output.

P: Start diltiazem or verapamil IV and then titrate to find the daily oral dose that controls ventricular rate and blood pressure. Once a daily dose is established, taper enalapril over 1 week.

Problem 3. Hyperlipidemia

S: Currently on step 1 diet and reports exercise 7 days a week.

O: Total cholesterol 240 mg/dL, LDL cholesterol 170 mg/dL, HDL cholesterol 34 mg/dL, triglycerides 180 mg/dL. Currently on gemfibrozil, 600 mg a day.

A: The use of gemfibrozil in SB is not the best choice because its action on the lipoprotein profile does not match the elevated lipoproteins in SB. Gemfibrozil mainly lowers triglycerides and raises HDL, but has little effect on total or HDL cholesterol. SB is at risk for coronary artery disease with risk factors of age, hypertension, and family history. Decreasing total and LDL cholesterol to below recommended levels is important in decreasing this risk. Other agents that may be considered are binding resins, niacin, and HMG-CoA reductase inhibitors. Both resins and HMG-CoA reductase inhibitors are very effective in reducing total and LDL cholesterol. In addition to these effects, niacin will also substantially raise HDL. However, niacin may potentiate the effect of warfarin, which would require increased monitoring. Furthermore, SB has a slightly elevated uric acid level, and niacin may exacerbate uric acid retention. An HMG-CoA reductase inhibitor, such as lovastatin would be well tolerated and requires only once daily dosing.

P: Discontinue gemfibrozil. Start lovastatin, 20 mg PO with dinner. Continue step 1 diet. Counsel SB to report muscle pain, tenderness, or weakness, especially if accompanied by fever or malaise.

Problem 4. Chronic Renal Failure

S: None

O: BUN 60, serum creatinine 3.5, calculated creatinine clearance 24 mL/min, calcium 6.5, phosphorus 6.3, hemoglobin 9.5, hematocrit 26%

A: SB's renal insufficiency is a direct result of long-standing hypertension. SB is experiencing alterations in calcium and phosphorus metabolism. Decreased production of the active form of vitamin D in the kidney leads to a decrease in the amount of calcium absorbed from the GI tract. Parathyroid hormone is increased, but resistance in the bone soon develops and the serum calcium level continues to drop. Serum phosphorous is increased secondary to decreased renal excretion. Treatment involves calcium and vitamin D supplementation, and aluminum antacids to bind phosphorous in the gut. However, we can potentially use calcium acetate (Phos-Lo) to replace calcium and lower serum phosphorous. Treatment also involves limiting phosphorous intake. Furosemide is a good choice in SB to prevent fluid overload and help control hypertension. Caution must be taken since loop diuretics can increase serum uric acid levels, especially since the patient is taking niacin. SB is also suffering from anemia of chronic disease, most likely caused by inadequate production of erythropoietin in the kidney. Erythropoetin supplementation is indicated to minimize any effects of anemia on the cardiac status of SB. Iron supplements should be given to ensure adequate response to erythropoetin.

P: Continue furosemide. Start calcitriol, 0.25 mcg by mouth daily. The dose may be titrated up to 1 mcg/day. Start Phos-Lo (calcium acetate, 667 mg/tab), 2 tabs with each meal. Start erythropoetin, 50 to 150 units/kg subcutaneously three times a week, and ferrous sulfate, 325 mg PO TID. Titrate to achieve a 2 to 4% increase in hematocrit every 2 weeks. Maintain hematocrit at 30 to 35% to prevent hypertension.

CASE 81 QUESTIONS

1. Should SB be given an antiarrhythmic agent before cardioversion to maintain sinus rhythm?
2. How should verapamil or diltiazem be given to control the ventricular rate in SB?
3. Can SB receive anticoagulation therapy with aspirin instead of warfarin?
4. What are the recommended levels of lipoproteins in SB?
5. Should SB be loaded on warfarin to achieve steady-state anticoagulation faster?

CASE 82

CC: BL is a man, age 60, brought to the emergency department by paramedics. He states that although he has not felt up to par over the last few days and has had a lot of nausea, vomiting, and chest pain, he did not seek medical help because he thought it was related to a recent drinking spree and usual heartburn. Yesterday while bending over to tie his shoes, "it" really hit him and he stayed home from work. Although he has only had a few drinks in the last 24 hours, his heartburn got worse and he took a whole bottle of antacid, which only made him more nauseated. This afternoon, when he couldn't breathe and felt like he was going to die, he called the paramedics. While in the emergency department, he becomes increasingly short of breath, produces frothy white sputum, is hemodynamically unstable, and requires endotracheal intubation. After transfer to the CCU a Swan-Ganz catheter is placed.

Past Medical History

BL has a 20-year history of gastroesophageal reflux disease (GERD) and has been seen occasionally with complaints of chest pain related to this disease. He has mild hepatic cirrhosis and hyperlipidemia, for which he has been treated for the past 5 years.

Social History

BL is a chronic alcoholic, who has bouts of heavy drinking that exceed his usual half bottle of scotch daily.

Medication History

Mylanta, 30 mL PO PRN for heartburn for 20 years
Cimetidine, 400 mg PO QHS for 3 years
Niacin, 2 g PO TID for 5 years
Multivitamins, 1 QD

Physical Examination

GEN: BL is an ashen-faced, lightly jaundiced, thin male in acute distress. Before intubation he complained of SOB, "heartburn," nausea, and feeling he was dying; he was productive of frothy white sputum and diaphoretic.

VS: BP 70/35, HR 120, RR 35 (shallow), T 37.8, Wt 66 kg

HEENT: WNL

COR: JVD 10 cm, PMI displaced laterally, positive S_3 and S_4 heart sounds

CHEST: Bilateral rales in lower two thirds of all lung fields

ABD: Palpable liver 4 cm below the costal margin

GU: WNL

RECT: Guaiac-negative

EXT: 3+ pitting edema to knees; decreased peripheral pulses; cyanotic, cold, and clammy

NEURO: Alert and oriented on initial presentation

Results of Laboratory Tests

Na 138 (138)   Hct 0.39 (39)   AST 1.06 (64)   Glu 13.3 (240)
K 3.5 (3.5)   Hgb 130 (13)   ALT 0.56 (34)   Ca 2.22 (8.9)
Cl 102 (102)   Lkcs 13.4×10^9 (13.4×10^3)   ALDH 12.45 (750) PO_4 1.36 (4.2)
HCO_3 12 (12)   Plts 230×10^9 (230×10^3)   Alk Phos 2.6 (155)   Mg 1.15 (2.3)
BUN 13.6 (38)   MCV 106 (106)   Alb 32 (3.2)   Uric Acid WNL
Cr 203 (2.3)   T Bili 34 (2)   Cholesterol 8.90 (345)
            Triglyceride 2.11 (186)
            CK 31.6 (1904)

Lkc differential: WNL, no bands

Urinalysis: WNL

Chest x-ray: cardiomegaly, diffuse infiltrates two thirds up from base, consistent with pulmonary edema

ECG: sinus tachycardia, PVCs 5/min, S-T segment elevations to 5 mm, and Q waves in leads II, III, aVF, V1–V4

ABG (room air): pH 7.21, PO_2 60, PCO_2 40

Results of Special Laboratory Tests

Day	Time	CK	CK-MB	CK-MB Fract
Adm	1500	31.6 (1904)	5.69 (343)	0.18 (18)
1	2300	25.3 (1524)	3.54 (213)	0.14 (14)
1	0700	20.2 (1217)	2.42 (146)	0.12 (12)

Day	Time	LDH	LDH_1 Fract	LDH_2 Fract
Adm	1500	12.45 (750)	0.49 (49)	0.27 (27)
1	2300	15.60 (940)	0.54 (54)	0.31 (31)
1	0700	23.66 (1425)	0.57 (57)	0.30 (30)

Hemodynamic Parameters

	BL	Normal	Units
Central venous pressure (CVP)	14	0–5	mm Hg
Right atrial pressure (RAP)	16	2–6	mm Hg
Pulmonary artery diastolic (PAP)	28	12	mm Hg
Pulmonary capillary wedge (PCWP)	27	5–12	mm Hg
Cardiac index (C.I.)	1.6	2.5–3.5	$L/min/m^2$
Systemic vascular resistance (SVR)	2200	800–1200	$dyne\text{-}cm\text{-}s^{-5}$

PROBLEM LIST

1. Gastroesophageal reflux disease (20 years)
2. Hyperlipidemia (12 years)
3. Hepatic cirrhosis (more than 5 years)
4. Acute myocardial infarction (MI)
5. Cardiogenic shock/congestive heart failure
6. Alcohol withdrawal syndrome (AWS)

CASE 82 SOAP NOTES
Problem 5. Cardiogenic Shock/Congestive Heart Failure

S: SOB, feeling of impending doom

O: General: signs and symptoms of MI, diaphoretic, HCO_3 12 mmol/L (12 mEq/L), cardiomegaly. Pump (heart) failure: BP 70/35, HR 120, PMI laterally displaced, S_3 and S_4 heart sounds, SCr 203 mmol/L (2.3 mg/dL), BUN 13.6 mmol/L (38 mg/dL), decreased peripheral pulses with cyanotic, cold, and clammy extremities. Venous congestion: JVD 10 cm, palpable liver 4 cm below the costal margin, 3+ pitting edema to knees. Pulmonary edema: SOB, frothy white sputum, RR 35, and shallow, bilateral rales lower two thirds, chest x-ray. Hemodynamic parameters (from Swan-Ganz catheter): CVP 14 mm Hg, RAP 16 mm Hg, PAP 28 mm Hg, PCWP 27 mm Hg, C.I. 1.6 $L/min/m^2$, SVR 2200 dyne-cm-sec^{-5}

A: BL has numerous signs of cardiogenic shock. Despite tachycardia (HR 120) and reflex vasoconstriction (SVR 2200), he cannot maintain adequate peripheral perfusion because of low cardiac output (C.I. 1.6), despite the inordinately high left ventricular filling pressures (PCWP 27). He is tachypneic, and the work of breathing has diverted a significant portion of the cardiac output to the respiratory muscles. As a consequence of his low cardiac output and blood pressure, his renal function is impaired. Venous congestion (CVP 14) results from right-sided heart failure and volume overload. The right ventricular failure is probably caused by back-up from the left ventricle (PAP 28), augmented by acidosis and hypoxemia. He has combined metabolic (HCO_3 12) and respiratory acidosis (PCO_2 40, should be lower with hyperventilation, RR 35) secondary to hypoperfusion and pulmonary edema, respectively. He is in severe respiratory compromise and requires intubation. BL is in great jeopardy, he meets the criteria for subset IV, which has a mortality rate of more than 50%. His condition is deteriorating rapidly and requires immediate treatment.

P: Begin therapy in the emergency department and transfer BL to the CCU as soon as possible. Start oxygen at 100% by way of endotracheal (ET) tube to treat hypoxemia and metabolic acidosis. He will be hyperventilated with pressure support to counteract respiratory acidosis and reduce or eliminate the work of breathing. BL has venous congestion, pulmonary edema, reduced renal function, and apparent volume overload; therefore, begin gentle diuresis with furosemide, 10 mg IV; repeat, and increase dose as necessary, titrating to PCWP of 18 to 20 mm Hg. Given the rapid progression of BL's heart failure, a combination of dopamine and dobutamine should be started to enhance myocardial contractility by stimulation of β_1 receptors. Initiate both dopamine and dobutamine drips at 5 mg/kg/min and titrate (increasing dobutamine first) to a maximum of 20 mg/kg/min as required to maintain a systolic blood pressure (SBP) of more than 90 mm Hg and HR of less than 100 bpm.

Problem 4. Myocardial Infarction

S: Chest pain, nausea, vomiting, SOB, and feeling of impending doom

O: ECG: S-T segment elevations to 5 mm with Q waves in leads II, III, aVF, V_1–V_4. Admission laboratory test results specific for MI: CK 31.6 mkat/L (1904 U/L), MB fraction 0.18, LDH 12.45 ukat/L (750 U/L); and nonspecific results: increased AST 1.06 mmol/L (64), Lkcs 13.4 × 10^9/L (13.4 × 10^3/mm^3) with no left shift, elevated blood glucose 13.3 mmol/L (240), and electrolyte abnormalities.

A: BL exhibits many signs and symptoms of a massive anterior/inferior transmural MI. His ECG showed S-T segment elevations, Q waves, and PVCs 5/min, and concurrent pump failure, which are evidence of location and extent of infarction. The history of chest pain ("heartburn") and the elevated, but decreasing CK levels with high MB fraction and increasing LDH levels (LDH$_1$ > LDH$_2$) indicate that the MI occurred at least 24 hours ago. However, the patient also related that he had ongoing chest pain, which may indicate continued or expanding ischemia.

P: Draw blood for baseline coagulation studies. Give a bolus of heparin, 5000 units IV, and start an infusion of 1000 units/hr. Titrate the infusion rate to maintain PTT at 1.5 to 2 times more than control. Continue the heparin infusion for 7 to 10 days. As soon as possible, start aspirin 160 mg (two 80-mg chewable tablets) and continue daily for at least 1 month. As soon as BL's blood pressure permits (SBP > 90 mm Hg), start captopril, 6.25 mg PO TID, increase to 12.5 mg TID, then to 25 mg TID, as tolerated. If chest pain recurs, give SL nitroglycerin, 0.4 mg. BL requires evaluation of the extent of occlusion of his coronary arteries and should undergo angiography when he is stable.

Problem 6. Alcohol Abuse/Withdrawal

S: Nausea and vomiting

O: Hct 0.34 (34), Hgb 110 g/L (11 g/dL), MCV 106 fl (106 um^3), K 3.5 mmol/L (3.5 mEq/L) PO$_4$ 0.58 mmol/L (1.8 mg/dL), Mg 1.15 mmol/L (2.3 mEq/L), and a history of alcohol abuse with little alcohol in the last 24 hours.

A: BL is at risk for alcohol withdrawal. He is known to use at least one half bottle of scotch per day and has had only "a few drinks in the last 24 hours." Withdrawal from alcohol causes severe agitation, which would increase the demand on the heart and the potential for further heart failure and ischemia. BL is thin and has a decreased hematocrit, hemoglobin, and increased MCV levels, which may indicate poor dietary intake and associated anemia. He is hypokalemic, hypophosphatemic, and hypomagnesemic, because of poor intake, use of aluminum-containing antacids, and/or recent vomiting. He should receive treatment for presumed vitamin and nutrient deficiencies and correction of any electrolyte abnormalities. BL should receive treatment for alcohol withdrawal. Proper management may prevent progression to more serious and potentially life-threatening levels of alcohol withdrawal syndrome, seizures, Wernicke's syndrome, and delirium tremens (DTs) (see Chapter 59, "Alcoholism").

P: For alcohol withdrawal syndrome, give diazepam 2.5 to 10.0 mg slow IV push (2.5 mg/min) Q6H. Monitor BL closely for signs and symptoms of alcohol withdrawal: agitation, tremors, diaphoresis, hallucinations, seizures, and autonomic hyperactivity. At the first sign of any of these findings, give additional diazepam, 2.5 to 10 mg, until he

is calm, and increase the maintenance dose. Before starting other treatments, additional laboratory test results should be obtained for evaluation of anemia (CBC count with reticulocyte count and iron, transferritin, and B$_{12}$ levels). Give thiamine, 100 mg, and folic acid, 1 mg IV, now. He should also be given injectable multivitamins, which must be infused over 8 to 10 hours, usually added to a liter of maintenance fluid (e.g., D5 1/2 NS 20 K at 125 mL/hr). However, BL's heart failure and reduced renal function make the administration of large volumes of fluid undesirable, and a smaller volume given more slowly may be required. Replacement of potassium (as in problem 4) and phosphate can be accomplished by infusing a solution containing 12 mmol phosphate and 40 mEq potassium over 4 hours. The volume used depends on the type of IV access (200 mL for central or 400 mL for peripheral). Magnesium replacement is required immediately in order to maintain myocardial function and intracellular potassium concentrations. BL is not severely hypomagnesemic, therefore infuse 1 g in 50 to 100 mL DSW over 30 to 60 minutes. Recheck magnesium levels after the infusion is completed.

Problem 3. Hepatic Cirrhosis

S: Nausea, vomiting, "heartburn"

O: General description: jaundiced and thin; palpable liver 4 cm below the costal margin; elevated LFTs: T Bili 34 μmol/L (2), Alk Phos 2.6 ukat/L (155), AST 1.06 μmol/L (64); decreased Alb 32 gm/L (3.2 gm/dL), and a history of cirrhosis

A: BL has a history of mild cirrhosis, most likely secondary to alcohol consumption. His only sign of liver damage is a slightly low albumin level, which may also be caused by poor diet associated with alcohol abuse. He does, however, have signs of alcoholic hepatitis; jaundice; and elevated bilirubin and liver enzyme levels. Assessment of BL's cirrhosis is complicated by his MI and heart failure (cardiac cirrhosis?), which also cause elevations in LFTs. He has no signs or symptoms of the complications associated with advanced cirrhosis.

P: BL should have further evaluation of his liver function. Get PT and PTT and watch for other signs of advancing disease. Educate him on the effects of continued alcohol use. Refer him to a social worker and to Alcoholic Anonymous after discharge.

Problem 2. Hyperlipidemia

S: None

O: Cholesterol 8.90 (345); triglycerides 2.11 (186)

A: Hyperlipidemia is a major risk factor for CAD, and now BL has suffered a massive MI. Current treatment of niacin 2 g TID for 5 years is inadequate, since his lipids are still elevated; more aggressive therapy is indicated. However BL has mild hepatic cirrhosis and caution is indicated.

P: It is questionable whether BL has complied with his niacin therapy, since alcohol aggravates the flushing seen with niacin. When BL is able to take oral medications, increase niacin to 3 g PO TID, given with meals. If after 8 to 12 weeks of therapy BL's cholesterol and triglycerides are still elevated, add gemfibrozil 600 mg PO BID, 30 minutes before morning and evening meals. Monitor cholesterol and triglycerides every 2 weeks initially, then every 1 to 3 months. Potential adverse effects should be followed with LFT, CBC, and serum uric acid determinations.

Problem 1. Gastroesophageal Reflux Disease

S: Heartburn, vomiting

O: None

A: BL smokes and uses alcohol, factors that predispose him to GERD. He did not get any relief with antacids, his usual medication. It is unlikely that the present symptoms are caused by GERD. BL is intubated, has severe hemodynamic compromise, reduced renal function, and mild hepatic cirrhosis, factors that must be considered when deciding on treatment.

P: Discontinue cimetidine, which is known to decrease hepatic blood flow and alter renal clearance. Discontinue antacids, which if aspirated may cause severe pneumonitis. Give ranitidine, 50 mg IV Q8H, change to oral ranitidine, 150 mg, or cimetidine, 400 mg BID when BL has recovered from cardiogenic shock. He should be reeducated about smoking and foods to avoid: coffee and other caffeine-containing drinks, alcohol, chocolate, and fatty foods.

CASE 82 QUESTIONS

1. What effect does acidosis have on the treatment BL may receive for cardiogenic shock? Should bicarbonate be administered to correct his metabolic acidosis?

2. BL is hypotensive. In addition to positive inotropes, should drugs with vasoconstricting effects be used to augment his blood pressure?

3. What adverse effect(s) can be expected from the use of positive inotropes in BL?

4. Since both dopamine and dobutamine are effective in increasing cardiac contractility, why were they used in combination instead of either agent alone?

5. Why is anticoagulation therapy appropriate for BL? Should he be treated with warfarin following heparin? If yes, how long?

6. BL has suffered an MI and is receiving anticoagulation therapy. Why wasn't he given metoprolol?

7. Diazepam is used for treatment of BL's alcohol withdrawal syndrome (AWS). Evaluate the use of diazepam in BL. What effects of diazepam may be desirable/undesirable in BL?

8. Why is BL's hepatic cirrhosis a cause for caution in the treatment of his hyperlipidemia?

CASE 83

CC: MB is a woman, age 68, who has been brought into the emergency department by her daughter after MB experienced the onset of right-sided weakness and an inability to speak.

Past Medical History

MB has a history of atrial fibrillation since 1990, first noted after an acute viral illness. She has rheumatoid arthritis and a history of hyperthyroidism s/p ^{131}I. She has mild osteoporosis.

Medication History

Digoxin, 0.125 mg daily
Naproxen, 375 mg twice daily
Levothyroxine, 0.2 mg daily
Calcium carbonate, 1250 mg daily
Conjugated estrogens, 0.625 mg daily

Allergies

None known

Physical Examination

GEN: Lethargic, weak-appearing elderly woman unable to speak, respond to questions, or walk

VS: BP 100/80, P 110 irreg irreg, R 18, T 36.5, Wt 58 kg

HEENT: Thin hair, patches of baldness

COR: Normal heart sounds, mildly displaced PMI

CHEST: Clear to P and A

ABD: Benign

GU: Deferred

RECT: Guaiac-negative

EXT: R-sided weakness, mild deformities hands/fingers

NEURO: Consistent with stroke

Results of Laboratory Tests

Electrolyte levels: within normal limits
CBC count: normal indices

CR 50 (0.6)
Ca 2.5 (9.4)
PO$_4$ 1.2 (3.75)
PT 11.4
INR 1.0
APTT 26 sec

ESR 65 mm/hr

Thyroxine (TT4) 150 nmol/L (12 ug/dL)

TSH 3 mU/L (3 uM/dL)

RT3U 0.3 (30%)

FT41 3.6

ECG: Irregularly irregular, consistent with atrial fibrillation

CT scan: evidence consistent with acute embolic stroke

Echocardiogram: large left ventricular thrombus

PROBLEM LIST

1. Atrial fibrillation
2. Rheumatoid arthritis
3. Hyperthyroidism

4. Osteoporosis
5. Acute stroke

CASE 83 SOAP NOTES
Problem 5. Acute Stroke
S: MB is unable to respond to questions.

O: Aphasia, muscle weakness; CT scan results consistent with stroke; weak-appearing; unable to walk or respond to questions

A: Embolic stroke, most likely secondary to atrial fibrillation and the presence of large thrombus in the ventricle.

P: Since the diagnosis has been confirmed as an embolic stroke, antithrombotic therapy is indicated. This diagnosis is crucial because the presence of hemorrhage would contraindicate antithrombotic therapy. Treatment with thrombolytic agents such as tissue plasminogen activator (TPA) is being investigated in some centers, but it remains investigational at this time. Therapy with heparin is indicated and it should be initiated with a bolus dose of 80 to 100 units/kg. For MB, this would be approximately 5000 to 6000 units. Before initiation of therapy, baseline coagulation studies, a CBC count, and platelet count should be obtained. A continuous infusion of 15 to 25 u/kg/hr should follow the bolus dose. This would be 900 to 1500 units/hr. She may be at slightly higher risk for bleeding because of her age and the fact that she is on NSAID therapy for her arthritis. The infusion should be started at the lower range. The therapeutic aPTT is 60 to 80 seconds, and the aPTT should be checked 4 to 6 hours after the bolus dose; the infusion should be adjusted according to the aPTT results. MB should be monitored closely for bleeding, and appropriate laboratory studies (e.g., CBC, platelets, stool guaiac, urinalysis) done daily for the first few days and every other day thereafter. Warfarin therapy should be started on the first day with a maintenance dose of 5 mg/day. The goal INR is 2.0 to 3.0. Factors in MB that may influence her response include the NSAID and hyperthyroidism. The NSAID will be discussed in the treatment of arthritis. Hyperthyroidism will potentiate warfarin effects by accelerating the clearance of the vitamin K-dependent clotting factors without influencing the pharmacokinetics of warfarin. Her coagulation study results are normal; therefore, it is unlikely that there will be an unusual response. The prothrombin time should be monitored closely. Even though the patient has a hisory of osteoporosis, heparin is not contraindicated. The osteoporosis associated with heparin occurs after prolonged therapy (6 months or longer). MB should receive physical therapy for stroke rehabilitation.

Problem 1. Atrial Fibrillation
S: MB cannot give history because of stroke.

O: ECG: irregularly irregular; physical examination reveals HR of 110 (also irregular); history

A: Atrial fibrillation of long standing, since 1983

P: Several factors may have predisposed MB to the onset of the dysrhythmia, including the acute viral illness, the history of hyperthyroidism, and possible coronary artery disease (un-

documented). Because the atrial fibrillation is of such long standing, it will probably not be converted to normal sinus rhythm. This is because the left atrium is more likely to be dilated, and subsequently, the conduction system is abnormal. The primary goal is thus rate control. Digoxin is a logical agent to use, but in MB it must be used with caution. MB's underlying thyroid status will not only alter the pharmacokinetics of digoxin but will also make it difficult to achieve adequate rate control, since one of the mediators of the increased rate is increased sympathetic tone. Hyperthyroidism increases the requirements for digoxin, secondary to an increased volume of distribution and increased clearance. The increased sympathetic tone is best controlled with a β-blocker. Before a β-blocker is started, left ventricular function must be assessed, to prevent exacerbation of heart failure. Other β-blocker-induced problems must be considered as well, including reactive airway disease, peripheral vascular disease, and diabetes. If a β-blocker is indicated, the selection of a hydrophilic one (atenolol, nadolol, or even metoprolol, which is mixed) is appropriate, to avoid CNS side effects. MB's renal function is adequate, although the age-adjusted creatinine clearance rate is mildly depressed. Digoxin dose must be adjusted for MB's low weight and renal function. Calcium-channel blockers, such as verapamil or diltiazem, may be considered because of their ability to decrease AV nodal conduction, but they may be limited by her relative hypotension. With rate control, her blood pressure may go up slightly because ventricular filling may be better, and therefore she may tolerate the agent. Since the only evidence of heart failure is a mildly displaced PMI, the best course would be to evaluate left-ventricular function by a wall motion study or further echocardiographic study. If function is well preserved, the digoxin could be stopped and β-blockers initiated with metoprolol, 25 mg BID, titrating up to a specific heart rate response (may require 100 to 200 mg/day), or atenolol, 25 to 50 mg QD (up to 100 mg/day). If left ventricular function is depressed, digoxin may be continued with appropriate dosage adjustment. As the thyroid function changes, careful attention must be paid to adjust dosages appropriately. Regular ECG and appropriate drug levels should be maintained. A heart rate of 80 to 90 bpm is a reasonable goal.

Problem 2. Rheumatoid Arthritis
S: MB is unable to give a history.

O: Finger and hand deformities, history, increased ESR

A: Rheumatoid arthritis

P: Therapy is difficult because of the need for concomitant anticoagulation. NSAIDs are relatively contraindicated because of their potential for gastric irritation, antiplatelet effect, and direct drug interactions with warfarin. In addition, they can lead to fluid retention and renal insufficiency. If MB's LV function is adequate, these may be lesser problems. If an NSAID is indicated, the two agents that appear to be the least offending are ibuprofen and naproxen. Direct drug interactions with warfarin are less likely to occur, and their antiplatelet effects are acceptable. They may cause GI irritation, and antacid therapy should be used. Because of MB's weight, start with naproxen, 375 mg BID, or ibuprofen, 400 mg Q6H. She should have stool guaiac tests performed regularly and her PT should be checked often as well. Since warfarin is being started at the same time, daily PT tests will help identify any accelerated response that may occur. Alternative agents for arthritis are not without risk. Steroids should be avoided because of their serious side effects, including osteoporosis. Gold and antimalarials are possible but not indicated at this time, and methotrexate is not indicated (see Chapter 28, "Rheumatoid Arthritis and Its Therapy").

Problem 3. Hyperthyroidism

S: MB is unable to give a history.

O: Decreased weight, abnormal thyroid function test results, TT4 150 (12), TSH 3 (3), RT_3U 0.3 (30), FT_4I 3.6, atrial fibrillation, thin hair, excessive dosage of levothyroxine

A: MB has a history of hyperthyroidism treated with [131]I. Since then she has been treated with levothyroxine, which is excessive. The correct dosage is approximately 1 to 2 μg/kg (average, 1.7 μg/kg), which in MB is approximately 0.1 mg/day. Levothyroxine has a half-life of 6 to 7 days, so it can be safely held for up to a week and then reinstituted at the lower, more appropriate dose. Symptoms must be followed carefully, and the laboratory test results reevaluated in 2 to 4 weeks. Remember that as the thyroid function corrects, the atrial fibrillation will improve, and the medications used for the treatment of atrial fibrillation may need adjustment.

P: Hold levothyroxine for 1 week, restart at 0.1 mg/day. Reevaluate thyroid function test results in 2 to 4 weeks.

Problem 4. Osteoporosis

S: MB is unable to give a history.

O: By medical history; MB taking calcium and estrogens

A: The use of estrogens in MB is controversial. She is postmenopausal, and estrogens may help decrease bone loss, but they will not replace bone loss. It is not clear how long she has been taking them. To assess the need for them, she should have appropriate bone density and x-ray studies performed. If bone density is well preserved, the estrogens should be continued, even in the face of atrial fibrillation. Estrogen therapy may be a contributing factor in deep venous thrombosis, pulmonary embolism, and stroke in some women, but it is unlikely to be a factor in a stroke associated with atrial fibrillation. Calcium therapy in conjunction with estrogens is advisable, although her dosage is low; it is equivalent to 500 mg of elemental calcium per day and should be increased to 1000 to 1500 mg/day or three tablets of calcium carbonate (1 tab TID with meals) daily.

P: As above

CASE 83 QUESTIONS

1. How long should anticoagulation therapy be continued in a patient with atrial fibrillation?
2. What is the recommended intensity of therapy with warfarin for atrial fibrillation?
3. Is there a role for β-blockers with intrinsic sympathomimetic activity in patients like MB?
4. How do conjugated estrogens interact with warfarin?
5. Does MB have any significant risk factors for bleeding with warfarin other than those already discussed in the case?

CASE 84

CC: JF is a man, age 29, seen in the hypertension clinic for follow-up of two previous high blood pressure readings. He has had diabetes since age 23. He states that he always takes his medication as prescribed but has been unable to comply with the low-salt, low-cholesterol diet that was recommended during the last visit.

Past Medical History

Type I (insulin-dependent) diabetes mellitus (DM) for 6 years. Mitral valve replacement 3 months ago, secondary to rheumatic heart disease. Iron deficiency anemia, secondary to heart surgery.

Hypercholesterolemia

Social History

JF smokes one pack of cigarettes per day. No alcohol intake.

Medication History

$FeSO_4$, 325 mg QD for 1 month

Warfarin, 7.5 mg QD

Insulin Reg and NPH, recently switched from pork to human

Ibuprofen, PRN for headache

Allergies

Sulfonamides; lovastatin (severe adverse reaction)

Physical Examination

GEN: Well-developed, well-nourished man, weight 80 kg, complaining of increasing headaches, dark stools, polyuria, polydipsia, and general weakness. He has had some spots of blood on the tissue after the last few bowel movements, but no other bleeding. He recently ran out of his Chemstrips, and thus has not checked his blood glucose levels for 1 week. He also mentions that his regular insulin is not its usual color.

VS: BP 190/98, HR 76, T 37, RR 18, Wt 80 kg, Ht 173 cm

HEENT: AV nicking; remainder of examination within normal limits

COR: NL S_1 & S_2

CHEST: NL

ABD: Soft without masses

GU: NL

RECT: Small external hemorrhoid

EXT: NL

NEURO: Oriented × 3

Results of Laboratory Tests

Na 143 (143)	Hct 0.34 (34)	ALT 0.37 (22)	Glu (Fasting) 22.2 (400)	INR 4.9	
K 4.5 (4.5)	Hgb 142 (14.2)	LDH 1.6 (95)	Ca 2.25 (9.0)	PTR 2.15	
Cl 103 (103)	Lkcs 9.0 × 10⁹ (9.0 × 10³)	Alk Phos 0.8 (45)	PO₄ 1.45 (4.5)	Hg 13.5	
HCO₃ 24 (24)	Plts 200 × 10⁹ (200 × 10³)	Alb 40 (4.0)	Mg 0.8 (1.6)	TG 3.6 (320)	
BUN 7.9 (22)	MCV 84 (84)	T Bili 17.1 (1.0)	Uric Acid 386 (6.5)	Chol 7.24 (280)	
CR 70.1 (0.8)	AST 0.5 (30)		PT 26.0; Control 12.0	LDL 1.81 (70)	
			PTT 47; Control 27.1	HDL 0.78 (30)	

Urinalysis: + 1 protein; – ketones; 0–1 RBCs/hpf; 2% glucose

Chest x-ray: Moderate cardiomegaly; bilateral fluffy infiltrates

ECG: WNL

PROBLEM LIST

1. Type I DM
2. Anticoagulation for mitral valve replacement
3. Anemia
4. Hypercholesterolemia
5. Hypertension

CASE 84 QUESTIONS

1. What if JF develops a severe persistent cough? What are the alternative antihypertensive agents?
2. Would addition of hydrochlorothiazide worsen JF's glycemic control? Could his hyperlipidemia worsen from a thiazide?
3. Should JF be asked about possible sexual dysfunction? Which antihypertensive drugs may cause or worsen sexual dysfunction?
4. Which antihypertensive drugs may actually worsen left ventricular hypertrophy (cardiomegaly)? What added risk is seen in hypertensive patients with LVH?
5. If JF were not taking iron, what would be the most likely cause of his melena?

CASE 85

CC: TA is a man, age 55, who is admitted from the clinic for workup and evaluation of a nonproductive cough, dyspnea, pleuritic chest pain, and a 4-kg weight loss.

Past Medical History

TA has a 30-year history of hypertension and a 10-year history of coronary artery disease, which were poorly controlled because of poor patient compliance. Two years ago, TA had an inferior wall myocardial infarction (MI) and developed sustained ventricular tachycardia (V-tach). Therapy with lidocaine, procainamide, and tocainide failed to prevent recurrences of V-tach. An electrophysiologic study (EPS), performed in the drug-free state, revealed sustained monomorphic V-tach that remained inducible during therapy with quinidine sulfate and flecainide acetate. Amiodarone therapy was instituted; after a loading of 18 g over a period of 10 days, a repeated EPS demonstrated nonsustained V-tach that was more difficult to induce, slower, and self-terminating.

There was no spontaneous recurrence of the V-tach on telemetry or 24-hour Holter monitoring. TA was discharged with a regimen of amiodarone, 400 mg daily. Subsequent to the MI, TA had symptoms of congestive heart failure (CHF), controlled on furosemide. Endoscopy 6 months ago showed a healed duodenal ulcer with moderate-to-severe gastritis. TA's angina has worsened over the past 6 months. Currently TA has 3 to 5 episodes of chest pain per week. TA presented with complaints of dyspnea, a nonproductive cough, and a 4-kg weight loss over the past 2 months.

Social History

TA has smoked one pack of cigarettes per day for 40 years. Currently he smokes 1 to 2 packs per week. On the average, he drinks a six-pack of beer per week.

Medication History

Amiodarone, 400 mg daily
Furosemide, 20 mg twice daily
Nitroglycerin, 0.4 mg as needed for chest pain
Cimetidine, 800 mg daily at bedtime
Ketoprofen, 75 mg three times daily

Allergies

No known drug allergies

Physical Examination

GEN: TA is an anxious man, appearing older than his stated age, who complains of pleuritic chest pain, dyspnea, and a nonproductive cough.
VS: BP 120/90, HR 105, T 38.2, RR 20, Wt 68 kg
HEENT: AV nicking and narrowing, corneal microdeposits
COR: Normal S_1, S_2, and + S_4
CHEST: Bilateral rales and pleural rub
ABD: WNL
RECT: Guaiac-positive
EXT: 1+ ankle edema, bluish-gray skin discoloration on sun-exposed areas

Results of Laboratory Tests

Na 134 (134)	Hct 0.32 (0.32)	ALT 0.64 (38)	Ca 2.22 (8.9)
K 3.3 (3.3)	Hgb 110 (11)	LDH 3.18 (192)	PO₄ 0.87 (2.7)
Cl 102 (102)	Lkcs 8.3 × 10⁹ (8.3 × 10³)	Alk Phos 0.8 (45)	Mg 1.15 (2.3)
HCO₃ 28 (28)	Plts 186 × 10⁹ (186 × 10³)	Alb 38 (3.8)	Uric Acid 400 (6.8)
BUN 6.1 (17)	MCV 70 (70)	T bili 14 (0.8)	PT 3.2 sec
Cr 106 (1.2)	AST 0.70 (42)	Glu 7.66 (138)	ESR 43 mm/hr

Lkc differential: WNL

Urinalysis: WNL

Chest x-ray films: Bilateral diffuse interstitial infiltrates

ECG: Shows evidence of old inferior wall MI; voltage changes consistent with LVH; currently is in sinus tachycardia with a rate of 100 bpm

Gallium scan: Increased lung uptake

Pulmonary function tests:

Baseline (2 years ago)
FEV$_1$ 81% predicted
TLC 105% predicted
DLCO 85% predicted
Current
FEV$_1$ 74% predicted
TLC 88% predicted
DLCO 45% predicted
Endoscopy: Moderate gastritis, no active ulcers, scarring from old ulcers

PROBLEM LIST
1. Hypertension for 30 years
2. Degenerative joint disease (DJD) for 10 years
3. Angina for 10 years
4. Peptic ulcer disease for 5 years
5. Congestive heart failure for 2 years
6. Ventricular arrhythmias for 2 years
7. Amiodarone toxicity
8. Anemia

CASE 85 QUESTIONS
1. TA is having difficulty swallowing the KCl tablet (K-Dur) because of its large size. The intern is considering switching to the liquid preparation. What recommendations do you have?
2. What patient education would you give TA about the proper use and storage of his nitroglycerin (NTG)?
3. Four months from now, TA returns to clinic complaining of a new-onset persistent cough that is extremely bothersome, especially at night. The cough prevents TA from sleeping. The intern feels this is still the amiodarone toxicity. What do you think?
4. The intern decides to discontinue the enalapril and would like you to suggest the medication TA should be started on for his CHF.
5. The intern wants to start TA on digoxin. What dose do you recommend? TA's current weight is 72 kg and current SCr is 106 (1.2 mg/dL).

CASE 86
CC: RS is a woman, age 58, who is in the clinic today for follow-up evaluation of angina pectoris. At her last visit, she was initiated on a nitroglycerin (NTG) transdermal patch, 0.4 mg/hr Q24H, and sublingual NTG, 0.4 mg PRN. She states that during the first week of this therapy the number of anginal episodes decreased from 4 to 5/week to 1 to 2/week; thereafter the episodes returned to 4 to 5 times/week. All of these anginal episodes occurred during physical exertion and were relieved by rest and administration of one sublingual NTG. RS is able to walk 4 to 5 blocks before developing chest pains. She denies fatigue, shortness of breath (SOB), orthopnea, and paroxysmal nocturnal dyspnea (PND).

Past Medical History
RS had a lateral myocardial infarction (MI) in November 1989. She also has a history of mild congestive heart failure (CHF); chronic atrial fibrillation resistant to quinidine, procainamide, and propafenone; and hypercholesterolemia.

Medication History
Digoxin, 0.125 mg QD
Furosemide, 40 mg QD
Warfarin, 5 mg QD
Lovastatin, 20 mg QPM
Captopril, 12.5 mg TID
KCl, 20 mEq BID
Nitroglycerin, 0.4 mg SL PRN
Nitroglycerin patch, 0.4 mg/hr Q24H

Physical Examination
GEN: Adult female in NAD
VS: BP 136/82, P-ventricular response 62 and irregular, RR 18, Wt 53.2 kg, Ht 165 cm
HEENT: PERRLA, EOM-I
COR: S$_1$, S$_2$, and S$_3$ heart sound, no JVD or HJR, no murmur
CHEST: Clear to auscultation and percussion
ABD: Soft, nontender with bowel sounds
GU: WNL
RECT: WNL
EXT: Normal pulses throughout, no peripheral edema
NEURO: Cranial nerves II-XII grossly intact, oriented × 3

Results of Laboratory Tests

Na+: 142 (142)	Hct: 0.40 (40.9)	RBC 4.64 × 1012 (4.64 × 10^6)
K+: 4.8 (4.8)	Hgb: 136 (13.6)	Chol 5.20 (200)
Cl: 103 (103)	Lkcs: 7.8 × 10^9 (7.8 × 10^3)	LDL 3.00 (115)
HCO$_3$: 25 (25)	Plts 333 × 10^9 (333 × 10^3)	VLDL 0.98 (38)
BUN: 60 (18)		HDL 1.2 (47)
SCr: 100 (1.1)		Trig 2.14 (190)
		Digoxin 1.8 (1.4)
		PT 18.8

Lkc Differential: Segs 0.64 (64), Bands 0.04 (4), Lymphs 0.29 (29), Monos 0.03 (3), Eos 0 (0) Baso 0 (0)

ECG: Atrial fibrillation with ventricular rate of 65 bpm

PROBLEM LIST
1. Atrial fibrillation
2. Congestive heart failure
3. Hypercholesterolemia
4. Coronary artery disease

CASE 86 QUESTIONS
1. While receiving counseling about her prescription medications from the pharmacist, RS asks about the use of ASA for the treatment of minor aches and pains. Would ASA be a safe OTC analgesic for RS to use on an occasional basis?

2. While reviewing RS's medication profile it is noticed that she is receiving a potassium supplement. What potential problems exist with regard to potassium homeostasis in RS, and how should they be managed?

3. RS returns to the clinic in 2 months with worsening CHF symptoms (pedal edema and dyspnea on exertion). What change in her maintenance medication regimen should be made to more effectively manage her CHF?

4. A random serum digoxin level from a sample drawn during one of RS's follow-up visits is reported as 5.76 nmol/L (4.5 ng/ mL). What is the most likely explanation for this elevated serum level, and how should it be handled?

5. During a routine clinic visit, a chemistry profile was obtained and an elevated uric acid level was noticed. RS does not have any symptoms of gout at this time. How should her hyperuricemia be managed?

CASE 87

CC: JO is a woman, age 28, who came to the emergency department complaining of intense pleuritic chest pain that came on suddenly. She also noted difficulty breathing and coughed up some bright red blood. She additionally states that before this time she had felt fine.

Past Medical History

JO has a history of palpitations and has been diagnosed as having mitral valve prolapse and paroxysmal supraventricular tachycardia (PSVT). This has not bothered her often, and she is currently controlling it with atenolol, 50 mg daily. She has a history of irritable bowel syndrome and iron deficiency anemia.

Medication History

Atenolol, 50 mg daily
Psyllium, 2 tablespoonsful daily
Ferrous fumarate, one tablet daily
Birth control pills (35 µg ethinyl estradiol □1 mg norethindrone, 21 days per month

Allergies

Bee stings cause generalized swelling; no known drug allergies

Physical Examination

GEN: Anxious-appearing young woman, sitting upright, complaining of shortness of breath and chest pain
VS: BP 155/95, P 110 reg, RR 25, T 37.8, Wt 62 kg
HEENT: WNL
COR: N1 S_1 mid-systolic click heard best along the left lower sternal border; negative S_3, S_4; increased P2

CHEST: Decreased breath sounds
ABD: Slight guarding
GU: Deferred
RECT: Guaiac-negative
EXT: Without clubbing, cyanosis, or edema
NEURO: Intact, alert, and oriented × 3

Results of Laboratory Tests

Na 141 (141)	Hct 0.33 (33)	AST 0.36 (27)	Glu 5 (95)
K 3.9 (3.9)	Hgb 110 (11)	ALT 0.38 (29)	Uric Acid 160 (3.0)
Cl 104 (104)	Lkcs 6 × 10⁹ (6 × 10³)	LDH 1.06 (75)	
HCO₃ 28 (28)	Plts 240 × 10⁹ (240 × 10³)	Alk Phos 1.88 (110)	
	MCV 85 (85)	Alb 42 (4.2)	
		T Bili 16 (0.9)	

Urinalysis: esterase +

Chest x-ray: Slight density in lower lobes

ECG: Sinus tachycardia with normal intervals.

ABGs: pO2 69, pCO2 36, pH 7.38

Ventilation perfusion scan (V/Q) shows a ventilation perfusion mismatch consistent with pulmonary embolism.

Pulmonary angiography confirms the diagnosis and localizes the clot to a large pulmonary artery.

PROBLEM LIST

1. Mitral valve prolapse
2. PSVT
3. Irritable bowel syndrome
4. Iron deficiency anemia
5. Pulmonary embolism
6. Contraception
7. Possible Urinary Tract Infection (UTI)

CASE 87 QUESTIONS

1. What are the nonhemorrhagic side effects of fibrinolytic agents?
2. How long should warfarin therapy be continued in the treatment of pulmonary embolism?
3. Is aspirin contraindicated in patients taking warfarin?
4. What is the risk to the fetus if a patient becomes pregnant when taking warfarin?
5. Is heparin a safe alternative to warfarin in a patient who wishes to become pregnant while taking warfarin?

CASE 88

CC: AR is a man, age 69, who presents to the cardiology clinic feeling nauseated and extremely fatigued.

Past Medical History

AR has a 6-month history of congestive heart failure (CHF) and was started on digoxin and furosemide at that time. At his last clinic visit 2 weeks ago, his digoxin dose was increased to 0.375 mg secondary to a level of 0.51 nmol/L (0.4 ng/ mL). AR was diagnosed with Addison's disease at age 30. AR has a 10-year history of hypertension.

Medication History

Digoxin, 0.375 mg PO QD
Furosemide, 40 mg PO QAM
Hydrocortisone, 20 mg PO QAM and 10 mg PO QPM
Fludrocortisone, 0.2 mg PO QD
Enalapril, 5 mg PO QAM
KCl, 10 mEq PO BID

Allergies

Contrast dye (rash)

Physical Examination

GEN: Well-developed, well-nourished, appearing pale and fatigued
VS: BP 160/95, HR 48, RR 18, Wt 70 kg, Ht 183 cm
HEENT: WNL
COR: Displaced PMI
CHEST: Clear
ABD: Positive bowel sounds
GU: Slightly enlarged prostate
RECT: Deferred
EXT: Ankle edema, excess skin pigmentation noted
NEURO: Oriented × 4

Results of Laboratory Tests

Na 145 (145)	Hct 0.39 (39)	AST 0.5 (30)	Glu 6.1 (110)
K 3.0 (3.0)	Hgb 140 (14)	ALT 0.5 (30)	Ca 2.2 (8.8)
Cl 96 (96)	Lkcs 8.5 × 10⁹ (8.5 × 10³)	LDH 1.7 (100)	PO₄ 0.97 (3.0)
HCO₃ 22 (22)	Plts 350 × 10⁹ (350 × 10³)	Alk Phos 1.5 (90)	Mg 1.0 (2.0)
BUN 3.5 (10)	MCV 80 (80)	Alb 50 (5.0)	Uric Acid 172 (2.9)
CR 106 (1.2)		T Bili 3.4 (0.2)	Digoxin 3.2 (2.5)

Lkc differential: WNL
Urinalysis: WNL
Chest x-ray: Enlarged cardiac silhouette
ECG: 1st-degree AV block, bradycardia

PROBLEM LIST

1. Addison's disease
2. Hypertension
3. CHF
4. Digoxin toxicity
5. Hypokalemia

CASE 89

CC: DA is a woman, age 57, who returns to the clinic for follow-up after being discharged from the hospital 3 days ago.

Past Medical History

DA came to the emergency department 10 days ago with an anterior wall myocardial infarction (MI). Immediately after MI, DA experienced intermittent bradycardia with occasional PVCs. DA was discharged with a 24-hour Holter monitor. Before DA's myocardial infarction, the frequency of anginal at-

tacks increased to 8 to 10 episodes per week. Previously she had an average of 2 episodes a week.

DA has experienced multiple episodes of Crohn's disease since age 25. Currently her Crohn's disease is in remission. Her last flare resolved 6 months ago. DA developed anginal pains 5 years ago. DA has had a long history of uncontrolled hypertension, which has resulted in congestive heart failure (CHF).

Past Surgical History

T and A, age 9
Appendectomy, age 22
Intestinal resection for enterocutaneous fistula, age 45

Social History

DA has smoked one and a half packs of cigarettes per day for 43 years. She continues to smoke. She drinks alcohol occasionally.

Family History

DA's mother died at age 55 of lung cancer, and her father died at age 61 of congestive heart failure. She has three children, all alive and well.

Medication History

Aspirin, 325 mg daily
Metoprolol, 25 mg twice daily
Nitroglycerin, 0.4 mg as needed for chest pain
Hydrochlorothiazide (HCTZ), 50 mg twice daily
KCl, 10 mEq daily
Sulfasalazine, 500 mg four times daily
Prednisone, 5 mg daily

Allergies

Allergic to penicillin and novocaine

Physical Examination

GEN: Slightly obese female with round face, in moderate distress, complaining of increasing palpitations, increased leg edema, nocturia, and SOB
VS: BP 150/100, HR 110, T 37.3, RR 24, Wt 70 kg, Ht 158 cm
HEENT: AV nicking and narrowing, retinal exudates
COR: Normal S₁, S₂, + S₃, and + S₄ with gallop, + JVD, - HJR
CHEST: Bilateral rales
ABD: Soft, nontender, hepatomegaly, abdominal striae
GU: Deferred
RECT: Guaiac-negative
EXT: 2+ ankle edema

Results of Laboratory Tests

Na 137 (137)	Hct 0.37 (37)	AST 0.42 (25)	Glu 7.05 (127)
K 4.7 (4.7)	Hgb 123 (12.3)	ALT 0.32 (19)	Ca 2.27 (9.1)
Cl 103 (103)	Lkcs 4.8 × 10⁹ (4.8 × 10³)	LDH 1.30 (78)	PO₄ 1.0 (3.2)
HCO₃ 23 (23)	Plts 220 × 10⁹ (220 × 10³)	Alk Phos 0.88 (53)	Mg 0.9 (1.8)
BUN 8.57 (24)	MCV 75 (75)	Alb 35 (3.5)	Uric Acid 320 (5.3)
SCr 177 (2.0)		T bili 17.1 (1)	PT 13.2

Lkc differential: WNL

Urinalysis: WNL

Chest x-ray: Not available

ECG: Shows evidence of anterior wall MI, voltage changes consistent with LVH, currently in sinus tachycardia at a rate of 110 bpm with occasional multiform premature ventricular contractions

Holter monitor: Tape shows that DA has multiform premature ventricular contractions at a frequency of approximately 100/hr.

PROBLEM LIST

1. Crohn's disease for 27 years
2. Hypertension for 20 years
3. Renal insufficiency for 5 years (result of uncontrolled hypertension)
4. Angina for 5 years
5. CHF for 2 years
6. S/P MI with arrhythmias

CASE 90

CC: SK is a man, age 45, brought to the emergency department Monday at 8 PM by two friends. Although confused and severely short of breath, he is able to complain loudly of crushing chest pain radiating to his neck, jaw, and left arm. His friends state that he was in his usual state of health when they arrived to watch the football game. They had pizza and shared a few six-packs of beer during the game. At halftime, SK complained of feeling sick, took a couple of swigs of antacid, stuck a tablet under his tongue and seemed better, although he spent most of the rest of the game in the bathroom. At the end of the fourth quarter, when his team failed to make the game-winning field goal, SK, red-faced and sweating, jumped out of his chair yelling, grabbed his chest, and fell back. His friends stuck two of his nitroglycerin tablets under his tongue and brought him to the emergency department.

Past Medical History

SK was admitted in 1989 for chest pain. Coronary angiography revealed 70% occlusion of the left anterior descending (LAD) artery, and 50 to 60% occlusion of the left circumflex arteries. ECG showed no ischemic changes. On his last clinic visit 6 months ago, he complained of increasing frequency of chest pain, i.e., 10 attacks per week. SK has moderately controlled insulin-dependent diabetes and 2 previous admissions for diabetic ketoacidosis. His past medical history is also significant for hypertension and hypercholesterolemia.

Medication History

Insulin Human Regular, 10 Units SC QAM and QPM
Insulin Human NPH, 10 Units SC QAM and QPM

Verapamil SR, 120 mg PO QD for 1 year
Furosemide, 40 mg PO BID for 6 months
Nitroglycerin, 0.4 mg SL PRN for chest pain for 2 years
Isosorbide dinitrate, 10 mg PO TID for 6 months
Cholestyramine, 4 g PO TID for 8 years
Lovastatin, 20 mg PO QD for 2 years

Physical Examination

GEN: SK is a confused, anxious, red-faced, well-developed, well-nourished man in moderate distress. He is tachypneic and diaphoretic and complains of severe (9 out of 10) chest pain radiating to his neck, jaw, and left arm.

VS: BP 180/100, HR 120, RR 45, T 38.3, Wt 78 kg

HEENT: AV nicking and narrowing

COR: Positive S_3 and S_4 gallop

CHEST: Clear to auscultation and percussion

ABD: Central obesity

GU: WNL

RECT: Guaiac-negative

EXT: Edema to midcalf

NEURO: Mildly confused, alert, and oriented × 3

ECG: Sinus tachycardia; S-T segment elevations to 6 mm in leads I, II, V_1 to V_6; flattened T waves.

Clinical presentation and ECG findings result in a diagnosis of evolving anterior wall myocardial infarction (MI). Appropriate therapy is started in the emergency department. SK is transferred to the coronary care unit (CCU); at 4:30 AM, multifocal premature ventricular contractions develop and rapidly deteriorate to ventricular fibrillation. SK becomes diaphoretic and loses consciousness. Systolic BP drops to 55 mm Hg and then becomes unmeasurable.

Results of Laboratory Tests

Na 135 (135)	Hct 0.40 (40)	AST 0.08 (48)	Glu 23.3 (420)
K 3.0 (3)	Hgb 130 (13)	ALT 0.38 (23)	Ca 4.15 (8.3)
Cl 105 (105)	Lkcs 12 × 10⁹ (12 × 10³)	LDH 7.3 (440)	PO₄ 1.03 (3.2)
HCO₃ 20 (20)	Plts 170 × 10⁹ (170 × 10³)	Alb 41 (4.1)	Mg 0.55 (1.1)
BUN 8.6 (24)			PT 11.5
Cr 110 (1.3)			PTT 34.8

Cholesterol 6.21 mmol/L (240)

Triglycerides 1.5 mmol/L (135)

ABG: pH 7.54, PO$_2$ 70, PCO$_2$ 25

Lkc differential: WNL, no bands

Urinalysis: 2% glucose, (−) ketones, (−) protein

Chest x-ray: WNL

Day	Time	CK	CK-MB	CK-MB Fract
Adm	2000	7.84 (472)	0.55 (33)	0.07 (7)
1	0400	15.5 (930)	1.86 (111)	0.12 (12)
1	1200	39.7 (2380)	7.93 (476)	0.20 (20)
		LDH	LDH₁ Fract	LDH₂ Fract
Adm	2000	7.33 (440)	0.43 (43)	0.28 (28)
1	0600	14.0 (840)	0.48 (48)	0.34 (34)
1	1200	22.0 (1320)	0.53 (53)	0.31 (31)

PROBLEM LIST

1. Insulin-dependent diabetes for 35 years
2. Hypertension for 20 years
3. Hypercholesterolemia for more than 10 years
4. Coronary artery disease (CAD) for more than 2 years
Added after admission:
5. Acute myocardial infarction (AMI)
6. Electrolyte abnormalities
7. Ventricular arrhythmias
8. Constipation

CASE 91

CC: WM is a male business executive, age 58, who recently returned from a trip to the Middle East. After arriving home, he noted swelling in his right calf and thigh accompanied by tenderness and redness. He has noted swelling in both legs recently, but this new episode is different, and the right leg is definitely more swollen than the left. He denies chest pain or shortness of breath. He exercises very little and is approximately 40 pounds overweight.

Past Medical History

WM was diagnosed as having Wolff-Parkinson-White (WPW) syndrome 6 years ago. He failed numerous antiarrhythmic drugs and is presently taking amiodarone. He has noted decreased exercise tolerance and that his shoes and pants are tighter than usual. A recent physical examination demonstrated abnormal liver function test results. He is overweight and admits to eating anything and everything he likes!

Social History

A heavy drinker, WM drinks several martinis with lunch and dinner plus two to three glasses of wine per day.

Medication History

Amiodarone, 200 mg daily for 5 years
Diphenhydramine, 25 to 50 mg Q6H PRN for itching
Alka Seltzer, PRN for headache pain

Physical Examination

GEN:	Obese male with smell of alcohol on breath
VS:	BP 110/70, HR 60, RR 16, Wt 125 kg, Ht 183 cm
HEENT:	Large neck, EOM intact, PERRLA, icteric sclera
COR:	Sustained impulse, nl S_1, S_2
CHEST:	Clear to P and A
ABD:	Obese, enlarged and palpable liver
GU:	nl
RECT:	Guaiac-negative
EXT:	Enlarged, red, painful R leg greater than L, 3+ pitting edema both lower extremities, decreased pulses bilaterally
NEURO:	Alert and oriented × 3, cranial nerves intact

Results of Laboratory Tests

Na 138 (138)	Hct 0.38 (38)	AST 7.26 (220)	Glu 6.1 (105)
K 3.5 (3.5)	Hgb 130 (13)	ALT 7.0 (200)	Ca 2.2 (8.8)
Cl 96 (96)	Lkcs 3.8×10^9 (3.8×10^3)	LDH 2.66 (150)	PO_4 0.8 (2.5)
HCO_3 24 (24)	Plts 200×10^9 (200×10^3)	Alb 35 (3.5)	Uric Acid 510 (8.5)
BUN 5.5 (18)	MCV 103 (103)	T Bili 78 (3.9)	
CR 110 (1.2)			

PT 13.2 sec INR 1.3 aPTT 30.2 sec (control 24–36)
Venogram: Consistent with filling defect in right calf and thigh
ECG: NSR 0.22/0.10/0.52 (PR/QRS/QT)
Chest x-ray: Slightly enlarged heart, normal lung fields

PROBLEM LIST

1. WPW syndrome
2. Obesity
3. Abnormal liver function test results
4. Deep venous thrombosis
5. Hyperuricemia
6. Alcohol abuse
7. Anemia

SKIN DISEASES

CASE 92

CC: BF is a woman, age 35, who complains of red, scaling skin on her elbows and knees. She is anxious and frustrated about not being able to stop smoking.

History of Present Illness

BF has noticed scaling plaques on her elbows and knees for several weeks, which seem to have become increasingly red and itchy. She notes no previous similar symptoms and admits that she has been afraid to put any lotions on the area for fear of making it worse. BF has attempted to quit smoking for the third time this year, but each time has returned to smoking after experiencing anxiety, insomnia, hunger, irritability, depression, and the craving for cigarettes.

Past Medical History

History of severe dysmenorrhea before initiation of oral contraceptives 10 years ago

Medication History

Ortho Novum 1/35 for 10 years

Allergies

Penicillin: rash

Social History

Tobacco: 2 packs/day for 10 years
Alcohol: drinks wine socially

Physical Examination

GEN: Well-developed, well-nourished female in no acute distress
VS: BP 120/70, HR 72, RR 16, T 37.1, Wt 50 kg, Ht 165 cm
HEENT: WNL
COR: RRR, S_1, S_2, no murmurs
CHEST: Clear to auscultation
ABD: Soft, nontender, nondistended
GU: WNL
RECT: WNL
EXT: Erythematous, dry, scaling psoriatic plaques on elbows and knees bilaterally
NEURO: Oriented X 3, CN II-XII intact

Results of Laboratory Tests

Na 142 (142)	Hct 0.4 (40)	AST 0.38 (23)	Glu 5.6 (100)
K 4.1 (4.1)	Hbg 130 (13.0)	ALT 0.43 (25)	Ca 2.3 (9.2)
Cl 98 (98)	Lkcs 6.0×10^9 (6.0×10^3)	LDH 1.2 (70)	PO_4 1.2 (3.6)
HCO_3 26 (26)	Plts 210×10^9 (210×10^3)	Alk Phos 1.17 (70)	Mg 1.1 (2.1)
BUN 4.3 (12)	MCV 85 (85)	Alb 40 (4.0)	
CR 76 (1.0)		T Bili 17.1 (1.0)	

PROBLEM LIST

1. Smoking cessation
2. Psoriasis
3. Contraception

CASE 92 SOAP NOTES
Problem 1. Smoking Cessation

S: Three failed attempts to quit smoking this year. BF experiences anxiety, insomnia, hunger, irritability, depression, and craving for cigarettes on trying to quit.

O: None

A: BF desires to quit smoking. BF has had made several attempts to quit smoking but has been unsuccessful because of bothersome symptoms. These symptoms (i.e., anxiety, restlessness, irritability, depression, insomnia, difficulty concentrating, and craving) are typical nicotine withdrawal symptoms. BF's desire to quit and the fact that she has experienced withdrawal symptoms when not smoking, make her a candidate for therapy. Many smokers can quit smoking without any therapy, but BF's failure to do so justifies initiating therapy. Her options include behavioral and/or pharmacologic treatment. Nicotine replacement decreases the withdrawal symptoms that are often responsible for the return to smoking after patients have tried to quit. Because BF's failed attempts to quit smoking seem largely a result of withdrawal symptoms, pharmacologic therapy is indicated. Group behavioral therapy may also aid BF; these programs often involve counseling, psychological support, and education.

Nicotine replacement in the form of nicotine gum seems less reliable in decreasing craving than does transdermal nicotine. This is likely because transdermal nicotine produces a more constant and higher level of nicotine. Also, the nicotine patch avoids the local oral adverse effects commonly associated with the gum (polacrilex); however, some patients feel they need to do something with their mouth and prefer the gum. Thus, the patch plus the gum may be beneficial in some patients.

P: BF should be started on a nicotine patch. Group therapy should also be encouraged. The higher dose patch (21 mg, Habitrol or Nicoderm; 15 mg, Nicotrol) should be used initially for 4 to 12 weeks, depending on the system used. If BF successfully abstains from smoking during this time, therapy should be continued at reduced doses. A

127

sample regimen would be Nicoderm, 21 mg for 4 to 6 weeks, then 14 mg for 2 to 4 weeks, followed by the 7 mg patch for 2 to 4 weeks. BF needs to be counseled to completely stop smoking while using the nicotine patch to avoid experiencing side effects from increased nicotine. BF should be told to apply the patch to a clean, dry, hairless area of skin on the trunk or upper outer arm, to rotate sites, and to avoid placing the patch on damaged skin (avoid areas with psoriatic plaques). BF should be monitored for symptoms of excess nicotine and the dose should be adjusted as necessary.

Problem 2. Psoriasis

S: Red, scaly, itchy skin on elbows and knees for several weeks: Erythematous, dry scaling psoriatic plaques on elbows and knees bilaterally

A: BF is experiencing a flare of psoriasis. This appears to be a new onset psoriasis as she recalls no previous similar symptoms. Although there is no cure for psoriasis, the goal is to achieve long periods of remission. Treatment options for psoriasis include topical therapy, phototherapy, and systemic therapy. In BF, who is experiencing relatively localized disease (elbows and knees), topical therapy is the first-line approach. Also, BF is newly diagnosed and thus has not yet failed topical therapy; therefore, more aggressive measures are inappropriate.

A common therapeutic agent for psoriasis is topical corticosteroids. They are thought to act by decreasing DNA synthesis and epidermal mitosis. Short courses of moderate to high potency topical steroids are often successful in clearing psoriasis, but in some individuals, may only lead to short remissions. In addition, the skin atrophy that may occur with long-term use of potent topical steroids is an important consideration. Thus, these agents should only be used during "flare-ups" to help decrease inflammation and irritation. Skin hydration with an emollient agent is often helpful, in that softening the skin decreases fissuring. Another option is salicylic acid, which acts as a keratolytic agent to promote desquamation of scales. A popular option is the use of salicylic acid in a hydrophilic base, applied under occlusion. This seems to help remove thick, adherent scales. Coal tar, another popular treatment option with a poorly understood mechanism of action, may have only mild antipsoriatic properties unless used in combination with UV radiation. Because of this and the added disadvantage of staining skin and clothing, it is not recommended as initial therapy for BF. Anthralin, another option for topical treatment, has a high incidence of skin irritation and staining of skin and clothing; thus, it is less often used.

P: For initial management of BF's psoriasis, 6% salicylic acid in 60% propylene glycol should be started. This will help both hydrate the skin and promote shedding of the scaling epithelial cells. In order to help remove the thicker scales, the ointment should be applied under occlusion at night. During the day, a midstrength topical steroid, e.g. triamcinolone acetonide 0.1% cream, can be applied twice daily to decrease inflammation and irritation. The steroid should only be applied during the "flare-up" and then discontinued to avoid local side effects, including striae and skin atrophy.

Problem 3. Contraception

S: None

O: None

A: BF has been using oral contraceptives for many years. She is now 35 years old and continues to smoke 2 packs of cigarettes per day. If she continues to smoke and use birth control pills, she may be at increased risk for cardiovascular side effects. While old data suggested an increased incidence of myocardial infarction, stroke, and thromboembolic disease for users of oral contraceptives, these adverse effects have been attributed to the high doses of estrogen and progestin contained in older formulations. With the newer formulations, the above risks are negligible in healthy women. The available data seem to indicate that in women over age 35, any increased risk of MI, thromboembolic disease, or stroke are related to concomitant risk factors, which include smoking, rather than to the use of oral contraceptives. Although some question remains as to the association between oral contraceptive use and breast cancer, the majority of studies show no association. There is a decreased risk of developing ovarian and endometrial cancer in oral contraceptive users. Because of these benefits associated with oral contraceptive use in addition to their potential bone-sparing effects and decrease in dysmenorrhea, as well as the lack of association with increased cardiovascular morbidity, the current recommendation is to continue oral contraceptives in healthy women over age 35 who do not smoke. BF also has a history of severe menstrual cramps, which have lessened during oral contraceptive use. Thus, BF seems to have derived some benefit from oral contraceptives. While she is healthy, with no history of hypertension, hyperlipidemia, or diabetes, she does continue to smoke. BF needs counseling in order to understand her increased risk of cardiovascular adverse effects if she continues to smoke and use oral contraceptives. Other options for BF include a diaphragm, intrauterine device, cervical cap, sponge, and condoms.

P: Because BF seems sincere in her desire to stop smoking, continue her oral contraceptives at this time. Explain to BF that failure to stop smoking will put her at increased risk for cardiovascular morbidity with continued oral contraceptive use. Encourage appropriate use of the transdermal nicotine and participation in group therapy. BF should be assessed in 3 to 6 months to determine whether her oral contraceptives should be continued or whether an alternate contraceptive method should be chosen.

CASE 92 QUESTIONS

1. If BF returns to the clinic in 5 days saying she is still experiencing withdrawal symptoms and has begun to smoke again, what can be done?

2. What dose and schedule of nicotine gum should be prescribed for BF, and how would you counsel her on the use of nicotine gum?

3. What symptoms would indicate nicotine excess in BF?
4. What is the incidence of systemic side effects with the use of topical steroids, and is there a concern in BF?
5. If BF returns to clinic with psoriasis on her scalp, what would be the best way to treat the scalp involvement?

CASE 93

CC: AM is a woman, age 54, who visits the clinic complaining of an itchy rash over her hands, arms, and forehead, which developed 2 days ago. She says that yesterday it began to appear on her abdomen and the front of her legs. AM indicates that she finished cleaning out brush and weeds along the fence 3 days ago. Two days ago, she worked on the garage in the afternoon wearing the clothes from the previous day because they were already dirty.

Past Medical History

AM has type II (adult-onset) diabetes that was identified over a year ago. She takes glyburide daily and has been stable. AM has had hypertension since age 45. She was controlled on hydrochlorothiazide but was switched to enalapril after her diabetes diagnosis. Peptic ulcer disease was detected by endoscopy 2 years ago. Treatment with cimetidine was successful, and she continues on a maintenance dosage.

Medication History

Glyburide, 2.5 mg PO QAM
Enalapril, 10 mg PO QAM
Cimetidine, 400 mg PO HS

Allergies

None known

Physical Examination

GEN: Obese female who appears restless and agitated and complains of itching
VS: BP 135/95, HR 85, RR 19, T 37.2, Wt 72 kg
HEENT: Several small patches of erythematous vesicles are located on the forehead, with a few vesicles on each side of the neck.
COR: WNL
CHEST: Clear
ABD: No masses or tenderness, areas of vesicles developing on skin
GU: WNL
NEURO: WNL
EXT: Arms and hands have numerous erythematous vesicular and bullous areas, some in a linear configuration. Several of these areas are weeping. The fronts of the thighs show erythematous areas with some swelling and beginning development of vesicles. No open, oozing areas are noted.

Results of Laboratory Tests

Glucose, fasting plasma (FPG) 6.4 (115), HbA$_{1c}$ 8% (both from clinic visit 1 month ago)

PROBLEM LIST

1. Hypertension
2. Peptic ulcer disease (PUD)
3. Type II (adult-onset) diabetes
4. Generalized vesicular pruritic rash

CASE 93 SOAP NOTES
Problem 4. Generalized Vesicular Pruritic Rash

S: AM complains of an itching rash that has developed over the last 2 days.
O: The rash involves both the inner and outer surfaces of the hands and arms. Vesicles and bullae are present with oozing. The abdomen and thighs are erythematous, with patches of vesicles developing. An estimated 25 to 30% of her skin surface is involved.
A: AM has developed contact dermatitis as a result of recent exposure to poison ivy while cleaning out weeds and brush. The extent of its development makes her quite uncomfortable due to the itching, and she requires relief.

AM requires systemic steroid treatment because of the amount of body surface area involved and the acute phase of the reaction. She has limited involvement of the facial area at this time. Concern about potential involvement of the eyes is another reason to use systemic steroids. In a patient with severe facial involvement only, systemic steroids would be used.

Topical steroids would not be appropriate for two reasons. First, topical steroids are not helpful in the acute phase with blistering (and weeping) because they do not penetrate well. Second, the extent of AM's lesions would make use of topical steroids expensive and difficult. Topical steroid products might be used later when the lesions have begun to dry. Since AM is to be treated with oral steroids, this is unnecessary.

The use of antihistamines (oral) in acute allergic contact dermatitis provides little if any benefit because histamine is not usually involved in type IV reactions. The primary benefit to AM would be the sedating properties of diphenhydramine in the acute phase. The choice of a less sedating antihistamine (e.g., terfenadine) would be inappropriate for AM.

Several concerns arise in placing this patient on prednisone because of her coexisting diseases or history. First, corticosteroids can cause hyperglycemia and may aggravate her diabetes. Second, corticosteroids can cause sodium retention, which may aggravate her hypertension. Third, corticosteroids cause GI irritation and have been implicated in the reactivation of peptic ulcers. Since AM will be on relatively short-term therapy and is receiving medication for each of these diseases, problems may not develop. She should be told how to take her prednisone (with meals) and be monitored carefully.

P: Start prednisone 60 mg/day for 10 to 14 days, with tapering by 5 mg/day thereafter. Apply Burow's solution to weeping areas, using compresses, for 30 min 4 to 6 times a day. Drain blisters, but do not remove tops. Take diphenhydramine, 50 mg PO Q6H PRN for itching, for the next few days. Discontinue use of the compresses as lesions dry and crust, which will occur over the next week. Continue monitoring blood glucose and blood pressure and report any significant stomach discomfort. If lesions do not begin to improve significantly within 5 days, AM should contact her physician.

Patient education: Prednisone should be taken with food or milk to decrease potential stomach irritation. AM may use gauze or strips of thin cloth for the compresses. Diphenhydramine will cause drowsiness, so she should not drive or undertake activity where this could be a hazard.

Problem 1. Hypertension

S: None

O: BP 135/95

A: AM's diastolic blood pressure is borderline. Her present illness may be contributory, since she is visibly aggravated by her symptoms. Her chart indicates that BP on last clinic visit 1 month ago was 130/85.

P: Check her compliance with medication (enalapril). Reevaluate on next visit after clearing of poison ivy. Have AM check her blood pressure three times per week and report any elevations above her current BP of 135/95.

Problem 2. Peptic Ulcer Disease

S: None

O: None

A: AM has had no signs or symptoms of the recurrence of her ulcer. (See discussion under problem 4 regarding use of corticosteroids in this patient.) Maintenance therapy is usually not required after a single episode of PUD.

P: Continue maintenance therapy with cimetidine until after prednisone is discontinued, then reassess the need for maintenance therapy.

Problem 3. Type II (Adult-Onset) Diabetes

S: None

O: AM reports daily blood glucose values in the 6.1 mmol/L (110 mg/dL) range with Visidex II.

A: AM's diabetes seems to be controlled with an oral hypoglycemic, as her last FPG was WNL and HgA$_{1c}$ at 8% is within normal range.

P: Have AM continue medication, check blood glucose daily, and watch diet carefully.

CASE 93 QUESTIONS

1. Why does the rash from poison ivy involve areas of unexposed skin?
2. Are drugs a possible cause of her condition?
3. How should increased glucose levels caused by steroids be managed?

4. What if the poison ivy involves her eyes or other areas?
5. What if the rash became infected?

CASE 94

CC: JD is a man, age 31, who is admitted to the Burn Center after being rescued from a house fire. JD was unconscious when found by a firefighter and removed from the burning house. JD suffered a 60% total body surface area (TBSA) burn, with approximately 40% TBSA full-thickness injury.

Before being admitted to the Burn Center, JD received the following treatments in the emergency department: (a) intravenous catheter inserted and lactated Ringer's solution infused at 500 mL/hr (1.5 L administered while in the emergency department); (b) endotracheal tube inserted during elective laryngoscopy and bronchoscopy that demonstrated inflammation, edema, and carbonaceous residue below the level of the vocal cords; (c) intramuscular injection of 0.5 mL diphtheria/tetanus toxoids; (d) intravenous injection of 100 mg thiamine; (e) insertion of an indwelling Foley catheter; (f) insertion of a nasogastric tube; and (g) application of mafenide acetate cream to all burned areas.

Past Medical History

Not significant. Date of last tetanus shot not known.

Social History

History of ethanol abuse.

Medication History

Occasional aspirin and antacid use.

Allergies

JD has no known drug allergies.

Physical Examination

GEN: Critically injured well-developed man

VS: BP 110/64, HR 142, RR 26, T 38, Wt 73 kg, Ht 178 cm

HEENT: Eyebrows, eyelashes, and nasal hair singed; corneas appear uninjured when examined using fluorescein stain; orotracheal tube in place.

COR: Tachycardic with normal S$_1$ and S$_2$, no murmurs or rubs

CHEST: Circumferential full-thickness injury; rales and rhonchi heard over all lung fields; inspiratory and expiratory wheezes

ABD: Absence of bowel sounds in all four quadrants

GU: WNL, Foley catheter in place. Total urine volume during ED stay is 42 ml. The urine is brownish red (evidence of hemochromogens).

RECT: Deferred

EXT: Left upper extremity (LUE) has blisters and burns that are pink and blanch to pressure. The right upper extremity (RUE) appears dry and leathery, with coagulated blood vessels visible under the eschar. Radial and ulnar pulses are absent in the RUE. Both lower extremities have intact blisters and are uninjured below the ankle.

NEURO: Does not respond to verbal stimuli. Responds to and localizes pain.

Results of Laboratory Tests

Na 143 (143)	Hct 0.51 (51)	AST 0.9 (54)	Glu 7.4 (134)
K 5.2 (5.2)	Hgb 175 (17.5)	ALT 1.04 (63)	Ca 2.05 (8.2)
Cl 110 (110)	Lkcs 4.5 × 10^9 (4.5 × 10^3)	LDH 4.08 (245)	PO_4 0.3 (0.9)
HCO_3 15 (15)	Plts 195 × 10^9 (195 × 10^3)	Alb 29 (2.9)	Mg 0.74 (1.8)
BUN 2.14 (6)	MCV 92 (92)	T Bili 24 (1.4)	
CR 80 (0.9)			

Lkc differential: Neutrophils 0.62, Bands 0.10, Lymphocytes 0.22, Monocytes 0.04

Urinalysis: Specific gravity 1.022, pH 6.2, protein-positive, leukocyte esterase-negative, blood-positive, glucose-negative, ketones-negative, urobilinogen normal.

Blood ethanol 45 mmol/L (206 mg/dL)

Arterial blood gas: pH 7.27, PO_2 9.6 kPa (72 mm Hg), PCO_2 4.4 kPa (33 mm Hg), HCO_3 14 mmol/L (14 mEq/L), FIO_2 0.4, Carboxyhemoglobin 0.37

Chest x-ray: Some minor peribronchial cuffing and the presence of an endotracheal tube (the tip is 3 cm from the carina), otherwise unremarkable

PROBLEM LIST

1. 60% TBSA flame burn
2. Arterial blood gas (ABG) abnormalities
   a. Carbon monoxide poisoning (37%)
   b. Metabolic acidosis
   c. Hypoxia
3. Hypovolemia
4. Hemochromogens in urine
5. Hypophosphatemia
6. Stress-related mucosal damage (SRMD) prophylaxis
7. Hyperkalemia
8. Absent peripheral pulses in the right arm

CASE 94 SOAP NOTES

Problem 1. Flame Burn

S: Critically injured male in acute distress

O: JD's chest has burns on the front, back, and both sides that are obviously full-thickness. LUE has blisters and burns that are pink and blanch to pressure. The RUE appears dry and leathery with coagulated blood vessels visible under the eschar. Both lower extremities have intact blisters and are uninjured below the ankle.

A: JD exhibits a 60% TBSA flame burn with approximately 40% TBSA full-thickness injuries. The LUE and both lower extremities appear to have partial-thickness injuries. The dry, leathery appearance of the RUE with visible coagulated blood vessels is pathognomonic for full-thickness injury.

P: Since only small areas of full-thickness burns can heal by contraction, JD's full-thickness injuries must be surgically removed (excised) and replaced with skin grafts (autograft). Because of the difficulty in differentiating partial-thickness from full-thickness burns on admission, the first surgery will take place on postburn day 2, 3, 4, or 5. This delay will allow areas of full-thickness injury to demarcate. In the interim, SSD will be applied twice daily, and eschar biopsies will be quantitatively analyzed for microbes every other day. Grafting of areas heavily colonized (ℓ 100,000 bacteria per gram of tissue) is usually delayed until the infection is controlled.

The prioritization for grafting of burned areas is to (1) maintain life, (2) preserve function (JD's burns of hands and joints), and (3) assure an optimal cosmetic result. In general, the limit for excision of burn wounds during a single operative procedure is 10 to 20% TBSA, since blood losses can average 200 to 500 mL for each 1% body surface excised. This limit can be increased to 20 to 35% TBSA when extremities are excised under tourniquet hemostasis. The technique used for full-thickness burns with deep subcutaneous tissue damage (JD's RUE) is fascial excision, in which the entire area of burned skin and subcutaneous fat is surgically removed. The technique used for deep partial-thickness and full-thickness burns is tangential (or sequential) excision, in which a dermatome is used to serially remove superficial slices of damaged tissue until a normal cutaneous tissue base is reached (as evidenced by uniform capillary bleeding) or normal subcutaneous tissue.

The excised burn wounds are closed with expanded autograft (using a skin-meshing device that makes patterned incisions into the graft) or temporarily closed with homograft or biosynthetic skin substitutes while waiting for donor sites to heal and be reharvested. Because of cosmetic considerations, excised facial burns are usually covered with full-thickness, nonmeshed autograft. Unless the burn depth can be accurately determined, excision of facial burns is usually delayed until postburn days 7 through 10.

Problem 2. ABG Abnormalities

S: None

O: Carbon monoxide is present in the blood in toxic amounts (37%). The arterial PO_2 is below normal (9.6 kPa, or 72 mm Hg) even with an increased FIO_2 of 0.4. The arterial pH is below 7.40, the PCO_2 is less than 40, and the HCO_3 is below normal. There is an anion gap metabolic acidosis of 23 ([143 + 5.2] − [110 + 15]).

A: JD was injured in an enclosed environment and suffered smoke inhalation. Carbon monoxide, the predominant gas in smoke, preferentially binds to hemoglobin, with an affinity approximately 200 times that of oxygen. By displacing oxygen from hemoglobin and shifting the oxyhemoglobin dissociation curve to the left, carbon monoxide poisoning produces tissue hypoxemia resulting in anaerobic glycolysis and lactic acidosis. Another possible explanation for the metabolic acidosis is cyanide toxicity. Burning plastic releases hydrocyanide, which when inhaled or absorbed through the skin, inhibits cellular oxidation. This poisoning of cellular oxidation produces hypoxemia and lactic acidosis. Three other possible contributors to lactic acidosis are inadequate oxygenation caused by impaired chest expansion, inadequate tissue perfusion because of hypovolemia, and shift of the oxyhemoglobin dissociation curve to the left because of hypophosphatemia.

P: Increase the FIO_2 from 0.4 to 1.0, which will increase the elimination rate of carbon monoxide. Increase the rate of fluid administration (see problem 3). Before administering sodium bicarbonate to normalize the arterial pH, wait until the effects of increased oxygen and fluids become evident. The metabolic acidosis may be resolved with increased tissue perfusion and oxygenation. As a general rule, bicarbonate is not administered unless the arterial pH falls below 7.20. Send a blood sample for cyanide determination. Have a cyanide antidote kit available for use. Assess the need for chest escharotomies by observing respiratory excursion and measuring tidal volume. Administer phosphorus intravenously (see problem 5). Finally, discontinue the application of mafenide acetate, which can produce metabolic acidosis by carbonic anhydrase inhibition. Use a different topical antimicrobial cream, such as silver sulfadiazine or nitrofurazone.

Problem 3. Hypovolemia

S: None

O: The best evidence for inadequate fluid resuscitation in JD is oliguria; current urine output 15 mL/hr. In addition, hemoconcentration, i.e., hematocrit .51 (51%), implies hypovolemia. Tachycardia could be the result of other factors.

A: The current fluid regimen is inadequate. The estimated fluid requirements for the first 24 hours after a burn can be calculated using the Parkland formula, where one half the total is administered over the first 8 hours and the other half during the next 16 hours.

Volume required (mL) = 4 mL × body weight (kg) × TBSA %.

For JD, this is: Volume = 4 × 73 × 60 = 17.520 mL

Since one half of this total should be administered over 8 hours, the rate of lactated Ringer's solution should be increased to:

(17.520 mL/2)/8 = 1095 mL/hr = 1100 mL/hr

P: Formulas to estimate burn resuscitation fluid requirements should not be relied on. Objective evaluation of resuscitation success and adequate organ perfusion is required. The most important parameter monitored is urine output. The usual goal for an adult is 0.5 to 1 mL/kg/hr. Definitive measurement of cardiac output can be accomplished by invasive monitoring with a Swan-Ganz catheter.

Problem 4. Hemochromogens in Urine

S: None

O: The urine is dark, and coagulated blood vessels are visible in the eschar.

A: The areas of full-thickness injury contain destroyed red blood cells that released free hemoglobin. It is also possible that some deeply burned areas contain destroyed muscle cells that released myoglobin. When excreted in urine, both hemoglobin and myoglobin will produce renal tubule necrosis and subsequent renal failure unless they are flushed through quickly.

P: Establish brisk urine flow in the range of 75 to 100 mL/hr, until the pigments gradually clear from the urine. Rapid urine flow rates can usually be produced with intravenous crystalloid alone, but an osmotic diuretic, such as mannitol, can be used. In a few hours, the pigments will clear and the rate of fluid administration can be reduced to the amount necessary to produce 0.5 to 1 mL/kg of urine per hour.

Problem 5. Hypophosphatemia

S: None

O: Blood sample demonstrates a low inorganic phosphorus concentration of 0.30 mmol/L (0.9 mg/dL).

A: The human body has great stores of phosphorus in bone but cannot extract phosphorus from these stores at a rate necessary to keep up with demand after an acute burn injury. Acute, severe hypophosphatemia is common after thermal injury, because of the increased demand for production of high-energy phosphate bonds. Ethanol abuse and malnutrition are also risk factors for the development of hypophosphatemia.

P: There is some concern about potential adverse reactions, such as metastatic calcification of calcium phosphate crystals, when administering phosphorus intravenously. These problems were reported during the 1960s, when massive doses of phosphorus were rapidly administered to patients with hypercalcemia. Since that time it has been demonstrated that intravenous administration of phosphorus is safe and effective in the treatment of acute severe hypophosphatemia. When administered to normocalcemic patients, doses up to 0.2 mmol/kg may be administered over a few hours.

Administer phosphorus, 0.2 mmol/kg over 2 to 3 hours intravenously, and obtain follow-up serum phosphorus concentrations. Repeat the dose until the deficit is corrected. Continued requirements can be met by adding phosphorus to parenteral nutritional fluids. When ileus resolves, oral phosphorus supplements, such as milk, may be administered.

Problem 6. Stress-related Mucosal Damage Prophylaxis

S: None

O: None

A: Diffuse superficial GI mucosal injury occurs quickly in patients with multiple trauma, closed-head injury, or burns.

The syndrome in burn patients is often called Curling's ulcer, based on the report of gastroduodenal lesions by T.B. Curling in 1842. The development of upper GI bleeding may often be prevented by early feeding or the administration of antacids, sucralfate, or H_2-receptor antagonists (H_2RA). Because this patient is severely ill and mechanically ventilated, there is some concern about the potential for bacterial colonization in the stomach, aspiration, and pneumonia when antacids or H_2RAs are used to buffer the stomach pH.

P: Because JD has an ileus, select an intravenous H_2RA rather than antacids or sucralfate. Famotidine offers the convenience of Q12H dosing, or continuous infusion of an H_2RA could be initiated. In addition to their beneficial effects in preventing SRMD, H_2RAs (specifically cimetidine) reduce the amount of fluid required for burn resuscitation.

Problem 7. Hyperkalemia

S: None

O: Laboratory report of potassium 5.2 (5.2)

A: This hyperkalemia could be the result of metabolic acidosis. Acidosis shifts K from the intracellular to the extracellular space. Hyperkalemia also could be caused by release of K from hemolyzed red blood cells in the full-thickness burns. Finally, this abnormal laboratory result could be an artifact of hemoconcentration/hypovolemia.

P: Continue to monitor serum potassium concentrations and ECG for evidence of uncorrected hyperkalemia. Do not administer intravenous insulin plus dextrose or sodium polystyrene sulfonate at this time.

Problem 8. Absent Peripheral Pulses in the Right Arm

S: Arm appears badly burned, swollen, and cyanotic.

O: Neither radial nor ulnar pulses can be identified by palpation or Doppler.

A: The edema and swelling caused by the circumferential burn has produced a compartment syndrome and compromised the circulation in the RUE. The pressure must be relieved by escharotomy.

P: Using an electrocautery or scalpel, surgeon will incise the eschar laterally through its entire depth. The incision is extended along the midlateral line of the arm until all circumferential eschar is cut and the constriction is relieved. Peripheral pulses are assessed following the procedure. If pulses continue to be absent, fasciotomy should be considered.

CASE 94 QUESTIONS

1. The surgical house officer suggests that JD should be placed on penicillin G, 2 million units IVPB every 6 hours, is this reasonable?
2. Should JD receive tetanus immune globulin?
3. If JD becomes more alert and attempts to remove his endotracheal tube or overrides and fights the ventilator, are

there preferred agents for sedation and neuromuscular blockade?

4. Since JD has a nasogastric tube attached to suction and absent bowel sounds, should nutritional support be delayed until ileus resolves?
5. The topical antimicrobial was changed from mafenide to silver sulfadiazine. If JD develops leukopenia (Lkc < 2.0 × 10^9/L) on postburn day 2 or 3, is it likely to be caused by sulfonamide hypersensitivity?

CASE 95

CC: SA, a woman, age 55, was admitted to the hospital 1 week ago in respiratory failure with pneumonia/bronchitis. Since admission she has been treated with a variety of medications including methylprednisolone (1 day), ampicillin/sulbactam, gentamicin, furosemide, theophylline, and phenytoin. Three days ago, she was begun on oral ampicillin (IV antibiotics discontinued) and continues to receive cimetidine, furosemide, and phenytoin. A diffuse erythematous, maculopapular rash is now noted on her back, buttocks, and thighs. The rash is pruritic.

Past Medical History

SA has a long history of chronic obstructive pulmonary disease (COPD) with restrictive lung disease secondary to kyphoscoliosis. On this admission for respiratory failure and infection, intubation was required. After intubation, she hyperventilated and experienced seizure activity. A computed tomographic (CT) scan showed a left frontal meningioma.

Medication History

Methylprednisolone, 75 mg IV Q6H (days 1 to 3)
Ampicillin/sulbactam, 3 g IV Q6H (days 1 to 4)
Furosemide, 20 mg IV QD (days 1 to 7)
Cimetidine, 300 mg IV BID (days 1 to 7)
Theophylline elixir, 150 mg Q6H (days 4 to 7)
Phenytoin suspension, 300 mg QHS (days 4 to 7)
Ampicillin, 500 mg PO Q6H (days 5 to 7)

Allergies

None known

Physical Examination

GEN: Patient has diffuse, erythematous, maculopapular rash over her back, buttocks, and thighs.

VS: BP 125/82, HR 80, RR 22, T 38

HEENT: WNL

COR: WNL

CHEST: Occasional rales, wheezes

ABD: Nontender, no masses

Results of Laboratory Tests

CBC (day 7): WNL except Lkcs differential
Lkcs 10.8×10^9 (10.8×10^3)
Eosinophils 8%

	Day 1	Day 7
PaO_2	44 mm Hg	60 mm Hg
$PaCO_2$	55 mm Hg	45 mm Hg

Theophylline level (day 6): 38.85 mmol/L (7 mg/mL)

Culture sputum: *Klebsiella pneumoniae*

PROBLEM LIST

1. COPD
2. Pneumonia/bronchitis
3. Seizures
4. Meningioma
5. Diffuse, erythematous maculopapular rash

CASE 95 QUESTIONS

1. What important drug interactions are possible in SA?
2. If SA's rash is still diffuse 4 days from now and has spread to her upper extremities, trunk, and face, what should be considered?
3. What are some of the issues that arise when the clear cause of an adverse drug reaction is not identified?
4. If SA cannot use inhalers correctly, would a spacer device be useful?

CASE 96

CC: LJ is a man, age 57, who presents to the clinic with generalized psoriasis on his trunk and upper and lower extremities. He has failed to respond to topical steroid therapy in the past, and also had an elevation in liver enzyme levels after a short course of methotrexate 4 months ago. He states that the plaques have progressively become more numerous and larger in size over the past few months, with only minimal itching and discomfort. He also complains of occasional episodes of substernal chest pains lasting approximately 5 minutes that abate with rest. He states that his asthma is mild and is controlled with occasional use of his inhaler.

Past Medical History

Psoriasis
Coronary artery disease for 3 years
Hypertension for 15 years
Asthma

Social History

Occasional ethanol consumption
Tobacco, one to two packs per day

Medication History

Children's aspirin, 81 mg, 2 tabs PO QD
Hydrochlorothiazide, 25 mg PO QD
Isosorbide dinitrate, 10 mg PO Q6H
Albuterol inhaler, 2 puffs PRN for shortness of breath

Allergies

Penicillin causes a rash.

Physical Examination

GEN: Well-developed, well-nourished male in no acute distress
VS: BP 153/94, HR 86, RR 14, T 37.3, Wt 73 kg
HEENT: Noncontributory
COR: RRR, S_1, S_2, no S_3, no murmurs
CHEST: Mild wheezing; otherwise clear
ABD: Soft, nontender, no masses; numerous well-marginated erythematous psoriatic plaques topped with gray scales.
GU: Noncontributory
RECT: Noncontributory
EXT: No edema, numerous well-marginated erythematous psoriatic plaques topped with gray scales located on upper and lower extremities bilaterally. Minimal pinpoint bleeding at the site where the scales are picked off. The patient states that he always tans, but only occasionally develops a sunburn upon exposure to sunlight.
NEURO: Orientated × 3, CN II-XII intact

Results of Laboratory Tests

Na: 136 (136)	Hct: 0.4 (40)	Glu (Random): 6.1 (110)
K: 3.9 (3.9)	Hgb: 140 (14)	Ca: 2.3 (9.2)
Cl: 98 (98)	Lkcs 6×10^9 (6×10^3)	PO_4: 1.3 (4)
HCO_3: 26 (26)	Plts: 179×10^9 (179×10^3)	Mg: 1.1 (2.2)
BUN: 6.8 (19)	MCV: 91 (91)	Uric Acid: 560 (9.4)
CR: 106 (1.2)		

Chest x-ray: WNL
ECG: Normal sinus rhythm

PROBLEM LIST

1. Hypertension
2. Coronary artery disease
3. Hyperuricemia
4. Psoriasis

CASE 96 QUESTIONS

1. What are indications and contraindications to PUVA (psoralen + ultraviolet light – A) therapy?
2. What are common patient counseling points to cover for patients receiving a prescription for calcipotriene (Dovonex)?
3. What are the common side effects of methoxsalen?
4. What patient education for PUVA therapy should be reviewed with LJ?
5. LJ presents to the emergency room 1 week later with severe pain in the big toe of his left foot, that began earlier in

the morning. An acute gouty attack is suspected, and colchicine is to be started. Suggest a dosage regimen for oral colchicine in the management of an acute gouty attack.

CASE 97

CC: LP is an 18-year-old woman who presents to the dermatology clinic complaining of worsening acne.

Past Medical History

LP states that she is in good health with no medical problems. She states that the acne on her face has worsened over the last 3 months. She is concerned because it is affecting her looks and would like something to make it better. Also of note, LP started taking birth control pills about 4 months ago.

Medication History

Ortho Novum 1/35

Allergies

None known

Physical Examination

GEN: Well-developed, well-nourished teenage female in NAD
VS: BP 115/70, HR 72, RR 18, Wt 47.3 kg
HEENT: PERRLA
COR: Nl S_1, S_2; no murmurs
CHEST: CTA
SKIN: Moderate acne over the forehead, chin, and cheeks

Results of Laboratory Tests

Na 140 (140)	BUN 7.14 (20)	Plts 250 × 10⁹ (250 × 10³)	Glu 6.6 (120)
K 3.7 (3.7)	CR 70.4 (0.8)	AST .167 (10)	Chol 2.8 (110)
Cl 104 (104)	Hct 0.4 (40)	ALT .12 (7)	
HCO₃ 25 (25)	Hgb 160 (16)	T Bili 1.7 (0.1)	

PROBLEM LIST

1. Acne
2. Oral contraception

CASE 98

CC: PP is a 55-year-old man with moderate psoriasis involving the scalp, elbows, knees, hands, and feet. He comes to the clinic because of worsening of his psoriasis for the past week.

Past Medical History

PP has a 20-year history of chronic obstructive pulmonary disease (COPD) that has been controlled with metaproterenol and ipratroprium inhalers with few exacerbations. Two weeks ago, PP developed a upper respiratory infection (URI) that was treated with a 2-week course of antibiotics. The URI exacerbated PP's COPD, and he required a 4-day course of oral prednisone with a rapid taper. When PP first developed the URI, his psoriasis worsened, but it improved dramatically when the oral steroids were added. Since tapering off the systemic steroids, PP's psoriasis has been troubling him, and he no longer gets relief with his current regimen of hydrocortisone 0.5% cream, diphenhydramine 25 mg PRN, and coal tar shampoo. PP also has gastroesophageal reflux disease (GERD), which only bothers him at night. PP gets heartburn when he lies down. He has been a heavy drinker and smoker all of his adult life.

Medication History

Hydrocortisone cream 0.5%, BID
Coal tar shampoo, every week
Diphenhydramine, 25 mg PRN for itch
Metaproterenol inhaler, 2 to 4 puffs PRN
Ipratroprium inhaler, 2 to 4 puffs PRN
Ranitidine, 150 mg PO QHS

Allergies

Cotrimoxazole causes a rash.

Physical Examination

GEN: Middle-aged male in no apparent distress, irritated by itchy, dry scaling skin.
VS: BP 120/80, HR 65, RR 23, T 37.0, Wt 75 kg
HEENT: WNL
COR: Nl S_1, S_2
ABD: Soft, nontender, positive bowel sounds
CHEST: Few expiratory wheezes, no rales or rhonchi
GU: WNL
RECT: WNL
EXT: Red lesions with silvery scales on elbows, knees, fingers, and toes; skin appears dry with scratch marks

Results of Laboratory Tests

Na 140 (140)	BUN 7.1 (20)	Lkcs 3.6 × 10⁹ (3.6 × 10³)	ALT 0.67 (40)
K 3.6 (3.6)	SCr 106.1 (1.2)	Plts 340 × 10⁹ (340 × 10³)	T Bili 20.5 (1.2)
Cl 96 (96)	Hct 0.42 (42%)	MCV 96 (96)	Ca 2.25 (9)
HCO₃ 25 (25)	Hgb 140 (14)	AST 0.75 (45)	PO₄ 1.19 (3.7)
			Mg 0.82 (1.6)

PROBLEM LIST

1. COPD
2. Psoriasis
3. GERD
4. Dry skin

DISEASES OF THE EYE AND EAR

CASE 99

CC: GT is a 78-year-old man who was brought to the clinic today by his daughter, the first time since his wife died 6 months ago. He complains of a painful red eye, with the eyelids sticking together upon awakening, and some visual disturbances.

Past Medical History

Hypertension for 20 years that is well-controlled. Nasal congestion for 3 days, which he is treating himself. Eye infection 2 years ago, which was treated with sulfacetamide eye drops.

Social History

GT lives by himself. He drinks alcohol but states that he does not abuse it. He does not smoke.

Medication History

Triprolidine and pseudoephedrine (Actifed), 2 tablets QID for 2 days
Hydrochlorothiazide, 25 mg daily.
Sulfacetamide eye drops, 2 drops Q6H (drops kept from his previous eye infection)
Potassium chloride tablets, 10 mEq 2 BID (he stopped taking it several months ago)

Allergies

Penicillin (rash)

Physical Examination

GEN: GT is a well-groomed gentleman who appears slightly wasted and dehydrated and has a red left eye with purulent discharge accumulated on the lashes.
VS: BP 144/96, HR 105, RR 23, T 37.2, Wt 57 kg, Ht 183 cm
HEENT: The left eye has a brilliant red appearance, more intense at the limbus, with a mucopurulent discharge. The right eye appears marginally red. Eyelids are moderately swollen. There is no evidence of trauma, but a gray, well-circumscribed corneal lesion can be seen with fluorescein stain. Pupils react mildly to light, slightly dilated.
COR: Sinus tachycardia
CHEST: WNL
ABD: Soft, tender
GU: Deferred
RECT: Deferred
SKIN: Dry and cool

Results of Laboratory Tests

Na 133 (133)	Hct 0.44 (44)	Glu 5.6 (101)
K 3.0 (3.0)	Hgb 2.3 (15)	
Cl 85 (85)	Lkcs 11.4 × 10^9 (11.4 × 10^3)	
HCO$_3$ 30 (30)	Plts 350 × 10^9 (350 × 10^3)	
BUN 8.5 (23.8)		
CR 150 (1.7)		

LFT: WNL

Chest x-ray: WNL

PROBLEM LIST

1. Hypertension
2. Cold and sinusitis
3. Visual disturbances
4. Conjunctivitis and keratitis
5. Fluid and electrolyte disturbances

CASE 99 SOAP NOTES
Problem 4. Conjunctivitis and Keratitis

S: GT complains of a painful, red left eye with the eyelids sticking together upon awakening. The redness started 2 days ago, but the pain had an acute onset this morning.

O: GT has a red left eye, with purulent discharge accumulating on the lashes; the right eye also appears slightly red. The conjunctiva of the left eye has a brilliant red appearance that is more intense at the limbus; the eye is also tearing and very sensitive to light. A small, gray, well-circumscribed corneal lesion is noticeable in the left eye. The eyelids are moderately swollen. Gram's stain of the discharge shows gram-positive lancet-shaped cocci in pairs.

A: This is an acute episode of *Streptococcus pneumoniae* conjunctivitis, which has progressed to keratitis in the left eye. The right eye appears to be contaminated as well. Keratitis is an ophthalmologic emergency because of the risk of rapid vision loss. The pain is caused by damage to the nerve endings in the cornea. Erythromycin ophthalmic ointment is indicated. Systemic antibiotics are also indicated because of the risk factors present (i.e., damage to the cornea, advanced age, and the cold and sinusitis that can develop into a secondary upper respiratory infection).

P: Stop the use of sulfacetamide immediately and begin with erythromycin, 0.5% ophthalmic ointment four times daily (Q6H) in the lower conjunctival sac. The eyelids must be massaged gently to spread the ointment, after 1 minute excess ointment can be wiped away with sterile cotton. The ointment should not be flushed from the eye following application. GT should be careful not to touch any part of the eye with tip of the tube, to prevent contamination of the ointment. The tube must be discarded after 30 days. Advise GT not to use any ophthalmic preparation that has been open for longer than 30 days.

Start with erythromycin, 250 mg PO Q6H for a course of 7 days. The tablets should be taken on an empty stomach, but taken with meals if GI irritation occurs.

Personal hygiene is very important. Use own towel to prevent contamination and spreading of the infection. Cotton balls can be used to clean the discharge from the eyes.

Problem 3. Visual Disturbances

S: GT complains of visual disturbance.

O: Slightly dilated pupils very painful on light stimulus

A: The visual disturbance may have two causes. Keratitis causes visual disturbance as a result of damage to the nerve endings. The very high dose of pseudoephedrine (480 mg/day) is double the maximum daily dose and can cause mydriasis due to contraction of the radial muscles of the iris by α_1-receptor formulation.

P: Decrease the doses of triprolidine and pseudoephedrine (Actifed) to 1 tablet TID (as discussed previously). Clean the discharge from the eye regularly and wear sunglasses to protect the eye from intense light.

Problem 2. Cold and Sinusitis

S: GT complains of nasal congestion and sinusitis.

O: GT has rhinorrhea and congestion, with a purulent discharge from the nose. No cough or lung involvement.

A: Pneumococcal conjunctivitis is often associated with a cold and sinusitis. GT is at risk for an upper respiratory tract infection, although it is not common for pneumococcal conjunctivitis to cause an upper respiratory infection. Continue with triprolidine and pseudoephedrine for symptomatic relief of the cold symptoms, but decrease the dosage, since the current dose is too high.

P: Decrease the doses of triprolidine and pseudoephedrine to 1 tablet TID. Warn GT that concurrent use of alcohol can cause drowsiness, and stress the importance of taking the recommended dose for OTC products.

Problem 1. Hypertension

S: None

O: BP 144/96

A: Hydrochlorothiazide had controlled GT's blood pressure well in the past, but it is not under control at present. Although oral administration of usual doses of pseudoephedrine to normotensive patients usually produces negligible effect on blood pressure, it is unlikely that GT's blood pressure will be under control with the high dose of pseudoephedrine.

P: Decrease the dose of triprolidine and pseudoephedrine to 1 tablet TID. Keep him on the same dose of hydrochlorothiazide and restart the potassium chloride tablets (10 mEq) 2 tablets BID. Reevaluate his therapy at the next visit within a week.

Problem 5. Fluid and Electrolyte Disturbances

S: GT complains of a dry mouth.

O: Poor skin turgor, skin cool and dry; Na 130 mmol/L, K 3.0 mmol/L, Cl 85 mmol/L, CO_2 30 mmol/L, BUN 8.5 mmol/L (23.8), SCr 150 mmol/L (1.7)

A: A dehydrated elderly gentleman with hyponatremia, hypokalemia, and hypochloremia probably caused by hydrochlorothiazide therapy and not taking his potassium supplementation.

Replace the fluid and electrolyte losses with an oral rehydration solution. It may take several months to completely correct a diuretic-induced total body potassium deficit, despite the fact that the serum potassium may return rapidly to normal. The development of hypokalemia in patients on diuretic therapy can be minimized by decreasing the dose of the diuretic and augmenting the potassium intake in the diet. Food and beverages rich in potassium (e.g., spinach, bananas, dried apricots, and orange juice) can be incorporated into the diet. The daily requirements of potassium, sodium, and chloride for adults are 50 to 150 mEq, 100 to 300 mEq, and 100 to 300 mEq per day, respectively. The sodium and chloride deficit will be quick to return to normal with some oral rehydration and a normal food and fluid intake.

P: Take 2 liters of an oral rehydration solution over a 2-day period. Encourage the intake of additional fluids. Restart with the potassium supplementation as discussed above. GT should return to the clinic next week to have his electrolyte status checked.

CASE 99 QUESTIONS

1. What organisms are most likely to cause corneal infiltrations, and with which topical antibiotic should you treat the infection? Are systemic antibiotics indicated?

2. How would you distinguish clinically between groups of microorganisms causing conjunctivitis (e.g., bacterial, viral, fungal)? What would be the appearance of allergic conjunctivitis?

3. Should you cover an infected eye with a patch? Is the use of corticosteroids indicated in this case?

4. The hydrochlorothiazide was changed to 12.5 mg during GT's visit to the clinic a week ago because his potassium level was still low. The following results were obtained with his visit today.
   BP 140/94, HR 90, Wt 64 kg
   Na 138 (138), Cl 103 (103), K 3.6 (3.6)
   How would you change GT's hypertension therapy?

5. When are lodoxamide tromethamine or levocabastine eye drops indicated?

CASE 100

CC: MC is a man, age 64, with a history of hypertension (HTN), angina, and gastroesophageal reflux disease (GERD) who came to the emergency department today with severe chest pain not relieved by nitroglycerin (NTG) sublingual (SL), two tablets. MC received one tablet NTG SL in the emergency department, with complete relief of his pain. MC also complains of increasing heartburn for 2 weeks, not relieved by antacids PRN. MC was admitted to rule out myocardial infarction (MI) and to work up his epigastric pain.

Past Medical History

MC has a history of exertional angina that is usually relieved by SL NTG. He has had 3 to 4 episodes in the last 2 years, with the last episode approximately 10 months ago. MC said the chest pain developed while he was working in his garden, so he took his last two NTG tablets, but they did not help. He also said that he has used the same bottle of NTG for the past 2 years. MC also has increasing epigastric pain, especially at night, not relieved by antacids PRN. He said the pain is so bad at night that he needs two shots of whiskey to sleep. MC's BP has been adequately controlled on propanolol, although he ran out of his medication last week and has not yet been able to get it refilled. MC does not have any major long-term complications from HTN; however, he mentioned that his vision has been blurred for the last couple of weeks.

Hospital Course

MI was ruled out in MC's case, on the basis of the level of CPK/isoenzymes and LDH and ECG findings. His endoscopy showed no ulcerations in the gastric mucosa. Two days after admission, MC had an ophthalmic examination of his fundus to work up his blurred vision. Atropine drops were used to dilate his eyes. Five minutes after administration of atropine, MC developed extreme eye pain, red steamy-appearing corneas, and an intraocular pressure (IOP) of 50 mm Hg.

Medication History

NTG, 0.4 mg SL PRN for chest pain
Maalox, PRN for heartburn
Propranolol, 20 mg PO BID

Social History

Alcohol: 2 drinks/day
Tobacco: 1 pack/day

Allergies

Sulfa (Stevens-Johnson syndrome)

Physical Examination

GEN: Well-developed, well-nourished man in moderate distress

VS: BP 150/95, HR 100, RR 20, T 37, Wt 80 kg
HEENT: Papilledema
COR: S-T depression consistent with ischemic changes
CHEST: Clear
ABD: Positive bowel sounds, slight tenderness without guarding
NEURO: Unremarkable

Results of Laboratory Tests

Na 140 (140)
K 3.8 (3.8)
Cl 101 (101)
HCO₃ 24 (24)
BUN 8.9 (25)

SCr 97.2 (1.1)
Hct 0.30 (30)
Hgb 143 (14.3)
Lkcs 7.0×10^9 (7.0×10^3)

CPK isoenzymes 0.95 (57)
MB fraction 0.01 (1)
LDH 1.25 (75)
UA: WNL

PROBLEM LIST

1. Coronary artery disease/rule out MI
2. Gastroesophageal reflux disease
3. Hypertension
4. Acute closed-angle glaucoma

CASE 100 SOAP NOTES

Problem 4. Acute Closed-Angle Glaucoma

S: MC experienced severe eye pain after administration of atropine eye drops.

O: Red, steamy-appearing corneas and an IOP of 50 mm Hg

A: Narrow-angle glaucoma developed from the use of atropine eye drops during MC's ophthalmic examination. Narrow-angle glaucoma is a painful and serious medical condition that needs immediate drug treatment to prevent blindness. Drug treatment with parasympathomimetics, carbonic anhydrase inhibitors, and hyperosmotic agents is aimed at decreasing the intraocular pressure. Acetazolamide, a carbonic anhydrase inhibitor, is contraindicated in MC because of his sulfa allergy. MC should receive immediate treatment with pilocarpine eye drops and intravenous mannitol. He should be closely monitored for resolution of glaucoma as well as drug-induced side-effects.

P: (a) Start pilocarpine 4%, 1 gtt Q 5 min × 6. Place finger on puncta to decrease systemic absorption. Monitor for cholinergic side-effects such as diarrhea and salivation; (b) Start mannitol, 1 to 2 g/kg IV (80 to 160 g = 400 to 800 mL of 20% mannitol). Monitor headache, nausea, vomiting, dehydration, pulmonary edema, CHF, and hypersensitivity reactions; (c) Although acetazolamide is a very effective agent for rapidly decreasing intraocular pressure, it is contraindicated in MC because of his severe sulfa allergy.

Problem 1. Coronary Artery Disease

S: MC has a history of CAD and came to the emergency department with severe chest pain not relieved by NTG SL.

O: S-T depression consistent with ischemic changes

A: MC's angina was probably precipitated by the combination of physical exertion and discontinuation of his β-blocker. Since he was well controlled on his previous regimen, he should remain on NTG SL and β-blockers. MC should be told the importance of medication compliance in relation to his diseases. Drug treatment for CAD is generally single or multiple drug regimens consisting of NTG, β-blockers, and calcium-channel blockers. These agents exert their pharmacologic effects by decreasing either preload or HR/contractility, which decreases work for the heart and ultimately decreases pain. Propranolol is a good drug choice in MC because it treats both HTN and CAD and simplifies his drug regimen. Calcium-channel blockers could also be used, although they lower esophageal sphincter pressure and may worsen GERD. Since MC has symptomatic GERD at this time, calcium-channel blockers should be avoided. Heart rate is the best indicator of clinical efficacy of β-blockers in the treatment of CAD. The propranolol should be titrated as necessary to adequately block MC's HR response to exercise. MC has a history of smoking and HTN, which are two major risk factors for the development of CAD. He should be advised about factors in his life that can be changed to improve his quality of life.

P: (a) Restart propranolol at 20 mg PO BID. Monitor HR and BP. Also, monitor CNS side-effects and impotence. Instruct MC on the importance of medication compliance in relation to his HTN and CAD. (b) Give MC a new prescription for NTG, 0.4 mg SL PRN for chest pain. Explain that NTG should be kept in a dry area and replaced 6 months after opening. Also, NTG should not be taken with alcohol, because it can cause severe hypotension. Review other important patient education issues regarding SL NTG (see Chapter 39). (c) Advise MC about the cardiovascular effects of smoking. Try to persuade MC to stop smoking.

Problem 2. Gastroesophageal Reflux Disease

S: MC has a 2-week history of increasing epigastric pain that worsens at night.

O: None

A: MC's 2-week history of increasing epigastric pain, which worsens at night, are typical signs of GERD. Since MC's epigastric pain is not relieved by antacids PRN, he should be started on an H$_2$-antagonist. He can still use antacids as needed for severe pain. Although alcohol helps him sleep at night, it decreases esophageal sphincter pressure and probably worsens the pain. Smoking can also exacerbate GERD by lowering esophageal sphincter pressure. MC should try to avoid alcohol and smoking.

P: Start cimetidine, 400 mg PO BID. Continue antacids as needed for severe pain. Avoid alcohol and smoking. Raise head of bed 6 to 8 inches.

Problem 3. Hypertension

S: MC has had blurred vision for the past few weeks

O: BP 150/95 and papilledema

A: MC has a long history of HTN that was adequately controlled on propranolol. His blood pressure on admission was slightly elevated, although he was in pain and had not been taking his medication. MC's papilledema and recent complaints of blurred vision may indicate end-organ damage associated with chronic HTN. Since MC's HTN is controlled on propranolol, he should continue on the same medication. Again, propranolol is a good drug for MC because it can treat his angina as well as his HTN. MC's elevated BP on admission may have resulted from the abrupt discontinuation of β-blockers, which should never be rapidly discontinued because of the possibility of rebound HTN. If compliance continues to be a problem for MC, then alternative antihypertensive medication should be started. Calcium-channel blockers should be avoided in MC because of his history of GERD. Also, thiazide diuretics should be avoided because of MC's sulfa allergy. Clonidine would not be an appropriate alternative agent, because it also causes rebound HTN if stopped abruptly. One possible alternative agent is an angiotensin-converting enzyme (ACE) inhibitor, although captopril is contraindicated by his sulfa allergy. MC should be educated on nondrug treatment for HTN (see Chapter 30).

P: Continue propranolol, 20 mg PO BID, and monitor BP and HR. If noncompliance continues, start enalapril 5 mg PO QD and again monitor BP. Also monitor for side effects of enalapril, such as dry cough, hyperkalemia, and hypotension. Continue propranolol for treatment of CAD.

CASE 100 QUESTIONS

1. How does omeprazole work for treatment of poorly responsive GERD? Recommend an appropriate dose, and list the monitoring parameters you would follow in a patient.
2. Explain the reasoning behind the idea of a nitrate-free period.
3. Would pindolol be an appropriate β-blocker to use in patients with CAD?

CASE 101

CC: KW is a woman, age 54, with a history of glaucoma, chronic obstructive pulmonary disease (COPD), non-insulin-dependent diabetes mellitus (NIDDM), chronic renal failure (CRF), and irritable bowel syndrome (IBS). She presents to the clinic with increasing fatigue, depression, polyuria, polydypsia, and polyphagia for 2 weeks and increasing shortness of breath (SOB) for 3 weeks.

Past Medical History

KW has a history of type II diabetes (NIDDM) that was well controlled, i.e., blood sugar 8.8 to 11.1 (160 to 200), on glipizide. She denies noncompliance, recent illness, fever, cough, or sputum production. KW was diagnosed with open-angle glaucoma 2 years ago and was started on pilocarpine. Approximately 3 weeks ago, timolol was added to her glaucoma medication because of poor control. KW admits to increasing her prednisone dose 2 weeks ago from 10 mg PO QD to 20 mg PO QD because of increasing SOB that was not controlled by her inhalers. Today KW has increasing SOB, signs and symptoms of hyperglycemia, and depression.

Medication History

Glipizide, 5 mg PO QD

Metaproterenol MDI, 2 puffs QID PRN for SOB

Ipratroprium MDI, 2 puffs QID PRN for SOB

Prednisone, 10 mg PO QD for 2 years (increased to 20 mg QD 2 weeks ago)

Chlorpheniramine, 4 mg PO QID PRN for sinus headache

Belladonna/phenobarbital, one tablet PRN for IBS

Timolol, 0.5% one gtt ou BID

Pilocarpine, 1% two gtts ou QID

Allergies

None known

Physical Examination

GEN: Obese, cushingoid-appearing woman in mild respiratory distress

VS: BP 140/90, HR 85, RR 26, T 37.5, Wt 100 kg

HEENT: IOP 45 mm Hg, moon facies, microaneurysms visible

COR: NL S1, S2; no murmurs

CHEST: Bilateral expiratory/inspiratory wheezes

ABD: Positive bowel sounds, abdominal striae, truncal obesity

SKIN: Facial acne lesions

GU: Unremarkable

NEURO: O X 3, intact

Results of Laboratory Tests

Na 144 (144)	BUN 14.3 (40)	Lkcs 5.8×10^9 (5.8×10^3)
K 3.6 (3.6)	CR 167 (1.9)	Ca 2.39 (9.6)
Cl 98 (98)	Hct 0.3 (30)	PO$_4$ 1.45 (4.5)
HCO$_3$ 24 (24)	Hgb 142 (14.2)	Mg 1.05 (2.1)

Urinalysis: specific gravity 1.020, pH 5.5, negative est. & nit., gluc 16.65 (3%), negative ketones

ABG: pH 7.35, PCO$_2$ 50, PO$_2$ 80

PROBLEM LIST

1. Diabetes/hyperglycemia
2. COPD exacerbation
3. Open-angle glaucoma
4. Chronic renal failure
5. Irritable bowel syndrome (IBS)
6. Steroid side-effects

QUESTIONS FOR CASE 101

1. If KW were started on insulin because of uncontrolled blood sugar levels despite maximum doses of glipizide, what would be an appropriate insulin regimen to use?

2. KW develops hyperphosphatemia and hypocalcemia secondary to CRF. How would you manage her electrolyte abnormality?

3. KW develops anemia of chronic disease, and the doctor wants to start erythropoietin. What dose would you recommend and what would you monitor?

4. Instruct KW on the proper technique for the instillation of eye drops.

CASE 102

CC: NK is an 8-month-old male infant who is brought to the outpatient clinic with a 2-day history of fever, runny nose, and intractable crying.

Past Medical History

NK is a previously healthy infant with no previous medical problems, who (according to his mother) began having a runny nose, sneezing, and a cough 5 days ago. Two days before this visit, NK developed a fever (37.7°C), was increasingly irritable, and often inconsolable.

Medication History

Acetaminophen liquid, PRN for fever

Immunizations are current

Allergies

None known

Physical Examination

GEN: Well-developed, well-nourished male infant who is crying and inconsolable

VS: BP 100/50, HR 96, RR 26, T 37.4, Wt 8 kg

HEENT: Normocephalic, atraumatic. Left tympanic membrane (TM) is erythematous, opaque, and slightly bulging. No discharge present. Rhinorrhea is present (clear in color). Mucous membranes are slightly dry, no pharyngeal erythema or lesions noted.

COR: Regular rate and rhythm. No murmurs or gallops noted.

CHEST: Tachypneic, otherwise clear to auscultation

ABD: Normoactive bowel sounds. Soft, nontender. No guarding appreciated.

GU: Normal external male genitalia; circumcised

RECT: Deferred

EXT: Moves all extremities, no cyanosis noted.

NEURO: Alert, responds to pain, otherwise unable to assess.

Results of Laboratory Tests

Na 141 (141)	Hct 0.40 (40)
K 3.6 (3.6)	Hgb 131 (13.1)
Cl 96 (96)	Lkcs 12.4×10^9 (12.4×10^3)
HCO$_3$ 22 (22)	
BUN 4.3 (12)	
CR 17.7 (0.2)	

Lkc differential: Segs 0.76 (76), Bands 0.12 (12), Monos 0.6 (6), Lymphs 0.6 (6)

Chest x-ray: Clear; no infiltrates noted.

PROBLEM LIST

1. Acute otitis media
2. Upper respiratory tract infection (URI)

CASE 102 QUESTIONS

1. Five days later, the mother calls and describes what appears to be a maculopapular rash on NK's trunk, which appeared 3 days after the antibiotic was started. Because she notes that her son appears to be better, she is anxious to discontinue the antibiotic. What is your recommendation to this mother? Justify your recommendation.
2. Three months later, NK exhibits symptoms that are identical to the earlier episode of otitis media. The mother brings her son into the clinic after a 3-day course of the antibiotic that was "left over" from the previous episode. How would you approach treatment of NK's second episode of otitis media?
3. What options are available to the physician should NK continue to have recurrent episodes of otitis media?
4. Should NK take an antihistamine/decongestant to improve his eustachian tube function?

CASE 103

CC: KL is an obese woman, age 60, who comes to the clinic for her monthly visit. She complains of a watery left eye and a sensation of something in the eye. She also complains of nausea, vomiting, dizziness, and a rapid heart rate.

Past Medical History

KL has a 30-year history of diabetes mellitus, controlled with diet and chlorpropamide; a history of chronic obstructive pulmonary disease (COPD); and rhematoid arthritis (RA). Two weeks ago she took a course of erythromycin for bronchitis.

Social History

IVDA (−); quit smoking 5 years ago after smoking for 20 years. She drinks one glass of wine a week.

Medication History

Chlorpropamide, 750 mg QD
Theophylline, 300 mg Q12H
Ibuprofen, 800 mg Q12H
Ipratropium inhaler, 2 puffs Q6H
Cimetidine, 400 mg Q12H

Allergies

NKDA

Physical Examination

GEN: Obese woman with a watery eye, nausea, vomiting, dizziness, and tachycardia
VS: BP 130/85, HR 120, RR 23, Wt 75 kg, Ht 165 cm
HEENT: Slightly red left eye with lid edema. Unilateral lacrimation and photosensitivity. A small, yellow elevation can be seen on the conjunctival side of the lid. Pupils equal, round, and reactive to light.
COR: HR 120, otherwise WNL
CHEST: Barrel chest, bilateral decreased breath sounds, midinspiratory crackles and wheezes, mild tachypnea, some sputum production and cough, but no SOB
ABD: Obese, no palpable masses
GU: WNL
RECT: Guaiac-negative.
EXT: Red, swollen MTP joints.
NEURO: WNL

Results of Laboratory Tests

Na 132 (132)	Hct 0.32 (32)	Glu 3.8 (68.4)
K 4.5 (4.5)	Hgb 100 (10)	RF neg
Cl 99 (99)	Lkcs 9.5×10^9 (9.5×10^3)	FANA diffuse pattern
HCO$_3$ 27 (27)	Plts 225×10^9 (225×10^3)	Theophylline 105 mmol/L (19 mg/mL)
BUN 6 (16.8)		
CR 80 (.9)		

ABG: pH 7.35, PO$_2$ 60, PCO$_2$ 55

Chest x-ray: Low flattened diaphragm, increased anteroposterior chest diameter.

Pulmonary function testing: FEV$_1$ 2 L, FEV$_1$:FVC < 70%.

PROBLEM LIST

1. COPD
2. RA
3. Questionable PUD
4. Lacrimation and foreign body sensation
5. Rule out theophylline toxicity
6. Diabetes mellitus, hypoglycemic episodes

CASE 104

CC: LR is a 16-year-old male who presents to his primary care physician complaining of a painful, "raw" left ear.

Past Medical History

LR has no significant past medical history. One week before admission, he complained of a feeling of water in his left ear, which he was unable to remove. Since then, his ear has become increasingly erythematous and painful, and 3 days ago he noted a clear fluid draining from his ear.

Medication History
Astemizole, 10 mg PO QD for seasonal allergies

Allergies
Ragweed

Social History
LR is an avid water skier who spends considerable time in the water during the summer months.

Physical Examination
GEN: Well-developed, well-nourished male in moderate distress secondary to pain; complains of pain and "weeping" of the left ear; otherwise, unremarkable

VS: BP 120/70, HR 86, RR 20, T 37.0

HEENT: NC/AT, PERRLA, EOMI. Left auricle is erythematous and tender to palpation. External auditory canal is macerated, with a small amount of serous fluid present. TMs are intact and normal in appearance. The remainder of the physical examination is unremarkable.

Results of Laboratory Test
Culture of fluid in left ear: pending

PROBLEM LIST
1. Acute otitis externa

NEUROLOGIC DISORDERS

CASE 105

CC: MJ is a man, age 42, who is brought to the emergency department experiencing a tonic-clonic seizure with loss of consciousness. The nurse at the skilled nursing facility (SNF) where MJ resides states that this is his third seizure in the last 30 minutes.

History of Present Illness

The nurse who brought MJ to the ER states that the first seizure occurred approximately 30 minutes ago and was characterized by jerking movements of his upper extremities, muscle rigidity, urinary incontinence and loss of consciousness that lasted approximately 2 minutes. This first episode was then immediately followed by another seizure lasting 4 minutes. The nurse reports that on the way to the hospital a third seizure occurred which lasted approximately 2 minutes.

Past Medical History

MJ has a 3-year history of generalized tonic-clonic seizures after a motor vehicle accident, which has left him a paraplegic, i.e., paralyzed from the waist down, and produced mild mental deficiency. He lives at a skilled care facility, which has taken good care of him since his accident. Approximately 3 months ago, MJ started to experience muscle aches and bone pain. Rib fractures were noted on chest films. MJ was also noted to have some overgrowth of his gums with easy bleeding upon brushing. His physician believed these events were related to his phenytoin therapy and reduced his dose from 400 mg at bedtime to 300 mg at bedtime. MJ's seizures were still well controlled; however he continued to experience the same symptoms. Approximately 2 weeks ago, his phenytoin dose was further reduced to 200 mg at bedtime.

Medication History

Phenytoin chewable tablets, 200 mg PO HS
Ibuprofen, 400 mg PO PRN for back pain
Chlorhexidine gluconate, 15 mL, swish and expectorate BID (started 2 weeks ago)
Acetaminophen 325 mg with codeine 15 mg, 1 tablet PO Q4-6H PRN for pain

Allergies

NKDA

Physical Examination

VS: BP 170/100, HR 105, RR 26, T 38, Wt 60 kg, Ht 175cm

HEENT: PERRLA, poor dentition
CHEST: Clear to auscultation
COR: Sinus tachycardia, S_1, S_2, no S_3 or S_4
EXT: Thin with minimal muscle development, especially lower extremities
NEURO: Unresponsive to deep pain

Results of Laboratory Tests

Na 140 (140)	Hgb 160 (16)	AST 0.5 (31)	Ca 1.95 (7.8)
K 5.2 (5.0)	Hct 0.4 (40)	ALT 0.4 (25)	Phos 0.80 (2.5)
Cl 100 (100)	Plts 150 × 10⁹ (150 × 10³)	Alb 44 (4.4)	Mg 1.1(2.5)
HCO₃ 20 (20)	WBC 8800/mm³	T Bili 9 (0.5)	Alk Phos 2.0 (120)
BUN 6.5 (18)	RBC 5.0 × 10¹²/L (5.0 × 10⁶/mm³)	Phenytoin 16 (4)	Cr 67 (0.8)

EKG sinus tachycardia
Glu 6.1 (110)
ABG 7.30/50/92/88% on room air

PROBLEM LIST

1. Status epilepticus
2. Osteomalacia
3. Generalized tonic-clonic seizures

CASE 105 SOAP NOTES
Problem 1. Status epilepticus:

S: Patient has had 3 tonic-clonic seizures within the past 30 minutes

O: Patient has had 3 seizures within the past 30 minutes that have been witnessed by his nurse. The seizures were described as jerking movements of the upper extremities, urinary incontinence, and muscle rigidity with loss of consciousness. MJ is unresponsive to deep pain, tachycardic, tachypneic, and acidotic by ABG. Phenytoin level reported as 16 (4.0).

A: The decrease in this patient's phenytoin dose over the last 2 weeks has probably accounted for the subtherapeutic level and lack of clinical benefit from the drug. The decrease in dosage from 400 to 300 mg at bedtime did not affect his seizure control; however, his pain and gingival hyperplasia persisted (see below). The decrease in dosage from 300 to 200 mg at bedtime resulted in inadequate seizure control. This patient's condition warrants immediate attention to prevent further clinical deterioration. Diazepam or lorazepam should be administered immediately for rapid termination of the seizures. Either agent can be used; however, lorazepam's longer duration of action (compared with diazepam) may provide a therapeutic advantage. In order to maintain seizure control, additional antiepileptic agents with longer duration of action need to be administered (i.e., phenytoin). Until the cause of the seizures is known and the initial laboratory test results are returned, dextrose and thiamine IV should be administered to correct any abnormalities that may be responsible for the seizures.

P: Give thiamine, 100 mg IV, and 25 gm of glucose (50 mL of D$_{50}$W) immediately. Start lorazepam, 0.075 mg/kg (4.5mg) IV at 2 mg/min, (or diazepam, 10 mg IV at 5 mg/min) immediately. Respiratory status and seizure control should be monitored. Phenytoin, 18 mg/kg (approximately 1100 mg) IV at a maximum rate of 50 mg/min, should be initiated at the same time. BP, HR, and ECG results should be monitored during the phenytoin infusion. Once the patient's condition has stabilized, revaluation of his antiepileptic regimen is warranted (see below).

Problem 3. Generalized Tonic-Clonic Seizures

S: Patient presents with status epilepticus on current regimen.

O: Patient has past medical history significant for generalized tonic-clonic seizures. Seizures observed to be tonic-clonic seizures. Phenytoin level is 16 (4).

A: This patient's current regimen of 200 mg at bedtime is insufficient to keep this patient seizure-free. At doses of 300 mg at bedtime, this patient is able to remain seizure-free, however the side effects of phenytoin remain (osteomalacia and gingival hyperplasia). There are two options in this patient with regard to his antiepileptic management. The first option is to increase this patient's phenytoin dose to 300 mg and attempt to manage the side effects (see below); the second option is to change to a different agent which will prevent the tonic-clonic seizures (i.e., carbamazepine). Switching this patient to carbamazepine would seem a reasonable alternative. Aplastic anemia and agranulocytosis have occured in association with carbamazapine therapy, and it is therefore recommended that a baseline CBC count be obtained before initiation of therapy. MJ's RBC, WBC, and platelet counts are all within normal limits. Carbamazepine should be initiated with low doses to help minimize dizziness, drowsiness, and GI effects and titrated against both therapeutic and toxic effects. Dosages can be increased every 3 to 7 days until serum concentrations between 5 and 12 ug/mL are obtained.

P: Initiate carbamezapine at 200 mg PO BID. The dosage can be increased by 200 mg every 3 to 7 days until a therapeutic response or target serum concentration is obtained. Once carbamezapine levels are therapeutic, phenytoin can be tapered by decreasing the dosage by one third every 1 to 2 weeks until discontinued. Monitor MJ for seizures and/or adverse drug reactions (i.e., GI upset, diplopia, drowsiness). A CBC count should be obtained at monthly intervals for the first 2 months and then yearly therafter. MJ should be taught to inform his nurses at the SNF of the first sign of sore throat or flu-like illness; in the event these symptoms occur, a CBC count should be checked.

Problem 2. Osteomalacia

S: MJ has complained of muscle aches and bone pain while on phenytoin.

O: Serum Ca 1.95 (7.8), phosphate 0.80 (2.5), Alk Phos 2.0 (120). Past medical history significant for rib fractures on chest films.

A: MJ's complaints of muscle aches, bone pain, and rib fractures and his laboratory test results, in conjunction with his taking phenytoin for more than 6 months, are all consistent with phenytoin-induced osteomalacia. Antiepileptic-induced osteomalacia has been most commonly associated with phenytoin use but may occur with long-term use of any antiepileptic agent. Since antiepileptic-induced osteomalacia is believed to be caused by decreased concentrations of effective vitamin D activity, the treatment of choice would be to administer vitamin D with or without calcium. Effective doses have ranged from 2,000 to 10,000 u/day of vitamin D or 0.25 to 0.75 ug/day of activated vitamin D (1,25 dihydroxyvitamin D3) for 4 to 6 months or until biochemical and radiologic findings return to normal. Changing this patient's regimen to a less implicated antiepileptic may also provide a benefit as well as help to manage this patient's gingival hyperplasia (see problem 3).

P: Change the patient's antiepileptic medication as above.

CASE 105 QUESTIONS

1. If MJ continues to experience seizures after the phenytoin loading dose has been administered, what therapy is recommended next?
2. Describe MJ's risk factors for phenytoin-induced osteomalacia.
3. What is the mechanism of action of phenytoin-induced osteomalacia?
4. If the physicians decided to keep MJ on phenytoin and increase his dose to 300 mg po HS, what techniques should be used to manage his gingival hyperplasia?

CASE 106

CC: JZ is a 38-year-old female brought to the emergency department by ambulance after her sister observed her to have 3 generalized tonic-clonic seizures at home.

History of Present Illness

Upon arrival at JZ's home, the paramedics noted that she was having a generalized tonic-clonic seizure characterized by loss of consciousness, tongue biting, urinary incontinence, and muscle rigidity and subsequent jerking movements of all extremities. The seizure lasted for 3 minutes and was quickly followed by another seizure that lasted 5 minutes. On the order of the base hospital, the paramedics administered diazepam, 10 mg IV. JZ's seizures were terminated, but she did not regain full alertness. While waiting to be seen by the medical resident in the emergency room, JZ had another generalized tonic-clonic seizure. JZ has a history of poor compliance with phenytoin therapy for epilepsy because the medication causes her gums to swell and bleed.

Past Medical History

JZ has had numerous episodes of recurrent epigastric pain with anorexia, vomiting, and weight loss over the past several years. She was last seen in the GI clinic 3 days ago, at which time she denied abdominal pain and other GI distress but reported a 3-week history of arthralgias, fatigue, and mild fever. JZ has a 7-year history of posttraumatic epilepsy. Her seizures are characterized by an aura described as a rising epigastric sensation followed by a tingling sensation that progresses from her neck to her head. This is then followed by loss of consciousness and a stereotypical generalized tonic-clonic seizure.

Current Medications

Phenytoin, 400 mg PO QD
Naproxen, 550 mg PO BID

Family History

Aunt had systemic lupus erythematosus (SLE) at age 27

Social History

Denies alcohol and tobacco use

Physical Examination

VS: BP 168/98, HR 110, RR 20, T 37.5, Wt 63 kg, Ht 160 cm
HEENT: Bite wound on tongue; erythematous malar rash; moderate gingival hyperplasia
CHEST: Clear
COR: Normal S1, S2; no S3 or S4
EXT: Moderate joint swelling of hands and feet
NEURO: Unresponsive to deep pain

Results of Laboratory Tests

Na 135 (135)	Hct 0.34 (34)	AST 0.5 (30)	Glu 6.8 (122)
K 4.8 (4.8)	Hgb 120 (12)	ALT 0.6 (36)	Amylase 3.67 (220)
Cl 95 (95)	Plts 45 × 10⁹ (45 × 10³)	Alb 42 (4.2)	Phenytoin <4.0 (<1.0)
HCO₃ 26 (26)		T Bili 17.1 (1.0)	ESR 50 (50)
BUN 13.6 (38)			ANA titer 1:480
CR 212 (2.4)			

PROBLEM LIST

1. Systemic lupus erythematosus for 12 years
2. Partial epilepsy with secondarily generalized tonic-clonic seizures for 7 years.
3. Chronic pancreatitis of unknown cause
4. Status epilepticus

CASE 106 SOAP NOTES
Problem 4. Status Epilepticus

S: Sister reports 3 seizures at home.

O: Recurrent generalized tonic-clonic seizures witnessed by paramedics and emergency room staff without recovery of consciousness between attacks. Bite wound on tongue, unresponsive to deep pain, increased BP, HR, Temp, and glucose level. PHT <4.0 (<1.0).

A: Phenytoin noncompliance is the most likely cause of status epilepticus in JZ, but other potential causes (e.g., metabolic abnormalities, other primary CNS disorders) should be investigated. Diazepam, 10 mg IV, administered by paramedics terminated seizures temporarily, but JZ had a recurrent seizure in the emergency department. This may be related to the short duration of diazepam's anticonvulsant effect. Another dose of diazepam may be administered for the immediate prevention of seizures, but additional anticonvulsant therapy (e.g., phenytoin) is necessary to maintain seizure control. Lorazepam is also effective for aborting repetitive seizures during status epilepticus and could have been used in place of diazepam for JZ. Lorazepam has a longer-lasting anticonvulsant effect than diazepam and may be preferred for this reason.

P: Give diazepam, 10 mg IV (or lorazepam, 4 mg IV) immediately. Monitor respiratory status and seizure recurrence. Without delay, initiate phenytoin, 20 mg/kg (1200 mg) IV at a rate of approximately 50 mg/min. BP, HR, and ECG should be monitored during IV phenytoin infusion. JZ should have a thorough neurologic evaluation to assess other possible causes of seizures.

Problem 2. Generalized Tonic-Clonic Seizure Disorder

S: Seizures characterized by rising epigastric sensation, tingling sensation and loss of consciousness, tongue biting, urinary incontinence, and muscle rigidity followed by jerking movements of all extremities; history of poor compliance with phenytoin due to bleeding and swelling of the gums

O: Moderate gingival hyperplasia

A: The adverse effects of JZ's phenytoin therapy are clearly unacceptable to JZ. Alternate antiepileptic drug therapy is therefore required. Carbamazepine is effective for partial and secondarily generalized tonic-clonic seizures and is not associated with gingival hyperplasia or other undesirable cosmetic changes.

P: Initiate carbamazepine, 100 mg PO BID, and increase the dose in 100 to 200 mg increments every 3 to 7 days as tolerated by JZ. Maintenance dosing of carbamazepine on a BID schedule is acceptable and may improve patient compliance. Dose escalation should be stopped when seizures are controlled or JZ experiences dose-limiting adverse effects. Gradually discontinue phenytoin therapy (e.g., over several weeks) once a therapeutic effect of carbamazepine is established. JZ should be referred for evaluation and treatment of her gingival hyperplasia. JZ should be counseled about the importance of compliance with her prescribed antiepileptic drug regimen and should be encouraged to discuss any adverse effects with her health care provider.

Problem 1. Systemic Lupus Erythematosus

S: Three week history of arthralgias, fatigue, and mild fever; family history of SLE (aunt).

O: Erythematous malar (cheek) rash; moderate joint swelling of hands and feet; BUN 13.6 (38), Cr 212 (2.4), Plat 45 × 109 (45 × 10³), (+) ANA (titer: 1:480), ESR 50

A: Clinical and laboratory data suggest that JZ is experiencing a mild exacerbation of her SLE. NSAIDs are effective for their analgesic, antiinflammatory, and antipyretic effects, but naproxen may be contributing to JZ's poor renal function. Sulindac may have a less pronounced effect on renal function. Although phenytoin has been implicated as a cause of lupus, JZ has a family history of SLE and probably has the idiopathic form of this connective tissue disorder.

P: Change NSAID therapy from naproxen to sulindac, 150 mg PO BID. Monitor BUN and Cr levels, urinalysis results, and BP for possible adverse effects of sulindac therapy and signs and symptoms of SLE for worsening of this condition. JZ should be counseled to avoid direct sunlight, as it may cause the rash to worsen. Hydroxychloroquine (200 to 400 mg daily) is also effective for treating the skin lesions of SLE and should be considered if the rash does not resolve.

Problem 3. Pancreatitis

S: None

O: Amylase 3.67 (220)

A: No clinical signs or symptoms of acute pancreatic inflammation; no evidence of pancreatic insufficiency (e.g., malabsorption or inability to maintain normal blood sugar levels)

P: There is no specific treatment for pancreatitis other than managing the symptoms of acute pancreatitis (e.g., abdominal pain, alterations in fluid balance, malnutrition) or the complications of chronic pancreatic insufficiency. JZ should be monitored for signs and symptoms of pancreatitis. A low-fat diet should be recommended, particularly when abdominal pain is associated with food intake.

CASE 106 QUESTIONS

1. JZ received an additional dose of diazepam (10 mg IV) and a full loading dose of phenytoin (1200 mg IV) in the emergency department, and her seizures were terminated. JZ was then admitted to the neurology service. The physician would like to continue maintenance anticonvulsant therapy by the intravenous route until JZ can be given oral medications. What anticonvulsant drugs are available for use in this setting and which would you choose for JZ?

2. How should JZ be monitored for the potential hematologic adverse effects of carbamazepine therapy?

3. After 1 week of carbamazepine therapy, JZ develops a pruritic erythematous rash on her trunk, arms, and thighs. What alternate antiepileptic drug would you recommend for the treatment of JZ's seizure disorder?

4. Two weeks after JZ is discharged from the hospital, she is readmitted with complaints of worsening arthralgias, weight loss, and fever of 104°F. A renal biopsy shows prolif-

erative lupus nephritis. How would you treat JZ's acute exacerbation of SLE?

5. During this hospitalization, JZ again develops anorexia, postprandial bloating, and greasy stools. The treating physician wishes to initiate pancreatic enzyme replacement. What would you recommend?

CASE 107

CC: DW is a 31-year-old woman with a history of low back pain and Crohn's disease who presents to clinic complaining of "colicky" right lower quadrant (RLQ) abdominal pain and increased back pain. Three weeks ago, she was seen for complaints of persistent bloody diarrhea, malaise, fever, anorexia, and a 20-pound weight loss. Total parenteral nutrition (TPN) was begun, and DW has since stopped losing weight. She is requesting meperidine for her pain, stating that she "always gets a shot when the pain gets this bad."

Past Medical History

DW's Crohn's disease began 15 years ago with frequent bouts of abdominal pain accompanied by low-grade fevers and diarrhea. The last exacerbation was 18 months ago, when prednisone and sulfasalazine were begun. Her low back pain has been present for 7 years, following an automobile accident. She has a history of frequent emergency department visits for meperidine injections, and one hospitalization for pain management. She has recently developed side effects from long-term glucocorticoid therapy. She also has a 1-year history of chronic depression that has not responded to the tricyclic antidepressants amitriptyline and doxepin.

Past Surgical History

DW underwent partial bowel resection and cholecystectomy 3 years ago, and last year she had a laminectomy performed on her lumbar spine, which decreased but did not eliminate her back pain.

Medication History

Prednisone, 30 mg PO QD for 18 months
Sulfasalazine, 500 mg PO QID
Phenelzine, 15 mg PO TID for 4 weeks for depression
Hydrocodone 5 mg/acetaminophen 500 mg, 2 tablets PO Q4-6H PRN for pain; DW takes 12 tablets per day

Allergies

Codeine produces nausea and vomiting.

Physical Examination

GEN: Disheveled, anorexic young woman in moderate distress; appears older than stated age

VS: BP 140/98, HR 100, RR 24, T 38, Wt 54 kg, Ht 168 cm

HEENT: Moon facies, aphthous mouth ulcers
COR: Normal S_1 and S_2
CHEST: Clear to auscultation and palpation, no rales or rhonchi
ABD: Distended abdomen with diffuse tenderness; marked tenderness in RLQ, with abdominal mass upon palpation; striae present
GU: WNL
RECT: Scarring due to healed perianal fistula
EXT: Mild bilateral LE edema; petechiae present
NEURO: O × 3

Results of Laboratory Tests

Na 150 (150)	Hct 0.35 (35%)	AST 1.14 (68)	Gluc 9.9 (180)
K 3.2 (3.2)	Hgb 110 (11)	Alk Phos 2.3 (135)	Ca 1.97 (7.9)
Cl 110 (110)	Lkcs 10.5×10^9 (10.5×10^3)	Albumin 30 (3.0)	PO_4 1.45 (4.5)
HCO_3 24 (24)	Plts 150×10^9 (150×10^3)	T Bili 17 (1.0)	Mg 1.0 (2.4)
BUN 7.1 (20)	MCV 100 (100)		B_{12} 221 (300)
Cr 84 (1.1)			Folate 9 (4.0)
			ESR 18 (18)

Stool guaiac-positive, bright red blood noted
Endoscopy negative for gastric ulceration

PROBLEM LIST

1. Crohn's disease with acute abdominal pain
2. Chronic low back pain
3. Anemia secondary to Crohn's disease
4. Electrolyte disturbances
5. Depression

CASE 107 SOAP NOTES
Problem 1. Exacerbated Crohn's Disease with Acute Abdominal Pain

S: DW complains of RLQ pain and is requesting opiates. She has had diarrhea, malaise, and anorexia with weight loss.

O: Diffuse and focal abdominal tenderness, mildly elevated leukocyte count, fistula scarring, aphthous mouth ulcers, and guaiac-positive stool. Vital signs are consistent with moderate distress, and patient exhibits low-grade fever. She has a 15-year history of Crohn's disease, with a partial bowel resection and healed perianal fistula. She also has decreased serum magnesium, calcium, folate, and B_{12} levels consistent with malabsorption and elevated AST and alkaline phosphatase levels. The right-sided tenderness and pain is characteristic of Crohn's disease, which can cause scarring and tissue masses at the ileocecal junction.

P: Increase sulfasalazine dose to a maximum of 4 g/day to induce remission. Larger doses produce a higher potential for adverse effects, including nausea, vomiting, anorexia, and hemolytic anemia. If unresponsive, a change to olsalazine, 500 mg twice daily, can be instituted. Olsalazine is bioconverted to 5-aminosalicylic acid (5-ASA), and approximately 95% of the ingested dose reaches the colon. Her prednisone dose should be increased to 40 to 80 mg/day in divided doses until remission, when she can be changed back to a single morning dose. Glucocorticoids produce a more immediate response than sulfasalazine, which often requires 3 to 4 weeks of treatment to induce remission. Glucocorticoid enemas, such as hydrocortisone, may re-

duce inflammation at the rectum and colon, but they are not necessary because of DW's systemic steroid use. Sulfasalazine or olsalazine can be discontinued upon remission of DW's Crohn's disease, since there is no evidence that they prevent recurrence. Once the symptoms of her Crohn's disease subside, systemic glucocorticoids should be decreased, as DW is suffering symptoms of prednisone-induced cushingoid syndrome and hypothalamus-pituitary-adrenal (HPA) axis suppression (e.g., moon facies, increased bruising, increased serum glucose concentration, mild lower extremity edema, and disturbances of sodium, potassium, and chloride levels). Prednisone should be decreased by 2.5 to 5 mg/day per week until a physiologic dose is reached (7.5 mg/day) and then by 1 mg/day per week. Morning cortisol levels should be checked monthly. When the level is more than 275.9 nmol/L (10 μg/dL), the glucocorticoid may be discontinued. While tapering the prednisone, monitor for an exacerbation of Crohn's disease, including bloody diarrhea, abdominal pain, or cramping, as well as for adrenal insufficiency, manifested by malaise, myalgia, hypotension, and altered glucose and electrolyte levels. DW should be counseled to report signs of recurring Crohn's disease or adrenal insufficiency.

While mild narcotics, such as codeine or meperidine, may be effective for the acute pain, chronic narcotic use should be discouraged to avoid opiate habituation. Narcotics may also exacerbate her depression and appetite loss by central nervous system depression. In addition, constipation induced by these agents may confuse monitoring of her Crohn's disease, as abrupt withdrawal of opiates can produce symptoms of pain and diarrhea that mimic those of an exacerbation of the illness. Acutely, opiates are acceptable, and morphine sulfate is a more potent analgesic with a longer duration of action than meperidine. She does not demonstrate a true allergy to codeine, as GI disturbance is a common side effect of this agent; emesis is common when codeine is used postoperatively because intraoperative anesthetics may still be acting upon the brain's central nausea centers. Further questioning of DW could determine whether her previous experience with codeine occurred in the immediate postsurgical period. Though DW reports meperidine has been effective in the past, it is contraindicated now because she is receiving phenelzine, a monoamine oxidase inhibitor (MAOI), that has been linked to both serious hypotension and life-threatening hypertensive crisis when administered with meperidine. In addition, meperidine has a short duration of action (2 to 3 hours), which leads to a more frequent need for the medication. Meperidine also has a higher potential for euphoria and possible habituation than other opiates. For moderate-to-severe pain, oral morphine, 20 mg every 4 to 6 hours, may be continued in the outpatient setting until DW's acute symptoms abate. Tapering of the opiate should begin within 24 to 72 hours of drug initiation, by reducing the amount of each dose. For example, morphine can be reduced to 15 mg for one day, then to 10 mg per dose for another 24 hours, and so on. An alternative taper consists of increasing the interval between doses, e.g., changing from a 4-hour interval to a 6-hour one, then an

8-hour one, and so on. A milder analgesic, such as 5 to 10 mg of either hydrocodone or oxycodone, may then be substituted. The latter agents have less propensity to induce nausea or emesis than either morphine or codeine. These medications should be discontinued as patient tolerance permits.

Problem 2. Chronic Low Back Pain

S: Current complaints of back pain

O: Vital signs consistent with moderate distress; 7-year history, with laminectomy 1 year ago; history of emergency department visits and one hospitalization for pain control

A: DW has chronic low back pain that is not responding to hydrocodone, a moderately potent opioid. The lack of response may be a result of tolerance induced by continued use of opiate agonists. She is also at risk for acetaminophen hepatotoxicity caused by ingestion of 6 g acetaminophen per day, and her elevated AST and alkaline phosphatase levels are consistent with a large acetaminophen load.

P: Her chronic low back pain is not responding to hydrocodone, probably because of opiate tolerance following long-term use of opiate agonists. She is also at risk for acetaminophen hepatotoxicity. After her acute pain problems have been controlled by morphine followed by a change back to hydrocodone or oxycodone (as above), a steady taper of her narcotic should be initiated (e.g., reduction by two tablets per day each week, until the medication is discontinued in approximately 6 weeks). This will allow endogenous pain control mechanisms to regain function and prevent the development of an abstinence syndrome. Continuous opioid use is not recommended for chronic low back pain, and nonpharmacologic treatments, such as physical therapy should be attempted. Further tests to elucidate the cause(s) of the back pain are required; nerve damage would best be treated with tricyclic agents or anticonvulsants, while degenerative joint disease or other musculoskeletal complaints would respond to acetaminophen. While taking acetaminophen, DW should be warned of the potential for hepatic toxicity with overcompliance, and instructed to keep her total daily dose of acetaminophen below 4 g. Since there is no current evidence of gastric ulceration, NSAIDs such as ibuprofen may be used to control her pain after the glucocorticoids have been discontinued. The two agents should not be used concomitantly, since they decrease platelet function, leading to greater risk of bleeding. If NSAIDs are begun, stool guaiac tests must be carefully monitored to detect gastric erosion, although her Crohn's disease may interfere. Renal function tests should also be monitored periodically, as NSAIDs reduce the glomerular filtration rate (GFR). A typical dose of ibuprofen for chronic pain management is 400 to 600 mg four times daily.

Problem 3. Anemia

S: DW's malaise may be a sign of her mild anemia.

O: Low Hct and Hgb, serum folate, and B_{12} levels, and increased MCV

A: The likely cause is a malabsorption syndrome caused by her exacerbation of Crohn's disease.

P: Multivitamins may be added to her TPN solution. Her Hgb, Hct, MCV, folate, and B_{12} levels should be monitored biweekly. After remission occurs and her TPN is discontinued, she may be given a multivitamin containing folic acid and B_{12}, and ferrous sulfate tablets, 325 mg PO TID. She should be told to take her ferrous sulfate with food if it causes stomach upset and that her stools may be darkened by iron supplements. Dairy products should be avoided during ferrous sulfate therapy to maximize absorption.

Problem 4. Electrolyte Disturbances

S: None

O: Increased serum sodium and chloride levels, decreased serum potassium, magnesium, and calcium levels

A: Abnormalities consistent with glucocorticoid use

P: Until steroids are discontinued, adjustments for potassium loss and sodium and fluid retention can be made in her TPN solution. Her electrolytes can be monitored as changes are instituted, until they are within normal ranges. In the outpatient setting, electrolyte and blood glucose levels can be monitored weekly. AST, albumin, alkaline phosphatase, and total bilirubin levels should be monitored monthly. Her infusion site should be observed for infection, and she should be warned of early signs of infection, such as elevated body temperature, redness, or discharge from the catheter site.

Problem 5. Depression

S: By history; complains of malaise

O: Disheveled appearance, anorexia

A: Depression refractory to tricyclic antidepressants may be worsened by chronic pain and by corticosteroids.

P: DW's dose of phenelzine can be optimized to a maximum of 60 mg/day. Should she continue to be unresponsive, she may be given a trial of trazodone, fluoxetine, or buproprion. Mood, appearance, and subjective reports of her depressive symptoms (e.g., lack of appetite, fatigue, malaise) should be monitored often and are expected to improve within 4 to 6 weeks. Further evaluation of her medication history should be performed, to determine why she failed previous trials of antidepressants. Often, these medications are discontinued before an adequate dose or duration of treatment is attained. However, they are safer to use than the MAO inhibitors, with less potential for drug-drug or food-drug interactions, and therefore are usually agents of first choice for treating depression. They also have analgesic effects and may decrease the intensity of DW's pain. Counseling and psychologic support should be provided for DW with medication. DW should be monitored for adverse reactions of medications, including sedation, increased heart rate, and changes in bowel or bladder function.

CASE 107 QUESTIONS

1. DW's sulfasalazine is increased. Three days later, she develops a rash on her torso. What action should be taken?

2. MRI is performed to evaluate DW's increased complaints of back pain. The study reveals nerve root damage. Select and outline a titration schedule for a drug to treat her neuropathic pain.

3. What would you monitor for this drug, and how often would you do this?

4. DW's physician wishes to use clonidine instead of continuing her hydrocodone with acetaminophen. How would you advise him to use this agent?

5. DW returns to the clinic for a 4-week follow-up. Her last four blood pressure measurements have been elevated. Her physician wishes to begin antihypertensive therapy and asks for your input.

CASE 108

CC: AJ is a 28-year-old black woman who presents to the hospital with a 2-day history of headache, vomiting, photophobia, and neck stiffness.

History of Present Illness

Two days PTA, AJ was taking a final exam in business school and experienced a sudden onset of a severe headache and a subsequent mild decrease in consciousness. AJ has complained of a 3-month history of an increased number of mild headaches, dizziness, and intermittent nausea and vomiting. AJ was admitted to the hospital; a head CT scan revealed a left intrafrontal hemorrhage with subarachnoid blood. Angiogram confirmed rupture of the left anterior communicating artery aneurysm and was negative for multiple aneurysms.

Past Medical History

Hypertension, most recent BP 155/101; angiogram (3.5 years ago): left anterior communicating artery aneurysm, 1 cm diameter; anxiety

Medication History

Hydrochlorothiazide, 50 mg PO QAM for 2 years
Valium, 5 mg PO BID for 5 years
Excedrin, 1 Q4H PRN

Allergies

Sulfa: rash; macrodantin: SOB; codeine: nausea

Social History

Smokes one pack of cigarettes/day. Drinks approximately 1.5 pots of coffee/day. Occasionally drinks alcohol

Review of Systems

Noncontributory

Physical Examination

GEN: Thin adult female with mild anxiety; easily arousable

VS: BP 180/110, HR 82, RR 16, T 37, Wt 60 kg, Ht 174 cm, ICP 14 mm Hg

HEENT: Mild nuchal rigidity, no adenopathy, oropharynx benign

COR: RRR, nl S1 and S2

CHEST: Clear to auscultation and percussion

ABD: NABS, soft NT, ND

GU, RECT, and EXT: WNL

NEURO: O × 3, speech fluent, facial sensation throughout, tongue midline, gait WNL, strength 5/5 throughout ext.

Results of Laboratory Tests

Na 142 (142)	Hct 0.33 (33)	Glu 5.8 (105)
K 3.8 (3.8)	Hgb 120 (12)	Ca 2.39 (9.6)
Cl 105 (105)	WBC 8 (8000)	Alk Phos 0.58 (35)
HCO$_3$ 23 (23)	Plts 290 (290)	Alb 44 (4.4)
BUN 6.4 (18)	MCV 85 (85)	T Bili 6.8 (0.4)
Cr 97.21 (1.1)	Mg 1.0 (2.0)	Uric Acid 499.6 (8.4)
	AST 0.1 (10)	

WBC diff, urinalysis, chest x-ray, ECG: all WNL

PROBLEM LIST

1. Subarachnoid hemorrhage
2. Hypertension
3. Anxiety

CASE 108 SOAP NOTES

Problem 1. Subarachnoid hemorrhage

S: AJ complains of sudden onset of a severe headache with mild deterioration of consciousness 2 days PTA, with a 2-day history of headache, vomiting, photophobia, and neck stiffness. AJ also has a 3-month history of an increased number of mild headaches, dizziness, and intermittent nausea and vomiting.

O: CT scan shows a left intrafrontal hemorrhage with subarachnoid blood. Angiogram 3.5 years ago revealed left ACA aneurysm; repeat angiogram shows rupture of aneurysm. AJ's BP is elevated at 180/110.

A: AJ has suffered a subarachnoid hemorrhage caused by rupture of a left ACA aneurysm. AJ's 3-month history of increased number of mild headaches, dizziness, and intermittent nausea and vomiting represent minor leaks or sentinel hemorrhage and are warning signs of subsequent major hemorrhage from the aneurysm. The sudden onset of severe headache is the hallmark of subarachnoid hemorrhage. Blood in the subarachnoid cerebrospinal fluid will cause meningism; AJ's symptoms of headache, photophobia, nuchal rigidity, and vomiting represent meningism. AJ's subarachnoid hemorrhage (SAH) is considered grade II according to the Hunt and Hess clinical grading scale. AJ's angiogram should be checked for multiple aneurysms, because multiple aneurysms occur in approximately 15% of cases.

P: Because AJ has grade II hemorrhage, she has a relatively good prognosis. Goal of treatment for SAH is to prevent complications, which are fatal in 25% of cases. The major neurologic complications are rebleeding of the aneurysm, hydrocephalus, and cerebral vasospasm. Hypothalamic dysfunction is another major complication. General preoperative medical management includes provisions for quiet bed rest with elevation of head of bed to 30° to facilitate intracranial venous drainage and pulmonary toilet to prevent atelectasis and pneumonia. AJ should be started on stool softeners (Colace, 100 to 250 mg PO BID) to prevent any strain, deep vein thrombosis (DVT) prophylaxis (heparin, 5,000 u SC BID and SCD's) and stress bleeding prophylaxis (H_2-blocker). Blood pressure is often elevated as a result of hypothalamic dysfunction, which leads to increased levels of circulating catecholamines. Systolic blood pressure should be lowered gently to avoid hypotension and cerebral ischemia. Short-acting antihypertensive agents, such as IV labetolol or SL nifedipine, should be used. Surgical clipping of the aneurysm is treatment of choice to prevent rebleeding. The International Cooperative Study Group findings show that patients with grade I to III presentations should undergo clip ligation via craniotomy and are candidates for early surgery (0–3 days). Surgery should be performed within 72 hours of the hemorrhage, to avoid the period of the highest incidence of vasospasm (3 to 14 days). If surgery is contraindicated or unavailable, antifibrinolytic agents, such as epsilon aminocaproic acid (EACA) or tranexamic acid, should be used. Use of antifibrinolytics is controversial because of the potential increased risk of vasospasm. Postoperative management includes anticonvulsant therapy for seizure prophylaxis, corticosteroids (dexamethasone, 4 mg IV Q6H) to control cerebral edema and inflammation, and adequate oxygenation. Dexamethasone is the corticosteroid of choice because of its relatively high antiinflammatory potency and low mineralocorticoid potency compared with hydrocortisone. Had AJ's CT scan revealed hydrocephalus, a ventricular drain would need to be surgically placed and intracranial pressure (ICP) gradually reduced to normal levels (12 to 15 mm Hg). Osmotic diuretics (mannitol, 0.25 to 1.0 g/kg over 15 to 20 minutes) may be used to lower ICP and alleviate cerebral edema. To prevent delayed cerebral vasospasm, hypervolemic-hypertensive-hemodilution or "triple-H" therapy should be instituted. The goal of therapy is to augment cerebral perfusion pressure to minimize cerebral ischemia from vasospasm. This is accomplished by raising systolic BP, cardiac output, and intravascular volume. In practice, hematocrit is reduced to 30 ± 3%, CVP elevated to 8 to 12 mm Hg, PCWP to 15 to 18 mm Hg, and systolic BP to approximately 150 to 170 mm Hg (up to as high as 200 to 220 mm Hg). Inotropic drugs (i.e., dopamine, norepinephrine, or phenylephrine) are used to keep systolic BP 20 to 40 mm Hg above pretreatment levels. Hypervolemia, or volume expansion, is accomplished with normal saline, nonprotein colloid, and/or albumin. Cerebral vasoselective calcium-channel blockers are used to reduce ischemic deficits associated with cerebral vasospasm. Nimodipine, 60 mg PO or through nasogastric tube every 4 hours for 21 days, should be initiated within 96 hours of SAH. If systolic BP is less than 110 mm Hg, give nimodipine 30 mg PO or NG every 2 hours.

Problem 2. Hypertension

S: No complaints

O: Recent BP 155/101; on admission 180/110. AJ's uric acid is elevated.

A: As mentioned above, hypertension can occur after SAH. However, AJ's most recent BP was 155/101, which indicates her underlying hypertension is not well controlled (age-related normal is less than 140/90 mm Hg). AJ's risk factors for hypertension include her race (black) and a modifiable risk factor, smoking. Her caffeine intake and anxiety are probably aggravating her hypertension. Her uric acid level is high, which may be caused by hydrochlorothiazide. Treatment for her essential hypertension should be delayed until SAH is controlled.

P: Once SAH is controlled, it would be reasonable to add a second agent to hydrochlorothiazide, such as a β-blocker or calcium-channel blocker. It would also be reasonable to stop the HCTZ and begin a β-blocker or calcium-channel blocker. Sodium restriction (to less than 2 g/day) and stress reduction need to be initiated. Also, AJ should be advised to stop smoking, and a smoking cessation program should be recommended.

Problem 3. Anxiety

S: No complaints

O: AJ is mildly anxious and easily arousable

A: AJ's primary physician started her on diazepam, 5 mg PO BID 5 years ago, when she started business school. Her anxiety may be exacerbated by her caffeine intake and stress from school. While AJ is hospitalized and in an ICU, therapy should be changed to a short acting IV benzodiazepine, such as lorazepam (2 mg/day, titrating for control of agitation). It is important to avoid benzodiazepine withdrawal because it may precipitate seizures.

P: Upon discharge, she should continue on diazepam and consider psychotherapy to improve coping abilities (such as stress from school). Dose of diazepam may be increased (up to 40 mg/day). Buspirone may be considered if symptoms do not improve on diazepam. The cause(s) of AJ's anxiety should be identified; biological anxiety should be distinguished from environmental anxiety-causing factors.

CASE 108 QUESTIONS

1. What are AJ's risk factors for development of an aneurysm and/or SAH?
2. What is the proposed mechanism of action for calcium-channel blockers for use in cerebral vasospasm?
3. How should anticonvulsant therapy (phenytoin) be initiated?
4. What are some considerations for use of antiemetic agents?
5. What is the Hunt and Hess grading scale?

CASE 109

CC: FF is a 14-year-old boy who is brought to the pediatric clinic for evaluation of recent onset of pain in the back and chest and a low-grade fever.

Past Medical History

FF's pain and fever began last night after returning from an all-day school field trip. He was able to sleep through the night, but this morning he is still in moderate pain. His complaints are similar to those of past exacerbations of his sickle-cell disease. His mother also reports that his teacher has been complaining that FF has been "daydreaming" in class more than usual, which is affecting his performance. FF's mother thinks these episodes are "petit mal" seizures; she has noticed that he has 6 to 7 brief episodes (3 to 5 seconds each) per week characterized by a blank stare and some eye blinking. He continues to use his inhaler 3 to 4 times daily and is compliant with all medications.

Current Medications

Ethosuximide, 250 mg PO TID
Sustained-release theophylline, 200 mg PO BID
Metaproterenol MDI, 1 to 2 puffs PRN for shortness of breath
Folic acid, 1 mg PO QD
Benzoyl peroxide cream 5%, applied once daily (first prescribed 1 week ago)

Allergies

ASA-induced bronchospasm

Physical Examination

GEN: Ill-appearing male exhibiting mild-to-moderate pain behavior during examination
VS: BP 100/76, HR 80, RR 18, T 37.4, Wt 44 kg, Ht 157 cm
HEENT: Mildly icteric sclera, erythematous skin with comedones and pustules on face and neck
CHEST: Mild expiratory wheezes, no rales or rhonchi
ABD: Hepatomegaly
NEURO: No nystagmus, steady gait

Results of Laboratory Tests

Na 142 (142)	BUN 3.6 (10)	Retic 0.01 (10)
K 4.0 (4.0)	CR 71 (0.8)	Theophylline 61 (11)
Cl 100 (100)	Hct 0.28 (28)	Ethosuximide 354 (50)
HCO$_3$ 25 (25)	Hgb 90 (9.0)	

PROBLEM LIST

1. Sickle-cell anemia with acute vasoocclusive painful crisis (4 admissions last year for parenteral narcotic treatment of vasoocclusive crises)
2. Asthma for 8 years (hospitalized once for exacerbation 3 years ago)
3. Generalized absence seizures for 4 years
4. Grade II acne

CASE 109 QUESTIONS

1. a. FF calls clinic 4 weeks later complaining that the benzoyl peroxide cream is "not working" despite applying the cream as directed each night. What would you recommend for treatment of FF's acne at this time?

b. FF responds by saying that he would like a prescription for Accutane (isotretinoin) because he has heard that this is the most effective medication for acne. How would you respond?

2. a. Several months later, FF is hospitalized for treatment of acute vasoocclusive crisis. Current medications include:
   Ethosuximide syrup, 750 mg BID by nasogastric tube
   Aminophylline, 25 mg/hr IV infusion
   Flunisolide MDI, 2 puffs BID
   Metaproterenol MDI, 1 to 2 puffs PRN for SOB
   Meperidine, 75 mg IV Q3-4H PRN for pain
   On hospital day 4, FF has a generalized tonic-clonic seizure. Identify 2 potential drug-related causes for FF's seizure. How would you assess whether these drugs might be implicated as a cause of this seizure?

b. On hospital day 6, FF has another generalized tonic-clonic seizure. Theophylline and meperidine have been ruled out as possible causes. A neurology consultation is obtained, and an idiopathic generalized-tonic seizure disorder is the diagnosis. What are your recommendations for chronic treatment of epilepsy in FF?

3. FF is seen in the pediatric clinic for evaluation 1 year later. He reports good control of absence seizures, but he has had 3 generalized tonic-clonic seizures in the past year, despite compliance with valproate, 750 mg PO TID. Attempts to further increase the dose of valproate resulted in intolerable dizziness and drowsiness. FF is very anxious about possibly having a seizure at school and would like to reduce the frequency of generalized tonic-clonic seizures even further. What change would you recommend for the treatment of FF's seizure disorder?

CASE 110

CC: SA is a woman, age 35, who presents to the emergency department complaining of sudden onset headache pain, nausea and vomiting, and chest pain for 3 days.

History of Present Illness

SA reports that she has 3 to 4 headache episodes per month, usually before the onset of her menses. This headache episode began 3 days ago. She describes her headache as bilateral, dull, throbbing pain. The pain has been so severe that she is not able to work. SA has been taking 2 to 3 ibuprofen 200 mg tablets every 6 hours without pain relief. SA also has noticed a worsening in her chest pain that is only mildly relieved by her antacid.

Past Medical History

SA was hospitalized 2 months ago for a distal vein thrombosis in her left lower calf for which she does not take any medication. She also has a history of gastroesophageal reflux disease (GERD), which began 5 years ago. Her reflux occurs at night just before lying down or when she bends over.

Medication History

Ibuprofen, 200 to 300 mg PO Q6H PRN for headache pain
Aluminum hydroxide gel (Amphojel®), 40 mL PO Q4-6H PRN
     for heartburn

Allergies

Sulfa drugs cause hives
Chlorpromazine causes dystonia

Social History

Tobacco: 2 packs per day
Caffeine: 4 cups of coffee per day

Review of Systems

Noncontributory

Physical Examination

GEN:	Obese female in moderate distress.
VS:	BP 128/82, HR 70, RR 30, T 36, Wt 90 kg, Ht 172 cm
HEENT:	PERRLA, photophobia, normocephalic, atraumatic, erythematous oropharynx
COR:	Normal S1 and S2, regular rate and rhythm
CHEST:	Moderate wheezing on inspiration
ABD:	Soft, nontender, no hepatosplenomegaly, no lymphadenopathy
RECT:	Guaiac-negative
EXT:	+ clubbing, no evidence of cyanosis; no evidence of swelling or erythema in lower extremities
NEURO:	Oriented to time, place and person; cranial nerves intact; normal deep tendon reflexes

Results of Laboratory Tests

Na 140 (140)	Hct 0.34 (34)	Glu 6.1 (110)
K 3.8 (3.8)	Hgb 120 (12)	Ca 2.2 (8.9)
Cl 109 (109)	Lkcs 5×10^9 (5×10^3)	PO₄ 0.64 (2)
HCO₃ 22 (22)	Plts 290×10^9 (290×10^3)	Mg 1.75 (3.5)
BUN 10 (30)	CR 88 (1)	

Chest x-ray: Normal
ECG: Normal

PROBLEM LIST

1. Acute migraine headache
2. Gastroesophageal reflux disease
3. Chronic migraine headache
4. Status post deep venous thrombosis

CASE 110 SOAP NOTES

Problem 1. Acute Migraine Headache

S: SA is complaining of sudden onset headache pain, nausea and vomiting for 3 days. She describes the headache as bilateral, dull, throbbing pain of sudden onset. SA states she experiences 3 to 4 headaches per month just before her menses.

O: SA is complaining of photophobia and emesis.

A: SA is symptomatic, with this migraine attack lasting 3 days.

She has not had any relief from maximum doses of ibuprofen, an NSAID. NSAIDs are effective in aborting acute onset migraines; however, SA continues to have migraine pain despite maximum dosing. For intractable migraines, products such as Cafergot BP®, dihydroergotamine (DHE), or narcotic analgesics may be used. Cafergot BP®, however, contains caffeine, which should be avoided in SA. SA has recently had a deep venous thrombosis, which is a contraindication for DHE therapy. The duration and severity of SA's headache and the accompanying symptoms warrant treatment. SA experiences dystonic reactions to chlorpromazine and although this is not an absolute contraindication, it should be avoided until SA is less anxious and her acute pain is controlled before attempting to rechallenge her. If a rechallenge of chlorpromazine is necessary, then an antihistamine with anticholinergic properties should be coadministered to prevent another dystonic reaction. Diphenhydramine and benztropine are two anticholinergic agents that are commonly used. For the treatment of SA's acute pain, a parenteral narcotic analgesic should be used since she has been vomiting and is nauseous.

P: Discontinue ibuprofen. Begin morphine sulfate, 3–5 mg every 2 hours intravenously, as needed to control her acute headache pain. SA should be switched to an oral medication as soon as possible. Acetaminophen with codeine tablets may be used. One to two tablets (containing 30 mg codeine per tablet) every four hours may be helpful, once SA is able to tolerate oral medication. Once SA's acute headache pain is controlled, SA should discontinue acetaminophen with codeine and begin prophylactic therapy.

Problem 2. GERD

S: SA is complaining of nausea, vomiting, and chest pain, which occurs at night just before lying down or while bending over.

O: SA has a history of GERD currently being treated with "as needed" aluminum hydroxide antacid. On physical examination, SA has evidence of an erythematous oral mucosa.

A: Since SA has a history of GERD, she should try to avoid or minimize any precipitating factors. Risk factors that may decrease lower esophageal sphincter pressure include smoking and obesity. SA has also been experiencing chest pain or heartburn just before lying down. Since SA has been managed with antacids with some success, an H₂-antagonist should be added to her regimen. In addition, SA should use an antacid with at least 80 mEq of acid buffering capacity 1 to 3 hours after meals and at bedtime. Amphojel® contains 10 mEq per 5 mL of acid buffering capacity. Since SA is taking 40 mL per dose, this is sufficient to neutralize stomach acids and prevent erosive esophagitis when reflux occurs. An H₂-blocker should added for acute relief. Her pain may also be relieved by the morphine sulfate used for her acute migraine headache pain.

P: Famotidine, 40 mg PO, should be given to SA along with an antacid that contains 80 mEq of acid-buffering capacity. SA should discontinue smoking. Since SA has been smoking for many years, it is likely that she is nicotine-dependent. SA should first attempt to decrease the quantity of cigarettes smoked per day, and enroll in a smoking cessation program. She should also receive dietary counseling in order to lose weight while maintaining adequate nutrition. SA should continue taking famotidine, 40 mg PO QD, to prevent further reflux symptoms. Her antacid may be used as needed for severe attacks.

Problem 3. Chronic Migraine Headache

S: SA reports she has 3 to 4 migraine headaches per month usually occurring before her menses.

O: Noncontributory

A: Since SA has more than 2 migraine attacks per month that are predictable and debilitating, she should receive prophylactic therapy. Caffeine containing products, such as Cafergot®, should be avoided because they may aggravate her GERD symptoms. Tricyclic antidepressants, which have anticholinergic effects, may also worsen GERD symptoms and therefore should be avoided. Propranolol (Inderal®) would be a good choice in SA, because it has been associated with a 70 to 80% response rate. A response may be seen within 4 to 6 weeks but may take up to 3 to 6 months.

P: Begin propranolol, 20 mg PO BID. The propranolol dose should be titrated to an average dose of 80 to 240 mg per day given BID to TID. Maximum doses should not exceed 320 mg/day. SA should be monitored closely for hypotension and bradycardia. In addition, she should have her cholesterol and blood glucose levels checked regularly.

Problem 4. Status Post Deep Venous Thrombosis

S: Noncontributory

O: SA has a history of deep venous thrombosis in her left calf, which required hospitalization. Currently SA has no evidence of erythema or swelling in either lower extremity.

A: Since SA had a distal deep venous thrombosis 1 month ago, long-term anticoagulation is not required.

P: Educate the patient on nondrug measures to prevent further clotting, such as walking, losing weight, and smoking cessation.

CASE 110 QUESTIONS

1. Besides narcotic analgesics, what other therapies may be used to control intractable migraine headaches?
2. What nondrug measures may help to relieve SA's chest pain?
3. What foods may precipitate migraine headaches?
4. Which antimigraine medications, if any, should be avoided in SA?

CASE 111

CC: HK is a man, age 59, who presents to the neurology clinic with recurrent seizures.

Past Medical History

HK has a 22-year history of idiopathic generalized tonic-clonic seizures. Seizures have occurred sporadically in the past; however, HK now reports about 4 seizures monthly.

Current Medications

Phenytoin, 500 mg PO QD for 22 years
Cimetidine, 800 mg PO QHS for 3 months
Captopril, 25 mg PO BID for 1 year

Social History

HK is a smoker (33 pack-years), drinks one pint of liquor daily, and was divorced 13 years ago. He lives alone.

Review of Symptoms

HK reports nausea, anorexia, occasional epigastric distress unrelated to food intake, and paroxysmal nocturnal dyspnea.

Physical Examination

GEN: Poorly groomed male appearing somnolent and with slurred speech
VS: BP 130/80, HR 80, RR 20, T 37, Wt 74 kg, Ht 175 cm
HEENT: Gingival hyperplasia
COR: Normal S1 and S2; (+) S3, (–) S4
RECT: Guaiac-positive
EXT: 1 + lower extremity edema
NEURO: (+) bilateral nystagmus on lateral gaze (at 45 degrees); unsteady gait; (+) Romberg sign

Results of Laboratory Tests

Na 144 (144)	BUN 5.0 (14)	MCV 108 (108)	T Bili 18.8 (1)
K 5.1 (5.1)	CR 97 (1.1)	AST 1.3 (78)	Glu 6.0 (108)
Cl 102 (102)	Hct 0.33 (33)	ALT 0.83 (50)	Phenytoin 130 (32.5)
HCO₃ 26 (26)	Hgb 110 (11)	Alb 32 (3.2)	

PROBLEM LIST

1. Idiopathic generalized epilepsy with tonic-clonic seizures (with phenytoin toxicity)
2. Alcoholism for 15 years
3. Peptic ulcer disease (PUD) (diagnosed by endoscopy 3 months ago) and gastritis
4. Congestive heart failure (CHF) caused by alcoholic cardiomyopathy

CASE 112

CC: FM is a 72-year-old man who presents to the geriatric outpatient clinic for a follow-up visit.

History of Present Illness

FM has been exhibiting signs of decreased mental status over the last few months. He has also had declining function over the past 6 weeks, since his last clinic visit.

Past Medical History

Hypertension
Non-insulin-dependent diabetes mellitus (NIDDM)
Decreased renal function
Chronic obstructive pulmonary disease (COPD)
Angina
Parkinson's disease
Constipation

Medication History

Levodopa/carbidopa, 25/250 mg, 1 tablet PO QID
Amantadine, 100 mg, 1 capsule PO BID
Tolbutamide, 500 mg, 1 PO TID
Triamcinolone inhaler, 3 puffs QID
Ipratropium bromide inhaler, 2 puffs Q6H
Albuterol inhaler, 2 puffs Q6H
Reserpine, 0.25 mg QD
Verapamil, 240 mg SR QD
Nitroglycerin, 9.0 mg, 1 capsule PO Q8H
Nitroglycerin SL, 0.4 mg every 5 minutes for 3 doses PRN for
   angina
Multivitamin tablet, 1 PO QD
Triamterene 50 mg/hydrochlorothiazide 25 mg, 1 capsule QD

Allergies

Penicillin

Physical Examination

GEN: Well-nourished male with decreasing mobility in no apparent distress
VS: BP 175/95, HR 100, RR 32, T 37.5, Wt 70 kg
HEENT: No evidence of trauma, PERRL, neck supple, no bruits, no JVD
COR: Irregular rhythm with occasional PVC, normal rate, normal S_1, S_2, no S_3 or S_4
CHEST: Diffuse expiratory wheezes bilaterally
ABD: Soft, distended, nontender, liver small 6 cm, no spleen palpable
GU: Normal male genitalia, prostate enlarged, nonnodular
SKIN: Purplish-red rash on thighs and lower extremities
RECT: Brown, heme-negative stool
EXT: Pulses decreased in lower extremities, (+) cogwheeled rigidity, (+) pill-rolling, (+) hypokinesis
NEURO: Strength 3/5, unsteady, sensory intact, alert and oriented for person and place, difficulty hearing, shakiness on standing

Results of Laboratory Tests

Na 135 (135)	CR 185.6 (2.1)	ALT .2 (12)
K 3.9 (3.9)	Hct 0.40 (40)	Alb 41 (4.1)
Cl 96 (96)	Lkcs 9.8 × 10⁹ (9.8 × 10³)	Glu 13.6 (245)
HCO₃ 27 (27)	Plts 305 × 10⁹ (305 × 10³)	Ca 2.3 (9.2)
BUN 13.6 (38)	AST .28 (17)	PO₄ 1.07 (3.3)
		Mg .75 (1.5)

PROBLEM LIST

1. Hypertension
2. NIDDM
3. Decreased renal function
4. COPD
5. Angina
6. Parkinson's disease
7. Constipation

CASE 113

CC: KM is a 60-year-old woman 3 days s/p total hip replacement. Immediately following her surgery, she was placed on meperidine, 10 mg/hr, with 10 mg rescue bolus doses every 15 minutes administered by means of a patient-controlled analgesia (PCA) device. This morning she experienced a tonic-clonic seizure that was treated with 500 mg IV phenytoin and 5 mg IV lorazepam. Her PCA was discontinued and the order changed to meperidine 75 mg IM Q4H PRN for pain. She is now complaining of headache and inadequate relief of her hip pain, and requests "something stronger."

Past Medical History

KM has a 25-year history of rheumatoid arthritis (RA) unsuccessfully treated with indomethacin, piroxicam, and aspirin because of premature discontinuation by the patient. She complained of gastric irritation with each medication. Before hospitalization, she was receiving acetaminophen 325 mg with codeine 60 mg, 10 to 12 tablets per day, and prednisone, 20 mg BID. She has had seizures for the past 4 years, after a fall down a flight of stairs during which her hip was dislocated, but before her hospitalization she was seizure-free for 6 months. She has hypertension, which is poorly controlled since KM stopped taking her propranolol, complaining that it made her feel "tired and slow." She also has hypothyroidism in conjunction with multinodular goiter, treated with levothyroxine.

Medication History (before admission)

Prednisone, 20 mg PO BID
Acetaminophen/codeine, 2 tablets every 4 to 5 hours
Phenytoin, 300 mg PO QHS
Thyroid, 1 grain PO QAM
Propranolol, 20 mg PO QID (discontinued 2 months ago)

Current Medications

Hydrocortisone, 100 mg IV Q6H
Heparin, 5,000 units SC Q8H
Meperidine, 75 mg IM Q4H PRN for pain
Phenytoin, 400 mg PO QHS
Levothyroxine, 0.1 mg PO QAM
Warfarin, 7.5 mg PO QHS for 2 days

Ketorolac, 60 mg IM Q6H, begun this AM
Hydrochlorothiazide, 50 mg PO QAM

Allergies
Penicillin causes a rash.

Physical Examination

GEN: Well-developed, obese female in severe distress
VS: BP 160/104, HR 110, RR 22, T 37, Wt 72 kg, Ht 165 cm
HEENT: WNL
COR: Nl S_1, S_2, positive S_3
CHEST: Clear, no rales or rhonchi
ABD: Soft, nontender, positive bowel sounds
GU: Foley catheter in place
RECT: Deferred
EXT: Bilateral inflamed, enlarged MTP, wrist, and knee joints

NEURO: O × 3, but exhibits slowed speech and memory impairment

Results of Laboratory Tests

Na 145 (145)	Hct 0.36 (36)	LDH 2.0 (120)	TSH 3
K 3.8 (3.8)	Hgb 115 (11.5)	Alk Phos 1.0 (60)	T4 64 (5)
Cl 108 (108)	Lkcs 10 × 10⁹ (10 × 10³)	Alb 38 (3.8)	Phenytoin 48 (12)
HCO₃ 22 (22)	Plts 250 × 10⁹ (250 × 10³)	Glu 11.1 (200)	INR 1.1
BUN 11.3 (30)	MCV 86 (86)	Ca 2.25 (9.0)	PT 15
Cr 115 (1.3)	AST 0.83 (50)	Mg 1.07 (2.6)	PTT 50

Urinalysis: WNL

Chest x-ray: Mild left ventricular hypertrophy

PROBLEM LIST

1. Rheumatoid arthritis
2. Seizures
3. Hypertension
4. Hypothyroidism
5. Chronic steroid use requiring stress coverage
6. Acute postsurgical pain
7. Postoperative antithrombotic therapy

PSYCHIATRIC DISORDERS

CASE 114

CC: TB is a 27-year-old female who presents to her primary care physician stating ''I feel that I am always on guard against something. I feel on edge.''

History of Present Illness

For the past three years TB has continually worried about success in her highly competitive career and the prognosis of her skin condition. During the past year her worry has increased, and she finds herself suffering from easy irritability, difficulty concentrating, shortness of breath (SOB), palpitations, and general nervousness. She also is suffering from fatigue, and the rash on her face and arms has worsened.

Past Medical History

TB has suffered from atopic eczema for the past 4 years. Her symptoms are mild, but she presents often to her physician for treatment and reassurance. The eczema did abate once when she was on a long vacation alone in the Rockies. She also has a history of dysmenorrhea and heavy menstrual periods.

Social History

TB drinks 4 cups of coffee per day. She does not drink alcohol.

Medication History

Hydrocortisone 0.5% cream, apply to affected areas on arms and face p.r.n.
Hydroxyzine HCl 25 mg PO q.i.d. p.r.n. nerves
Ibuprofen 600 mg PO q.i.d. p.r.n.

Allergies

None known

Physical Examination

GEN: Slender female, mildly anxious, hypervigilant, diaphoretic
VS: BP 110/65, HR 85, RR 20, T 37, wt 47 kg
HEENT: WNL except for pale conjunctiva
COR: RRR without murmurs
CHEST: CTA
ABD: WNL
GU and
RECT: WNL, stool guaiac-negative
EXT: Several mild eczematous lesions on R and L anticubital fossae and face; pale nail beds

Results of Laboratory Tests

BUN 2.5 (7)	Lkcs 5.5×10^9 (5.5×10^3)	Glu 4.7 (85)	TSH 3 (3)
CR 61 (0.8)	Plts 270×10^9 (270×10^3)	TIBC 82 (460)	T_3 2.3 (150)
HCT 0.32 (32)	MCV 70 (70)	Ferritin 110 (110)	T_4 23 (1.8)
Hgb 90 (9)	RBC 3.1×10^{12} (3.1×10^6)		

PROBLEM LIST

1. Atopic eczema
2. Iron deficiency anemia (IDA)
3. Generalized anxiety disorder (GAD)

CASE 114 SOAP NOTES
Problem 3. GAD

S: TB complains of constant worry (often unfounded), easy irritability, lightheadedness, difficulty concentrating, SOB, palpitations, and ''feeling always on guard against something. I feel on edge.''

O: TB is tremulous, anxious, perspiring, hypervigilant.

A: TB is suffering from generalized anxiety disorder based on her symptoms. The symptoms are causing her moderate distress, but her functioning is not severely impaired. Her IDA may be mildly exacerbating her anxiety (palpitations, lightheadedness). Anxiety also may be exacerbated by caffeine. The efficacy of hydroxyzine is not well-established in the treatment of GAD.

P: The goal of treatment is to reduce the anxiety symptoms to a manageable level; total amelioration of the symptoms may not be possible. Since her symptoms are causing her moderate distress, pharmacotherapy may be warranted concurrent with supportive counseling and relaxation therapy. Start supportive counseling and reassure TB about her physical health. Discontinue the hydroxyzine and start benzodiazepine therapy. Start diazepam 5 mg PO b.i.d. Continue therapy for 2 weeks and then attempt to taper the dose and discontinue the medication. If symptoms persist, buspirone may be considered. TB should be advised to switch to decaffeinated coffee. Educate TB about the expectations of treatment and advise her that short-term pharmacotherapy is the plan. TB should be advised of the sedative effects of benzodiazepines and their effects on cognition (use care when driving or when engaged in other potentially hazardous activity).

Problem 2. IDA

S: TB complains of fatigue, palpitations, and lightheadedness.

O: TB is a pale female in NAD. Laboratory findings are consistent with IDA: decreased RBC, ferritin, HCT, and Hgb levels. Peripheral blood smear shows hypochromic, microcytic RBCs. Slight tachycardia is noted.

A: Iron deficiency anemia is based on physical examination, laboratory findings, and history of heavy menstrual blood losses. No other evidence of blood loss (stool guaiac-negative).

P: The goal in the treatment of IDA is to normalize hemoglobin and hematocrit levels by repleting iron stores. Begin iron sulfate 325 mg PO t.i.d., and continue for 3–6 months after the normalization of the CBC. TB should be advised to keep the iron preparation away from children to avoid accidental ingestion, as iron is toxic in overdoses. The iron should be taken on an empty stomach if possible, since food may decrease absorption by 40%–50%. If gastric intolerance does develop (nausea, epigastric pain, constipation, abdominal cramps, diarrhea), she can take the iron with meals, but this may require a longer duration of therapy. Begin counseling to improve her dietary habits. Monitor subjective complaints, reticulocyte count (expect an increase in 7 days and return to normal in 2–3 weeks), hematocrit (expect a 0.6 [6%] increase in 3 weeks and return to normal in 6 weeks), hemoglobin (expect increase of 2 g/ liter [2 mg/100 ml] in 3 weeks and return to normal in 6 weeks), and peripheral blood smear.

Problem 1. Atopic Eczema

S: TB complains of a progressively worsening rash with itching. This exacerbation has been concurrent with increasing stress at work and worsening of anxiety.

O: TB has eczematous patches on face and R and L anticubital fossae. Patches on her arms appear crusted, hyperkeratotic, and inflamed.

A: TB has atopic ezcema exacerbated by stress and anxiety. She is at risk of developing a secondary infection as a result of her continuous scratching of the affected areas. Drug therapy is, therefore, justified.

P: Discontinue hydrocortisone 0.5% cream, as this preparation strength is inadequate for the initial management of the rash. Begin betamethasone 0.1% cream, and apply to lesions t.i.d. to alleviate itching and inflammation. Reevaluate lesions in 2–3 weeks, and adjust topical steroid therapy appropriately. Maintenance therapy should consist of a low-strength corticosteroid preparation (e.g., hydrocortisone 1%) applied once or twice daily. Therapy should be discontinued gradually to reduce the chance of rebound flares of the topical lesions.

QUESTIONS FOR CASE 114

1. What are some potential advantages of buspirone over benzodiazepines in the treatment of GAD?
2. What are the disadvantages associated with buspirone treatment, especially in patients with GAD previously treated with benzodiazepines?
3. Why was hydroxyzine discontinued?
4. What is the role of nonpharmacologic approaches in the treatment of GAD?

5. When TB returns to clinic in 2–3 weeks for reevaluation of her dermatologic condition, the lesions have improved significantly. How would you recommend adjusting her topical steroid therapy?

CASE 115

CC: RF is a 36-year-old female who comes to the general medicine clinic for refills of imipramine, ampicillin, and tetracycline. She also complains of frequent painful urination, lower abdominal pain, foul-smelling urine, intense vulvar burning, and flu-like symptoms.

History of Present Illness

RF has a history of recurrent UTI (four UTIs this year). She was recently treated with ampicillin 250 mg PO q.i.d. for 10 days. She missed her follow-up appointment because she was asymptomatic and she thought that "her urinary infection was cured." Now, 4 weeks later, RF returns to the clinic complaining of frequent, painful urination. She also reports that despite the fact that she was treated with acyclovir for her recurrent genital herpes last month, she is now experiencing the same symptoms (vulvar burning and white vaginal discharge) again.

Past Medical History

RF has a long history of recurrent UTI, recurrent genital herpes, and chronic acne. She also goes through frequent episodes of binging and purging. Last year she was diagnosed with bulimia and started on imipramine. She has a history of noncompliance with her medications. The only medication that she takes on a regular basis is her imipramine because it also helps her insomnia.

Medication History

Ampicillin 250 mg PO q.i.d. × 10 days (last dose was taken 4 weeks ago)
Acyclovir 200 mg PO q.i.d. × 5 days (admits that she did not finish the 5-day course)
Imipramine 200 mg PO q. h.s.
Tetracycline 250 mg PO b.i.d.
Ortho-Novum 7/7/7 q.d.

Allergies

None known

Social History

Tobacco-negative
Alcohol-heavy consumption during weekends
Has had several sex partners in the past year, now monogamous

Review of System
Noncontributory

Physical Examination
GEN: Thin and anxious female in no acute distress
VS: T 38, BP 120/76, HR 89, wt 51 kg, ht 150 cm
COR: Normal
ABD: Soft and nontender
RECT: Guaiac-negative, perianal pain
EXT: Normal
Pelvic: Multiple papules and vesicles, "cottage cheese"-like vaginal discharge

Results of Laboratory Tests
Na 135 (135)
K 3.9 (3.9)
Cl 99 (99)
HCO_3 25 (25)
BUN 5.3 (15)
CR 0.9 (79.5)

HCT 36 (36)
Hgb 190 (19)
Plts 190×10^9 (190×10^3)
Alb 49 (4.9)

Urinalysis: Gram's stain—gram-negative rods (consistent with previous Gram's stain), cloudy, pH 8.0, SG 1.015, WBC 10–15/mm^3, RBC 0–1/mm^3, WBC esterase +

Urine culture: Pending
Culture of vesicles: Pending
Microscopic exam of lesion exudate: + herpes infection

Problem List
1. UTI
2. Genital herpes
3. Acne
4. Bulimia

CASE 115 SOAP NOTES
Problem 1. UTI
S: RF complains of frequent, painful urination and foul-smelling urine.
O: RF has a history of recurrent UTI. UA is positive for UTI and is cloudy. She has a low grade temperature (T 38).
A: RF is experiencing an uncomplicated UTI. She could be experiencing a relapse to her previous therapy (ampicillin). A high incidence of ampicillin resistant E. coli has been reported in the literature. Therefore, another alternative should be considered. Also, her history of noncompliance to medications put her at a higher risk to fail therapy or develop resistant pathogens. Since her urine culture is still pending, she should be treated empirically with an alternate agent. Treatment may be streamlined once the culture and sensitivity results are available.
P: Most of the pathogens found in UTI are susceptible to trimethoprim-sulfamethoxazole (TMP/SMX) and cephalosporins. RF should be started on TMP/SMX DS PO b.i.d. for 7–14 days. A follow-up urine culture should be obtained 2–4 weeks after the completion of therapy. If the urine culture reveals pathogens resistant to TMP/SMX, then

cephalexin, nitrofurantoin, or ciprofloxacin may be considered. RF should also be instructed that antibiotics (such as TMP/SMX) can interact with her birth control pills and decrease their efficacy. She should use other methods of contraceptions while taking antibiotics.

Problem 2. Genital Herpes
S: RF complains of painful urination, abdominal pain, and vulvar itching.
O: Vaginal "cottage cheese" discharge, vesicles on pelvic exam, + herpes infection on microscopic exam, T 38, and perianal pain. RF has a history of recurrent herpes.
A: Genital herpes tends to recur in almost all patients afflicted by the infection. Genital HSV infections are usually diagnosed based on the history and clinical presentation. RF is experiencing classic signs and symptoms of genital herpes. Her history of noncompliance and her sexual activity may have contributed to failure of the therapy. RF is now symptomatic and should be treated to prevent further complications. Recurrent HSV episodes are shorter and milder compared to the initial infection. Therapy of recurrent infections should be initiated within 2 days of onset of symptoms. Since RF experiences recurrent episodes of genital herpes, prophylactic administration of acyclovir can be considered.
P: Before initiating the therapy for HSV infection, RF should be educated about her disease state and should be counseled about the importance of compliance with her medication (refer to the answer to question 3). Acyclovir, while not particularly effective, is currently considered the treatment of choice for initial and recurrent cases of HSV infections. Since recurrent episodes are generally milder, the effect of acyclovir to treat recurrent episodes is questionable. Treatment of recurrent herpes infection with acyclovir is only recommended for patients with more than six episodes per year with severe symptoms. The dose is 200 mg PO q.i.d. Prophylaxis should be continued only for a period of 1 year. Warm sitz baths may also help alleviate pain and discomfort.

Problem 3. Acne
S: RF is not currently experiencing a significant outbreak of acne.
O: RF has history of chronic acne.
A: Tetracycline is commonly used to treat chronic acne. The use of oral contraceptive could be associated with appearance, disappearance, or improvements in acne. Progestins can stimulate the production of sebum and estrogens can suppress the production of sebum. RF is on Ortho-Novum which has more estrogenic activity and can therefore improve RF's acne problem. It is well-documented that stress can trigger acne. Therefore, it should be explained to RF that her current UTI and recurrent HSV infection may worsen her acne.
P: As long as RF is tolerating tetracycline, she should continue taking it daily. Tetracycline is usually well-tolerated and has a low incidence of side effects. RF should be told

SECTION 14: PSYCHIATRIC DISORDERS

that she should not take tetracycline with antacids, dairy products, and iron compounds. RF should also be counseled about the importance of skin hygiene.

Problem 4. Bulimia

S: Binging episodes

O: RF is diagnosed with bulimia.

A: Bulimia and anorexia are classified as psychiatric illnesses. There is no satisfactory treatment for bulimia (refer to the answer to question 5). Bulimia is characterized by binge eating which is usually followed by a form of purging (self-induced vomiting, laxative abuse, extensive exercise, etc.). Patients with bulimia do not usually experience severe weight loss unless they have an anorexic component to their eating disorder. RF is underweight and therefore she could also have anorexia. In general, half of anorectics have bulimia as well.

P: RF should continue taking her imipramine. Studies have shown that, in general, there is an association between major depressive illnesses and eating disorders. Some bulimic patients respond to anticonvulsant therapies if their binge behavior is secondary to a neurological disorder analogous to epilepsy. Since RF drinks alcohol, she should be notified about the possibility of oversedation with concomitant use of alcohol and imipramine.

QUESTIONS FOR CASE 115

1. What are the most common pathogens that cause UTIs?
2. Is RF a candidate for UTI prophylaxis?
3. What is the role of counseling for patients with genital herpes?
4. Name the most common treatments for acne.
5. What are the differences between anorexia and bulimia? What are the treatment options?

CASE 116

CC: MK is a 34-year-old man who has attempted suicide and is being evaluated for treatment.

History of Present Illness

MK was a successful aerospace engineer who was laid off from his job and has been unemployed for 8 months. He began to drink heavily recently and has lapsed into deep depression, often contemplating suicide. After MK's wife left him, he ingested an unknown number of Darvocet N-100 tablets (propoxyphene/acetaminophen) and was treated successfully for the propoxyphene overdose in the emergency department (ED). He is now admitted to the hospital for observation and further treatment.

Social History

Drank a bottle of gin each day for the past 3 days
Smoked 1 pack of cigarettes per day × 10 years (quit 2 years ago)

Medication History

Alupent inhaler (metaproterenol) 2–4 puffs q4h p.r.n.

Allergies

Sulfa drugs (rash)

Physical Examination

GEN: Thin, lethargic male complaining of mild nausea
VS: BP 110/80, HR 80, RR 18, T 37.4°C, wt 68 kg
HEENT: Unremarkable
COR: Percusses at midclavicular line without murmur or gallop
CHEST: Clear to percussion and auscultation
ABD: Thin and soft without masses, tenderness, or organomegaly
GU: WNL
RECT: WNL
EXT: Pulses intact and palpable
NEURO: Alert and oriented × 3

Results of Laboratory Tests

Na 140 (140)	HCT 0.40 (40)	AST 1.0 (60)	Glu 6.11 (110)
K 4.0 (4.0)	Hgb 160 (16)	ALT 1.17 (70)	PT 14.0
Cl 106 (106)		LDH 3.33 (200)	Acetaminophen 2 hours
HCO₃ 25 (25)		Alk Phos 1.67 (100)	postingestion 330 (5)
BUN 6.43 (18)		T Bili 17.1 (1.0)	
CR 70.7 (0.8)			

Lkc differential, urinalysis, chest x-ray, ECG: all WNL

PROBLEM LIST

1. Mild asthma in good control
2. Suicidal ideation secondary to depression

CASE 116 SOAP NOTES
Problem 2. Suicidal Ideation Secondary to Depression

S: MK has been depressed and contemplated suicide after losing his job.

O: MK has actually attempted suicide by ingesting an unknown number of Darvocet N-100 tablets.

A: MK requires immediate pharmacologic treatment for his depression. Psychotherapy and counseling would also be appropriate initial treatment for MK. Tricyclic antidepressants (TCAs) should be avoided in a patient contemplating suicide because overdoses from TCAs can be fatal. In addition, the use of alcohol may exacerbate MK's depression, and he should be encouraged to stop drinking.

P: Initiate psychotherapy and counseling. Nontricyclic antidepressants, such as trazodone or fluoxetine, may be appropriate (note that reports of fluoxetine contributing to increased suicidal tendencies have not been substantiated). Begin with a low dose and titrate to effect; clinical efficacy may not be observed for 4–6 weeks. For example, start MK on 20 mg PO fluoxetine q. AM. If no clinical improvement is observed after 3–4 weeks, increase the dose to 20 mg PO b.i.d., but do not exceed the maximum dose of 80 mg/day. Monitor for the efficacy as well as for the side effects of the drug selected. Common adverse effects associated with fluoxetine include anxiety, nervousness, drowsiness, sweating, nausea, and diarrhea.

Problem 1. Mild Asthma
S: No evidence of distress
O: Lungs appear to be clear on examination.
A: MK requires no treatment for his asthma. His condition appears to be in control with metaproterenol.
P: Continue metaproterenol and monitor for efficacy and for side effects of the drug.

QUESTIONS FOR CASE 116
1. MK has been started on fluoxetine, and the new medical resident wants to add L-tryptophan to augment the response to fluoxetine. How do you respond to this?
2. During rounds, MK's attending physician asks you how long MK should be treated with fluoxetine if he is responding to the drug. What is your response?
3. In addition, the resident wants to know what to do if MK is not responding to the drug. What is your recommendation?
4. It is now 4 days since MK has been treated for his Darvocet-N overdose. Except for complaints of nausea, he has done well. However, this morning, he has been vomiting, confused, and lethargic. He complains of upper quadrant pain and appears jaundiced. What could account for these symptoms?
5. Upon questioning, MK states that he does not remember how many Darvocet-N tablets he ingested. The attending asks you how many tablets MK would have had to ingest in order to observe the signs and symptoms of hepatotoxicity?

CASE 117
CC: MJ is a 62-year-old woman who is experiencing side effects from her therapy for schizophrenia.

History of Present Illness

MJ presented to the ambulatory care clinic for a refill of her medications. She complained to the pharmacist of thirst, lethargy, and constipation that began a month ago. Her speech was slurred, with her tongue sticking out of her mouth. Her eyes appeared to blink frequently, and her arms and legs moved in a writhing, involuntary manner. She states that she has been hearing some "voices" again the past 2 weeks and needs some ear plugs to "shut them out."

Family History

Mother has history of depression

Medication History

Haloperidol 4 mg PO t.i.d. × 20 years (dose recently decreased)
Benztropine 1 mg PO b.i.d.
Docusate sodium 100 mg PO q.d.
Phenytoin 100 mg PO t.i.d.
Ibuprofen 200 mg PO q4-6h
Conjugated estrogens 0.625 mg PO q.d.
Multivitamins 1 PO q.d.

Allergies

Chlorpromazine (rash)

Physical Examination
GEN: Lethargic, thin, anxious, and depressed-looking woman
VS: BP 100/60, HR 70, RR 18, T 38
HEENT: PERRLA; EOMs intact
COR: Regular, without murmurs or extra sounds
CHEST: Lungs clear bilaterally to auscultation and percussion
ABD: Soft, tender, no palpable masses
GU: Deferred
RECT: Deferred
EXT: No clubbing, cyanosis, or edema
NEURO: Normal

Results of Laboratory Tests
Cr 62 (0.7)
Alb 20 (2)
Phenytoin 27.7 (μmol/liter (7 mg/ liter)

PROBLEM LIST
1. Schizophrenia × 30 years
2. History of generalized tonic-clonic seizures secondary to head injury 5 years ago (1–2 seizures per year)
3. Tardive dyskinesia (TD)
4. Anticholinergic side effects (sedation, constipation)

CASE 117 SOAP NOTES
Problem 1. Schizophrenia
S: MJ is depressed and has been hearing "voices" again for the past 2 weeks.
O: None
A: MJ's schizophrenia appears to be in poor control and requires immediate treatment to enable her to function normally. She is experiencing adverse effects from her neuroleptic therapy (see problems discussed below). Haloperidol has a low affinity for lowering seizure thresholds and is an appropriate drug for MJ given her history of seizures; in addition, the drug has low sedative, orthostasic, and anticholinergic effects, which are desirable properties when selecting a neuroleptic for a 62-year-old. However, despite the low risk of these side effects, they can nonetheless be manifested with long-term therapy. Haloperidol also has a high risk for extrapyramidal syndrome (EPS) effects. MJ's haloperidol dose was decreased recently, which has resulted in her now hearing "voices" (as well as causing TD).
P: Determine from MJ what dose of haloperidol she was on before the recent decrease, and increase the haloperidol dose accordingly. Monitor MJ for decreased auditory hallu-

cinations and clinical improvement. Follow improvements in TD, EPS, and anticholinergic effects closely per problems discussed below.

Problem 3. Tardive Dyskinesia

S: None

O: MJ is showing clinical features of the buccolinguomasticatory triad. Her speech is slurred, with her tongue protruding from her mouth. She has choreiform and athetoid movements (involuntary moving of arms and legs).

A: MJ is showing signs of tardive dyskinesia (TD) from her treatment with neuroleptics and may require some form of therapy to prevent progression of these symptoms. Her gender, age, and duration of neuroleptic therapy puts her at risk for developing TD. Because MJ has also been on haloperidol for over 20 years, it is likely that this condition is irreversible. Since her schizophrenia appears to be worsening, her neuroleptic dose cannot be further decreased (problem 1). Drug therapy for TD may provide temporary relief of symptoms, but it should not be used for long-term treatment. In this case, consider the use of amantadine, which has been used in conjunction with neuroleptics in patients with TD to "desensitize" the dopamine receptors.

P: Start amantadine 100 mg PO b.i.d. Monitor for improvements in the symptoms of TD, which should be seen in about a week. Advise MJ on the side effects of amantadine, such as nausea, dizziness, anxiety, livedo reticularis, or confusion. Assess for early signs of TD semiannually or quarterly, and note that prevention is probably the best treatment.

Problem 4. Anticholinergic Side Effects

S: None

O: MJ is lethargic, thirsty, and constipated.

A: MJ is experiencing anticholinergic side effects from her therapy and requires treatment to alleviate these signs. Although haloperidol is less likely to cause anticholinergic effects, they can occur with chronic therapy. Constipation is the more serious concern because of the potential fecal impaction, megacolon, etc.

P: For thirst, recommend increased fluid intake and sucking on sugarless gum or candy. For constipation, start docusate 100 mg PO b.i.d., with high-fiber diet. Review carefully the other clinical symptoms of anticholinergic effects, such as blurry vision and urinary hesitancy. Monitor anticholinergic side effects; if improvement is not noted in 2–4 weeks, MJ should return to clinic for assessment.

Problem 2. Tonic-Clonic Seizures

S: None

O: None

A: MJ has 1–2 seizures per year. She is currently on phenytoin and requires no other treatment. Phenytoin is the appropriate drug for this type of seizure. While the level of phenytoin appears to be low (27.7 mmol/liter [7 mg/liter]), it is important to note that when adjustments are made for MJ's low albumin level, the phenytoin level will be within therapeutic range

$$\text{adjusted } Cp = \frac{\text{observed } CP}{(1-\alpha)}\left(\frac{\text{observed albumin}}{\text{normal albumin}}\right)+\alpha$$

$$\text{adjusted } Cp = \frac{7 \text{ mg/liter}}{(1-0.1)(2 \text{ g/dl}/4.4 \text{ g/dl})+0.1}$$

$$\text{adjusted } Cp = 13.8 \text{ mg/liter } (54.7 \text{ mmol/liter})$$

Note that phenytoin could have possible drug interactions with some of the medications that MJ is taking: (a) a loss of seizure control may occur when phenytoin and estrogens are used together, (b) the serum haloperidol level may be decreased with phenytoin and result in loss of control of psychiatric symptoms, and (c) the pharmacologic effects of phenytoin may be increased with ibuprofen and possibly result in toxicity characterized by nystagmus, ataxia, etc. Also note that MJ's neuroleptic, haloperidol, has low seizure activity.

P: Continue with phenytoin. Monitor for seizures and the possibility of drug interactions (as above). Educate MJ on the side effects of phenytoin (e.g., nystagmus, ataxia, slurred speech, confusion, gingival hyperplasia).

QUESTIONS FOR CASE 117

1. Is it possible that MJ is suffering from neuroleptic withdrawal instead of tardive dyskinesia?
2. MJ is noted to be "depressed-looking." Would it be appropriate to start her on an antidepressant?
3. MJ has an allergic reaction to chlorpromazine. Explain why she can take haloperidol.
4. Educate MJ on other drug interactions that are clinically significant with haloperidol.
5. Would MJ be a good candidate for clozapine?

CASE 118

CC: KR, an 8-year-old asthmatic patient, has poor academic performance in his second-grade class.

Past Medical History

KR was taken to the ED during winter recess for shortness of breath and "blueness" of skin color. What appeared to be a fainting spell occurred on the way to the hospital, but no other episodes were observed. ED personnel told the parents to contact their family physician to rule out asthma. KR's parents decided, on their own, to initiate a treatment regiment using over-the-counter (OTC) asthma inhalers. Prior to that episode, KR had a history of atopic dermatitis in the antecubital and popliteal fossae. These latter episodes have responded to OTC topical hydrocortisone and Keri lotion.

Social History

KR's problem was brought to his family's attention by his second-grade teacher. She was concerned that KR was falling further and further behind. KR's parents agreed to a school-based educational evaluation that identified significant speech and language problems, thought to be secondary to KR's recurring bouts with chronic bilateral serous otitis media. KR's cognitive potential measured well within the average range; however, a discrepancy of more than 20 standard score points was noted between reading comprehension achievement scores and his cognitive potential, indicating learning disabilities. KR's distractibility and impulsivity are also contributing to his academic limitations and worsening social status with his peers.

Medication History

Primatene Mist p.r.n.
Hydrocortisone cream 0.5% p.r.n.
Keri lotion applied after bath/shower

Allergies

Ragweed pollen (hay fever)

Physical Examination

GEN: Male child (8 years old), normal physical development, adequate diet/nourishment
VS: BP 104/64, HR 72, RR 20, T 37, wt 23.1 kg (50th percentile), ht 132 cm (75 percentile)
HEENT: Normocephalic, bilateral myringotomy with P.E. tubes, language therapy initiated for frontal lisp and concept formation
COR: Normal S_1 and S_2, no murmurs, rubs, or gallop
CHEST: Clear to auscultation and percussion, but sl. indication of hyperinflation
ABD: Soft, nontender, with no masses
EXT: WNL
NEURO: Oriented × 3; DTRs and cranial nerves normal

Results of Laboratory Tests

Na 137 (137)	HCT 0.49 (49)	Glu 8.1 (145)
K 3.7 (3.7)	Hgb 160 (16)	Ca 2.3 (9.4)
Cl 103 (103)	Lkcs 8.5 × 10⁹ (8.5 × 10³)	PO₄ 1.1 (3.5)
HCO₃ 22 (22)		Chol 3.95 (152)

Pulmonary function tests: RV 3.1 liter, $FEV_{1.0}$ 1.9 liter, FVC 3.4 liter, $FEV_{1.0}/FVC(\%)$ 65%
Lkc differential: Eos 700/mm³
Urinalysis: WNL

PROBLEM LIST

1. Asthma
2. Eczema
3. Attention deficit hyperactivity disorder (ADHD) suspected

CASE 118 SOAP NOTES

Problem 1. Asthma

S: No recent complaints; KR has used Primatene on 3 occasions in the past 4 months
O: Pulmonary function test results are consistent with diagnosis of bronchial asthma, but no wheezing is present.

A: No need for any change in therapy
P: Continue to monitor for any exacerbation of respiratory symptoms.

Problem 2. Eczema

S: KR has had some scaling and itching.
O: KR indicated that he has not used Keri lotion consistently and has been out of hydrocortisone for at least 6 months. "Mom keeps forgetting to buy it."
A: Eczema was formerly controlled but is now flaring as a result of patient noncompliance.
P: Recommend consistent use of Keri lotion as previously used and 0.5% hydrocortisone to reduce rash when it flares.

Problem 3. Attention Deficit Hyperactivity Disorder

S: KR's teacher has indicated that he is not progressing at the educational rate of his peers. He is disruptive in class and his social interaction and self-esteem are both suffering as a result.
O: KR has increased motor activity, short attention span, excessive impulsivity, and reading comprehension limitations in the presence of normal IQ results.
A: Achievement testing by the special education consultant confirmed a significant reading discrepancy. Behavior rating scales showed limited hyperactivity but significant shortness of attention with significant impulsive behaviors, particularly touching other children (hugging and hitting) in an aggressive manner. A diagnosis of attention deficit hyperactivity disorder was made. Therapy should focus on increasing attention span, increasing response to appropriate stimuli, and increasing reflectivity before acting.
P: Give pemoline tablets 75 mg per day. (This drug was selected based on anecdotal experience of the consulting neurologist. Since there are no clinical studies that identify any significant advantage for one CNS stimulant over another, this agent was selected for an initial trial.) Advise parents to place KR in special education classes for reading remediation with participation in regular second-grade classroom activities for all other subjects and activities. Urge education and/or counseling of teachers about his disorder and the pharmacologic treatment. Encourage participation in therapy for all members of the family, not just isolated counseling for KR.

QUESTIONS FOR CASE 118

1. As pemoline therapy is initiated, KR's parents want to know how long he will need medication.
2. What are the appropriate monitoring parameters for pemoline therapy?
3. KR returns to the clinic in 6 weeks, but has not responded well to his medication. Should his dose of pemoline be increased or should alternative therapy be considered?
4. KR usually uses an antihistamine/decongestant combination (Actifed) for his hay fever. Will there be any problem with using this agent concurrently with pemoline?

5. KR's asthmatic attacks have been more frequent now that he has been on pemoline therapy for approximately 9–10 months. Is there any problem with the concurrent usage of theophylline and pemoline?

6. If pemoline dosage is increased to 112.5 mg/day with no effect on KR's behavior, what therapeutic alternatives are available?

CASE 119

CC: RS is a 25-year-old female who is well-known to the county ED for her drug-seeking behavior and frequent "run-ins" with the police. A history by her girlfriend, with whom RS was "partying," revealed that during the previous night RS shot "an eight ball of snow," drank vodka, and ingested large amounts of oral diazepam. RS's friend reports that RS has had two incidents of "blacking out" after "partying" within the past week.

Social History

RS is a single parent and lives with her 4-year-old son in a motel located downtown. RS smokes one pack of cigarettes per day (× 12 years), drinks alcohol almost daily (mostly vodka and gin), and uses intravenous cocaine "whenever I can afford it." RS also takes oral diazepam 5 times a week, usually consuming between 5–30 mg at any given time. The diazepam was originally prescribed for RS when she was a teenager in psychotherapy. RS had a single grand mal seizure 12 years ago and has a history of noncompliance with her seizure medication.

Allergies

Cherries cause itchy hives

Medication History

Diazepam 5–30 mg PO q.d. p.r.n. anxiety
Phenytoin 300 mg PO q. AM

Physical Examination

GEN: Skinny, emaciated adult female in acute distress
VS: BP 80/50, HR 55 Reg, RR 6, T 37.6, current wt 54 kg, dry wt 52 kg, ht 152 cm
HEENT: Pupils fixed and dilated to 7 mm
COR: Normal S_1 and S_2, no S_3 or S_4 or murmurs
CHEST: BS decreased, no rales, rhonchi, or wheezes
ABD: Distended, nontender, bowel sounds decreased but audible
GU: WNL
RECT: Guaiac-positive
EXT: Decreased DTRs, + asterixis
NEURO: Oriented × 0, responsive only to painful stimuli

Results of Laboratory Tests

Na 132 (132)	HCT .35 (35)	AST 1.75 (105)	Glu 3.8 (70)
K 3.7 (3.7)	Hgb 115 (11.5)	ALT 7.8 (470)	PT 13.5
Cl 100 (100)	Lkcs 10 × 10⁹ (10 × 10³)	Alk Phos 2.5 (150)	INR 1.3
HCO₃ 27 (27)		Alb 25 (2.5)	Ethanol 20.6 (95)
BUN 6.8 (19)		T Bili 27.4 (1.6)	Phenytoin <4 (<1)
CR 88.4 (1.0)			

Urinalysis: + EtOH, + cocaine, + ecgonine, + benzodiazepine

Chest x-ray: Clear, no signs of pneumonia, mild cardiomegaly

PROBLEM LIST

1. Benzodiazepine overdose
2. Guaiac-positive
3. Alcohol dependence
4. Cocaine abuse
5. Seizure disorder

CASE 119 SOAP NOTES

Problem 1. Benzodiazepine Overdose

S: RS has a history of taking oral diazepam 5–30 mg PO q.d. for stress relief.

O: VS reveal decreased BP 80/50, HR 55, RR 6, O × 0, responsive only to painful stimuli.

A: RS has a polydrug abuse problem (diazepam, ethanol and cocaine). Diazepam is a long-acting benzodiazepine that can last 50–150 hours. RS is likely to have a diazepam duration of action closer to the 150 hr range because of her decreased liver function and because of the quantity she ingested (30 mg). RS has increased LFT's and an increased PT (and INR) and most likely has decreased synthetic live function and a decreased ability to metabolize benzodiazepines. Flumazenil is a competitive benzodiazepine receptor antagonist (brand name Romazicon, formerly called Mazicon). Recently, flumazenil has become available and is very effective for the reversal of the signs and symptoms of benzodiazepine overdose. Flumazenil is administered in dosages of 0.2 mg IV administered over 15–30 seconds. Flumazenil only reverses the effects of benzodiazepines and does not affect opiates, cocaine or alcohol. Contraindications to flumazenil include an allergy to benzodiazepines or flumazenil, history of seizure, head trauma and the reversal of benzodiazepine(s) administered for status epilepticus or the control of intracranial pressure. RS has a relative contraindication to flumazenil—seizure history. However, it is unlikely that RS will experience an adverse reaction, specifically a seizure, because she only had one seizure in the past 12 years and has a history of noncompliance with her seizure medication. Other adverse reactions to flumazenil include: nausea, dizziness, agitation and pain at the injection site. The duration of action of flumazenil ranges from 15 minutes to 2.5 hours (average 53 minutes). Onset of action if 1–2 minutes and peak effect for flumazenil occurs within 6–10 minutes. Because the reversal of benzodiazepines with flumazenil is a competitive inhibition at the receptor site and because the average duration of action of flumazenil is 53 minutes, it may be necessary to re-administer flumazenil until the insulting benzodiazepine has beeen metabolized by the liver. Most patients will respond to a cumulative dosage of 1–3 mg (10–30 ml) of flumazenil. If a patient does not respond within 5 minutes of receiving a total dosage of 5 mg (50 ml), the major cause of sedation is probably not due to a benzodiazepine.

P: Administer flumazenil 0.2 mg IV over 15 seconds. After the initial dosage, if the desired level of consciousness is not obtained, give a second dose. Continue monitoring RS for at least four hours after the last dose of flumazenil to insure that competitive inhibition at the benzodiazepine receptor sites has occurred.

Problem 3. Alcohol Dependence

S: RS has had frequent blackouts.

O: RS is a binge drinker (two bottles of wine before this ED visit). LFT results reflect chronic liver disease and decreased nutritional status:
Alb 25 g/liter (2.5 g/dl)
ALT 7.8 ukat/liter (470 u/liter)
AST 1.75 ukat/liter (105 u/ liter)
Alk Phos 2.5 ukat/liter (150 u/liter)
PT 13.5
INR 1.3
PE: guaiac-positive and distended, nontender abdomen (wt increased by 2 kg)

A: RS has a serious binge-drinking habit and has some signs and symptoms of chronic alcohol damage. RS's alcohol consumption is causing liver disease that could progress to cirrhosis. RS is guaiac-positive, which may be secondary to esophageal varices attributed to portal hypertension from cirrhosis. RS is at risk for alcohol withdrawal, even though she is a binge drinker. Alcohol withdrawal is most likely to occur 24–72 hours after discontinuing alcohol, but it may occur up to 7 days after discontinuing alcohol. RS has already taken diazepam, which may be contributing to her decreased mental status (O × 1). It is difficult to assess for Wernicke-Korsakoff psychosis because RS is only oriented to person.

P: Monitor electrolyte, vital signs (BP, RR, HR, T), and for signs and symptoms of alcohol withdrawal (nausea, vomiting, sweating, agitation, tremors, and possibly seizures). After systolic blood pressure is above 110 mm Hg, give furosemide 40 mg IV and monitor BP. Begin thiamine 100 mg IV q.d. for Wernicke-Korsakoff psychosis induced from chronic alcohol use/dependence. Avoid intramuscular injections in RS since she has increased PT and INR and is at risk for hematoma development. Rehydrate RS with D5W and monitor blood glucose, since RS is at risk for hypoglycemia after alcohol consumption and possibly decreased nutritional intake. Give phytonadione 10 mg SQ q.d. × 3 and begin a multivitamin q.d. Monitor PT and INR.

Problem 5. Cocaine Overdose

S: RS's friend states that RS was shooting an "eight ball of snow" before coming to ED.

O: Urinalysis is positive for cocaine and ecgonine (cocaine metabolite); CXR shows mild cardiomegaly.

A: RS has used intravenous cocaine by history and has a cocaine-positive urinalysis. RS is not exhibiting any physical signs or symptoms of cocaine abuse at present, most likely because of the polydrug abuse. (Alcohol and diazepam cause CNS depression, and cocaine causes CNS stimulation, but of much shorter duration.) RS's mental status is not assessable at present. RS has mild cardiomegaly on her ECG and needs education about the dangers of cocaine abuse, intravenous drug abuse, and the effects of cocaine on the myocardial muscle.

P: RS should receive drug counseling and information about the physical dangers of cocaine use. Defer giving an antidepressant to RS until she is more arousable and can be assessed for depression contributing to her illegal drug use. If RS has depression as a component of her drug-seeking behavior, consider Trazodone 50 mg at bedtime every night (in conjunction with therapy) for 6 weeks. RS should also be counseled on the risks of HIV infection from intravenous drug abuse and shared needles.

Problem 1. One Grand Mal Seizure (by History)

S: History of a single seizure 15 years ago and history of noncompliance with phenytoin

O: PHT < 4 (μmol/liter (<1 mg/dl)

A: RS is noncompliant with phenytoin. Her only seizure was 15 years ago. RS's need for antiepileptic medication is questionable because she has a history of noncompliance with phenytoin and the last seizure was 15 years ago.

P: Discontinue phenytoin. Monitor RS for seizures.

Problem 4. Guaiac-Positive

S: None

O: Rectal physical examination: guaiac-positive

A: RS is most likely guaiac-positive secondary to esophageal varices attributed to an increase in portal-venous hypertension from her alcohol-induced hepatotoxic liver damage. RS is additionally at risk for gastrointestinal bleeding because of her increased PT and INR (decreased synthetic function of the liver), also most likely caused by alcohol-induced hepatotoxicity. RS's binge drinking may have contributed to her guaiac-positive stool because alcohol acts as a gastric irritant.

P: Give RS stress ulcer treatment with ranitidine 50 mg IV q8h, and when she can take oral medication, change to ranitidine 300 mg PO q. h.s. Monitor RS's HCT and Hgb levels, stool guaiac test results, PT, INR, and vital signs. Educate RS about peptic ulcer disease, risk factors, and the need to discontinue alcohol consumption. Encourage RS to join Alcoholics Anonymous or a similar alcohol-abstinence therapy group.

QUESTIONS FOR CASE 119

1. RS's ED doctor vaguely remembers reading about clonidine in relation to drug abuse in a medical journal and asks you the role for this drug with narcotic-abuse patients.

2. How common is use/abuse with CNS stimulants?
3. What are the signs and symptoms and treatment of cocaine overdose?
4. What are the pharmacologic actions of cocaine?
5. If RS were to begin to suffer alcohol withdrawal, what treatment would you recommend?

CASE 120

CC: TR is a 64-year-old male who is admitted through the ED of his community hospital for workup of a 1-month history of anorexia, nausea, abdominal distress, fatigue, and what he describes as "a swollen belly and knees." He also notes redness on the palms of his hands.

Past Medical History

TR has a history of drinking a fifth of bourbon several times weekly, since his wife's death 5 years ago. He has been admitted to alcohol treatment programs on two occasions in the past, but has been unable to complete these programs and stay "dry." Two years ago, he fell off a ladder while painting his house and sustained a right frontal lobe hematoma and basilar skull fracture. One month later, he experienced two generalized seizures and has been on phenytoin since that time. He has been seizure-free for the past year.

TR has suffered from mild chronic bronchitis and emphysema for 15 years, which he currently manages with a metered-dose inhaler.

He developed a gastric ulcer 4 years ago and has since had one episode of GI bleeding. He currently takes cimetidine to prevent recurrence.

He also has degenerative joint disease (DJD) of his hips, but this has not been severe enough to interfere with his daily activities.

TR has a 20-year history of Type II diabetes mellitus (AODM), which is diet-controlled.

Past Surgical History

Craniotomy for drainage of subdural hematoma after fall 2 years ago

Social History

Ethanol—as above
Cigarettes—1 pack per day (quit 10 years ago)

Allergies

None known

Medication History

Phenytoin 300 mg PO b.i.d.
Cimetidine 400 mg PO q. h.s.
Albuterol inhaler two puffs q4-6h p.r.n. wheezing
Theophylline elixir 2 tbsp p.r.n. severe wheezing

Ibuprofen 200 mg (OTC) 2 tabs p.r.n. hip pain (2–3 times weekly)

Review of Systems

Significant for blurred vision, abdominal tenderness, mild cough, and heme-positive stools

Negative for fever, chest pain, diarrhea, weight loss, emesis, and hemoptysis

Physical Examination

GEN: Obese, lethargic male in no apparent distress
VS: BP 130/75, HR 85 reg, RR 16, T37, wt 98 kg
HEENT: PERRLA: sclera anicteric
NECK: Supple; no nodes or thyromegaly
CHEST: Faint rales and rhonchi
COR: RRR
ABD: Taut, obese; positive liver edge; positive spleen tip; positive fluid wave
RECT: Guaiac-positive
EXT: 1–2+ pitting edema of knees bilaterally
NEURO: AO × 3; speaks slowly: CN II-XII intact; motor: LEs 5/5 bilaterally; UEs 4+/5 bilaterally

Sensory grossly intact: DTRs normal, negative for asterixis
SKIN: Spider angiomas on chest; palmar erythema

Results of Laboratory Tests

Na 132 (132)	HCT 0.296 (29.6)	AST 0.67 (40)	Glu 13.9 (250)
K 3.4 (3.4)	Hgb 102 (10.2)	ALT 0.28 (17)	Ca 2.15 (8.6)
Cl 98 (98)	Lkcs 2.7 × 10⁹ (2.7 × 10³)	Alk Phos 10.6 (638)	Mg 0.7 (1.7)
HCO₃ 27 (27)	Plts 76 × 10⁹ (76 × 10³)	Alb 30 (3.0)	Phenytoin 99 (25)
BUN 3.2 (9)	MCV 82 (82)	T Bili 10 (0.6)	PT INR 1.5 (14)
CR 80 (0.9)		GGT 29.17 (1750)	

PROBLEM LIST

1. Type II DM, diet-controlled
2. Chronic obstructive pulmonary disease
3. Peptic ulcer disease (PUD); S/P GI bleeding
4. Seizure disorder; S/P hematoma/skull fracture
5. DJD
6. Chronic alcoholic cirrhosis, portal hypertension, ascites, splenomegaly, and R/O varices
7. Leukopenia, thrombocytopenia, and splenomegaly

CASE 120 SOAP NOTES
Problem 6. Chronic Alcoholic Cirrhosis, Portal Hypertension, Ascites, Splenomegaly, and R/O Varices

S: TR is admitted to hospital complaining of anorexia, nausea, fatigue, "a swollen belly and knees," and red palms.
O: TR has a 5-year history of alcohol abuse with previous admissions to treatment programs (none completed). Findings include a tender abdomen, enlarged liver edge and spleen tip, positive fluid wave, and 1–2 + edema of the knees. He shows no asterixis. He has increases in alkaline phosphatase and GGT (γ-glutamyl transpepdidase) and protime, and decreases in albumin, hemoglobin, hemato-

crit, and potassium. Stool guaiac shows occult blood.

A: TR has many of the common manifestations of alcoholic liver disease. The primary problem is cirrhosis with portal hypertension. His anorexia, nausea, fatigue, tender abdomen, and positive liver edge, and his social and previous detoxification history support this diagnosis. The increases in alkaline phosphatase, GGT, and protime are a manifestation of the disease, while the hypoalbuminemia may be caused by the disease or poor diet, and his decreased serum potassium may reflect increased urinary excretion of potassium.

Complications of cirrhosis include splenomegaly, ascites, esophageal or gastric varices, hepatic encephalopathy, and hepatorenal syndrome. TR exhibits several of these (in addition to those cited above), including palmar erythema, spider angiomas, and peripheral edema (cirrhosis and portal hypertension); positive spleen tip (splenomegaly); and positive fluid wave (ascites). The heme-positive stools and decreased Hgb and HCT may indicate slowly oozing esophageal varices, an exacerbation of his PUD, or even a new GI lesion such as cancer. He is alert and oriented to person, place, and time, tests negative for asterixis (no hepatic encephalopathy), and maintains normal BUN and Scr (no evidence of hepatorenal syndrome).

P: TR requires abstinence from alcohol, proper nutrition, supportive care, maintenance of fluid and electrolyte balance during detoxification, and rehabilitation. Drug therapy is required for the complications of liver disease. Many modes of therapy will be initiated simultaneously.

Nutrition: Some of the laboratory results indicate that TR may be suffering from a folate deficiency anemia (decreased Lkcs, Hgb, HCT, platelets) so supplementation is advised, after determining folate and vitamin B_{12} levels. Thiamine is routinely supplemented in alcoholics because Wernicke's encephalopathy may be caused by a deficiency of this vitamin. Pyridoxine can be added if peripheral neuropathies are a problem (not in this patient). TR has a protime INR of 1.5, which may indicate a lack of vitamin K, and 1–3 doses are advisable for reversal of coagulopathy. Because TR has an elongated protime, subcutaneous (rather than intramuscular) injection is the preferred route of administration. Daily monitoring of the protime is essential. In addition, multiple vitamin supplementation is advisable until a better diet can be achieved.

Fluid and electrolyte balance should include monitoring electrolytes frequently, monitoring intake and output ("Is and Os"), and electrolyte replacement therapy. Hypokalemia and/or hypomagnesemia may contribute to delirium tremens. Water restriction should be considered if the serum sodium concentration decreases further because water retention and excess antidiuretic hormone may contribute to dilutional hyponatremia.

TR will probably experience a significant course of alcohol withdrawal symptoms with delirium tremens (DTs), and his safety and care must be ensured. The goal is to keep the patient calm but awake, experiencing fairly normal wake-and-sleep cycles. Benzodiazepines are the drugs of choice, and lorazepam, chlordiazepoxide, and diazepam

have all been used. As elimination of the chosen agent may be decreased in patients with liver disease, it would seem prudent to select an agent with a relatively short elimination half-life and without psychoactive metabolites. Lorazepam is a sound choice and may be given intravenously or orally. Doses should be titrated based on patient response. After the initial 7- to 10-day detoxification, drug therapy can be adjusted downward and the rehabilitation process begun.

TR's hospital course may be prolonged while treatment for ascites (and possible varices) is considered. The drug of choice for treatment of ascites is the antialdosterone, potassium-sparing diuretic spironolactone, but higher-than-usual doses are usually needed with ascitic fluid. Monitoring parameters include serum and urine electrolyte levels, "Is and Os," weight, abdominal girth, and BUN. TR's presentation is more indicative of an exacerbation of PUD than of acutely bleeding varices, but it is necessary to monitor for signs of varices including hematemesis, a precipitous drop in Hgb and HCT levels, and hypovolemic shock. If any of these were to occur, drug therapy includes immediate volume repletion, possible transfusion, cold saline irrigation of the stomach to cause vasoconstriction, sclerotherapy, and/or intravenous vasopressin.

Drug Therapy for Problem 6
Folate 1 mg PO q.d. × 3 weeks
Thiamine 100 mg PO q.d. × 10 days
Vitamin K 10 mg SQ q.d. × 1–3 doses
Multiple vitamin 1 PO q.d.
Potassium replacement therapy PO or IV for a serum K < 3.5 mmol/liter
> IV rate should not exceed 10 mEq/hr, diluted in D5W or NS; usual dose is 30–40 mEq given over 3–4 hours; recheck serum K level 3–4 hours after completion of infusion and repeat until serum K is 3.8–4.0 mmol/liter.
> Then begin oral liquid or tablets 20–60 mEq/day in divided doses.

Magnesium replacement therapy PO or IV
> IV 1 g diluted in D5W or NS and infused over a minimum of 2 hours; recheck serum magnesium level 3–4 hours after completion of infusion

Lorazepam 1–4 mg PO or IV q4-6h p.r.n. agitation/DTs; may titrate up or down; continue for 7–10 days before tapering off
Spironolactone 100 mg PO q.d. titrate up to 400 mg q.d. at 3- to 5-day intervals, based on patient response

Problem 7. Leukopenia, Thrombocytopenia, and Splenomegaly

S: None
O: Positive spleen tip; Lkcs 2.7×10^9/liter (2.7×10^3/mm^3), Plts 76×10^9/liter (76×10^3/mm^3)
A: Splenomegaly itself may cause leukopenia and thrombocytopenia. Leukopenia is frequently found in congestive splenomegaly caused by portal vein hypertension. However, TR's leukopenia and thrombocytopenia may be caused by

folic acid deficiency anemia or be drug-induced. Current drug therapy for TR that could be contributing to this process includes phenytoin, ibuprofen, and (rarely) cimetidine. However, since TR has been stabilized on phenytoin for 2 years and cimetidine for 4 years, and only rarely takes ibuprofen, it seems unlikely that the leukopenia and thrombocytopenia that have developed within the last 2 months are caused by his drug therapy. The decreased counts are probably secondary to progression of his primary disease.

P: Institute folate replacement therapy per problem 6. Because drug therapy seems an unlikely cause of the leukopenia and thrombocytopenia a "watch-and-wait" strategy is appropriate.

Problem 4. Seizure Disorder; S/P Hematoma-Skull Fracture

S: Blurred vision; anorexia and nausea

TR states he has been seizure-free for 1 year.

O: Phenytoin level 99 μmol/liter (25 mg/liter)

A: TR is adequately controlled on phenytoin for seizure prophylaxis but may be experiencing toxic effects of blurred vision, anorexia, and nausea. TR's phenytoin dose may need to be lowered. However, two drug-drug interactions and one drug-disease interaction must be considered. Cimetidine decreases the hepatic metabolism of phenytoin, potentially causing a rise in phenytoin levels. Folic acid may increase the metabolism of phenytoin, thus predisposing the patient to an increased risk of seizures. TR's hepatic disease may prevent phenytoin elimination and cause increased phenytoin levels.

P: Hold 1 or 2 doses of phenytoin. Recheck phenytoin levels daily. Restart phenytoin at new maintenance dose of the equivalent dose of 550 mg/day. This can be achieved most easily by continuing to use the sustained-release capsules and dosing 200 mg every other morning, alternating with 300 mg every other morning, and continuing to give 300 mg every evening. The daily doses will then be 500 mg q.o.d. alternating with 600 mg q.o.d., averaging 550 mg/day. (See calculations for new maintenance dose below.) Monitor phenytoin levels at frequent intervals. Observe TR for seizures. Consider decreasing his phenytoin dose further if his cimetidine dose is increased and/or if phenytoin levels indicate.

Phenytoin Calculations

For ease in calculation, convert 99 μmol/liter to 25 mg/liter so that the answer will be in mg/day.

There is no need to adjust phenytoin level for hypoalbuminemia until albumin is less than 30 g/liter (3.0 g/dl).

$$(S)(F)(Dose/\tau) = \frac{(V_m)(Cp_{SSave})}{K_m + Cp_{ssave}}$$

$$V_m = \frac{(S)(F)(Dose/\tau)(K_m + Cpssave)}{Cp_{ssave}}$$

$$V_m = \frac{(0.92)(1)(600 \text{ mg/day})(4 + 25 \text{ mg/liter})}{(25 \text{ mg/liter})}$$

$$V_m = 640 \text{ mg daily}$$

$$Dose = \frac{(V_m)(\text{desired Cpssave})(\tau)}{(K_m + \text{desired Cp}_{ssave})(S)(F)}$$

$$Dose = \frac{(640)(15 \text{ mg/liter})(1 \text{ day})}{(4 + 15)(0.92)(1)}$$

$$Dose = 550 \text{ mg/day}$$

Phenytoin can be given 200 mg every other morning, alternating with 300 mg every other morning. Maintain 300 mg every evening.

Problem 3. PUD

S: Abdominal distress

O: Heme-positive stools; decreased Hgb and HCT levels

A: Hopefully, TR is just experiencing an exacerbation of his PUD. The ibuprofen that he takes for the arthritis in his hips may contribute to this bleeding. The other disease that must be ruled out is progression of his portal hypertension to esophageal varices. At this point he is not critically ill because of this process.

P: Discontinue ibuprofen. MD to perform an endoscopy to determine the exact location of bleeding. Increase cimetidine dose to the full therapeutic treatment dose of 800 mg PO q. h.s. × 4–6 weeks. Monitor guaiac test results, daily Hgb and HCT levels, and for signs and symptoms of esophageal varices.

Problem 2. COPD

S: TR states "slight, chronic cough."

O: Vital signs stable (VSS); TR in NAD; mild cough with faint rales and rhonchi

A: TR has controlled his mild bronchitis and emphysema for 15 years with the use of an albuterol inhaler and an occasional dose of his favorite theophylline elixir. From his history it appears that his COPD stabilized when he stopped smoking 10 years ago. His COPD is under control at this time. Albuterol is effective, but the use of theophylline is not advised. P.r.n. dosing of theophylline will not maintain a therapeutic drug level and will be of no benefit to TR. In addition, there is a potential drug-drug interaction between cimetidine and theophylline, and theophylline elixirs contain alcohol, which may cause a problem for TR during his rehabilitation therapy. TR should be able to manage exacerbations of his COPD with a slight increase in the frequency of use of his albuterol inhaler.

P: Discontinue theophylline. Continue to manage COPD with albuterol.

Problem 5. Degenerative Joint Disease of the Hips

S: TR states he takes two ibuprofen approximately three times weekly, with relief, for arthritic hip pain.

O: Heme-positive stools; low Hgb and HCT

A: DJD of the hips appears to be of minor concern to TR. Of greater concern is the fact that he is using a nonsteroidal antiinflammatory drug (NSAID) and is experiencing bleeding. Since his hip pain does not seem to be important, a medication with analgesic, rather than antiinflammatory, effect may suffice. Acetaminophen, although not a perfect alternative, may be effective if the dose is held low (because of his hepatic problems).

P: Discontinue ibuprofen. Suggest acetaminophen in doses of 650 mg at a time, with the goal of limiting the intake to two tablets daily or every other day.

Problem 1. Type II Diabetes Mellitus (AODM), Diet-Controlled

S: TR states that his diabetes is diet-controlled and that he does not routinely conduct fingerstick blood glucose or even urine glucose tests at home.

O: Blood glucose 13.9 mmol/liter (250 mg/dl)

A: TR is most likely NOT a diet-controlled diabetic but has neglected to monitor his glucose to come to this conclusion. Since his immediate course of therapy includes detoxification he may not be eating well for a few days and may need to be managed with q6h fingersticks and sliding-scale insulin for the short term. The next phase of his diabetic program will be diet education and stabilization on insulin if necessary. An oral hypoglycemic agent is not the regimen of choice for TR because even some of the second-generation oral hypoglycemics have been reported to cause disulfiram-like reactions when mixed with alcohol.

P: Monitor q6h fingerstick glucose levels and q.d. blood glucose levels for the immediate future. Consider ordering a sliding-scale of regular human insulin for subcutaneous administration if levels remain above 11.1 mmol/liter (200 mg/dl). (See example below.) Initiate a diet education program and insulin in the future.

Sliding Scale Insulin Regimen

Blood glucose or fingerstick glucose conc. in mmol/liter (mg/dl)	Regular human insulin (subcutaneously)
<3.9 (70)	give orange juice and call MD
3.9–11.1 (70–200)	no insulin
11.1–13.9 (200–250)	2 units
13.9–16.7 (250–300)	4 units
16.7–19.4 (300–350)	6 units
19.4–22.2 (350–400)	8 units
>22.2 (400)	10 units and call MD

QUESTIONS FOR CASE 120

1. Are phenothiazines used in the management of alcohol detoxification?
2. What is the current role of sclerotherapy in the treatment of esophageal varices?
3. If TR experienced esophageal varices (and failed sclerotherapy), how would you recommend that vasopressin be administered?
4. Discuss the advisability of the use of disulfiram in recovering alcoholics.

5. Would you recommend that TR be given an injection of pneumococcal vaccine before discharge?

CASE 121

CC: JM is a 35-year-old female who complains of shortness of breath, a smothering sensation, trembling, lightheadedness, rapid pounding of the heart, and a fear she might die. These complaints had a sudden and dramatic onset and lasted 15 minutes. On presentation to the ED, the symptoms were completely resolved. She gives a history of knee and wrist pain. She had been brought in by a friend after becoming afraid she was "losing control" while they were shopping. JM's symptoms had been occurring over the past 6 months with increasing frequency (about once weekly at present). She was seen in a different ED 3 weeks previously and was told she was physically healthy and now desires a second opinion. Her initial "attack" came 6 months ago while driving her car on the expressway. She has found these experiences so terrifying that she lives in dread of their recurrence. In the last few months she has become more confined to her home (e.g., has groceries delivered, shops by mail) to avoid situations in which help may be unavailable or where she may be embarrassed. JM ventured out today at the coaxing of her close friend.

Past Medical History

JM has no previous hospitalizations. For 4 years, her local MD has treated her on a nonregular basis for mild rheumatoid arthritis, with symptoms fairly well-controlled on ibuprofen in the past. She has also suffered from chronic migraine headaches for 7 years (previously diagnosed by a neurologist). She describes the frequency of her headaches as about 1 every month.

Social History

JM is married and has three children in elementary school. She has smoked 1 pack of cigarettes per day for 14 years. She describes herself as having been a social drinker in the past. She also consumes 4–5 cups of coffee each day. She has no family history for suicide or alcohol abuse.

Medication History

Ergotamine tartrate with caffeine 1 mg/100 mg (Cafergot) 2 tablets at onset of migraine attack and 1 every 30 minutes until relief of headache, not to exceed 6 tablets total
Ibuprofen 600 mg t.i.d. p.r.n. arthritis pain
OTC: BC powders, pseudoephedrine

Allergies

Penicillin
"Sulfa" drugs
Pine pollen

Physical Examination

        VS: BP 140/85, 145/87, 145/90, HR 85, RR 27, T
            37.5
    HEENT: WNL
    CHEST: Clear to auscultation
      COR: WNL
      ABD: WNL
       GU: Deferred
     RECT: Deferred
      EXT: Skin pale, diaphoretic; wrists and knees are pain-
            ful on flexion
    NEURO: WNL, alert and oriented × 3

Results of Laboratory Tests

Na 138 (138)	HCT 0.37 (37.2)	AST 0.17 (10)	Glu 4.1 (73)
K 3.7 (3.7)	Hgb 112 (11.2)	ALT 0.40 (24)	PO₄ 0.97 (3.0)
Cl 98 (98)	Lkcs 8 × 10⁹ (8 × 10³)	Alk Phos 0.7 (40)	Mg 0.6 (1.2)
HCO₃ 25 (25)	Plts 158 × 10⁹ (158 × 10³)	Alb 30 (3.0)	Uric Acid 360 (6)
BUN 3.6 (10)	MCV 86 (86)	T Bili 5 (0.3)	PT 14.2
CR 70 (0.8)	MCHC 310 (31)		PTT 39.2

Lkc differential: WNL

Urinalysis: WNL

Chest x-ray: WNL

ECG: WNL

Urine drug screen: negative

PROBLEM LIST

1. Chronic migraine headache × 7 years
2. Rheumatoid arthritis × 4 years
3. Panic disorder with agoraphobia

QUESTIONS FOR CASE 121

1. What common cardiac condition has been linked to panic disorder?
2. If JM experiences intolerable side effects to amitriptyline used in migraine prophylaxis, what other agents could be used?
3. Should JM's apparent mild hypertension be addressed pharmacologically at this point? Justify your answer.
4. What are the advantages of alprazolam over imipramine and phenelzine?
5. What is the average maintenance dose of alprazolam in treatment of panic? What is the appropriate duration of alprazolam treatment?

CASE 122

CC: DR is a 65-year-old woman with multiple medical problems who has become very depressed over the last several months.

Past Medical History

DR has a history of Type I diabetes for 40 years and is complaining of depression and numbness/tingling in her left foot, which began 4 months ago. She denies any current signs and symptoms of hyper- or hypoglycemia but admits to occasional hypoglycemic episodes when she does not "eat on time." DR has been noncompliant with checking her blood glucose levels. She has had no chest pains for the past 6 years.

Family History

Her father, mother, and brother all have a history of Type I diabetes.

Past Surgical History

Cataract surgery 10 years ago

Medication History

Regular human insulin 20 units SQ q. AM and 10 units SQ q. h.s.

NPH human insulin 20 units SQ q. AM and 10 units SQ q. h.s.

Nitroglycerin 0.4 mg SL p.r.n. chest pain

Levothyroxine 0.1 mg PO q.d.

Conjugated estrogen 0.625 mg PO q.d.

Docusate sodium 100 mg PO b.i.d.

Clonidine 0.1 mg PO b.i.d.

Hydrochorothiazide (HCTZ) 50 mg PO b.i.d.

Cholestyramine 4 g PO b.i.d.

Allergies

Aspirin ("stomach pain")

Physical Examination

      GEN: Nervous, thin, depressed female
       VS: BP 100/60, HR 70, RR 18, T 37, wt 60 kg
    HEENT: WNL, except for complaints of blurred vision
      COR: Normal S1, S2; no S3, S4, or murmurs
    CHEST: WNL
      ABD: Soft, no palpable masses
       GU: WNL
     RECT: Guaiac-negative
      EXT: Tingling/numbness, left foot
    NEURO: Cranial nerves intact; alert and oriented × 3

Results of Laboratory Tests

Na 142 (142)	HCT 0.38 (38)	AST 0.83 (50)	Glu 5.6 (100)
K 5.2 (5.2)	Hgb 130 (13)	ALT 0.66 (40)	HgA₁C 10
Cl 108 (108)	Lkcs 4 × 10⁹ (4 × 10³)	LDH 2.0 (120)	TG 40 (350)
HCO₃ 28 (28)	Plts 300 × 10⁹ (300 × 10³)	Alk Phos 1.67 (100)	TSH 0.4 (0.4)
BUN 7.14 (20)			Free T₄ Index 1.2
CR 310 (3.5)			Chol 3.9 (150)
			HDL chol 0.52 (20)

Lkc differential, chest x-ray, ECG: all WNL

Urinalysis: pH 1.020, glucose (−), protein (3+), casts (+)

PROBLEM LIST

1. Type I diabetes
2. Depression
3. Angina
4. Hypothyroidism

5. Hypertriglyceridemia
6. Hypertension

QUESTIONS FOR CASE 122

1. If DR had been diagnosed with the following depressions, suggest how she should be treated:
   a. Dysthymia
   b. Double
   c. Delusional
   d. Atypical
2. DR has been started on amitriptyline, and you are asked to comment on a possible drug interaction between amitriptyline and levothyroxine.
3. One month later, DR's depression appears to be responding to amitriptyline, and the attending wants to take her off amitriptyline since depression is now "no longer a problem." How long should DR be continued on drug therapy?
4. It is now 8 months into therapy, and DR's depression remains in control on a daily dose of 50 mg amitriptyline. How should the drug be discontinued?
5. Assuming that DR had not responded to amitriptyline, assess whether the following therapeutic options would have been appropriate for her:
   a. Phenelzine
   b. Methylphenidate
   c. Electroconvulsive therapy (ECT)

CASE 123

CC: SF is a 47-year-old man admitted to the hospital for cardiac catheterization and coronary arteriography resulting from increasing angina. While in the hospital, he complains of extreme difficulty sleeping. He states that he always has a difficult time falling and staying asleep whenever he is in a new environment.

Past Medical History

SF has a history of multiple medical problems (see below). With respect to sleep, he reports that he generally falls asleep fairly easily at home and sleeps 6–7 hours/night, waking up refreshed and alert. Occasionally, he has had difficulty sleeping in the past, usually if he is in a new environment or if some stressful event (e.g., a job interview) is about to occur. He has used flurazepam in the past, but complains that it makes him feel too drowsy the next morning. His wife confirms his difficulty sleeping in unfamiliar environments and reports that he has no observable limb twitches, snoring, or respiratory pauses during the night. He describes recent onset of occasional vise-like chest pain while exercising. The pain centers over his sternum and subsides within 3 minutes with rest and the use of nitroglycerin.

Social History

SF has a smoking history of two packs per day for 28 years.

Family History

His father died of a heart attack at age 56.

Medication History

Allopurinol 300 mg PO q.d.
Nitroglycerin 0.4 mg SL p.r.n.
Isosorbide dinitrate 20 mg PO q6-8h
Verapamil SR 240 mg PO q.d.
Hydrochlorothiazide 50 mg PO q.d. × 20 years
Ipratropium inhaler 2 puffs q4-6h
Albuterol inhaler 2 puffs q4-6h
Theophylline 200 mg PO b.i.d.

Allergies

Cholestyramine and colestipol—severe nausea and vomiting

Physical Examination

GEN:	Moderately obese, somewhat anxious male
VS:	BP 140/90, HR 70 regular, RR 12, wt 90 kg
HEENT:	WNL
COR:	Normal S1, S2; no S3, S4, or murmurs
CHEST:	Bilateral rales and rhonchi
ABD:	Absence of splenomegaly, bruits, or masses
GU:	WNL
RECT:	Deferred
EXT:	No peripheral edema; nicotine stains on fingers
NEURO:	WNL

Results of Laboratory Tests

Na 138 (138)	HCT 0.48 (48)	ALT 0.5 (30)	Glu 8.3 (150)
K 5.0 (5.0)	Hgb 160 (16)	LDH 3.34 (200)	Ca 2.25 (9)
Cl 102 (102)	Lkcs 6 × 10⁹ (6 × 10³)	Alk Phos 1.3 (80)	PO₄ 1.3 (4)
HCO₃ 24 (24)	Plts 300 × 10⁹ (300 × 10³)	Alb 40 (4)	Mg 1 (2)
BUN 6.4 (18)			Uric Acid 416 (7)
CR 115 (1.3)			Chol 8.3 (320)
			TG 1.35 (120)

Lkc differential: WNL
Urinalysis: WNL
Chest x-ray: WNL
ECG: NSR
Theophylline: Pending
24-hour uric acid excreted: 900 mg
Pulmonary function tests: WNL, with reversible component

PROBLEM LIST

1. Angina
2. Hypercholesterolemia
3. Hyperuricemia
4. Hypertension
5. Chronic obstructive pulmonary disease (COPD)
6. Insomnia

QUESTIONS FOR CASE 123

1. Why would you not select quazepam for SF?
2. Describe rebound insomnia. What is the risk in SF?
3. Would temazepam or estazolam have been equally good choices in treating SF?
4. Why is it important to rule out the presence of sleep apnea insomnia in SF?
5. If SF were to receive triazolam for 14 consecutive nights, how would you plan to deal with the possible rebound insomnia associated with discontinuation?

CASE 124

CC: TD is a 16-year-old female high-school student admitted to the hospital with complaints of fatigue and weakness. She appears markedly underweight but denies any eating problems.

History of Present Illness

Over the past several months, TD has been involved with a rigorous exercise program (daily 3–5 mile runs and aerobics) to get in shape for cheerleading try outs and to "fit in more with her friends." She has lost a total of 20 kg over the last month and is concerned about not making the cheerleading squad because she thinks she is "too fat." Her parents have noticed a progressive decrease in the amount of food intake and an increased amount of time spent by herself. TD also states that she occasionally vomits after eating and her last menses was over 4 months ago.

Past Medical History

Unremarkable

Medication History

TD admits to taking her mother's water-pill (hydrochlorothiazide) and various non-prescription laxatives to help maintain her weight. She denies the use of alcohol, tobacco or any other medications.

Allergies

No known allergies

Physical Examination

GEN: The patient is a quiet, emaciated young female with noticeable hip, knee and elbow joints. Despite her pronounced weight loss she perceives herself as being overweight.

VS: BP 85/60, HR 54, RR 24, T 37, Wt 36.5 kg (less than 35% ideal body weight), ht 165 cm

HEENT: Dry mucous membranes, mild acne on face and back

COR: Bradycardia; hypotension

CHEST: Clear to auscultation and percussion

ABD: Soft, non-tender with no masses found

EXT: Dry, flaky skin; cold extremities

NEURO: Alert and oriented × 3 (person, time & place)

Results of Laboratory Tests

Na 121 mmol/L　　　　　BUN 18.5 mmol/L (52 mg/dL)
K 2.7 mmol/L　　　　　Cr 53 mmol/L (0.6 mg/dL)
Cl 70 mmol/L　　　　　WBC 4×10^9 (4×10^3)
HCO$_3$ 36 mmol/L

Thyroid screen (TSH, T$_4$, T$_3$ Uptake, FTI) WNL
Amylase WNL
Catecholamine levels WNL

Arterial Blood Gases

pH 7.58; PCO$_2$ 40; PO$_2$ 90; HCO$_3$ 36; BE +11

Problem List

1. Significant weight loss
2. Dehydration
3. Electrolyte disturbances (hypokalemia, metabolic alkalosis)
4. Amenorrhea
5. Acne

CASE 124 SOAP NOTES

Problem 1. Significant Weight Loss

S: Pronounced emaciation; intense exercising and restrictive diet; self-image of being overweight despite weight loss; progressive weakness and fatigue.

O: Significant weight loss of 20 kg (56 kg down to 36 kg) over past month; elevated BUN consistent with muscle/protein wasting.

A: TD is diagnosed with anorexia nervosa having a >35% weight loss in a short period of time secondary to her desire to fit in with friends and make the cheerleading squad. An advanced stage of the disease is present as indicated by the extent of muscle wasting and the progressive fatigue and weakness. Tests evaluating thyroid function, pancreatic enzymes and catecholamine levels were all within normal limits suggesting that metabolic or endocrine abnormalities such as hyperthyroidism, pancreatic dysfunction and pheochromocytoma, were not likely causes for the weight loss.

P: The management of TD involves correction of nutritional deficiencies and increased weight gain at a slow but gradual rate (approx. 0.1–0.3 kg/day). A nutritional/dietary service should become involved to closely follow progress. TD should be encouraged to take food orally but if she refuses, tube feeding should be started. Supervision of meals is recommended initially and daily weights should be closely monitored. Positive incentives or privileges should be awarded contingent upon weight gain. Supportive and behavioral therapy (individual, group and family) represents the mainstay of therapy and should be implemented as soon as TD is stable. Strong emphasis should be placed on overcoming TD's negative self-image and self-esteem, and the patient must understand that overcoming the illness requires a great deal of effort and perseverance. The danger of starvation and its consequences (sudden death) should be carefully explained to TD. Therapeutic intervention with antidepressants do not appear to offer significant benefits unless depression exists as a contributing factor. More recently, serotonergic agents have also been evaluated and their role in the treatment of anorexia nervosa is unclear at this time. Regular follow-up appointments should be scheduled after discharge to monitor progress (body weight and electrolytes).

Problem 2. Dehydration

S: Reduced intake of fluids in conjunction with diet; use of diuretics and laxatives to lose weight; complaints of fatigue and weakness.

O: Poor skin turgor and dry mucous membranes; reduced blood pressure (BP 85/60); electrolyte abnormalities consistent with dehydration; reduced body weight.

A: Dehydration secondary to problem 1. The use of diuretics, laxatives, and the occasional vomiting after meals further depletes TD's fluid and electrolyte status.

P: Formulas for calculating fluid deficit have been established; however, because TD's weight loss is not due entirely to fluid loss, utilizing these deficit calculations may result in significant overhydration. TD should be started on a standard maintenance IV solution of D_5WNS supplemented with KCl 20 mEq/L at a rate of 50–100 ml/hr. Continue IV rehydration until TD's blood pressure increases to within an acceptable level, electrolyte imbalances begin to correct and a marked improvement in skin turgor and mucous membranes is present. Again, encourage TD to utilize the oral route of fluid administration if possible. Instruct TD to discontinue using her mother's diuretics and the non-prescription laxatives. Similar to problem 1, educating the patient on the importance of proper nutrition is essential. Monitor TD's electrolytes and blood pressure.

Problem 3. Electrolyte Disturbances

S: None

O: K 2.7 mmol/L
Cl 70 mmol/L
pH 7.58; PCO_2 40; PO_2 90; HCO_3 36; BE +11

A: Hypokalemia and hypochloremia with associated metabolic alkalosis secondary to diuretic abuse and vomiting. The hypokalemia is primarily due to reduced dietary intake and enhanced elimination through gastric loss (vomiting); hypochloremia is more associated with misuse of diuretics. Arterial blood gas results reflect a metabolic alkalosis as shown by the increased pH, HCO_3, and base excess.

P: This form of metabolic alkalosis (diuretic-induced) responds favorably to administration of normal saline (NaCl). Control of vomiting and rehydration of TD with the above mentioned IV solution and potassium supplementation (D_5WNS with KCl 20 mEq/L) should help resolve the metabolic alkalosis. To acutely increase serum

potassium, a series of 3 to 4 parenteral potassium "bumps", in the form of 10 mEq KCl in 50 ml of D_5W, can be administered each as a 60 minute infusion. Serum potassium levels obtained 3 to 4 hours after administration of the potassium bumps should reflect a noticeable rise in serum potassium. In severe situations, administration of hydrochloric acid solutions can rapidly correct acid/base abnormalities if necessary. However, this approach is reserved for severe or refractory cases. Close monitoring of TD's electrolytes, especially during initial therapy, is critical in order to avoid overcompensating the imbalance. Potassium supplementation with oral tablets or increased dietary intake of food rich in potassium (i.e., bananas, orange juice) may be appropriate for TD as follow-up therapy.

Problem 4. Amenorrhea

S: None

O: Absence of menses for over 4 months

A: Amenorrhea is a manifestation frequently seen in patients with anorexia nervosa, and is one of the criteria used to diagnose the condition. With severe weight loss, basal levels of luteinizing hormone and follicle stimulating hormone are diminished. This hormonal reduction is believed to contribute to the development of amenorrhea.

P: There is very little drug therapy available for the treatment of amenorrhea. In most situations, as body weight is regained menses returns to a normal cyclical pattern. TD should be instructed to note when menses returns and to contact her physician with any subsequent changes that may occur.

Problem 5. Acne

S: None

O: Presence of comedones on the face and back

A: TD is currently at an age where *Propionibacterium acnes* tends to be a common problem. In addition, the psychological burden being experienced by TD may also be contributing to her acne problem. She denies using any medicated preparations for managing the acne but wants to clear up the acne.

P: Considering TD's acne problem is fairly mild, proper skin cleansing followed by topical application of 5% benzoyl peroxide cream twice daily should produce a noticeable improvement in the acne within a 5–7 day period. Existing blemishes should begin to dry up and there should be a significant reduction in the number of new comedones. After completing one week of therapy, if satisfactory results are not obtained, more potent preparations may be required. A 10% cream, and 5 and 10% gel formulations are available and tend to be effective, especially against severe or refractory acne. In addition, topical preparations of antimicrobial agents are available (i.e., clindamycin). If the response to more potent dosage formulations are unsatisfactory, TD should be seen by a dermatologist.

CASE 124 QUESTIONS

1. Should TD's anorexia nervosa be treated with total parenteral nutrition?

2. Which of the DSM III-R criteria for anorexia nervosa were evident in TD?
3. What is the primary concern, in addition to nutritional imbalance, associated with the severe emaciation frequently encountered in patients with anorexia nervosa?
4. Describe the common patient characteristics and behaviors associated anorexia nervosa that can often times be recognized by the pharmacist.

CASE 125

CC: LB is a 34-year-old male who was brought to the ED by ambulance after his wife found him unresponsive on the bathroom floor. A history given by LB's wife reveals that he has enrolled in a methadone detoxification program for a week and a half and that LB started shooting ``Mexican tar'' after an old friend of his came into town 2 days ago.

Past Medical History

LB had a revision of a right hip arthroplasty 4 weeks ago. LB had his first hip arthroplasty at age 17, when he broke his hip in a fall from a dune buggy. LB has had asthma since he was 5 years old and has a history of noncompliance with his medications. LB has been involved in a methadone maintenance program continuously for the last 15 years. A week and a half ago, LB began a methadone detoxification program.

Social History

Nondrinker; smokes 1 pack/day × 20 years; IV drug abuse of heroin, last was 2 days ago

Allergies

Codeine n/v

Medication History

Methadone via detoxification program 80 mg p.o. q.d.
Theophylline 300 mg p.o. b.i.d.
Albuterol 2-mg tablets p.o. b.i.d.

Physical Examination

GEN: LB is a comatose male; he is cyanotic and has respiratory depression and pinpoint pupils.
VS: BP 80/50, HR 45, RR 8, T 38.5, Wt 75 kg, Ht 183 cm
HEENT: Pupils are symmetrically pinpoint in size.
COR: Sinoatrial bradycardia (no S3, S4, or murmurs)
CHEST: Decreased RR; no rales, rhonchi, or wheezes
EXT: Cyanotic, cold, clammy skin, several needle-track marks on right arm with slight erythema and inflammation
NEURO: Unresponsive; oriented × 0

Results of Laboratory Tests

Na 140 (140) | HCT 0.45 (45) | AST 0.58 (35) | Glu 4.4 (80)
K 3.7 (3.7) | Hgb 160 (16) | ALT 0.58 (35)
Cl 96 (96) | Lkcs 12.4 × 10⁹ (12.4 × 10³) | Alk Phos 2.2 (133)
HCO₃ 23 (23) | Plts 140 × 10⁹ (140 × 10³) | Alb 24 (2.4)
BUN 7.1 (20) | | T Bili 20.5 (1.2)
CR 71 (0.8)

Urinalysis: WNL
Theophylline: <5.5 (m/liter (<1 mg/liter)
Tox screen: (+) morphine

PROBLEM LIST

1. Asthma
2. S/P right THA revision, 4 weeks ago
3. Thrombophlebitis
4. Acute pain management
5. Heroin overdose
6. Risk for opioid withdrawal

QUESTIONS FOR CASE 125

1. Why is LB at greater risk for narcotic overdose than someone who abuses only IV heroin?
2. What is meant by narcotic dependence?
3. LB shows signs and symptoms of narcotic side effects. Which side effects are not characterized by tolerance?
4. What is the maximum dose of naloxone that can be given for LB's narcotic overdose?
5. Why is methadone used for heroin detoxification (as in LB) or methadone maintenance?
6. LB suddenly complains of tenderness and pain in his right calf. Objectively, his right calf is larger than the left calf, and LB has a positive Homan's sign but a negative VQ scan. What problem is LB most likely experiencing and what treatment would you recommend?

CASE 126

CC: RS is a 30-year-old obese man who was brought to the ED by the police after he was found walking on the freeway, shouting obscenities at the oncoming traffic. He is both belligerent and hyperactive.

History of Present Illness

RS is a graduate student with a 6-year history of bipolar disorder, which appeared to be under control until approximately 2 weeks ago. At that time, RS's colleagues noted that he spent several sleepless nights in the laboratory and was obsessed with the idea that the results of his research would earn him the Nobel prize.

Social History

Mother has a history of chronic depression.
RS drinks 4 cans of beer every evening and eats a 6.5-oz bag of potato chips every evening with beer.

Medication History

Lithium carbonate 300 mg p.o. t.i.d.
Cimetidine 400 mg p.o. b.i.d. for only 2 weeks
Generic NaHCO3 tablets—ingests "handful" after each meal
Imipramine 50 mg p.o. t.i.d.

Allergies

None known

Review of Systems

RS has ulcer pain that is not relieved by sodium bicarbonate.

Physical Examination

GEN:	Obese, well-developed, well-nourished, agitated male
VS:	BP 140/80, HR 80 regular, RR 20, T 38, Wt 100 kg (IBW 75 kg)
HEENT:	PERRLA. EOMI
COR:	Regular, without murmurs or extra sounds
CHEST:	Clear to auscultation.
ABD:	Soft, tender, no palpable masses
GU:	WNL
RECT:	Guaiac-negative
EXT:	WNL
NEURO:	Cranial nerves intact. Muscle strength is 5/5 and bilaterally symmetrical.

Results of Laboratory Tests

Na 137 (137)	HCT 0.42 (42)	AST 1.0 (60)	Glu 6.7 (120)
K 3.4 (3.4)	Hgb 150 (15)	ALT 1.33 (80)	Cholesterol 7.7 (300)
Cl 100 (100)		LDH 2.5 (150)	Lithium 0.5 (0.5)
HCO₃ 26 (26)		Alk Phos 1.67 (100)	Imipramine pending
BUN 7.14 (20)			
CR 88.4 (1.0)			

Lkcs differential, urinalysis, chest x-ray, ECG: all WNL
Cholesterol 4 months ago 7.5 (290)

PROBLEM LIST

1. Bipolar disorder
2. Depression
3. Peptic ulcer disease (PUD)
4. Alcoholism
5. Hypercholesterolemia
6. Anticholinergic side effects

CASE 127

CC: JR is a 56-year-old male with an acute episode of schizophrenia caused by noncompliance with medications.

History of Present Illness

JR has a 7-year history of schizophrenia, was acting suspiciously all week, and constantly complained of the radio and television "talking to him." At one point, JR called two local television stations and threatened to kill the news anchorpersons if they continued to "talk to him." On the day of admission, he became so furious at the news anchors' continued attempts to "speak" to him that he picked up his TV set and threw it out the window. Fortunately, nobody was hurt. He was placed immediately in four-point restraints in the locked unit of the hospital.

Family History

Father committed suicide.
Both brother and sister have histories of depression.

Medication History

Trifluoperazine 10 mg p.o. q.i.d.
Trihexyphenidyl 15 mg p.o. b.i.d.
Diazepam 5 mg p.o. b.i.d.
Amitriptyline 25 mg p.o. t.i.d.
Fluocinonide 0.05% cream applied b.i.d.-q.i.d.
Pilocarpine HCl 2% ophthalmic solution 1–2 gtts q.i.d.

Allergies

Thorazine "upsets stomach"

Physical Examination

GEN:	Agitated, belligerent, disheveled, and hallucinating male with flat, anxious affect
VS:	BP 130/90, HR 80, RR 20, T 37.6
HEENT:	Visual acuity (without correction) 20/60 OD and 20/ 80 OS. IOP 36 mm Hg OU. Ophthalmoscopy and gonioscopy consistent with open-angle glaucoma. No evidence of cataracts or pain.
COR:	WNL
CHEST:	WNL
ABD:	WNL except for complaints of nausea
EXT:	Erythematous, thick plaques with silvery scales on knees and legs
NEURO:	Cranial nerves intact; alert and oriented × 3

Results of Laboratory Tests

Na 142 (142)	HCT 0.45 (45)	Glu 6.7 (120)
K 4.0 (4.0)	Hgb 150 (15)	
Cl 110 (110)	Lkcs 5 × 10⁹ (5 × 10³)	
HCO₃ 28 (28)	Plts 300 × 10⁹ (300 × 10³)	
BUN 7.1 (20)		
CR 79.6 (0.9)		

PROBLEM LIST

1. Schizophrenia
2. Psoriasis
3. Chronic open-angle glaucoma

CASE 128

CC: MC is a 64-year-old man who comes to the clinic and complains of extreme difficulty sleeping. "I haven't slept well for many years." He states that he can fall asleep pretty well after drinking one-half pint of whiskey, but within a few hours he "tosses and turns" for the remainder of the night. He gets up in the morning feeling unrefreshed. He reports no chest discomfort but has recently felt "palpitations in his heart."

History of Present Illness

MC reports that he has tried all hypnotics for his insomnia, but although they sometimes help for a few nights, they stop working and his insomnia returns to being as bad as ever.

Social History

MC has a smoking history of one pack per day for 44 years. Ethanol use is two six-packs of beer and up to one pint of whiskey per day for 40 years.

Medication History

Digoxin 0.25 mg p.o. q.d.
Acetaminophen 650 mg p.o. q.i.d.
Multivitamins 1 p.o. q.d.
Docusate sodium 100 mg p.o. b.i.d.

Allergies

None known

Physical Examination

GEN:	Thin, anxious male, looking 10 years older than his stated age
VS:	BP 130/90, HR 100 regular, RR 20, T 38
HEENT:	No jaundice in the eyes. PERRLA. EOMI
COR:	WNL
CHEST:	Clear, but breathing is not very deep
ABD:	Liver slightly enlarged
EXT:	Intermittent pain in left hip and knee, with moderate stiffness
NEURO:	All pulses palpable; no tenderness over either ankle; both calves soft

Results of Laboratory Tests

Na 142 (142)	HCT 0.32 (32)	AST 1.5 (90)	Glu 4.4 (80)
K 3.5 (3.5)	Hgb 100 (10)	ALT 1.3 (80)	Folate 11.3 (5)
Cl 105 (105)	Lkcs 2.8×10^9 (2.8×10^3)	LDH 5 (300)	Vitamin B$_{12}$ 192 (260)
HCO$_3$ 25 (25)	Plts 120×10^9 (120×10^3)	Alk Phos 2.5 (150)	
BUN 5.4 (15)	MCV 110 (110)	Alb 25 (2.5)	
CR 159 (1.8)		T Bili 34.2 (2)	

Rheumatoid factor (−)
Lkc differential: WNL except for hypersegmented neutrophils on smear

PROBLEM LIST

1. Alcohol abuse
2. Chronic insomnia
3. Paroxysmal ventricular tachycardia (PSVT)
4. Degenerative joint disease (DJD)
5. Increased liver enzyme levels secondary to alcohol abuse

CASE 129

CC: MO is a 23-year-old female presenting to the outpatient clinic seeking professional advice to assist her efforts at controlling her weight.

History of Present Illness

MO has made several unsuccessful attempts at weight reduction through various diets. She reluctantly presents to the clinic concerned about her inability to lose weight. She admits to frequent, uncontrollable urges to consume large quantities of sweet foods over a relatively short period of time. Often, this "binge-eating" is followed by self-induced vomiting. She is uncomfortable discussing her binge-and-purge problem but wants to overcome it. MO appears noticeably depressed about her condition and she has a very negative self-image and low self-esteem.

Past Medical History

In past clinic visits, MO has frequently complained of fatigue and "being sick and run down." Based on her previous clinic visits, there is a marked fluctuation in her body weight.

Social History

MO is socially withdrawn and spends the majority of her weekends and free time alone at her apartment. She is apprehensive about dating secondary to her diminished self-image. She admits to using alcohol and marijuana on a regular basis, especially when she is depressed.

Medication History

MO admits to using Ex-Lax after her meals to help reduce absorption of food. She denies taking anti-depressants or any other medications.

Allergies

No known allergies

Physical Examination

GEN:	MO is a modestly obese female who appears depressed about her inability to lose weight. Several small ulcerations are present in her oral cav-

ity and gums, dentation is poor and parotid
glands appear slightly enlarged.

VS: BP 110/80, HR 68, RR 24, T 37, Wt 73 kg (previous clinic visits as low as 61 kg), Ht 165 cm

Laboratory Results
Standard electrolytes were WNL except:
K 3.0 mmol/L

Problem List
1. Bulimia
2. Depression
3. Hypokalemia

CASE 129 SOAP NOTES
Problem 1. Bulimia
S: History of fluctuating body weight; laxative abuse.
O: MO frequently relies on a binge-and-purge method to reduce her body weight; presence of hypokalemia (K 3.0 mmol/L); enlarged parotid glands; oral ulcerations and dental caries secondary to frequent vomiting.
A: The diagnosis of bulimia is made based on the above clinical findings. With the exception of hypokalemia, characteristic laboratory and physical findings are usually not evident. Frequently bulimia is difficult to recognize due to the non-specific presentation and secretive behavior of those afflicted by the illness. Fortunately, MO was willing to admit her eating disorder which made establishing the diagnosis of bulimia less difficult.
P: Supportive care and behavior therapy represent the most effective approach to managing bulimia. MO should be assured that her eating disorder is a common illness and that effective therapy exists. MO should be encouraged to keep a record of her binge-and-purge episodes to try and identify triggering factors. In addition, she should work closely with her behavioral therapist to restrict her eating to 3–4 planned meals. Group behavioral therapy may also be beneficial. On average effective therapy lasts 6–8 months and may extend up to 2 years. Discourage MO from misusing non-prescription laxatives. The use of tricyclic antidepressants (i.e., imipramine) and monoamine oxidase inhibitors (i.e., phenelzine) have demonstrated some usefulness in managing bulimic patients. More recently, investigations involving serotonin reuptake inhibitors (i.e., fluoxetine) have also shown promise in the treatment of eating disorders (see problem 2).

Problem 2. Depression
S: Complaints of being depressed; anti-social behavior; low self-image
O: Alcohol and marijuana use
A: Bulimic patients frequently present with signs and symptoms of depression and diminished self-esteem. The depression appears to be greatest following an eating binge.
P: Behavioral therapy as mentioned above will prove useful for M.O.'s depression. Additionally, MO could also be started on oral imipramine (100–200 mg/day in 4 divided doses) which is a preferred tricyclic anti-depressant agent for managing patients with bulimia. Imipramine should be continued for 6–8 weeks and the importance of compliance should be strongly emphasized. As an alternative, the anti-depressant fluoxetine (60 mg/day) has been shown to be very effective at decreasing the frequency of binge-and-purge episodes in both depressed and non-depressed individuals. In addition, compared to tricyclics and mono-amine oxidase inhibitors, fluoxetine tends to be associated with fewer adverse events. An approved indication for the treatment of bulimia is anticipated sometime in 1995. The monoamine oxidase inhibitor phenelzine has also been shown to be effective, but should be avoided due to MO's present dietary indiscretion which may put her at potential risk for significant food-drug interactions. Encourage MO to restrict the use of alcohol and marijuana because of their additional depressive effects.

Problem 3. Hypokalemia
S: None
O: K 3.0 mmol/L
A: Hypokalemia secondary to frequent vomiting.
P: Explain the importance of proper nutritional intake. If MO is unable to resolve her self-induced vomiting, oral supplementation of potassium (10–20 mEq/day) should be prescribed. Follow-up appointments should include periodic electrolyte levels to avoid the complications of electrolyte imbalance.

CASE 129 QUESTIONS
1. What are the primary differences between anorexia nervosa and bulimia?
2. Should patients with bulimia be hospitalized?
3. Which pharmacologic agents can be use to manage patients with bulimia?
4. Can bulimia be successfully treated with medication alone?

CASE 130
CC: PM is an 18-year-old male who presents to clinic with multiple complaints. He complains of cramping and abdominal pains for the past 2 years and states that the pain is usually relieved after passage of flatus or stool. PM states that he feels constipated every day and takes bisacodyl tablets at least 5 x/week. PM describes his stool as "pencil-thin" alternating with cramping diarrhea that comes and goes irrespective of bisacodyl ingestion. PM admits to drinking 3–6 beers/day and eating a diet consisting solely of fast-food hamburgers and french fries. PM also admits to smoking one to two "joints" per day. PM states that he really wants to change his lifestyle and increase his energy level before beginning college.

Past Medical History

Not significant

Social History

PM is a high school senior with a 4.0 GPA who has been accepted into a very prestigious college. Marijuana "joint" unknown purity and adulterants
Ethanol: 3–6 beers per day

Allergies

Penicillin—anaphylaxis

Medication History

Bisacodyl 2 mg p.o. q.d. 5 ×/week p.r.n. constipation

Physical Examination

GEN: Lethargic-appearing male complaining of abdominal pain and bloating, decreased energy, and constipation for the past 2 years
VS: BP 120/75, HR 70 reg, RR 18, T 37.2, Wt 65 kg, Ht 168 cm
HEENT: WNL
CHEST: No rales, rhonchi, or wheezes, normal BS bilaterally

ABD: Soft, tender, +RUQ pain
GU: WNL
RECT: Guaiac-negative

Results of Laboratory Tests

Na 142 (142)	HCT 0.39 (39)	AST 0.8 (48)	Glu 5.3 (95)
K 4.0 (4.0)	Hgb 120 (12)	ALT .9 (54)	TIBC 86 (480)
Cl 102 (102)	Lkcs 4.0 × 10^9 (4.0 × 10^3)	Alb 23 (2.3)	Fe 5.4 (30)
HCO$_3$ 25 (25)	Plts 210 × 10^9 (210 × 10^3)	T Bili 32.5 (1.9)	
BUN 3.6 (10)	MCV 70 (70)		
CR 50 (0.6)	MCHC 310 (31)		
	MCH 24 (24)		

U/A: positive for cannabinoids (marijuana)
Sigmoidoscopy: WNL
Stool: Negative for O+P and for *Clostridium difficile* toxin

PROBLEM LIST

1. Irritable bowel syndrome (IBS)
2. Chronic stimulant laxative abuse
3. Anemia
4. Marijuana abuse
5. Alcohol abuse

INFECTIOUS DISEASES

CASE 131

CC: OM is a 43-year-old man who presents to the hospital with fevers, night sweats, malaise, abdominal pains, and a persistent sore throat. OM also complains of a 2-week history of acute vision loss with headaches and occasional ``floaters'' in the left eye.

Medical History

OM has a medical history of seizures since childhood, stabilized on phenytoin (last seizure 1 year ago). OM was diagnosed HIV(+) 2 years ago when he was treated for oral candidiasis. He was hospitalized 6 months ago for *Pneumocystis carinii* pneumonia (PCP) and was successfully treated with trimethoprim/sulfamethoxazole. OM has been in stable health prior to his recent presentation.

Social History

OM is a marine biologist. He is homosexual and has been in a monogamous relationship for the past 4 years. He denies multiple partners and at present his lover is HIV negative. OM denies intravenous drug use and does not drink or smoke.

Medication History

Zidovudine 200 mg po TID
Trimethoprim/sulfamethoxazole DS po QD
Multivitamin with Iron 1 tab po QD
Rifabutin 150 mg po QD
Phenytoin 300 mg po HS

Allergies

None known

Physical Examination

GEN: Thin, ill-appearing man
VS: BP 110/60, HR 70, T 39.3°C, RR 14, Wt 77 kg
HEENT: (−) exudate, (−) oral thrush, (+) cervical lymphadenopathy
COR: Normal S_1 and S_2; no murmurs, rubs, or gallops
CHEST: WNL
ABD: (+) Bowel sounds, diffuse tenderness
GU: WNL
RECT: WNL; (−) guaiac
EXT: WNL
NEURO: Alert and oriented × 3

Results of Laboratory Tests

Na 141 (141)	Cl 97 (97)	BUN 5.7 (16)
Hct 0.28 (28)	LKCS 0.6×10^9 (0.6×10^3)	ANC 408
Glu 4.96 (90)	ALT 1.54 (92)	Alb 28 (2.8)
K 4.1 (4.1)	HCO_3 23 (23)	SrCr 88.4 (1.0)
Hgb 82 (8.2)	Plts 98×10^9 (98×10^3)	MCV 118 (118)
AST 1.96 (118)	ALK Phos 4.02 (240)	T bili 34.2 (2.0)
		Amylase 81 (81)

CD_4 count 44 cells/mm^3
CD_4/CD_8 ratio 12%
Blood cultures (+) CMV (+) MAC
Ophthalmic examination (+) white exudates with hemorrhage in left eye

PROBLEM LIST

1. HIV (+)
2. CMV retinitis
3. Neutropenia
4. MAC

CASE 131 SOAP NOTES
Problem 1. Cytomegalovirus (CMV) Retinitis

S: Patient complains of acute vision loss with headaches.

O: (+) fundoscopic examination, white exudate with hemorrhage in left eye. (+) CMV blood cultures, CD_4 lymphocytic count 44 cells/mm^3.

A: OM is severely immunocompromised (CD_4 count 44 cells/mm^3). His ophthalmic examination is consistent with CMV retinitis. He needs to be treated to prevent further loss of vision and ultimately blindness. Treatment consists of induction for 14–21 days followed by maintenance therapy indefinitely to prevent or decrease time to relapse. The two currently approved agents for treatment are ganciclovir (GCV) and foscarnet. Both agents are equally efficacious; therefore, patient specific indications must be considered. A greater survival benefit has been demonstrated with the use of foscarnet; however, this fact alone does not necessarily make it the best choice. The most common adverse effect of foscarnet is nephrotoxicity. OM has a calculated creatinine clearance of 94.3 ml/min and is not renally compromised. OM does, however, have a history of seizures, and seizures have been reported with the administration of foscarnet. GCV is myelosuppressive and may not be an appropriate choice in this patient with an ANC <500 cells. OM also has a platelet count of 98,000. A platelet count less than 30,000 is an absolute contraindication to use of GCV. If zidovudine is held and G-CSF is given, GCC may be tolerated. GCV should be the preferred agent in patients with a history of seizures.

P: Hold zidovudine and reassess antiretroviral therapy. Start

G-CSF (see problem 3. Neutropenia). Induce GCV IV 5 mg/kg every 12 hours for 14–21 days. Dose adjustments should be made based on renal function, and duration of treatment should be based on response to treatment. Plan to monitor CBC and platelets at baseline and twice weekly. Continue maintenance therapy post induction, at a GCV dose of 5 mg/kg IV Q24h indefinitely. With the availability of oral GCV, maintenance therapy can be initiated at 1 gm po TID.

Problem 2. HIV (+)

S: See social history.

O: Decreased CD_4 cell count (44 cells/mm^3). Mild anemia (decreased Hct and Hgb) with macrocytosis (increased MCV 118). Progression of disease (CMV retinitis and disseminated MAC).

A: OM has been on zidovudine therapy for more than 1 year. The benefit of continuing therapy or decreasing the dose to 300 mg/day is controversial. He has significant progression of his disease (decreased CD_4, CMV, and disseminated MAC) and now presents with neutropenia (ANC 408) and borderline anemia. Zidovudine is a bone-marrow suppressive agent. Patients receiving GCV for CMV have additive bone marrow suppression. Switching to a less myelosuppressive antiretroviral agent is a reasonable consideration. DDI 200 mg po BID is an appropriate alternative. DDI is not as effective as zidovudine for monotherapy. One study has shown some survival advantages with zalcitabine (DDC) vs DDI, but more data and clinical experience are available for DDI. Stavudine (d4T) is indicated for patients intolerant to AZT, DDI and DDC.

P: Plan to switch to DDI 200 mg po BID (for patients who weigh more than 60 kg with no history of alcohol use and normal amylase levels). Consider decreasing trimethoprim/sulfamethoxazole for PCP prophylaxis from one DS tablet QD to one single-strength tablet daily or one double-strength tablet three times a week. Plan to monitor serum amylases, LFTs, and electrolytes. Patient should be educated about the risks and benefits of therapy.

Problem 3. Neutropenia

S: Patient complains of persistent sore throat.

O: OM has a WBC of 0.6 and an ANC of 408.

A: This patient has been on zidovudine therapy 600 mg/day for more than 1 year. Zidovudine is a bone-marrow suppressive agent. He has severe neutropenia (ANC 408), sore throat, fevers, and is at increased risk for infection. Concomitant use of bone-suppressive drugs (trimethoprim/sulfamethoxazole, zidovudine, GCV) increases the risk for neutropenia. This patient's zidovudine will be discontinued because he also has active CMV retinitis and will be treated with GCC. OM should be treated with a colony stimulating factor G-CSF such as filgastrim (Neupogen).

P: The goal of treatment is to prevent further infection in a severely neutropenic patient and restore the ANC between 500 and 1,000. An additional goal is to increase the WBC to a maximum of 10,000. Plan to start G-CSF 150–300 mcg SQ (three times weekly or titrate based on ANC/WBC). The ANC will begin to increase 2 to 4 days after beginning G-CSF. Monitor CBC with differential daily to prevent excess bone marrow stimulation. Plan to educate the patient about the risk from severe neutropenia. Plan to teach the patient aseptic techniques for self-administration of G-CSF when discharged.

Problem 4. Disseminated MAC (D-MAC)

S: Patient complains of malaise, night sweats, and abdominal pains.

O: Fevers (T 39.3°C), anemia (Hgb 8.2, Hct 28), (+) MAC blood cultures, increased AST, ALT, T bili, ALK Phos and CD_4 of 44 cells/mm^3.

A: This is a 43-yr-old patient with AIDS who has a CD_4 count of 44 cells/mm^3. Disseminated MAC usually occurs in patients with CD_4 counts less than 100. The patient has subjective and objective complaints consistent with disseminated MAC disease and must be treated because it is a major cause of morbidity and mortality in patients with AIDS. This patient was treated with a subtherapeutic MAC regimen (rifabutin 150 mg po QD instead of the recommended dose of 300 mg po QD) and this may be one of the reasons for his symptomatic presentation of disseminated disease. Therapy includes combinations of various compounds, two to five drug combinations. No therapy currently available will eradicate the organism from the host, and the selection of compounds for the treatment is institution- and practitioner-specific. However, combinations usually are a macrolide plus ethambutol alone with one or two of the following: rifabutin, clofazamine, ciprofloxacin, rifampin, or amikacin. The occurrences of optic neuritis secondary to ethambutol is a caution in this patient with CMV retinitis. This patient was on rifabutin prophylaxis for MAC and developed D-MAC; therefore, he may have rifabutin-resistant organisms and may not respond to rifabutin or rifampin.

P: Plan to discontinue rifabutin and start two-drug therapy, clarithromycin 500 mg po BID and ethambutol 1200 mg po QD (15 mg/kg/day). If no response (resolution of symptoms) addition of a third drug may be warranted (ciprofloxacin or clofazamine). If ciprofloxacin and DDI are administered concomitantly, dosing should be staggered dose by 2 hours. Plan to add amikacin if patient becomes very septic and severely ill. Resolution of symptoms generally are observed within 2 weeks to 1 month of treatment. Plan to decrease the number of drugs when symptoms improve. Continue full-dose therapy for rest of patient's life. Monitor for therapeutic efficacy (decreased symptoms) and toxicities with agents used.

QUESTIONS FOR CASE 131

1. How important is treatment for CMV retinitis? What quality-of-life issues influence choice of agents?
2. Give 5 patient education points for didanosine (DDI).
3. What patient education is necessary for HIV patients with neutropenia who self-administer G-CSF?

4. What are five health care maintenance issues all HIV (+) patients should know and how do they affect patient care?
5. Identify six common agents and their dose and toxicities used in the treatment of disseminated MAC.

CASE 132

CC: TC is a 57-year-old woman who is planning a 3-month trip around the world. She will be traveling through areas where conditions are unsanitary, water may be contaminated, and malaria and hepatitis are endemic. She realizes that she may be exposed to many different diseases and requests a shot to minimize her risk for becoming infected.

Medical History

TC is postmenopausal and has some difficulty sleeping through the night.

Medication History

Conjugated estrogens 0.625 mg QD × first 21 days of each month
Calcium carbonate p.r.n.
Flurazepam HCl 15 mg p.r.n.

Social History

Tobacco: negative
Alcohol: socially

Physical Examination

GEN: Well-developed, well-nourished, slightly obese woman in no apparent distress
VS: BP 125/80, HR 75, RR 25, T 37.3°C, Wt 86 kg, Ht 168 cm
HEENT: Normal
COR: RRR, no murmurs
CHEST: Clear to auscultation
ABD: Soft, nontender, no palpable masses, bowel sounds present
GU: Normal woman
RECT: Normal, stool guaiac-negative
EXT: Normal
NEURO: Alert and oriented to time, place, and person; deep-tendon reflexes WNL

Results of Laboratory Tests

None performed

PROBLEM LIST

1. Failure to understand the implications of diseases that she is likely to encounter
2. Exposure to unsanitary conditions with potential for hepatitis A, hepatitis B, cholera, and typhoid infection
3. Likely exposure to chloroquine-resistant malaria

4. Lengthy absence from the United States with potential difficulty obtaining prescription and over-the-counter (OTC) medications

CASE 132 SOAP NOTES
Problem 1. Failure to Understand Implications of Diseases

S: TC asks for a shot so she will not become ill during her extended trip around the world.
O: None
A: TC obviously does not understand that she may be exposed to some potentially serious infections and must take the appropriate precautions.
P: TC must be counseled about the likelihood of encountering unsanitary conditions during her travels and the potential for contracting serious infectious diseases such as cholera, typhoid, malaria, and hepatitis. She should be advised on the need for specific immunizations and prophylactic measures, including nondrug interventions such as use of mosquito nets while sleeping, wearing long sleeves and long pants, use of insect repellants, boiling any water that may be contaminated, not eating raw vegetables that have been washed in contaminated water, and not eating foods that may not have been adequately refrigerated. TC may want to take an antibiotic for prophylaxis against traveler's diarrhea. In addition, the Centers for Disease Control (CDC) must be contacted about immunization requirements for specific countries included in her itinerary.

Problem 2. Potential for Hepatitis A, Hepatitis B, Cholera, and Typhoid Infections

S: TC requires preexposure prophylaxis to hepatitis A or possibly vaccination against hepatitis A, vaccination against hepatitis B, and typhoid vaccination.
O: None
A: Ideally, the CDC should be contacted about endemic diseases in specific countries. The CDC can also provide information about the risk for hepatitis A and B. The WHO no longer recommends cholera vaccination, and no country currently requires evidence of cholera vaccination prior to entry.
P: To prevent hepatitis B, TC should be vaccinated with a recombinant hepatitis B vaccine. Ideally, the series of three immunizations will be initiated 6 1/2 months prior to departure to allow 2 weeks between the hepatitis B vaccination and administration of IGIM for hepatitis A prophylaxis. After the initial 1-ml immunization, the second and third immunizations should be administered 1 and 6 months later.

As a hepatitis A prophylactic measure, TC should receive IGIM 0.02 ml/kg i.m. immediately prior to travel but 2 weeks after the final immunization for hepatitis B and typhoid fever.

Typhoid is spread by contaminated food and water, and typhoid immunization results in immunity in up to 90% of individuals. An orally administered vaccine is as effective as the parenteral products. TC should take one capsule every other day for four doses. TC should be advised to avoid taking antibiotics during the time she is taking the oral typhoid vaccine.

Problem 3. Exposure to Chloroquine-resistant Malaria

S: TC will be exposed to chloroquine-resistant malaria.

O: None

A: TC will require chemoprophylaxis for chloroquine-resistant malaria. TC is postmenopausal, so there are no concerns about potential teratogens. Travel to areas with chloroquine resistance places a person at high risk for development of malaria. Sulfadoxine will be prescribed in the event of an acute febrile illness; therefore, a history of hypersensitivity to sulfonamides should be elicited.

P: Malaria can be caused by any one of four different *Plasmodium* organisms that are transmitted to humans by the Anopheles mosquito. Symptoms of malaria may not occur until months after exposure to the organisms, so it is important to be compliant with the medication used for prophylaxis. If TC will be exposed only to organisms that are not resistant to chloroquine, this is the medication of choice. The dose of chloroquine is 300 mg (base), and therapy should begin 1 week before she plans to arrive in the area and should continue with weekly doses until she has been away from the area for 4 to 6 weeks. In addition, one dose (3 tablets) of pyrimethamine-sulfadoxine should be prescribed in case TC experiences an acute febrile illness in an area that does not have adequate medical care available. A negative history of hypersensitivity to sulfonamides should be elicited.

If TC is going to an area where there is known resistance, mefloquine (228 mg base) should be administered 1 week before she plans to arrive in the area and should continue with weekly doses until she has been away from the area for 4–6 weeks. TC is not taking any β-blockers or calcium-channel blockers, which are known to interact with mefloquine.

Adverse effects with chloroquine and mefloquine include gastrointestinal disturbances and dizziness. Stevens-Johnson syndrome has been associated with pyrimethamine-sulfadoxine, and any rash noted after taking this medication should be reported to a physician.

Problem 4. Difficulty in Obtaining Prescription and OTC Medications

S: TC will be away from the United States for 3 months.

O: None

A: TC's prescription medication may be provided in 1-month supplies, and there is the potential for running out of necessary medications.

P: TC should be advised about the need for continuing the prescription medication and consulting with the prescriber so the appropriate measures can be taken to allow for purchase of sufficient prescription and OTC medications prior to departure.

QUESTIONS FOR CASE 132

1. What is the risk for transmission of HIV with hepatitis B immunization?
2. What potential problems should TC be counseled about if a sulfa-containing medication is prescribed?
3. Why should TC not take antibiotics at the same time she is taking the oral typhoid vaccine?
4. What is the risk of HIV transmission with IgG?
5. TC is going to travel for 3 months. Will the IgG last for 3 months?

CASE 133

CC: JS is a 60-year-old man with chronic obstructive pulmonary disease (COPD) and a history of heavy alcohol use who presents to the emergency room with fevers, severe right-sided chest pain, increasing shortness of breath (SOB), and an increased heart rate.

Medical History

JS has a long history of COPD, which strongly correlates with his smoking history of 25 years. JS carries two inhalers, metaproterenol and ipratropium, and uses them when he becomes short of breath. JS had not been admitted to the hospital for a COPD exacerbation since 1994, but subsequent to his last COPD hospitalization 2 months ago, JS has been taking prednisone 30 mg po every day. He admits that it upsets his stomach so he "misses a few doses here and there." JS's alcohol problem has been complicated by several alcohol withdrawal seizures, the most recent occurring 2 years ago. JS currently takes phenytoin for seizure prophylaxis. Because of the seizure episodes, JS enrolled in Alcoholics Anonymous and has not had a drink for more than 1 year. Approximately 3 years ago, JS was diagnosed with degenerative joint disease (DJD) for which he takes acetaminophen with no complaints. JS presents to the ER today after 2 days of increasing malaise, SOB, spiking fevers, chest pain, rigors, and tachycardia.

Medication History

Phenytoin 400 mg po HS
Ipratropium inhaler 2–4 puffs when needed
Metaproterenol inhaler 2–4 puffs when needed
Prednisone 30 mg po QD
Acetaminophen 650 mg po TID

Allergies

Ampicillin (rash)

Physical Examination

GEN: Diaphoretic, agitated, weak-looking man with obvious SOB
VS: BP 140/90, RR 28, HR 125, T 39.5°C, Wt 65 kg
HEENT: Purulent, rust-colored sputum × 2 days
COR: Nl S_1, S_2; no murmurs
CHEST: Prolonged expiratory phase, bilateral rales and rhonchi, RLL dullness

ABD: Gastric pain
RECT: Guaiac-positive stools
GU: WNL
NEURO: Oriented × 3, appropriate affect, lethargic

Results of Laboratory Tests

Na 145 (145)   Hct .49 (49)   AST 0.67 (40)
K 3.7 (3.7)   Hgb 180 (18)   ALT 0.53 (32)
Cl 101 (101)   Lkcs 18.6 × 10⁹ (18.6 × 10³)   Alb 42 (4.2)
HCO₃ 33 (33)   Plts 300 × 10⁹ (300 × 10³)   Phenytoin 80 (20)
BUN 59 (21)
CR 106.1 (1.2)

Lkc differential: PMN 0.88 (88%), Bands 0.10 (10%),
  Lymphs 0.02 (2%)
ABG (on room air): PO_2 70, PCO_2 47, pH 7.35
PFTs: FEV_1-60% (pre-β_2-agonist), FEV_1/FCV-70%
  (post-β_2-agonist)
Sputum Gram's stain: >50 Lkcs/HPF; 0-5 epithelium
  cells/HPF; gram-positive cocci in pairs (many)
Blood cultures: Pending
Chest x-ray: RLL consolidation consistent with right
  lower lobe pneumonia

PROBLEM LIST

1. COPD
2. Alcohol abuse
3. Seizure disorder
4. Degenerative joint disease
5. Steroid side effects
6. Pneumococcal pneumonia

CASE 133 SOAP NOTES
Problem 6. Pneumococcal Pneumonia

S: JS presents to the ER with a 2-day history of fever, chest
pain, chills, and increased purulent rust-colored sputum
production. JS also complains of increased shortness of
breath and malaise and lethargy.

O: Chest x-ray shows consolidation and he has poor ABGs. JS
also has an elevated Lkc with left shift and bands present.
His temperature is elevated to 39.5°C and HR and RR are
above normal. The Gram's stain of the sputum suggests
Streptococcus pneumoniae, and blood culture results are
pending.

A: JS appears to have pneumonia, and based on the initial
Gram's stain, the likely organism is S. pneumoniae. Empiric therapy must be initiated immediately, and JS should
be admitted to the hospital. The antibiotic selected should
cover S. *pneumoniae* empirically, but it may need to be
changed after definitive culture results are available. Pneumococcal pneumonia is common in patients with underlying risk factors such as COPD, cardiovascular disease, diabetes mellitus, and chronic alcoholism, and in splenec-
tomized patients. JS has two risk factors (COPD and alcoholism) that predispose him to this infection. His chest x-
ray is also consistent with pneumonia (lobal consolidation), and his Lkcs have a predominance of PMNs with
bands present. This shift to the left is a sign of an ongoing

infection. Penicillin G is the drug of choice for pneumococcal infections. In adults, 600,000 units of procaine penicillin G intramuscularly every 12 hr is effective therapy. JS
has a mild allergy to ampicillin (GI upset), but this "allergy" does not preclude the use of penicillin. If JS had
had a mild allergy to ampicillin such as a maculopapular
rash without urticaria or shortness of breath, a cephalosporin could be used instead of penicillin. Penicillins have
an 8%–15% cross-sensitivity pattern with cephalosporins.
Given JS's allergy history, penicillin is still the drug of
choice and should be initiated empirically.

P: Begin procaine penicillin G 600,000 units i.m. every 12 hr.
Therapy should be continued for 10 days. If JS responds
to parenteral penicillin therapy, oral penicillin may replace
the parenteral therapy after approximately 5–7 days. JS
could complete his 10-day antibiotic course with penicillin
V 250 mg po every 6 hr. JS will require monitoring of
his temperature, Lkcs, chest x-ray, and sputum and blood
cultures. After the culture results are final, sensitivities must
be checked to ensure that the correct antibiotic choice
was made.

Problem 1. COPD Exacerbation

S: JS complains of increasing shortness of breath, dyspnea,
and lethargy.

O: JS has a slightly elevated PCO_2, a slightly decreased PO_2,
mild respiratory acidosis, decreased FEV_1, and an FEV_1/
FCV ratio <0.8.

A: JS is experiencing an exacerbation of his COPD secondary
to his acute respiratory infection. Although it is difficult
to discern whether a patient with COPD has chronic bronchitis or emphysema, an attempt should be made to characterize the disease. Chronic bronchitis ("blue bloater")
patients have a chronic cough and heavy sputum production, are commonly overweight, have altered ABGs, and
have frequent exacerbations of their disease. Conversely,
emphysema patients ("pink puffers") typically have increasing dyspnea, have lost weight, and have an extensive
smoking history. Additionally, patients with emphysema do
not have marked sputum production or cough. JS recently
began to produce sputum (2 days ago), and his ABGs are
close to normal. Based on these findings, it appears that
JS may be characterized as having emphysema. His current
respiratory compromise is probably secondary to his infectious process. The immediate goal of therapy for JS is to
correct air flow obstruction and to improve his functional
status. After the acute episode is treated, subsequent goals
include (1) optimizing drug therapy, (2) preventing or
minimizing future disease exacerbations, (3) altering environmental influences such as smoking, and (4) improving
his nutritional status. Nebulized or metered-dose inhaled
metaproterenol every 4 hr should be initiated. Additionally, although controversial, parenteral or oral corticosteroids can be given. Patients with severe airway obstruction
seem to respond better to steroids than do more stable
patients. Overall, 15%–25% of patients with severe COPD
will show improvement in FEV_1 with corticosteroids. The
use of anticholinergics may be beneficial, especially during

the acute exacerbation. JS has been using ipratroprium at home, and this should be continued. Combination therapy of ipratroprium and β-agonists produces greater increases in FEV_1 than either agent used alone. JS must learn the proper use of inhalers before discharge from the hospital. Finally, because patients with emphysema experience weight loss secondary to poor nutrition, his nutritional status should be evaluated.

P: 1. Begin methylprednisolone 60 mg IV every 6 hr with a rapid taper down to oral prednisone 30 mg po QD within 3 days. JS is experiencing steroid side effects from his chronic steroid use, so the need for the continuation of this therapy should be reevaluated after the acute exacerbation resolves. Inhaled steroids should be considered if it is felt that JS responds to this treatment.

2. Begin nebulized metaproterenol 0.3 ml of a 5% solution diluted in 2.5 ml of normal saline every 4 hr. Continue ipratroprium inhalations 2 puffs four times a day. Monitor arterial blood gas levels, chest examination, heart rate, respiration rate, and breathing patterns to assess efficacy of treatment. JS has been using his metaproterenol inhaler p.r.n. but probably would benefit from a regimen change to scheduled inhalations plus p.r.n. use. JS also uses his ipratroprium on a p.r.n. basis, which is not effective and should also be changed to a scheduled administration regimen.

3. Begin maintenance fluids (D5W1/2NS at 75–100 ml/hr) to ensure that JS is adequately hydrated. A nutritional consultation should be sought before discharge.

4. Because drug therapy is sometimes ineffective in the treatment of emphysema, patients need education about the negative impact that smoking has on their disease. Cessation of smoking will not recover lost lung function, but it may decrease the rate of further lung damage. Because JS's condition is not terminal, he should be advised to stop smoking immediately.

Problems 2 and 3. Alcohol Abuse and Seizure Disorder

S: JS has a long history of alcohol use with subsequent withdrawal seizures.

O: History. His last documented seizure was 2 years ago.

A: JS has been attending Alcoholics Anonymous meetings and has been sober for approximately 1 year. JS is still taking phenytoin prophylactically. His most recent phenytoin level was 80 (20). JS has no evidence of gingival hyperplasia, nystagmus, drowsiness, diplopia, rash, or ataxia. Phenytoin is not used to treat alcohol withdrawal seizures unless there are focal neurologic deficits, head trauma, or an underlying chronic seizure disorder. Some clinicians prescribe phenytoin prophylactically, as is the case with JS. If JS continues to abstain from drinking, his phenytoin therapy could also be discontinued. Discontinuation of therapy is sometimes advantageous for psychologic and financial reasons. Discontinuation of anticonvulsants should be attempted slowly (over 2–3 months) in patients with an underlying seizure disorder to avoid precipitating an episode.

JS's phenytoin should be tapered over 1 month because his seizures were secondary to alcohol withdrawal.

P: Continue to monitor JS for adverse reactions to phenytoin and consider discontinuation of therapy.

Problem 4. Degenerative Joint Disease

S: None

O: None

A: Drug therapy of degenerative joint disease (DJD) should be aimed at relieving the symptoms. The exact etiology of the ailment is not known. Intermittent inflammation contributes to the pain of DJD, so nonsteroidal antiinflammatory drugs (NSAIDs) may provide an antiinflammatory effect. Acetaminophen controls the pain in many cases and does not subject the patient to the undesirable side effects of NSAID therapy. Systemic glucocorticosteroids are rarely indicated, but intra-articular injections may provide symptomatic relief; however, steroids should always be used judiciously.

P: Maintain current therapy with acetaminophen. JS has no active symptoms at this time. JS must have his liver function test results monitored for baseline comparison purposes. JS should be questioned about his acetaminophen intake. If his analgesic requirement is increasing (greater than 3–4 g per day), his treatment plan must be reevaluated.

Problem 5. Steroid Side Effects

S: JS reported gastric pain during his physical examination.

O: JS has subjective findings and guaiac-positive stools.

A: Chronic steroid therapy is often associated with a myriad of adverse effects, one of which is gastric ulceration (see chapter 16). JS has been taking prednisone for approximately 2 months and admits that he is not always compliant with the therapy. Patients should not be placed on chronic steroid therapy unless they have severe disease. From JS's medical history, it appears that steroid therapy should not have been initiated at that time. Now JS is experiencing gastric pain and guaiac-positive stools. His hematocrit and hemoglobin levels are stable, so his GI ulceration is probably minimal and should resolve on removal of the steroid or changing to every-other-day administration. There is no need to initiate H_2-antagonist therapy at this time, although antacid therapy may alleviate JS's gastric pain. After a rapid taper from parenteral steroid, JS should begin to taper off prednisone completely, because the drug is not indicated and it is causing an adverse reaction in this patient.

P: Begin taper after acute exacerbation resolves and JS is taking po prednisone. An example of a taper is as follows:

Prednisone 30 mg po QD × 5 days
Prednisone 20 mg po QD × 5 days
Prednisone 10 mg po QD × 5 days
Stop prednisone

JS was not compliant with his prednisone regimen to begin with, so the taper can be achieved over 15 days. Because we do not know exactly how much of the prednisone JS was taking PTA, this taper is conservative. Monitor for signs of adrenal insufficiency such as flu-like symptoms, diaphoresis, and electrolyte abnormalities. Also monitor for an exacerbation of his COPD.

QUESTIONS FOR CASE 133

1. After receiving the first dose of penicillin, JS developed hives and a total body rash and became even more short of breath. Epinephrine was administered. Since JS had an anaphylatic reaction to penicillin, what alternative therapy would you suggest to treat his pneumococcal pneumonia?

2. The medical team wants to begin theophylline therapy in JS. Calculate an appropriate oral loading and maintenance dose. (Remember to consider concurrent drug therapy in your calculations.)

3. Describe the side effects of phenytoin (i.e., which are dose-related and which are non-dose-related).

4. Instruct JS on the proper use of his inhalers.

5. A year has passed since JS's pneumonia hospitalizations. JS now presents to the ER with nausea, vomiting, drowsiness, jaundice, and liver tenderness. A toxicity screen is ordered and JS has an acetaminophen level of 118 µg/ml (taken 13 hr after ingestion). JS admits that he has been taking an increased amount of acetaminophen over the past few months and that today his pain was so bad that "he just wanted to end it all." How would you treat this acetaminophen overdose?

CASE 134

CC: MS is a 42-year-old man who presents to the emergency department with a 2-day history of fever, chills, and abdominal pain. He also has been tired and has not had much of an appetite for weeks.

Medical History

MS was found to have abnormal liver function tests and thrombocytopenia during a routine clinic visit 3 years ago. At that time he was found to be positive for hepatitis C virus. One year later MS had a liver biopsy positive for chronic active hepatitis. MS has had intermittent symptoms of fatigue, right upper quadrant pain, jaundice, weakness, and anorexia during the last 3 years. He has ascites that fluctuate in size. He also has gum bleeding when he brushes his teeth and occasional epistaxis.

MS has a history of posttraumatic seizures since he suffered head trauma in an automobile accident 8 years ago. His seizures are characterized by loss of consciousness, muscle rigidity, and then jerking movements of the extremities, urinary incontinence, and tongue-biting. MS has been taking phenytoin since the first seizure and was averaging one seizure every 4 to 6 months. He has not had a seizure for the past 26 months.

Social History

Denies alcohol or tobacco use.

Medication History

1. Spironolactone 100 mg po QD
2. Furosemide 40 mg po QD
3. Phenytoin 300 mg po QHS

Allergies

No known drug allergies.

Physical Examination

GEN: Tired-looking man in moderate distress

VS: BP 144/84, HR 84, RR 22, T 39°C, Wt 75 kg, Ht 183 cm

HEENT: PERRLA, EOMI, anicteric, + nystagmus on far lateral gaze

COR: No S_3 or S_4, no murmurs

CHEST: Lungs clear to auscultation and percussion

ABD: Increased girth, + hepatosplenomegaly, + fluid wave, + abdominal pain, + diffuse tenderness

RECT: Guaiac-negative

EXT: 2+ edema

NEURO: WNL, no asterixis

Results of Laboratory Tests

Na 136 (136)	Cl 105 (105)	MCV 96 (96)
Hct 0.42 (42)	WBC 12.1 × 10⁹ (12,100)	Alb 35 (3.5)
AST 3.72 (223)	PO₄ 2.4 (0.77)	PT 13.7⁹
Glu 6.4 (115)	HCO₃ 24 (24)	Cr 88.4 (1.0)
K 3.7 (3.7)	Plts 84 × 10₉ (84 × 10₉)	T bili 36 (2.1)
Hgb 120 (12)	Alk Phos 0.48 (29)	INR 1.4
ALT 2.87 (172)	Mg 0.9 (1.8)	PTT 34⁹
Ca 9.3 (9.3)	BUN 5.7 (16)	Anti-HCV +

Phenytoin 49.5 µmol/L (12.5 mg/dL)

Wbc differential: PMNs 82%, bands 9%, lymphocytes 8%

Urinalysis: WNL

Chest x-ray: WNL

EKG: WNL

EEG: WNL

Paracentesis + cloudy ascitic fluid, white cell count 540 cells/m³, Gram's stain positive for gram-negative rods

Ascites bacterial culture pending

Blood cultures: Pending

PROBLEM LIST

1. Spontaneous bacterial peritonitis
2. Chronic active hepatitis
3. Thrombocytopenia
4. Posttraumatic seizure disorder

CASE 134 SOAP NOTES

Problem 1. Spontaneous Bacterial Peritonitis

S: Two-day history of fever, chills, and abdominal pain.

O: Temperature elevated, abdominal pain, diffuse abdominal tenderness, increased white count with left shift, paracentesis with cloudy fluid and high white cell count.

A: MS's presentation is consistent with primary or spontaneous bacterial peritonitis (SBP). It is called "primary" or "spontaneous" peritonitis because there is no evident source for the infection. Patients with ascites are at risk for developing SBP, and MS presented with the classic symptoms (fever, chills, abdominal pain and tenderness, diagnostic paracentesis). Blood cultures were obtained to rule out systemic infection. The gram stain from the paracentesis is positive for gram negative rods, which account for about 70% of SBP infections. Empiric antimicrobial treatment should also cover for gram-positive cocci, especially nonenterococcal streptococci. Enterococci and anaerobes are rarely pathogens in SBP. Empiric antibiotic therapy with an aminoglycoside and ampicillin or a second- or third-generation cephalosporin should be initiated; specific antibiotic therapy can be selected after bacterial culture results are available. Treatment duration is usually 10 to 14 days. Most patients show clinical improvement within 24 to 48 hours, otherwise other medical causes should be investigated. The mortality rate associated with SBP is about 40%, and the reinfection rate at 1 year is approximately 70%.

P: Start empiric antibiotic treatment with ceftizoxime 1 g intravenously every eight hours. Monitor signs and symptoms for clinical improvement, laboratory findings, ascites, and blood cultures, and for adverse effects of ceftizoxime (rash, hypersensitivity reactions, nausea, diarrhea).

Problem 2. Chronic Active Hepatitis

S: History of chronic active hepatitis and intermittent symptoms of fatigue, RUQ pain, jaundice, weakness, and anorexia, ascites, and bleeding.

O: Positive evidence on liver biopsy, anti-HCV +, elevated AST and ALT, hypoalbuminemia, elevated PT/INR, increased girth, hepatosplenomegaly, and fluid wave.

A: MS has been diagnosed with chronic active hepatitis, presumably triggered by hepatitis C. Liver biopsy is required to establish a diagnosis of chronic active hepatitis. It is unlikely that phenytoin caused GN's hepatitis. Hepatitis secondary to phenytoin is an idiosyncratic adverse effect that usually occurs within the first 8 weeks of treatment and presents with fever, rash, and lymphadenopathy. MS started phenytoin 8 years ago without incident. The clinical spectrum of the chronic active hepatitis ranges from asymptomatic illness to fatal hepatic failure, and the course is variable. MS has signs and symptoms of the disease plus complications from cirrhosis (ascites, spontaneous bacterial peritonitis, hepatosplenomegaly, thrombocytopenia). When chronic active hepatitis is not caused by hepatitis B virus or non-A, non-B viruses, glucocorticoids are the therapy of choice. However, in chronic active hepatitis that is caused by non-A, non-B hepatitis virus, long-term glucocorticoid therapy is not beneficial and may be detrimental. Generally, supportive care is the therapy of choice. One therapeutic modality that shows promise is interferon alfa,

which has had some success at reducing liver enzyme levels and improving hepatic histology.

P: Continue supportive treatment of complications. Consider interferon alfa treatment if current exacerbation of chronic active hepatitis does not resolve.

Problem 3. Thrombocytopenia

S: Gum bleeding, epistaxis.

O: Platelet count is 84×10^9/L, hepatosplenomegaly.

A: Thrombocytopenia is probably the result of hypersplenism secondary to liver disease. The spleen normally stores about one third of the circulating platelets and removes nonfunctional platelets, but when the spleen is enlarged, it can sequester and destroy up to 80% of the circulating thrombocytes, causing thrombocytopenia. Clinical manifestations such as bleeding generally do not occur until the platelet count is less than 50×10^9/L, and severe spontaneous bleeding not until the platelet count is less than 20×10^9/L. Trauma, intramuscular injections, rectal examinations, suppositories, enemas, and medications that affect platelet function should be avoided to minimize the risk of bleeding.

P: Monitor bleeding and platelet count and transfuse platelets if MS starts to hemorrhage or the platelet count falls below about 25×10^9/L. Avoid trauma, intramuscular injections, rectal examinations, suppositories, enemas, aspirin, nonsteroidal antiinflammatory drugs.

Problem 4. Posttraumatic Seizure Disorder

S: History of posttraumatic generalized tonic-clonic (GTC) seizures, characterized by loss of consciousness, tonic-clonic movements, urinary incontinence, and tongue-biting. MS has not had a seizure for 26 months.

O: Phenytoin serum level is 49.5 μmol/L (12.5 mg/dL). The therapeutic range of phenytoin is 40–80 μmol/L (10–20 mg/dL). EEG normal.

A: MS's posttraumatic GTC seizures are presently well controlled by phenytoin with no seizures in 26 months. He is tolerating the medication without reports of ataxia, diplopia, dizziness, drowsiness, gingival hyperplasia, or peripheral neuropathy. MS has nystagmus, which is a dose-related adverse effect that may occur at therapeutic serum levels and does not require a reduction in dose. Phenytoin is primarily eliminated by hepatic metabolism, therefore MS's liver disease warrants more frequent monitoring for adverse effects.

P: Continue phenytoin 300 mg orally at bedtime. Continue to monitor seizure character and frequency, and for adverse effects.

QUESTIONS FOR CASE 134

1. Is MS a candidate for withdrawal of anticonvulsant drug therapy?
2. What type of patient education should MS receive regarding his thrombocytopenia?
3. How is hepatitis C transmitted?

4. In 6 months, MS presents to clinic with mental status changes, drowsiness, and asterixis. How would you treat his hepatic encephalopathy?

5. Which laboratory tests are the most reliable for evaluating the "function" of the liver?

CASE 135

CC: MG is a 24-year-old woman who presents to the hospital with progressive weakness, poor appetite, fevers, shaking chills, diarrhea, and abdominal cramps.

History of Present Illness

MG has a long history of intravenous heroin abuse and prostitution. She has had a 20-pound weight loss, debilitation, and low-grade fevers over the last month. Her last use of IV heroin was the morning prior to admission. The cramping, diarrhea, and shaking chills began the morning of admission, when her mother brought her to the emergency room.

Medical History

MG has a history of multiple urinary tract infections, the last one occurring 2 months prior to admission.

Medication History

Trimethoprim/sulfamethoxazole DS once daily for 3 days, 1 month PTA; history of poor compliance

Allergies

No known drug allergies

Social History

Tobacco: 1.5 packs/day
Alcohol: 6 beers daily (none for 2 weeks)
HIV risk factors: prostitution and IVDA

Review of Systems

Noncontributory

Physical Examination

GEN: Pale, ill-appearing, cachectic, and combative woman in distress
VS: BP 120/70, HR 90, RR 15, T 38.5°C, Wt 45 kg, Ht 160 cm
HEENT: Oral mucous membranes appear without exudate or erythema; she exhibits excessive rhinorrhea and sialorrhea, PERRLA.
COR: III/VI systolic ejection murmur lower sternal border
CHEST: Clear to ascultation and percussion
ABD: Soft, moderately tender, positive bowel sounds, no hepatosplenomegaly

GU: WNL
RECT: Guaiac-negative
EXT: Severe sclerosis of visible veins in arms and legs, distal muscle wasting of right leg; splinter hemorrhages seen on finger tips.
NEURO: Right-sided weakness, oriented to person, normal deep-tendon reflexes, cranial nerves intact

Results of Laboratory Tests

Na 130 (130)	Hct 0.35 (35)	AST 0.18 (11)	Glu 5.2 (94)
K 4.5 (4.5)	Hgb 100 (10)	ALT 0.22 (13)	Ca 1.77 (7.1)
Cl 97 (97)	Lkcs 18.4 × 10^9 (18.4 × 10^3)	LDH 1.42 (85)	PO$_4$ 1.03 (3.2)
HCO$_3$ 20 (20)	Plts 200 × 10^9 (200 × 10^3)	Alk Phos 0.92 (55)	Mg .95 (1.9)
BUN 17.8 (50)	MCV 90 (90)	Alb 30 (3)	Uric Acid 416 (7)
CR 106 (1.2)		T Bili 17 (1)	ESR 60

Urinalysis: Cloudy, gram-positive cocci in clusters, pH 7, specific gravity 1.020, RBC 0, Lkcs 0

Chest x-ray: Negative

HIV: Negative (completed 1 month prior to admission)

Blood culture: Pending

PROBLEM LIST

1. Endocarditis
2. Heroin withdrawal

CASE 135 SOAP NOTES
Problem 1. Endocarditis

S: MG complains of weakness, anorexia, and low-grade fevers for 1 month prior to admission.

O: The physical examination reveals a murmur, fever, tachycardia, and splinter hemorrhages. Her laboratory results are consistent with an infection: a high sedimentation rate and an elevated white blood cell count with a shift to the left.

A: Probable infective endocarditis. Most likely cause is *Staphylococcus aureus* given his long history of IV drug abuse. Further evidence for *S. aureus* as the causative organism is the presence of gram-positive cocci in clusters in his urine. Seeding of the kidneys is commonly found as a consequence of *S. aureus* bacteremia. Other possible organisms include *Pseudomonas aeruginosa*, other enteric gram-negative bacilli and occasionally, *Candida* species.

The location of the murmur and the history are consistent with tricuspid valve involvement, but this should be confirmed with echocardiography, preferably transesophageal. Empiric therapy should be started to cover *S. aureus* and gram-negative bacilli. Usual regimens include a penicillinase-resistant penicillin (oxacillin or nafcillin) usually given for a total of 4–6 weeks, plus gentamicin for a brief course at the onset. Since her case appears uncomplicated, she may be a candidate for short-course or oral therapy or both. Consider the addition of rifampin, if response is not seen within the first week. One exception to the standard regimen is avoidance of aminoglycoside in a patient at high risk for developing toxicity (elderly, preexisting renal insufficiency) and therefore, a broad-spectrum β-lactam should be used for coverage of gram-negative bacilli. The addition of an aminoglycoside for synergy with the penicillin for a brief period at the beginning of the therapy is generally recommended for more rapid clearance of the bacteremia and is unlikely to result in significant renal toxicity. The second exception is to use vancomycin rather than a penicillin only if there is known to be a high prevalence of methicillin-resistant staphylococci in the community or in the drug-abusing population. Vancomycin is necessary if the organisms cultured are methicillin-resistant.

Tricuspid valve excision with or without replacement is effective and appropriate for signs of valve failure or failure to respond or both despite adequate therapy.

P: Transesophageal echocardiogram for detection of valvular vegetations should be performed. Nafcillin or oxacillin 2 gm q6h (200 mg/kg/day) plus gentamicin 60 mg IV q12h should be initiated. Monitor vital signs, blood cultures, susceptibility tests, ESR, urinalysis, renal function, complete blood counts, pulmonary function tests, chest examination for possible pulmonary embolism, signs and symptoms of drug allergy (e.g., rash, interstitial nephritis).

Problem 2. Heroin Withdrawal

S: MG complains of shaking chills, abdominal cramps, and diarrhea.

O: MG is combative, with significant sialorrhea and rhinorrhea. Her last dose of heroin was 24 hr prior to admission, with symptoms occurring 16 hr after her last injection. On physical examination, she is tachycardic and exhibits abdominal tenderness.

A: MG is experiencing heroin withdrawal. Her symptoms and the timing of the last heroin dose are consistent with this diagnosis. Excessive shaking, sweating, abdominal cramping, and diarrhea are some hallmark symptoms. These symptoms should subside within 5–10 days of abstinence, without treatment. Generally these symptoms are self-limiting and non-life-threatening; however, cardiovascular collapse has occurred in rare cases. Clonidine has been used with some success in lessening the symptoms of opiate withdrawal.

P: Begin clonidine tablets 0.4 mg BID for 2 days. Then apply 2 clonidine-2 transdermal patches. The patches should be replaced once, for a total of 14 days. Monitor MG's echocardiogram for arrhythmias. Administer alprazolam 0.5 mg when needed for anxiety and combativeness and diphenhydramine 50 mg for insomnia. Administer belladonna alkaloids with phenobarbital 4–8 tablets daily for suppression of diarrhea and abdominal cramping. The anticholinergic effects will also help alleviate the excessive rhinorrhea and sialorrhea. Prochlorperazine 25-mg suppository or 10 mg IV may be given if vomiting occurs. Will taper the above medications over 2 weeks, and encourage patient to join a drug abuse program.

QUESTIONS FOR CASE 135

1. What is the pathogenesis of endocarditis in intravenous drug abusers and why are they more likely to have tricuspid valve involvement?
2. What are splinter hemorrhages and the other lesions associated with endocarditis? Why do they occur?
3. What if the transthoracic echocardiogram results are negative? Are there other more specific tests that may be used? If so, which ones? If not, is endocarditis automatically ruled out?
4. What organism(s) is or are most likely to produce endocarditis in the intravenous drug abuser, and why?
5. What alternative antibiotic(s) might be used if MG were to develop a sensitivity to penicillin?

CASE 136

CC: FT is a 59-year-old man on a 14-day vacation cruise who comes to the ship's infirmary complaining of 3 days of diarrhea, abdominal cramps, headache, and malaise. He has been feeling feverish for about 24 hr. The diarrhea, which looked clear at the start, began to get bloody and more voluminous.

Medical History

FT has a 9-year history of angina and coronary artery disease, for which he has undergone two coronary artery bypass surgeries, the last being performed 6 months ago. Since becoming ill on the cruise, he has been experiencing frequent episodes of chest tightness and shortness of breath with exercise, despite using the new medication the doctor gave him for this problem.

He has a history of congestive heart failure (CHF), first diagnosed 4 years ago after he experienced shortness of breath, dyspnea on exertion, and needing two pillows at night to breathe while sleeping.

Social History

Tobacco: 1 pack per day since age 17, none in past year
Alcohol: Social drinking only
Coffee: 8 cups per day
Occupation: Vice president of a marketing firm

Medication History

Digoxin 0.25 mg po QD
Dipyridamole 75 mg po TID
Aspirin 325 mg po TID
Furosemide 40 mg po BID
Verapamil 80 mg po TID (started 1 week ago)
Isosorbide 10 mg po q8h
Nitroglycerin 0.4 mg s.l. p.r.n.
Ibuprofen 200 mg po p.r.n. (takes for headaches or pain)

Physical Examination

GEN: Well-developed, well-nourished man in mild distress

VS: BP 150/85, HR 100, RR 24, T 38.6°C, Wt 95 kg (97 kg before the cruise)

HEENT: Dry mucous membranes, mild jugular venous distention

COR: Normal S_1, S_2, presence of an S_3 gallop

ABD: Soft, nontender, positive hepatojugular reflux

EXT: 1+ ankle edema, nicotine stains on fingers

Results of Laboratory Tests

Na 129 (129)   Ca 2.5 (10)
K 2.9 (2.9)
Cl 95 (95)
HCO₃ 18 (18)
BUN 10.7 (30)
CR 124 (1.4)

Fecal Lkcs: Positive

Stool culture: Comma-shaped gram-negative rods identified as *Campylobacter jejuni*

PROBLEM LIST

1. Angina
2. CHF
3. Diarrhea

CASE 136 SOAP NOTES
Problem 3. Diarrhea

S: Three-day history of diarrhea, headache, malaise, and abdominal cramps; feverish feeling for 1 day

O: Elevated temperature at 38.6°C; isolation of *Campylobacter jejuni* from stool sample; low sodium, potassium, and bicarbonate levels; dry mucous membranes; positive fecal Lkcs.

A: FT is suffering from *Campylobacter* gastroenteritis, which is ruining his vacation. Management of the gastroenteritis is necessary to prevent dehydration and electrolyte disturbances. He currently shows some signs of hypovolemia and electrolyte disturbances such as hyponatremia, hypokalemia, low bicarbonate level, tachycardia, and an increased BUN-to-CR ratio. The hypokalemia may cause an increased risk of digoxin toxicity. Erythromycin is considered the drug of choice for this infection. It is indicated for FT, because he is showing signs of significant infection such as bloody diarrhea and hypovolemia. The addition of erythromycin to FT's drug regimen may result in increased bioavailability and serum levels of digoxin. This may be of little clinical significance though; treatment with erythromycin will last for only 5 days. His diarrhea may be controlled by using a bulk-forming agent such as kaolin-pectin or attapulgite. Antiperistaltic agents such as loperamide or diphenoxylate with atropine may be of some use also, but the use of atropine in FT should be discouraged because the anticholinergic effects may worsen his angina by causing tachycardia. He will need to supplement his fluid and electrolyte intake to help replace what has been lost.

P: Begin erythromycin 250 mg po QID for 5 days. Add attapulgite 1200 mg po after each loose stool. Monitor frequency and consistency of stools, blood pressure and heart rate, symptoms such as headache and malaise, temperature, and serum sodium, potassium, and bicarbonate levels. FT should be advised to replace GI fluid losses with the oral rehydration solution recommended by the World Health Organization or equivalent solutions. When the diarrhea abates, he should revert to his sodium-restricted diet for CHF. He should be cautious about drinking water or milk on the cruise and eat only well-cooked poultry. In addition, he should be advised to separate his attapulgite from his other medications, especially digoxin.

Problem 2. CHF

S: Presence of two-pillow orthopnea, dyspnea on exertion, shortness of breath

O: S_3 gallop, mild hepatojugular reflux, mild jugular venous distention, 1+ ankle edema

A: FT is mildly symptomatic of both right- and left-sided CHF. The verapamil may be contributing to the CHF by causing a decrease in myocardial contractility, and it should be discontinued. Discontinuation of the verapamil may cause a sudden decrease in serum digoxin levels, because its coadministration with digoxin results in a decreased volume of distribution and clearance. Ibuprofen should be avoided because it may cause sodium and water retention, thereby increasing intravascular volume and cardiac workload. FT may have been experiencing tachyphylaxis to the isosorbide. The preload reducer isosorbide should be taken TID and not every 8 hr, so that there is a nitrate-free interval. Adequate preload reduction is necessary, because he is showing congestive symptoms. If the discontinuation of verapamil and ibuprofen does not result in symptomatic improvement, an afterload reducer may be warranted. Hydralazine may cause a reflex tachycardia and worsen his angina, so it would not be the first choice. An angiotension converting enzyme (ACE) inhibitor such as captopril will reduce both preload and afterload. It would not be wise to start captopril at this time because FT has a low serum sodium level, indicating a very high renin state, and the administration of captopril under these conditions could result in a precipitous fall in blood pressure.

P: Discontinue verapamil and ibuprofen. Check FT's digoxin level. Hold furosemide until FT is rehydrated. Increase isosorbide to 20 mg po TID. Monitor digoxin levels, serum sodium and potassium levels, blood pressure and heart rate, and the patient's symptoms. When FT's serum sodium level is greater than 130 mmol/liter (130 mEq/liter), start captopril 6.25 mg po TID. FT should be counseled on nondrug treatments for CHF, such as a low-sodium diet and adequate bed rest. The use of nonsteroidal antiinflammatory drugs (NSAIDs) for pain relief should be avoided, and acetaminophen used instead. FT should be advised to take captopril on an empty stomach to optimize bioavailability.

Problem 1. Angina

S: FT complains of chest tightness with exercise.

O: History of coronary artery disease for which he has had two coronary artery bypass grafts

A: FT has serious coronary artery disease, as evidenced by his need for bypass surgeries. His risk factors for CAD include being male, smoking, obesity, and being middle-aged. He is currently experiencing some chest tightness with exercise. His diarrhea may be causing the tachycardia that could be contributing to an increase in myocardial oxygen demand and causing his chest tightness. Other contributing factors may include tachyphylaxis to the isosorbide (as discussed in the previous problem), excessive caffeine intake, and stress from his job. Increasing the isosorbide for CHF may help prevent his chest tightness. The dipyridamole and aspirin may be useful for maintaining graft patency and should be continued.

P: Continue dipyridamole, aspirin, and sublingual nitroglycerin at current doses. Change his isosorbide regimen as in CHF section. Check cholesterol levels. Monitor frequency of anginal episodes. Counsel FT on a low-cholesterol diet, suggest relaxation techniques, and suggest that he find help to quit smoking and lose weight. He should be informed about proper storage and use of nitroglycerin.

QUESTIONS FOR CASE 136

1. If FT does not tolerate erythromycin, what alternatives are there for treating *Campylobacter* infection?
2. What questions should a health care provider ask a patient who complains of diarrhea?
3. FT asks you to recommend an OTC agent for his heartburn. He points to Maalox, Tums, Mylanta, and Alka-Seltzer. Which would you recommend or not recommend and why?
4. Are any of FT's medications photosensitizing, putting him at risk for severe sunburn?
5. What factors predispose a patient to digoxin toxicity?

CASE 137
CC: RC is a 24-year-old woman who comes to the city health clinic with a chief complaint of itching and redness around the pelvic and thigh area.

Medical History

RC is a 24-year-old prostitute well known to the clinic, where she has been treated for multiple sexually transmitted diseases. Most recently, she was treated for primary syphilis (12 months ago). She now has progressing itching and redness around the pelvic area. She states that the symptoms worsen at night. Currently, she has no other complaints. RC was diagnosed with alcoholic cirrhosis 1 year ago, secondary to heavy alcohol use since age 16. Her disease is mild and has not progressed. RC denies any recent weight gain, edema, or abdominal girth enlargement. RC uses heroin on a daily basis. Her current habit is $75.00/day (approximately 90 mg heroin). She has attempted rehabilitation for her drug abuse problem several times, without success. RC was last seen in the clinic 12 months ago, at which time she had an HIV antibody test performed. RC is noncompliant and does not take her spironolactone.

Social History
Intravenous drug user (heroin 90 mg/day)
Alcohol (1 pint vodka/day)
Smoker (1 ppd × 10 years)

Medication History
Spironolactone 25 mg po BID

Allergies
None known

Physical Examination
GEN: Pale, cachectic ill-appearing woman, in no apparent distress
VS: BP 104/70, HR 105, RR 13, T 37.5°C, Wt 55 kg (0.5 kg water gain), IBW 65 kg
HEENT: Pinpoint pupils, drooping eyelids
COR: S_1, S_2, no S_3, no murmurs
CHEST: Clear to auscultation
ABD: Slight ascites with a mild fluid wave, no pitting edema
GU: Unremarkable, except for small areas of erythema on pelvic area
EXT: Several areas of induration and needle punctures along arms
NEURO: Slightly lethargic, but O × 3

Results of Laboratory Tests

Na 131 (131)	Hct 0.28 (28)	AST 0.98 (59)	Glu 6.1 (110)	Fe 7.2 (40)
K 4.3 (4.3)	Hgb 80 (8)	ALT 0.77 (46)	Ca 2.2 (8.8)	Folate 2.3 (1.0)
Cl 108 (108)	Lkcs 4.5 × 10⁹ (4.5 × 10³)	Alb 32 (3.2)	PO₄ 0.81 (2.5)	B₁₂ 221 (300)
HCO₃ 26 (26)	Plts 125 × 10⁹ (125 × 10³)		Mg 0.85 (1.7)	CD₄ 723 (723)
BUN 3.6 (10)	MCV 76 (76)		PT 12.7	
CR 70.7 (0.8)	Retic .008 (8)		INR 1.1	

Urine electrolytes: Na 40 (40), K 20 (20)
Serology: VDRL: 1:64 (last VDRL titer-posttreatment: 1:4)
HIV-antibody: Positive
Pregnancy test: Negative

PROBLEM LIST
1. Alcohol abuse
2. Alcoholic cirrhosis
3. Heroin abuse
4. Syphilis
5. *Pthirus pubis* (crab louse)
6. HIV infection
7. Mixed anemia

CASE 137 SOAP NOTES
Problem 4. Syphilis
S: None
O: RC has an elevated VDRL titer.
A: Syphilis is an infection caused by the spirochete *Treponema pallidum*. It is transmitted sexually and from mother to fetus. Syphilis is divided into several stages depending on clinical manifestations and serologic findings. Primary

syphilis occurs after a 3-week incubation period, when a painless indurated ulcer called a chancre appears. The center of this ulcer is filled with spirochetes. The chancre is usually missed in women because it is asymptomatic and resolves spontaneously after 2–6 weeks. Secondary syphilis occurs approximately 6 weeks after the appearance of the chancre and typically presents as generalized lymphadenopathy and maculopapular rash over the soles of the palms and feet. Patients who are asymptomatic but have positive serologic studies are categorized as having early latent (positive serologic tests for less than 1 year) or late latent (positive serologic tests for more than 1 year or for an unknown duration) syphilis. The clinical manifestations of tertiary syphilis may involve several organs, including the central nervous and cardiovascular systems. It usually develops several years after asymptomatic syphilis infection.

The diagnosis of syphilis is usually based on serologic testing. The only definitive diagnosis is observation of *Treponema pallidum* on dark-field examination, but this is difficult because specimens yielding spirochetes rarely can be collected, except when a primary chancre is present. Nontreponemal tests (VDRL, RPR) are nonspecific and inexpensive tests used for screening large populations. Treponemal tests (FTA-ABS, MHA-TP) are antibody tests specific for treponemal infection. Neither of these tests confirms or excludes a diagnosis of syphilis, because once a patient is infected with the spirochete, serologic test results remain positive, despite appropriate treatment. However, there is a correlation between reactive disease and nontreponemal serologic titers. Nontreponemal testing can be used to indicate reactive disease (baseline titers required) or demonstrate successful treatment (4-fold decrease in titers). The results of RC's VDRL test indicate a 4-fold increase (1:4 to 1:64) in titer, compared with her baseline value. Therefore, RC is diagnosed with early latent syphilis, because she is asymptomatic and has been infected for less than 1 year. The drug of choice for syphilis infection is penicillin. The treatment of primary, secondary, or early latent infection is identical. Because RC does not have an allergy to penicillin, she should be treated with benzathine penicillin i.m. for one dose. This will provide the low continuous levels of penicillin required to treat syphilis infections.

P: RC should receive one dose of penicillin G benzathine 2.4 million units i.m. She should return to the clinic for follow-up VDRL titers at 3, 6, and 12 months. If VDRL titers fail to decrease or increase 4-fold, RC should be retreated. RC should be educated in preventing transmission of syphilis and other sexually transmitted diseases.

Problem 5. *Pthirus pubis* (Crab Lice)

S: RC complains of itching and redness around the pelvic area. She describes a progression of symptoms and complaints, especially at night.

O: On physical examination, RC has some small erythematous areas around the pelvic area.

A: RC has the clinical manifestations of crab lice. In addition to the erythema and pruritus caused by crab lice, the worsening of symptoms at night is typical, because the lice become more active at night. The crab lice lay eggs, which can be deposited in bedclothes, clothing, or furniture. The recommended treatment for crab lice is either lindane or pyrethrin with piperonyl butoxide. Both affect the central nervous system of the lice, causing death. Lindane is a synthetic agent; pyrethins are made from natural substances and are considered to be less toxic. This is usually the agent of choice in children. Both agents are effective in eradicating crab lice.

P: RC should receive 30 ml of 1% lindane for the treatment of crab lice. She should be instructed on the proper use of lindane and educated on methods that will completely eradicate crab lice infection. RC should receive education about the proper use of lindane to eradicate crab lice:

1. Shampoo: apply to body and lather for 4–5 min, then rinse. Lotion: apply to body and leave for 8–12 hr, then shower.
2. May repeat in 1 week if crab lice are again detected (eggs may hatch over this period of time).
3. May cause some local irritation and pruritus. Do not apply more than once in 24 hr.
4. Treat any family members, sexual partners, or roommates.
5. Wash all bedclothing, clothes, and furniture that may be infected.

Problem 2. Alcoholic Cirrhosis

S: RC denies recent weight gain, edema, or abdominal girth enlargement.

O: On physical examination, RC demonstrates a mild fluid wave, ascites, and a 0.5-kg weight gain. Her liver function test results are slightly elevated, but her albumin level and prothrombin time are within normal limits. The spot urine electrolyte levels are within normal limits (normal urine sodium is diet-dependent).

A: RC has mild cirrhosis secondary to long-term alcohol use. Her symptoms are mild, as indicated by physical examination and liver function test results. She also continues to retain good synthetic function. The urine electrolyte levels do not indicate hyperaldosteronism common in cirrhotic patients. She states that she is noncompliant with her spironolactone, and therefore the urine electrolytes do not reflect a reversal of the Na/K urine concentrations as a result of spironolactone therapy. Since the drug is not adding any therapeutic benefit, it should be discontinued. RC's cirrhosis is otherwise stable.

P: Discontinue spironolactone. Attempt rehabilitation to prevent further deterioration of liver function. Monitor liver function test results and synthetic function test results. Also, monitor weight gain, edema, or abdominal girth size, which may indicate a worsening of her disease.

Problem 7. Mixed Anemia

S: None

O: RC has decreased hemoglobin, hematocrit, reticulocyte count, iron, and folate levels, but her MCV is normal. On physical examination, RC appears pale.

A: Typically, iron deficiency anemia presents as a hypochromic, microcytic anemia. It is usually asymptomatic and found by routine clinical laboratory testing. Conversely, folate deficiency anemia is normochromic, macrocytic anemia, but it also may be asymptomatic. When a mixed anemia occurs, as in RC, laboratory indicators such as the mean corpuscular volume (MCV) may appear normal. Diagnosis is usually confirmed by folate, iron, and vitamin B_{12} levels and a microscopic viewing of a blood smear. Alcoholic patients commonly have mixed anemia secondary to poor dietary intake. Folate deficiency is more common than vitamin B_{12} deficiency, because body stores of folate are depleted faster. RC has a mixed iron and folate deficiency anemia, because her vitamin B_{12} levels are within normal limits. She should receive iron and folate replacement.

P: RC should be started on iron sulfate 325 mg po TID and folate 1 mg daily. The duration of folate replacement should be 3 weeks, while iron replacement should continue for 3–6 months. RC should return to clinic for follow-up and repeat of laboratory tests. She should receive counseling on the side effects of iron and methods that alleviate these adverse effects. She should be encouraged to improve her dietary intake to prevent long-term complications of anemia.

Patient Education

1. Iron may cause feces to turn black-brown; this does not indicate a problem. Also, iron may cause constipation. An over-the-counter (OTC) agent such as docusate sodium may be used to help this problem. Stimulant agents such as senna or Ex-Lax should not be used long-term.

2. Iron should be taken on an empty stomach, but it may cause stomach upset. If this occurs, RC can take her medication with food.

3. Normally, anemia is not a symptomatic disease. RC may feel well, but her laboratory values indicate anemia. She should be told this and instructed on compliance with her medications.

4. Iron should be kept out of the reach of children.

Problem 3. Heroin Abuse

S: RC states that she uses heroin ($75.00) on a daily basis.

O: RC has symptoms of acute heroin intoxication: droopy eyelids, pinpoint pupils, lethargy, and hypotension.

A: Addictive disease is characterized by physical and psychologic addiction. Several factors contribute to the development of this disease, including environmental factors, genetics, underlying psychiatric disease, and social difficulties. Treatment of addictive disease involves two stages: medical treatment of acute withdrawal, and intense long-term psychotherapy. RC has attempted rehabilitation several times, without success. It is common for patients with addictive disease to have multiple relapses. Often, several attempts are made before rehabilitation occurs. RC should continue to attempt rehabilitation and she should be guided to appropriate programs for counseling. However, she can receive medical management for detoxification on an outpatient basis.

The treatment of heroin addiction may include symptomatic and maintenance treatment. The medical management of heroin withdrawal can involve a nonnarcotic detoxification or the use of methadone. The treatment of choice depends on the philosophy of the clinic. The nonnarcotic approach to detoxification focuses on the four major symptoms of heroin withdrawal: anxiety, insomnia, gastrointestinal symptoms, and musculoskeletal symptoms. Increased sympathetic outflow from the locus ceruleus produces the symptoms associated with heroin withdrawal. Clonidine can be used to alleviate withdrawal symptoms, because it acts centrally to decrease sympathetic outflow from the locus ceruleus. The dosing of clonidine depends on the ability of the patient to tolerate the effects of this drug on blood pressure. Typically, a single test dose of 0.1 mg is given by mouth, and the blood pressure is measured after 1 hr. Additional agents can be used to manage symptoms not fully alleviated by clonidine. Diphenhydramine or flurazepam can be used to treat insomnia, while the symptoms of anxiety are usually controlled with phenobarbital or chlordiazepoxide. Propoxyphene or cyclobenzaprine can be used to manage the musculoskeletal symptoms. Gastrointestinal symptoms (diarrhea abdominal cramping, and vomiting) can be managed by loperamide, dicyclomine, prochlorperazine, or belladonna alkaloids.

Methadone can be used to prevent heroin withdrawal symptoms and was once thought of as a "cure" for heroin addiction. However, methadone is a long-acting fully addictive narcotic with an abuse potential similar to that of heroin. Multiple daily dosing is used to decrease the euphoric effects of large doses of methadone, in an attempt to discourage abuse. Methadone is dosed based on the daily use of heroin. Generally, 1 mg of methadone is used for each 2 mg of heroin, then divided into four doses if the dose is greater than 40 mg per day. The dose can then be reduced on a daily basis by 5 mg per day or titrated to the patient's symptoms. Methadone also can be used as maintenance therapy. Patients who cannot live without opioids sometimes require maintenance therapy to prevent relapse. Long-term management of heroin abuse by this method has been replaced with psychotherapy that emphasizes a drug-free state, because methadone maintenance leads to drug diversion and continued abuse. Clonidine is not an appropriate choice for RC, because she will require alcohol detoxification. Clonidine can mask the hypertension seen with uncontrolled alcohol withdrawal. RC may receive methadone or symptomatic treatment without clonidine for heroin withdrawal.

P: Based on RC's daily heroin use, she should receive 40 mg of methadone daily, given in four divided doses. She should be tapered 5 mg per day or as tolerated. The rate of taper should be based on objective information rather than patient desire. RC should be monitored for objective and subjective symptoms of heroin withdrawal such as nausea, vomiting, abdominal cramping, muscle spasms, hypertension, and anxiety. Detoxification cannot take the place of supportive counseling. RC should receive counseling on a daily basis from persons experienced in the treatment of addiction. She should also be educated on the medical complications of intravenous drug use.

Problem 1. Alcohol Abuse

S: RC admits to drinking 1 pint of vodka daily. She has been drinking since she was 16 years old.

O: RC demonstrates long-term effects of alcohol abuse, including mixed anemia and alcoholic cirrhosis.

A: Alcoholism is an addictive disease characterized by psychologic and physical addiction. The long-term sequelae of alcoholism are significant and include cardiomyopathy, endocrine and central nervous system disorders, and gastrointestinal toxicity. RC already has hepatic complications associated with long-term alcohol ingestion. Therefore, she should receive treatment for alcohol dependency. Withdrawal from alcohol occurs in four stages. The severity of the symptoms depends on the amount of physical dependency the patient has developed. The first stage begins approximately 6–8 hr after the last drink, because alcohol levels begin to fall. It is characterized by anxiety, hyperflexia, hypertension, nausea, vomiting, insomnia, tachycardia, and diaphoresis. Stage 2 occurs 24 hr after the last drink and lasts approximately 2–3 days. Symptoms include auditory or visual hallucinations, tremor, and hyperactivity. Stage 3 includes characteristics of stages 1 and 2, but is more severe and also includes seizures. Delirium tremens, fever, illusions, confusion, and seizures characterize stage-4 withdrawal. Stage 4 is associated with the highest mortality rate, because aspiration, shock, hyperthermia, and arrhythmias may occur.

Alcohol withdrawal can be treated on an outpatient basis with careful monitoring. Therapy includes the use of phenobarbital or chlordiazepoxide. Patients with excessive alcohol intake will have high tolerance to benzodiazepines and barbiturates, because all of these agents are thought to interact with γ-amino butyric acid (GABA) receptors. Therefore, relatively high doses may be required. Generally, a phenobarbital dose is based on the amount of alcohol used daily: 30 mg of phenobarbital for every 2 ounces of hard liquor. Additionally, supportive treatment with fluids and vitamins is important in the treatment of alcoholic patients. Fluids high in electrolytes (e.g., Gatorade) are appropriate for this purpose.

P: Based on RC's daily alcohol consumption, she should receive phenobarbital 100 mg po QID, with 15 mg given on an "as-needed" basis for breakthrough symptoms. RC should then be tapered 15–30 mg every 3 days. She should be monitored for symptoms of withdrawal or barbiturate intoxication. RC should be given nutritional supplementation and counseled to increase her fluid intake with high electrolyte solutions. She should return to clinic daily for evaluation and counseling. RC should be informed about the long-term effects of alcohol.

Problem 6. HIV Infection

S: None

O: RC has a recent positive HIV antibody test result, although her CD_4 count is within normal limits.

A: RC has asymptomatic HIV infection. Because her CD_4 count is within normal limits, she is at low risk for opportunistic infections. RC should return to clinic for periodic assessment to enable early detection of progressive HIV infection.

P: Monitor clinical laboratory test results and assess the need for treatment if infection progresses. RC should receive counseling about the implications of being HIV-positive and changes in her lifestyle that could help prevent transmission as well as improve her quality of life. It should be emphasized to RC that this virus is transmitted sexually and by sharing used needles. She should be educated on the use of condoms to prevent transmission to sexual partners.

QUESTIONS FOR CASE 137

1. How is syphilis treated in HIV-infected patients and patients with AIDS?
2. How is neurosyphilis diagnosed and treated?
3. How is syphilis treated in a patient with a penicillin allergy?
4. When should RC be started on zidovudine? Discuss the dosing and monitoring parameters.
5. RC returns to clinic 8 months later with a CD_4 count of 154 mm^{-3}. She continues to be asymptomatic. Discuss any additional treatment that RC should receive.

CASE 138

CC: OB is 24-year-old woman seen in the AIDS clinic for complaints of poor appetite and a 4.4-kg weight loss since her last clinic visit 1 month ago. She also complains of fatigue, weakness, and inability to do her daily activities. She says she is not depressed, she just does not feel like eating.

Medical History

OB became HIV (+) 3 years ago. Since then she has had recurrent oral candidiasis, responsive to clotrimazole troches. She had one *Pneumocystis carinii* pneumonia (PCP) episode last year, for which she was hospitalized and treated successfully with pentamidine. She has also experienced an episode of vaginal candidiasis, diagnosed at her last clinic visit 1 month ago.

Social History

OB is a college student in her freshman year. She is a heterosexual and lives with parents and one sibling. OB has had only one sexual partner (she is currently not sexually active). She has no history of intravenous drug use, does not drink and smokes occasionally, one pack of cigarettes every 3 months.

Medication History

Clotrimazole troches 10 mg po 5 × /day
Zidovudine 200 mg po TID
Dapsone 100 mg po QD

Allergies

Sulfa (hives/rash)

Physical Examination

GEN: Cachetic, frail-looking young woman in no apparent distress
VS: BP 75/50, T 37.8, HR 80, RR 22, Wt 39 kg (4.4-kg loss)
HEENT: Few patchy white plaques in oral cavity
COR: RRR, nl S_1 S_2
CHEST: Clear to auscultation
ABD: Soft, nontender, positive bowel sounds.
GU: Unremarkable
RECT: WNL, guaiac negative
EXT: WNL
NEURO: Intact, alert, oriented, cooperative.

Results of Laboratory Tests

Na 138 (138)	Cl 100 (100)	MCV 115 (115)
Hct 0.28 (28)	LKCS 3.1×10^9 (3.1×10^3)	Ca 2.4 (9.7)
Alk Phos 1.72 (103)	T bili 8.5 (0.5)	CR 70.7 (0.8)
K 3.5 (3.5)	HCO_3 26 (26)	AST 0.46 (28)
Hgb 90 (9)	Plts 170×10^9 (170×10^3)	PO_4 1.07 (3.3)
Alb 28 (2.8)	Glu 6.1 (110)	ALT 0.38 (23)
	BUN 3.6 (10)	Mg 1.0 (2.1)

Blood cultures negative for MAC × 3; fungal cultures negative

Stool negative for parasites

CD_4 lymphocyte count 80 cells/mm^3 (last count 120 cells/mm^3)

PROBLEM LIST

1. MAC prophylaxis
2. Antiretroviral therapy
3. Nutrition
4. Poor appetite

CASE 138 SOAP NOTES

Problem 1. MAC Prophylaxis

S: None
O: HIV (+), CD_4 count of 80 cells/mm^3
A: OB has a CD_4 lymphocyte count less than 100 cells/mm^3 (80) and is at increased risk for developing disseminated MAC. At present, rifabutin is the only agent approved for the prevention of disseminated MAC in AIDS patients with advances HIV infection.
P: Start rifabutin 300 mg po QD. The dose may be administered as 150 mg po BID, because she has poor appetite and may be noncompliant from nausea. Rifabutin reduces the incidence of bacteremia by 50% in patients with CD_4 cell counts less than 50 to 100 cells/mm^3. Plan to monitor LFTs, because rifabutin is a potent hepatic P-450 enzyme inducer, and elevated bilirubin and alkaline phosphatase

levels and hepatitis have been associated with this drug. Rifabutin is well tolerated, but uveitis has been noted in patients on dosages greater than 300 mg/d and in patients receiving concomitant clarithromyin and fluconazole therapy. Clarithromycin increases serum levels of rifabutin and can lead to rifabutin toxicity, including severe anterior uveitis. Educate the patient that rifabutin may cause red-orange discoloration of body secretions, including urine and tears.

Problem 2. Antiretroviral Therapy

S: History of HIV infection
O: HIV (+), decrease in CD_4 lymphocyte count from 120 cells to 80 cells/mm^3. Progression of disease (recurrent oral candidiasis, PCP 1 year ago, and vaginal candidiasis a month ago), and mild anemia (decreased Hgb and Hct) with macrocytosis.
A: OB has been on antiretroviral therapy (zidovudine) for more than 3 years, and demonstrates signs of disease progression. The duration of zidovudine benefit is somewhat controversial. Because the patient has no history of drinking, no signs of pancreatitis (nl amylase) or peripheral neuropathy, she may benefit from a change in therapy to ddi. DDI may have activity against zidovudine resistant strains of HIV.
P: Start DDI 125 mg po BID. Monitor serum amylase and advise patient to report any abdominal pain. Plan to restart zidovudine if further disease progression occurs. Consider combination antiretroviral therapy if a further decrease in CD_4 cell count occurs.

Problem 3. Nutrition

S: OB complains of fatigue, weakness, and inability to perform daily activities.
O: Weight loss of 4.4 kg in a frail cachectic woman. Albumin 2.8.
A: HIV and many HIV related conditions can cause weight loss, fatigue and weakness; therefore, repeated tests to determine the cause are important. OB has three negative blood cultures for MAC, negative fungal cultures, negative stool for parasites and no fever. OB has a poor appetite, significant weight loss (4.4 kg over 1 month) and a negative workup for other conditions. She may need nutritional and vitamin supplementation.
P: Start multivitamin with iron tablets one po QD. Consider nutritional supplements (Ensure, Advera, Nutren and Resource). Refer OB to the clinic dietitian or nutritionist to design an individualized nutritional strategy. An aggressive nutritional and exercise program may help prevent wasting and malnutrition.

Problem 4. Poor Appetite

S: The patient complains of a poor appetite.
O: Weight loss of 4.4 kg over 1 month. Frail-looking, cachectic woman.
A: OB's medication profile needs to be reviewed to determine if any drugs are affecting her appetite and food intake. Dapsone and zidovudine may contribute to her decreased

appetite. OB needs aggressive intervention. Malnutrition increases her risk for opportunistic infections. There are two drugs approved for appetite stimulation which may lead to weight gain: megestrol acetate and dronabinol. The fatigue, insomnia, and loss of coordination associated with dronabinol make it a less favorable option for this patient.

P: Start megestrol acetate (Megace) 80 mg po TID (titrate up to 800 mg po QD if needed). Monitor for nausea, vomiting, and edema. Closely monitor weight.

QUESTIONS FOR CASE 138

1. What other agents may soon be indicated for MAC prophylaxis?
2. Give four reasons when it is appropriate to switch from zidovudine to DDI.
3. How effective is combination antiretroviral therapy?
4. What is HIV wasting?
5. Does nutrition correlate with death in the HIV positive patient?

CASE 139

CC: AH is a 50-year-old man who presents to the general medicine clinic with 2-day history of fever, productive cough, shortness of breath, and pleuritic chest pain.

History of Present Illness

AH started to have productive cough 5 days ago for which he took OTC cough medicine without relief. Three days later, he developed fever, difficulty in breathing, pleuritic chest pain, and increased rusty-colored sputum production.

Medical History

AH has a history of congestive heart failure secondary to rheumatic heart disease, diagnosed 20 years ago. He was started on hydrochlorothiazide and captopril at the time of diagnosis. He also developed chronic renal insufficiency due to the progression of his heart failure. One month ago, he felt severe pain in his left great toe after jogging for 30 minutes. His serum uric acid was found to be elevated and allopurinol was started. He also has had chronic insomnia for 6 months for which he takes diphenhydramine without relief.

Medication History

Captopril 12.5 mg po TID
Hydrochlorothiazide 25 mg po QD
Allopurinol 300 mg po QD
Diphenhydramine 50 mg po QHS
Robitussin 1 tbsp Q6H p.r.n. cough

Allergies

Penicillin (anaphylaxis)

Social History

Tobacco: 1 1/2 pack per day for 10 years
Alcohol: none

Review of Systems

Noncontributory

Physical Examination

GEN: Well developed well-nourished man in mild distress
VS: BP 135/88, HR 101, RR 20, T 38.5°C, Wt 68 kg, Ht 162 cm
HEENT: PERRLA
NECK: Supple, (+) JVD 12cm
COR: Normal S_1 and S_2, positive S3, no murmurs
CHEST: Bilateral crackles and rales at the lower lung base
ABD: Soft, nontender, no hepatosplenomegaly
RECT: Guaiac-negative
EXT: 1+ pitting edema bilaterally, no clubbing or cyanosis
NEURO: Oriented to time, place and person, normal deep tendon reflexes

Results of Laboratory Tests

Na 125 (125)	Ca 2.3 (9.1)	Alk Phos 0.83 (50)
Hct 0.37 (37)	Cl 101 (101)	Mg 0.98 (2.4)
AST 0.25 (15)	Lkcs 18 × 10⁹ (18 × 10³)	BUN 12.1 (34)
Glu 7.7 (140)	LDH 1.4 (84)	MCV 90 (90)
K 4.5 (4.5)	PO₄ 0.8 (2.5)	Alb 46 (4.6)
Hgb 110 (11)	HCO₃ 26 (26)	Uric Acid 446 (7.5)
ALT 0.42 (25)	Plts 180 × 10⁹ (180 × 10³)	CR 185.6 (2.1)
		T Bili 10.3 (0.6)

Sputum: Gram's stain: gram-positive cocci in pairs, moderate polymononuclear cells, few epithelial cells

Culture: Pending

CXR: Right lower lobe infiltrates, left side unremarkable

EKG: PR 0.13, normal axis, sinus tachycardia with HR 101

PROBLEM LIST

1. Pneumonia
2. Congestive heart failure
3. Chronic renal insufficiency
4. Gout
5. Chronic insomnia

Use SOAP for the above problems.

CASE 139 SOAP NOTES

Problem 1. Pneumonia

S: AH complains of fever, productive cough, shortness of breath, pleuritic chest pain, and increased rusty-colored sputum production.

O: AH has a temperature of 38.5°C. He is also tachypneic, in sinus tachycardia, and has bilateral crackles and rales in lower lung base. He has leukocytosis and positive chest x-ray consistent with pneumonia.

A: AH suffers from community-acquired pneumonia. His risk factors for pneumonia include congestive heart failure, uremia, smoking, and old age. Preliminary sputum Gram's stain suggests that it is probably a pneumococcal pneumonia. Because AH is only in mild distress, he can be treated as an outpatient. Penicillin is the drug of choice for pneumococcal pneumonia. Other empiric antimicrobial therapies include cephalosporins such as cephalexin or cefuroxime axetil, trimethroprim/sulfamethoxazole, or erythromycin. AH has an anaphylactic reaction to penicillins, so cephalosporins should be avoided due to potential cross-reactivity with penicillins. Erythromycin or trimethoprim/sulfamethoxazole may be used. Erythromycin may be a better choice for community-acquired pneumonia because it also covers atypical pathogens such as *Legionella pneumophilia*, *Chlamydia pneumoniae*, and *Mycoplasma pneumoniae*.

P: Start erythromycin 500 mg po QID for seven days. Inform AH about possible gastrointestinal upset and instruct him to finish the full course of antibiotics even if he feels better after a few days.

Problem 2. Congestive Heart Failure

S: None

O: AH has a S_3 gallop and JVD of 12 cm. He also has 1+ pitting edema bilaterally.

A: AH has signs of heart failure despite captopril and hydrochlorothiazide. Congestive heart failure is associated with significant morbidity and mortality and it is essential to optimize AH's therapy to prevent the progression of his disease. He has a positive S_3, which is an indication for digoxin. Captopril is a good choice for AH because it has been shown to decrease mortality in patients with mild to moderate heart failure. Consider increasing the captopril dose in the next clinic visit if his symptoms persist after the addition of digoxin.

P: Start digoxin 0.125 mg po QD. Check digoxin level in 1 week. Monitor for signs of digoxin toxicity (nausea, vomiting, arrhythmias, bradycardia). Monitor serum creatinine, electrolytes (especially magnesium and potassium), and for symptoms of congestive heart failure (peripheral edema, JVD, shortness of breath).

Problem 3. Chronic Renal Insufficiency

S: None

O: AH has elevated BUN and CR.

A: AH has chronic renal insufficiency secondary to congestive heart failure. He currently has no signs of acute renal failure and his renal function is stable. His estimated creatinine clearance is 40.5 ml/min.

P: Continue to monitor serum creatinine and urine output. Avoid nephrotoxic drugs. Need to reduce dose of allopurinol to 200 mg/day based on renal function (see gout problem below).

Problem 4. Gout and Hyperuricemia

S: AH had severe pain at his left toe 1 month ago.

O: AH's serum uric acid is mildly elevated.

A: The causes of AH's gouty attack are trauma to his left toe, renal insufficiency, and hydrochlorothiazide. Acute gouty attacks may be treated with colchicine or nonsteroidal anti-inflammatory agents such as indomethacin. NSAIDs are best avoided because of AH's renal dysfunction.

Therapy for hyperuricemia includes allopurinol and probenecid. Although allopurinol is a better choice for patients with renal dysfunction than probenecid, the dose of allopurinol is too high for AH because his creatinine clearance is <50 mL/minute. Because AH has had only one gouty episode, therapy for hyperuricemia can be withheld unless he has persistent attacks and continued hyperuricemia.

P: Discontinue allopurinol. Give colchicine 0.6 mg to be taken at the onset of an acute gouty attack and repeated hourly until pain relief is achieved or AH experiences nausea, vomiting, or diarrhea. If AH continues to experience frequent acute gouty attacks, monitor AH's uric acid level and consider uricosuric therapy.

Problem 5. Insomnia

S: AH has insomnia for more than 6 months unrelieved by diphenhydramine.

O: None.

A: AH's chronic insomnia is probably due to his medical disorders such as congestive heart failure and chronic renal insufficiency. Diphenhydramine is a sedating sleeping aid that is effective in the treatment of short-term insomnia. However, it has not been shown to be effective in the treatment of chronic insomnia. Benzodiazepines such as triazolam may be helpful to AH, although they also should be used for long-term therapy. Flurazepam is not recommended because of the potential accumulation of active metabolites due to AH's renal function.

P: Start triazolam 0.125 mg po QHS. Instruct AH not to take triazolam with alcohol. If AH's insomnia continues to progress or is not relieved, AH should seek counseling to determine if there is a depressive component to his insomnia.

QUESTIONS FOR CASE 139

1. What are the most common pathogens causing community-acquired pneumonia?
2. What is the incidence of cross-reactivity between penicillins and cephalosporins?
3. Which medications have been shown to reduce mortality in patients with congestive heart failure?
4. How should asymptomatic hyperuricemia be managed?
5. What are the causes of chronic insomnia?

CASE 140

CC: BF is a 55-year-old man diagnosed with acute lymphocytic leukemia (ALL) 2 weeks PTA. He is currently receiving day 10 of his induction chemotherapy regimen. On day 7 of therapy, he became febrile, was pancultured, and empirically started on ceftazidime and tobramycin. Despite this aggressive antibiotic therapy, last evening he spiked a temperature to 39.8°C. He also complains of nosebleeds, fever, and painful oral lesions.

Medical History

BF was diagnosed with rheumatoid arthritis (RA) 2 years ago and has been managed with nonsteroidal antiinflammatory drug (NSAID) therapy. BF has been otherwise healthy prior to the diagnosis of ALL (bone marrow biopsy (+), peripheral Lkcs 55 × 10^9 (55 × 10^3).

Medication History

Daunorubicin 100 mg IV D1-3
Vincristine 2 mg IV D1,8,15,22
Prednisone 50 mg po BID D1-28
Asparaginase 10,000 U s.q. D17-28
TMP/SMX DS po BID Fri, Sat, Sun
Ranitidine 50 mg IV q.8
Prochlorperazine 10 mg IV/i.m. q6 p.r.n. N/ V
Naproxen 500 mg po BID
Allopurinol 300 mg po QD

Allergies

None known

Physical Examination

GEN: Thin, ill-appearing man
VS: BP 130/82, HR 90, RR 26, T 39.8°C, Wt 57.0 kg, Ht 147 cm, BSA 1.68 m^2
HEENT: Neck supple, (-) conjunctival hemorrhage, (+) white plaques on oral mucosa
COR: RRR, nl S$_1$S$_2$
CHEST: Clear
ABD: Soft nontender, positive bowel sounds, Hickman catheter site erythematous
GU: WNL
RECT: Deferred 2° thrombocytopenia
EXT: Multiple ecchymosis and petechiae
NEURO: Intact, nonfocal examination

Results of Laboratory Tests

Na 139 (139)	Hct 0.28 (28)	AST 1.13 (68)	Glu 6.44 (116)
K 4.1 (4.1)	Hgb 94 (9.4)	ALT 0.3 (19)	Ca 2.5 (10.1)
Cl 100 (100)	Lkcs 0.1 × 10^9 (0.1 × 10^3)	Alk Phos 8.9 (532)	PO$_4$ 0.97 (3.0)
HCO$_3$ 26 (26)	Plts 13 × 10^9 (13 × 10^3)	Alb 41 (4.1)	Mg 1.0 (2.1)
BUN 5.7 (16)			Uric Acid 535 (9.0)
CR 88.4 (1.0)			

Lkc differential: N 0.6 (60%), Promyeloblasts present
Urinalysis: WNL
Chest x-ray: WNL, no infiltrates
Blood culture: Negative
Oral scraping culture: Candida albicans

PROBLEM LIST

1. Rheumatoid arthritis
2. ALL
3. Fever with neutropenia
4. Thrombocytopenia
5. Oral candidiasis

CASE 140 SOAP NOTES
Problem 2. Acute Lymphocytic Leukemia (ALL)

S: None

O: (+) Bone marrow, Lkcs >50 × 10^9 (50 × 10^3) 2 weeks prior to therapy

A: BF is currently undergoing induction chemotherapy for ALL. The regimen of prednisone, vincristine, asparaginase, and daunorubicin is reported to be >80% effective in inducing a complete remission. BF is currently experiencing bone-marrow toxicity manifested by decreased platelets and decreased absolute neutrophil count (ANC).

P: Continue remaining induction therapy and supportive care for the decreased platelet and Lkcs levels. Repeat bone marrow biopsy to assess response to therapy.

Problem 3. Fever with Neutropenia

S: BF complains of fever.

O: BF's absolute neutrophil count (ANC) is <100, with a temperature of 39.8°C. Culture results are negative to date, but the Hickman catheter site is erythematous.

A: BF is profoundly neutropenic, which places him at an increased risk of infection from bacterial, fungal, and viral pathogens. The most common bacterial pathogens are gram-negative rods such as *Escherichia coli*, *Klebsiella pnuemoniae*, and *Pseudomonas aeruginosa* as well as gram-positive cocci, including *Staphylococcus aureus* and coagulase-negative staphylococci. BF is currently on ceftazidime and tobramycin, which are both very active against aerobic gram-negative bacilli including *P. aeruginosa*. The regimen lacks significant activity against gram-positive isolates and anaerobes. The erythematous Hickman site is a possible source of infection, and the therapy should be broadened to provide coverage against staphylococci. BF should receive vancomycin, rather than an antistaphylococcal penicillin or first-generation cephalosporin, because these agents are less reliable against coagulate-negative staphylococci such as *S. epidermidis*. The vancomycin peaks should be 20–35 mg/liter, and the troughs from 5–15 mg/liter.

P: Start vancomycin:

$$CrCl = \frac{(140 - 55)57kg}{(72)(1.0)} = 67.3 \text{ ml/min} = 4.04 \text{ liter/hr}$$

$$Cl_{vanco} = 0.65 × 4.04 \text{ liter/hr} = 2.62 \text{ liter/hr}$$

$$Vd = 0.7 × 57 \text{ kg} = 39.9 \text{ liter}$$

$$k = 0.066 \text{ hr}^{-1} \quad t_{1/2} = 10.5 \text{ hr}$$

$$Dose = \frac{Cpdes × Vd}{FS} (1 - e^{-0.66(12)}/e^{-0.66(12)}) = 488 \text{ mg}$$

Recommend >500 mg IV q.12

$$\text{Predicted peak} = \frac{500}{39.9} (e^{0.66(2)}/1 - e^{-0.066(12)})$$

$$= 20 \text{ mg/liter}$$

$$\text{Predicted trough} = 20 \text{ mg/liter} (e^{-0.066(10)})$$

$$= 10.3 \text{ mg/liter}$$

Vancomycin infusions should be administered over 1 hr to minimize the potential for the red-man syndrome. Monitor vancomycin peaks (around the fourth dose), BUN, and Cr while on therapy. If BF remains febrile, consider resistant gram-negative pathogens or a fungal infection, especially as BF has oral candidiasis (see problem 5).

Problem 4. Thrombocytopenia

S: BF complains of nosebleeds.

O: Plts 13; ecchymosis and petechiae were noted on examination of the extremities.

A: The thrombocytopenia is secondary to the cytotoxic ALL induction chemotherapy. BF is also receiving naproxen, which can inhibit platelet aggregation. BF requires platelet transfusions, and all antiplatelet and i.m. injections should be discontinued, to decrease the risk of hemorrhage.

P: The naproxen should be discontinued. Prochlorperazine and morphine should be administered IV rather than i.m. BF should receive platelet transfusions to maintain his platelet count $>20 \times 10^9$ (20×10^3).

Problem 5. Oral Candidiasis

S: BF complains of painful oral lesions.

O: White plaques, *Candida* present on oral mucosa.

A: BF has oral candidiasis secondary to immunosuppressive therapy and recent initiation of broad-spectrum antibacterial therapy. He requires treatment, because he is symptomatic and is at risk for systemic dissemination. The treatment alternatives for oral-pharyngeal candidiasis (thrush) include either topical or systemic therapies. Topical therapy with nystatin suspension (500,000 Units "swish and swallow" q6h) or clotrimazole troches (10 mg 5 ×/day) is usually effective. Patient compliance with therapy often is suboptimal because nystatin suspension has a bitter taste and clotrimazole troches require contact time for dissolution, which can be painful in patients with mucosal ulceration secondary to stomatitis. Even with optimal compliance, relapses with topical therapy are common in immunocompromised patients, and systemic therapy is often necessary. The available agents include ketoconazole, fluconazole, and amphotericin B. The imidazoles are preferred over amphotericin B, because they are better tolerated and are without renal toxicity. Both ketoconazole (200–400 mg/day) and fluconazole (100–200 mg/day) are effective in treating oral candidiasis. Ketoconazole requires an acidic environment for absorption; thus patients on concomitant H_2-antagonist, antacid, or omeprazole therapy may have a decreased clinical response. Fluconazole absorption does not appear to be pH-dependent, and thus it would be the preferred agent for BF, because he is currently receiving ranitidine. If BF is unable to tolerate oral medications, alternatives include fluconazole (100–200 mg IV) or low-dose amphotericin (15 mg IV QD).

P: BF should be treated with fluconazole 200 mg po now, and then 100 mg po QD for 7–10 days.

Problem 1. Rheumatoid Arthritis

S: History of RA for 2 years

O: No obvious findings at present

A: BF is without symptoms at present. The induction regimen contains prednisone 100 mg per day, which would alleviate RA symptoms. Naproxen has antiplatelet effects and should be discontinued while BF is thrombocytopenic, to reduce the risk of hemorrhage.

P: Discontinue naproxen.

QUESTIONS FOR CASE 140

1. What is the role of monotherapy in the treatment of febrile neutropenia?
2. When should empiric antifungal therapy with amphotericin B be initiated in the treatment of febrile neutropenia?
3. What is the duration of antimicrobial therapy in patients with neutropenia and fever?
4. What is the role of TMP-SMX in the treatment of ALL?
5. Should BF receive a colony-stimulating factor?

CASE 141

CC: BG is a 6 1/2-year-old boy who presents to the clinic with a complaint of inability to sleep through the night and perianal itching. Mom reports that BG tires easily and complains of earaches.

Medical History

BG was born at 38 weeks' gestation; birth weight was 2.9 kg. Mother received no prenatal care. BG received the first diphtheria and tetanus toxoid and pertussis (DTP) vaccine and oral polio vaccine (OPV) at 6 months of age, when he was seen in the clinic with mild symptoms of an upper respiratory infection. He has received no further immunizations.

Medication History

None

Social History

Diet: high carbohydrate, low protein
Attends kindergarten and daycare after school

Physical Examination

GEN: Well-developed, small for age, pale boy in no acute distress

VS: BP 90/70, HR 110, RR 20, T 37°C, Wt 16 kg (5th percentile), Ht 115 cm (25th percentile)

HEENT: Normocephalic, pale conjunctiva, hyperemic, opaque, bulging tympanic membrane on left, nose and throat normal

COR: Normal

CHEST: Clear to auscultation

ABD: Soft, nontender, bowel sounds present

GU: Normal male

RECT: Perianal area reddened and excoriated; microscopic examination of tape applied to perianal skin reveals *Enterobius vermicularis* eggs.

EXT: Pale nail beds, thin extremities

NEURO: Alert and oriented to time, place, and person; normal DTRs (deep tendon reflexes)

Results of Laboratory Tests

Hgb 97 (9.7)
Hct 0.297 (29.7)
MCV 77 (77)

Peripheral smear: Microcytic, hypochromic red blood cells

PROBLEM LIST

1. Immunizations not up to date
2. Itching around perianal area
3. Anemia
4. Probable frequent otitis media

QUESTIONS FOR CASE 141

1. What are the routinely seen adverse effects associated with DTP administration?
2. How should the response to iron therapy be evaluated?
3. What further interventions may be indicated to treat otitis media that fails to respond to ampicillin or amoxicillin, or recurs?
4. What immunizations should be administered to BG if he does not return for the second round of immunizations until he is 7 years old?
5. If BG had sickle cell disease, how would his immunization(s) or the schedule be changed?

CASE 142

CC: ME is a 56-year-old man seen in clinic. He is a recent immigrant who has never been fully treated for TB and also has a parasitic infection, iron deficiency anemia, hyperuricemia, and hypertension (HTN).

Medical History

ME is a 56-year-old man who recently immigrated to the United States from a Third World country. He has recently finished a 20-day course of metronidazole and Iodoquinol, after intestinal amebiasis was diagnosed in an extensive workup of chronic intermittent diarrhea and weight loss. His diarrhea has markedly improved, and ME is symptomatically better. He denies any history of fevers or night sweats. He does have a 10- to 15-pound weight loss over 1 year. ME has a history of tuberculosis 7 years ago. He describes having taken "medicine" for 3 months, then he stopped. He also has iron-deficiency anemia, hyperuricemia, and hypertension (HTN) for 10 years.

Social History

ME is married and has farmed. He smokes cigarettes, 1 pack/day for 40 years. He does not drink alcohol.

Family History

ME's wife is alive and well. He has four children, living at home, who are also alive and well.

Allergies

Penicillin, which the patient describes as causing a difficulty in breathing.

Medication History

Triamterene (75 mg)/Hydrochlorothiazide (50 mg) 1 po q. day
Iron sulfate 325 mg po BID

Review of Systems

Negative

Physical Examination

VS:	BP 150/92, HR 84, RR 16, T 37.2°C, weight and height not done
HEENT:	Fundi normal; edentulous; no lymphadenopathy
COR:	Regular rate and rhythm without murmur
CHEST:	Diffuse wheezing, decreased breath sounds throughout
ABD:	Liver 8 cm, spleen not palpable
EXT:	No clubbing, cyanosis, or edema
GU:	WNL
RECT:	Prostate WNL, stool heme-positive, no masses

Results of Laboratory Tests

Na 139 (139)	Hct 0.364 (36.4)	AST 0.58 (35)	Glu 6.1 (110)
K 3.5 (3.5)	Hgb 112 (11.2)	AST 0.58 (35)	Ca 2.5 (10.1)
Cl 108 (108)	Lkcs 8.6 × 10⁹ (8.6 × 10³)	ALT 0.67 (40)	PO₄ 1.1 (3.4)
HCO₃ 24 (24)	Plts 296 × 10⁹ (296 × 10³)	LDH 3.3 (200)	Mg 1.05 (2.1)
BUN 6.8 (19)	MCV 77 (77)	Alb 42 (4.2)	Uric Acid 725.6 (12.2)
CR 141 (1.6)		T Bili 8.6 (0.5)	Chol 5.7 (220)
			PT 12
			PTT 34

Lkc differential: Lymphs 0.2 (20), Eos 0.03 (3), Monos 0.04 (4)

Chest x-ray: Right apical scarring; hyperinflation consistent with COPD

KUB: No air fluid levels

Skin tests: PPD (+), Candida skin test (+); mumps skin test (+).

PROBLEM LIST

1. Hypertension
2. Hyperuricemia
3. Partially treated tuberculosis
4. Parasitic infection
5. Iron-deficiency anemia

QUESTIONS FOR CASE 142

1. What if ME refused to comply with taking his medication? Would a twice-a-week regimen be reasonable?
2. What if ME returns to the clinic in 3 months with increased levels of liver enzymes (e.g., increased AST, ALT)?
3. What if discontinuing ME's hydrochlorothiazide only decreased his uric acid level by 59.5 μmol/liter (1 mg/100 ml)?

4. What factors contribute to the rising incidence of tuberculosis in this country?
5. What other diseases can produce an microcytic anemia besides iron deficiency anemia?

CASE 143

CC: DL is a 72-year-old woman transferred to the hospital from a nursing home, with fever, anorexia, nausea, vomiting, and flank pain of 2 days' duration.

Medical History

DL has multiple medical problems and therefore was placed in the nursing home 2 years ago. DL has a long history of rheumatoid arthritis and has been on steroid therapy for years. DL also has a long history of hypertension that had been controlled with propranolol for the past 2 years. DL also has angina, for which she receives nitroglycerin sublingually p.r.n. chest pain. Recently, the incidence of anginal attacks has increased to several episodes of chest pain per week.

DL suffered a stroke 4 months ago, which left her with a partial paralysis on her left side, a neurogenic bladder requiring intermittent catheterization, and a speech impairment. In the past 2 weeks, DL was having more difficulty voiding, so a continuous Foley catheter was placed. The nursing home also states that DL is depressed and started her on amitriptyline 3 weeks ago.

Medication History

Prednisone 20 mg po QD × 4 years
Propranolol 20 mg po BID × 2 years
Nitroglycerin 0.3 mg s.l. p.r.n. CP; MR q. 5 min × 3
Aspirin 325 mg po QD × 4 months
Amitriptyline 100 mg po BID × 3 weeks

Physical Examination

GEN: Thin, ill-appearing elderly woman in moderate distress
VS: BP 163/94, HR 89, RR 28, T 39°C, Wt 55 kg, Ht 166 cm
HEENT: Moon facies
COR: Sinus tachycardia
CHEST: Clear
ABD: CVA tenderness, striae
GU: Foley catheter in place
RECT: Deferred
EXT: Thin, tissue-paper skin, mild swelling of MCP and MTP joints
NEURO: Alert and oriented × 3

Results of Laboratory Tests

Na 140 (140)	Hct 0.33 (33)	AST 0.63 (38)	Glu 15.5 (280)
K 4.2 (4.2)	Hgb 117 (11.7)	ALT 0.6 (36)	Ca 2.2 (8.9)
Cl 102 (102)	Lkcs 18 × 10⁹ (18 × 10³)	LDH 2.1 (126)	PO₄ 0.97 (3)
HCO₃ 26 (26)	Plts 200 × 10⁹ (200 × 10³)	Alk Phos 1.85 (111)	Mg 0.9 (1.8)
BUN 11.4 (32)	MCV 82 (82)	Alb 38 (3.8)	Uric Acid 178 (3)
CR 124 (1.4)		T Bili 18.8 (1.1)	

Lkc differential: P 76%; B 10%; L 13%; E 1%
Urinalysis: >20 bacteria/HPF; > 15 Lkcs/HPF
Chest x-ray: WNL; no infiltrates

PROBLEM LIST

1. Hypertension
2. Rheumatoid arthritis
3. Angina
4. Stroke
5. Neurogenic bladder
6. Depression
7. Prednisone toxicity
8. Pyelonephritis

QUESTIONS FOR CASE 143

1. When DL came into the hospital, she had a Foley catheter in place. If the nursing home had placed her on prophylactic antibiotics, would DL's infection have been prevented?
2. Why is it preferable to remove the catheter?
3. In patients who are catheterized, what guidelines can be followed to minimize the risk of infection?
4. One day later, DL's urine culture returns with *Pseudomonas aeruginosa* as the causative organism. What antibiotics would provide adequate coverage? Should DL's therapy be changed?
5. After 5 days of antibiotic therapy, DL has been afebrile for 48 hr. Would you recommend a change to oral therapy? If so, what options are available?

CASE 144

CC: SF is a 65-year-old woman who presents to the hospital with fevers, chills, night sweats, weakness, headaches, and a decreased appetite.

History of Present Illness

SF has a history of mitral valve replacement 2 years prior to admission, secondary to severe mitral valve regurgitation. Four weeks prior to admission, she underwent a dental procedure. 1 hour prior to this, ampicillin 2 g was administered with a 1-g dose repeated 6 hr later. Immediately thereafter, she began flossing daily. Two weeks later (2 weeks prior to admission) she developed fevers to 38°C, chills, night sweats, malaise, headache, and decreased appetite that resulted in a 7-pound weight loss.

Medical History

SF had a long history of mitral valve regurgitation, discovered in childhood. Two years prior to admission, the valve damage had become severe, and she underwent mitral valve replacement with a synthetic valve. Since this time, she has always taken prophylactic antibiotics prior to any high-risk procedure and has had no history of endocarditis or other infections. She has been taking warfarin daily since her valve replacement.

Medication History

Warfarin 2.5 mg QD
Diazepam 5 mg TID
Flurazepam 15 mg q.HS p.r.n. sleep

Allergies

None known

Social History

Tobacco: negative
Alcohol: negative

Review of Systems

Noncontributory

Physical Examination

GEN: Pale, elderly-appearing woman in no acute distress
VS: BP 120/70, HR 75, RR 13, T 39°C, Wt 60 kg, Ht 160 cm
HEENT: PERRLA, oral cavity without lesions or erythema, tympanic membranes normal without signs of inflammation. Roth spots seen upon ophthalmologic examination
COR: Systolic ejection murmur III/VI at the left sternal border, normal S_1 and S_2
CHEST: Clear to ascultation and percussion
ABD: Soft, nontender, no hepatosplenomegaly
RECT: Guaiac-positive
EXT: Embolic lesions seen on finger tips of both hands. Bruising noticed on both legs from thigh to ankle and upper arms.
NEURO: Oriented to time, place, and person; cranial nerves intact; normal deep tendon reflexes

Results of Laboratory Tests

Na 138 (138)	Hct 0.30 (30)	AST 0.58 (35)	Glu 5.55 (100)
K 4.2 (4.2)	Hgb 120 (12)	ALT 0.33 (20)	Ca 2.4 (9.7)
Cl 98 (98)	Lkcs 12 × 10⁹ (12 × 10³)	LDH 1.7 (101)	PO₄ 1.07 (3.3)
HCO₃ 22 (22)	Plts 170 × 10⁹ (170 × 10³)	Alk Phos 1.08 (65)	Mg 1 (2)
BUN 3.6 (10)	MCV 65 (65)	Alb 51 (5.1)	PT 29
CR 106 (1.2)		T Bili 13.7 (0.8)	ESR 55

Urinalysis: No organisms seen, clear, pH 7.5, SG 1.020, no RBC/Lkcs/casts
Chest x-ray: Normal
Transesophageal echocardiogram: Vegetation 1 × 2 cm found on mitral valve
Blood cultures: Pending

PROBLEM LIST

1. Prosthetic valve bacterial endocarditis
2. Anemia
3. Benzodiazepine addiction

QUESTIONS FOR CASE 144

1. Discuss the development of endocarditis in this patient despite the administration of antimicrobial prophylaxis for the dental procedure. Could this recur and what should be done in the future?
2. Why are serum bactericidal titers appropriate when the minimal inhibitory/bactericidal concentrations are already known?
3. Are there any antibiotics that should be avoided while SF is taking warfarin?
4. What is the antimicrobial therapy for streptococci that are moderately or fully resistant to penicillin?

CASE 145

CC: DA is a 17-year-old previously healthy boy who presents to a local emergency room with fever and altered mental status.

History of Present Illness

DA has had a 2-day history of intermittent fever and a painful headache unrelieved by extra-strength acetaminophen tablets. This morning DA complained of increasing lethargy and slept much of the remaining day. Six hours prior to admission, DA was difficult to arouse and had three documented episodes of vomiting.

Medical History

DA has a 3-year history of intermittent atrial fibrillation, associated with Wolff-Parkinson-White syndrome, which has improved on procainamide, which has not fully suppressed the arrhythmia.

Medication History

Procainamide 750 mg po q6h

Allergies

None known

Physical Examination

GEN: Male disoriented to person, place, and thing, in mild respiratory distress
VS: BP 135/72, HR 95 and regular, RR 30, T 40.5, Wt 62.5 kg (usual Wt 65 kg), Ht 170 cm
HEENT: Head was without trauma, ears clear, PERRLA, normal vessels without papilledema, normal dentition
NECK: Decreased mobility, positive Brudzinski's sign
COR: NL heart sounds, RRR
CHEST: Rales could heard on the right side, decreased breath sounds and dullness to percussion: right greater than left.

ABD: WNL
EXT: WNL
NEURO: Lethargic, not oriented to person, place, or thing, reflexes were 3+ throughout and symmetrical, motor was intact.

Results of Laboratory Tests

Na 145 (145)	Scr 80 (0.9)	Mg 1.05 (2.1)
K 4.0 (4.0)	HCT 0.46 (46.0)	Alb 45 (4.5)
Cl 105 (105)	Hgb 148 (14.8)	Glucose 5.0 (90)
HCO$_3$ 24 (24)	Lkcs 16.5 × 10^9 (16.5 × 10^3)	
BUN 6.4 (18)	Plt 285 × 10^9 (285 × 10^3)	

Cerebrospinal fluid: Lkcs 1.8 (1.8 k), 90% PMN
Glu 1.7 (30)
Protein 1.25 (125)
Gram's stain: gram-positive diplococci
Arterial blood gases: Room air; pH 7.48 pCO$_2$ 35 mm Hg pO$_2$ 90 mm Hg HCO$_3$ 24 mmol/liter O$_2$ Sat 90%

PROBLEM LIST

1. Wolff-Parkinson White syndrome with intermittent atrial fibrillation
2. Pneumococcal meningitis
3. Aspiration pneumonia

QUESTIONS FOR CASE 145

1. Could DA's current symptoms be caused by his intermittent atrial fibrillation?
2. What organism(s) is/are the leading cause of meningitis in this age group?
3. What drug therapy might have altered DA's clinical presentation?
4. What factors predisposed DA to aspiration pneumonia?
5. Should DA's aspiration be treated at this time?

CASE 146

CC: JC is a 25-year-old woman who is admitted to the hospital with fever, abdominal pain, and pain in the right index finger and wrist. She has complained of generalized pain and aches and loss of appetite for the past 3 days. JC also presents with anxiety and diaphoresis.

Medical History

JC was diagnosed 6 months ago in the outpatient clinic for pelvic inflammatory disease (PID) secondary to gonorrhea. At that time, she was successfully treated with the standard regimen of ceftriaxone 250 mg i.m. × 1 and doxycycline 100 mg po twice a day for 7 days. JC also admits to daily crack cocaine use. She has had two previous episodes of gonococcal disease, which were also treated.

Medication History

Norethindrone 0.5 mg, ethinyl estradiol 35 μg daily
Ibuprofen 200 mg q6h

Social History

JC admits to prostitution as the sole source of income. Averages 6–8 sex partners a day. Smokes approximately one pack of cigarettes per day. Drinks alcoholic beverages regularly. JC is a daily crack cocaine user.

Allergies

None known

Physical Examination

GEN: Well-developed woman complaining of fever, pain in abdomen and right index finger and wrist.
VS: BP 100/80, HR 98, T 39.2°C, Wt 55 kg
HEENT: Negative
COR: Heart rate regular with no murmurs
CHEST: WNL
ABD: Slight-to-moderate pain with rebound tenderness and guarding
GU: Slight vaginal discharge
RECTO: WNL
NEURO: Anxiety with feelings of weakness
EXT: Painful swollen joint in right index finger and pain in right wrist with limited range of motion
SKIN: Indurated needle puncture marks on antecubital fossa of left arm

Results of Laboratory Tests

Na 142 (142)	Hct 0.38 (38)	AST 0.167	Glu 6.5 (118)
K 4.8 (4.8)	Hgb 105 (10.5)	ALT 0.25 (15)	Ca 2.7 (10.8)
Cl 101 (101)	Lkcs 33 × 10^9 (33 × 10^3)	LDH 1.8 (110)	PO$_4$ 1.03 (3.2)
HCO$_3$ 24 (24)	Plts 260 × 10^9 (260 × 10^3)	Alk Phos 1.6 (95)	
BUN 4.3 (12)		Alb 35 (3.5)	
CR 79.6 (0.9)		T Bili 13.7 (0.8)	

Lkc differential: 85P
Urinalysis: WNL
Joint fluid, right index finger: purulent aspiration with many PMNs, Gram's stain shows gram-negative diplococci, blood cultures also positive
HIV: Negative

PROBLEM LIST

1. Probable disseminated gonococcal infection with infectious arthritis and tenosynovitis
2. Pelvic inflammatory disease
3. Cocaine abuse

QUESTIONS FOR CASE 146

1. What advantage does cefoxitin have over ceftriaxone in the treatment of JC?
2. Is there a difference in the cefoxitin dose for this patient?
3. Why was JC also started on doxycycline therapy?
4. What is the relationship of tenosynovitis in the diagnosis of this case?
5. What is the alternative drug therapy for PID in a patient who gives a history of β-lactam allergy?

CASE 147

AM is an anorexic 28-year-old woman who presents to clinic with complaints of lower abdominal pain and brown foul-smelling vaginal discharge. She also complains of frequency and burning upon urination, which she complained of 4 days ago and for which she was given a prescription for amoxicillin. This was her fourth urinary tract infection (UTI) in a year.

Medical History

Recurrent urinary tract infections
Gonorrhea × 2, Chlamydia × 1
Severe acne with scarring
Anorexia
Gravida IV, para III, s/p tubal ligation

Social History

AM is unmarried, with a history of multiple sexual partners. She currently lives with her new boyfriend and 3 children.
Denies smoking, alcohol use, and IVDA.

Medication History

Amoxicillin 500 mg orally three times a day for 7-day course
Tetracycline 250 mg orally twice a day as needed for acne flares

Allergies

Trimethoprim (TMP)/sulfamethoxazole (SMX)—rash

Physical Examination

GEN:	Thin woman in moderate distress
VS:	BP 100/80, HR 80, RR 16, T 99.7°F, Wt 50 kg, Ht 170 cm
HEENT:	Deep acne scars on face with whiteheads and blackheads
COR:	WNL
CHEST:	WNL
ABD:	Soft, tender bilaterally, increased suprapubic tenderness
GU:	Cervical motion tenderness, adnexal tenderness, foul-smelling drainage, and tampon in place × 1 week.
RECT:	WNL
EXT:	WNL
NEURO:	WNL

Results of Laboratory Tests

Na 136 (136)	Hct 0.38 (38)	ALT 0.58 (35)	Glu 5.6 (101)
K 4.2 (4.2)	Hgb 126 (12.6)	LDH 2.66 (150)	Ca 2.2 (8.8)
Cl 102 (102)	Lkcs 6 × 10⁹ (6 × 10³)	Alk Phos 2.0 (120)	PO₄ 1.28 (4.0)
HCO₃ 27 (27)	Plts 350 × 10⁹ (350 × 10³)	Alb 40 (4.0)	Mg 1.0 (2.0)
BUN 3.9 (11)	MCV 86 (86)	T Bili 18 (1.0)	Uric Acid 357 (6.0)
CR 80 (0.9)			

Lkcs differential: Neutrophils 0.68 (68), bands 0.07 (7), lymphs 0.13 (13), monos 0.08 (8), eos 0.02 (2)

Urinalysis: straw, clear, 1.005, 5.0 pH, prot-, gluc-, ket-, bact 0, Lkcs 0-1, RBC 0-1
Vaginal discharge: gram-negative diplococci, *Neisseria gonorrhoeae*—sensitivities pending
Positive monoclonal AB for *Chlamydia*, KOH preparation, wet preparation, and VDRL-negative

PROBLEM LIST

1. Severe acne
2. Anorexia
3. Urinary tract infection, recurrent UTIs
4. History of sexually transmitted diseases (STDs)
5. Pelvic inflammatory disease (PID)

QUESTIONS FOR CASE 147

1. If you had to treat AM's PID on an inpatient basis, outline a treatment plan for her PID including goals, monitoring parameters, and patient education.
2. What are the potential complications of PID and how can they be prevented?
3. Outline a treatment plan for AM's boyfriend.
4. How would you counsel AM and her boyfriend on safe sex and the proper use of condoms?
5. What other possible regimens are available to AM for prophylaxis of recurrent UTIs? List one advantage and one disadvantage of each regimen.

CASE 148

CC: YK is a 42-year-old woman who presents to the medical clinic with complaints of severe headaches, blurred vision, and pain in her eyes in sunlight, which had started 2 days ago. YK also complains of poor appetite due to pain on eating and swallowing.

Medical History

HIV-positive from IVDA, diagnosed 3 years ago
Oral candidiasis
Heroin overdose × 2

Surgical History

T & A at age 12
Appendectomy at age 23

Social History

Unemployed taxi driver
IVDA: heroin and cocaine × many years
Ethanol: occasional
Smoking: quit 6 months ago

Medication History

Zidovudine 200 mg po q4h
Clotrimazole troches 5 × daily

Trimethoprim/sulfamethoxazole (TMX/SMX) DS BID
Ketoconazole 200 mg po QD

Allergies

Penicillin—rash

Physical Examination

GEN: Ill-looking woman looking older than stated age, recent weight loss 5 kg since last visit to the clinic 6 weeks ago

VS: BP 105/60, HR 120, RR 28, T 38.5°C, Wt 50 kg, Ht 170 cm

HEENT: Fundi: yellow-white exudates with focal hemorrhages; oral cavity: white patchy plaques throughout the cavity and throat

COR: Rapid, normal heart sounds

CHEST: Clear

ABD: No pain or tenderness on examination

GU: WNL

RECT: Guaiac-negative

EXT: Thin, but WNL

NEURO: WNL

Results of Laboratory Tests

Na 138 (138)
K 4.1 (4.1)
Cl 98 (98)
HCO₃ 29 (29)
BUN 7.1 (20)
Cr 114 (1.3)
Hct .32 (32)

Hgb 108 (11)
Lkcs 2.1 × 10⁹ (2.1 × 10³)
Plts 220 (220)
MCV 110 (110)

Culture: Blood—CMV (+); oral and esophageal brush–Candida (+)

PROBLEM LIST

1. AIDS
2. CMV retinitis
3. Esophageal candidiasis

QUESTIONS FOR CASE 148

1. What if YK develops severe diarrhea?
2. What is the regimen for foscarnet in the treatment of YK's CMV retinitis?
3. Is there an alternative to intravenous drug therapy for the treatment of YK's CMV retinitis?
4. If YK were to request assistance to stop her heroin abuse, what would be an appropriate detoxification regimen for her?
5. What analgesics can you use for YK's headaches as well as AIDS-related generalized myalgia?
6. If YK should require prolonged intravenous home antibiotic therapy, what risks should you consider?

CASE 149

CC: RT is a 32-year-old woman S/P CRT for ESRD secondary to type I diabetes mellitus (DM), who presents with fevers, malaise, and worsening SOB. She reports flank pain in addition to scant urine production and increasing lower extremity edema over the past week. RT was admitted to the hospital to rule out transplant rejection and evaluate her fevers. A chest x-ray revealed RLL infiltrates, and on hospital day 2, RT underwent bronchoscopy to determine the cause of her pulmonary infiltrates.

Medical History

Transplant rejection 1 month PTA (treated with pulse high-dose steroids)

Type I DM × 19 years (blood glucose well-controlled on NPH and regular insulin)

ESRD × 1 year (secondary to DM; received hemodialysis 3 × / week prior to transplant)

Hypertension × 3 years (secondary to ESRD)

Peptic ulcer disease × 1 month (diagnosed at last hospitalization, currently on therapy for active disease)

Hyperlipidemia × 6 years. RT has a H/O hypercholesterolemia 9.8 (380) and hypertriglyceridemia (>4.5 [400]). She was initially managed with diet modification, and 6 months PTA she was started on gemfibrozil therapy.

Surgical History

S/P CRT 2 months PTA

Medication History

Cyclosporine 200 mg po BID
Prednisone 30 mg po q.AM
Acyclovir 800 mg po QID
Famotidine 40 mg po BID
Insulin 20 Units NPH s.q. q.AM/10 Units Regular s.q. q.AM/q.PM
Isradipine 5 mg po BID
Azathioprine 50 mg po q.h.s.

Allergies

None known

Physical Examination

GEN: Ill-appearing woman in apparent respiratory distress

VS: BP 170/94, HR 80, RR 26, T 39.2°C, Wt 58.2 kg (50.4 kg 2 weeks PTA), Ht 168 cm

HEENT: WNL
  COR: SR, nl S_1, S_2
CHEST: Decreased breath sounds RLL, diffuse rales
  ABD: Soft nontender, positive bowel sounds
   GU: Pain on palpation over graft site on left side
 RECT: Guaiac-negative stool
  EXT: 2+ edema bilat LE
NEURO: Alert, O × 4

Results of Laboratory Tests

Na 136 (136)	Hct 0.24 (24)	AST 0.5 (30)	Glu 18.9 (342)
K 4.8 (4.8)	Hgb 80 (8.0)	ALT 0.32 (19)	Ca 2.1 (8.6)
Cl 103 (103)	Lkcs 21.8 × 10^9 (21.8 × 10^3)	Alk Phos 1.45 (87)	PO$_4$ 1.2 (3.9)
HCO$_3$ 18 (18)	Plts 363 × 10^9 (363 × 10^3)	Alb 31 (3.1)	Mg 1.0 (2.0)
BUN 24.6 (69)		T Bili 6.8 (0.4)	Chol 8.84 (342)
CR 371 (4.1)			TG 1.89 (168)

Lkc differential: N 0.908 (90.8%), bands present, L 0.07 (7%), M 0.013 (1.3%), E 0.003 (0.3%), B 0.006 (0.6%)

Urinalysis: 3+ protein, (+) casts, 3+ glucose

Chest x-ray: RLL infiltrate

Bronchoscopy Cx: Aspergillus fumigatus

Renal biopsy: Lymphocytic infiltration of tubulointerstium (c/w acute rejection)

PROBLEM LIST
1. Type I DM
2. Hyperlipidemia
3. HTN
4. ESRD
5. Renal transplant rejection
6. PUD
7. Aspergillus pneumonia

QUESTIONS FOR CASE 149
1. What toxicities are associated with amphotericin B therapy?
2. How can the toxicities associated with amphotericin B therapy be managed?
3. Should the dosage of amphotericin B be reduced for renal insufficiency?
4. What adjunctive therapies can be used in combination with amphotericin B in the treatment of aspergillosis?
5. What is the role of fluconazole in the treatment of aspergillosis?

CASE 150
CC: KC is a 25-year-old man admitted to the Burn Unit 1 week ago following an explosion in the pharmacy where he worked in which he suffered burns over 70% of his body, with lung involvement. KC is intubated. He has been afebrile since admission, but for the past several days, KC has become increasingly disoriented. Today his temperature spiked to 40°C.

Medical History
Unremarkable

Medication History
Ringer's lactate 175 ml/hr
Enrich via jejunostomy tube (JT) 60 ml/hr
Metoclopramide 10 mg via JT q8h
Cimetidine 300 mg IV q8h
Silvadene to burn wounds QID

Allergies
Penicillin

Physical Examination
  GEN: Well-developed man with third-degree burns over 70% body surface area
   VS: BP 90/60, HR 100, RR 20, T 40°C, Wt 70 kg (admit) 75 kg (now), Ht 180 cm
HEENT: Facial burns, singed nasal vibrissae, singed eyebrows
  COR: No murmurs, rubs, or gallops
CHEST: Wheezes, bilateral rales
  ABD: Blood-tinged nasogastric aspirate, good bowel sounds, gastric residuals <10 ml
   GU: WNL, urine output 40 ml/ hr
 RECT: WNL
  EXT: Full-thickness burns of arms, partial-thickness burns of legs
NEURO: Oriented to person and place, decreased mental status

Results of Laboratory Tests

Na 155 (155)	CR 110 (1.2)	Alb 19 (1.9)	PO$_4$ 1.32 (4.1)
K 3.6 (3.6)	Hct 0.29 (29)	Glu 5.3 (96)	Mg 0.8 (1.7)
Cl 110 (110)	Hgb 110 (11)	Ca 2.0 (8.0)	Osm 275 (275)
HCO$_3$ 22 (22)	Lkcs 19 × 10^9 (19 × 10^3)		
BUN 5.4 (15)	Plts 322 × 10^9 (322 × 10^3)		

Lkc differential: Bands 0.13 (13%), Segs 0.82 (82%), Lymphs 0.015 (1.5%)

Chest x-ray: Interstitial edema and infiltrate throughout all lung fields

PROBLEM LIST
1. Burn
2. Fluid replacement/hypoalbuminemia
3. Nutrition
4. Stress ulcer
5. Sepsis

QUESTIONS FOR CASE 150
1. Blood and sputum cultures were obtained prior to starting antibiotics. Blood cultures grew *Enterobacter cloacae* sensitive to ciprofloxacin, imipenem, SMX/TMP, and gentamicin, but resistant to cefazolin, cefotetan, and ceftriaxone; and *Staphylococcus aureus* that is methicillin-resistant but vancomycin-sensitive. Sputum cultures also grew *Enterobacter cloa-*

cae with the same susceptibility pattern. How would these culture results change the antibiotic regimen KC is receiving?

2. There is a nationwide shortage of albumin, and the staff is asked to conserve the use of albumin. What are the alternative agents that can be used?

3. KC does not tolerate his enteral feedings at 100 ml/hr, but tolerates them at 80 ml/hr. What can be done to meet his nutritional requirements?

4. KC develops a severe rash, resembling exfoliative dermatitis. Reviewing his medication profile, what drug is most likely to cause this rash and what should be done? Medication profile includes:
   Cimetidine
   Vancomycin
   Metoclopramide
   SMX/TMP
   Gentamicin

5. It is now day 21 postburn, and KC has been receiving total parenteral nutrition for 7 days. His temperature has spiked again. This time blood cultures grew the same organisms as before with the same sensitivity patterns. However, sputum cultures now reveal gram-negative aerobes and anaerobes. What is the likely source of the new pathogen and what antibiotic(s) can be used to empirically treat this bacteria?

CASE 151

CC: LW is a 12-month-old, 15-kg girl who is brought to the clinic by her mother with a 3-day history of a "cold," lethargy, and irritability.

Medical History

LW has had a mild, nonproductive cough and runny nose, with increasing lethargy and irritability over the past 3 days. She began pulling on her right earlobe this morning. Her appetite is very poor, and she felt slightly warm to the touch. LW had one bout of otitis media 2 weeks ago. LW also has a history of chronic diaper rash.

Social History

LW lives with her mother and father, who are both recovering from the "flu."
LW has no siblings and does not attend daycare.

Medication History

Vitamin supplement 1 ml po QD
Amoxicillin 250 mg po TID (50 mg/kg/day)—completed a full 10-day course 3 days ago
Immunizations: DPT and TOPV at 2, 4, and 6 months of age

Physical Examination

GEN: Well-developed, well-nourished girl, crying, in moderate distress, tugging on right earlobe

VS: BP 100/68, HR 124, RR 30, T 39°C, Wt 15 kg
HEENT: Pale skin; right tympanic membrane red and bulging, no exudate seen; neck supple; scant clear, watery nasal discharge
COR: WNL, no murmur
CHEST: Good breath sounds, no rales or rhonchi
ABD: Soft, nontender, no distention, positive bowel sounds
GU: Erythema, tenderness, and inflammation over entire diaper area, vesicular satellite lesions on periphery of redness
RECT: Deferred
EXT: WNL
NEURO: Awake and alert with no focal findings

Results of Laboratory Tests

Na 140 (140)	Hct 0.42 (42.0)
K 4.5 (4.5)	Hgb 130 (13.0)
Cl 99 (99)	Lkcs 12 × 10⁹ (12 × 10³)
HCO₃ 26 (26)	Plts 230 (230)
BUN 2.9 (8)	Glu 4.4 (80)
Cr 53.0 (0.4)	

Lkc differential: Pending

PROBLEM LIST

1. Scheduled immunizations
2. Chronic diaper rash
3. Viral upper respiratory tract infection
4. Acute otitis media

CASE 152

CC: AG is a 33-year-old woman admitted for a severe flare-up of ulcerative colitis. Her PPD test result recently converted to positive. She has iron deficiency anemia, mitral valve prolapse, and arrhythmia, and is a problem pain patient.

Medical History

AG is a 33-year-old woman with a 15-year history of idiopathic ulcerative colitis (IUC) admitted to hospital after a 5-day history of increasing diffuse crampy abdominal pain, bloody stools, fevers, chills, and lightheadedness. Last flare of UC was 2 months ago, at which time she was begun on prednisone. She recently changed jobs and 1 month ago was noted to have a positive PPD reaction on a screening physical examination. PPD reaction 2 years earlier was negative. She has no pulmonary symptoms or signs. She was diagnosed with IUC 15 years ago. She also has iron-deficiency anemia and mitral valve prolapse, diagnosed 9 years ago by ECHO. She has recurring episodes of paroxysmal ventricular tachycardia (PSVT) with the initial diagnosis made 9 years ago. She presently is being treated with propranolol.

Social History

AG is married. She is employed as a nurse at a local teaching hospital. She denies tobacco or IV drug use. She admits to occasional alcohol use.

Family History

AG's father and mother are both alive and well. She has two young boys, ages 2 and 5, both in good health.

Allergies

NKDA

Medication History

Sulfasalazine 1 g po TID
Folate 1 mg po QD
Prednisone 15 mg po QD
Propranolol SR 60 mg QD
Iron sulfate 300 mg po BID

Review of Systems

Per HPI

Physical Examination

VS: (Supine) BP 120/70, HR 108; (Sitting) BP 100/60, HR 124, RR 22, T 38°C
HEENT: No lymphadenopathy, normal icterus, oropharynx dry
CHEST: Clear
COR: Tachycardic, regular, II/VI systolic flow murmur
ABD: Positive bowel sounds, moderate left lower quadrant tenderness, no rebound, no hepatosplenomegaly
EXT: No clubbing, cyanosis, or edema
RECT: Gross blood, no masses
GU: Normal genitalia, normal adnexa, normal cervix

Results of Laboratory Tests

Na 147 (147)	Hct 0.358 (35.8)	AST 0.63 (38)	Glu 5.77 (104)
K 4.2 (4.2)	Hgb 102 (10.2)	ALT 0.7 (42)	Ca 2.5 (10.2)
Cl 114 (114)	Lkcs 15.5 × 10⁹ (15.5 × 10³)	LDH 3.5 (210)	PO₄ 1.1 (3.4)
HCO₃ 21 (21)	Plts 695 × 10⁹ (695 × 10³)	Alk Phos 1.3 (76)	Mg 1.15 (2.3)
BUN 11 (31)	MCV 81 (81)	Alb 39 (3.9)	Uric Acid 250 (4.2)
CR 141 (1.6)		T Bili 15.4 (0.9)	Chol 3.88 (150)
		T Protein 85 (8.5)	PT 12.5
			PTT 34
			ESR 75

Lkc differential: Segs 0.75 (75), Band 0.12 (12), Lymph 0.08 (8), Eos 0.01 (1), Mono 0.02 (2)
Chest x-ray: No infiltrates or cavities, cardiac shadow normal
KUB: No air fluid levels
ECG: Tachy, sinus rhythm

PROBLEM LIST

1. Ulcerative colitis
2. Mitral valve prolapse
3. Arrhythmia
4. Iron-deficiency anemia
5. Recent PPD conversion
6. Abdominal pain secondary to UC

CASE 153

CC: HP is a 75-year-old black man admitted to the hospital for progressive abdominal discomfort and spiking fevers that started 1 week ago. HP also complains of chronic anorexia and back pains.

Medical History

HP has been on continuous ambulatory peritoneal dialysis (CAPD) since 1980 because of chronic renal failure secondary to uncontrolled hypertension. His dialysis has been efficiently performed without complications at home by his daughter until recently, when his daughter left for a vacation. HP has had the diagnosis of essential hypertension since age 35. His hypertension (HTN) has been poorly controlled because of noncompliance with his medication regimens. End-organ damage has been noted from HTN.

HP was diagnosed as having open-angle glaucoma in 1975, when he complained of visional field changes including loss of peripheral vision.

HP has a history of osteodystrophy and osteomalacia secondary to his chronic renal failure.

HP has also had chronic constipation because of his low-fiber diet and water intake, in addition to his aluminum and calcium therapies. His symptoms usually include mild anorexia and back pain.

HP has allergic rhinitis that is usually seasonal. "Allergy season will be starting soon according to my past experience."

Social History

Tobacco or cigarettes: none
Alcohol: occasional beer; 2 six-packs of cola per day
Lives alone, immobile most of the day

Surgical History

Placement of CAPD catheter 1980 without complication

Medication History

Epinephrine 2% 2 gtts OU BID
Captopril 25 mg QD
Furosemide 20 mg po BID
Ferrous sulfate 325 mg po TID
Aluminum hydroxide (Alucaps) 1 capsule with each meal
Calcium carbonate (oyster shell preparation) one tablet QD
Fleet enema QD for constipation

Allergies

Penicillin VK (rash on arms and legs 1987, denies SOB), was used to treat "strep throat."

Physical Examination

GEN: Man in moderate distress with fevers, chills, and acute abdominal discomfort

VS: BP 140/95, no orthostatic changes; HR 95, RR 25, T 40°C, Wt 80 kg (dry weight is 70 kg), Ht 157 cm (was 165 cm)

HEENT: Stable visual field deficits; IOP measurements— OD 45 mm Hg, OS 36 mm Hg; bilateral corneal and conjunctival pigmentation; gonioscopic examination reveals bilateral open angles; no cataracts; bilateral AV nicking

COR: Normal S_1 and S_2; no murmurs, rubs, or gallop

CHEST: Clear to auscultation and percussion

ABD: Diffuse tenderness upon palpation, guarding and rebound tenderness; erythema and exudate at exit site of CAPD catheter; no bowel sound

GU: Reduced urine output—approximately 5 ml/day

RECT: Guaiac-negative, no hemorrhoids, black stool

EXT: 2+ pedal edema

NEURO: Oriented to time, place, and person: cranial nerves intact; normal deep tendon reflexes (DTRs)

Results of Laboratory Tests

Na 143 (143)	Hct 0.35 (35)	AST 0.25 (15)	Glu 4.96 (90)
K 5.5 (5.5)	Hgb 120 (12)	ALT 0.33 (20)	Ca 1.75 (7.0)
Cl 102 (102)	Lkcs 20.8 × 10⁹ (20.8 × 10³)	LDH 1.5 (90)	PO₄ 2.68 (8.3)
HCO₃ 17 (17)	Plts 250 × 10⁹ (250 × 10³)	Alk Phos 6.67 (400)	Mg 2 (4)
BUN 25 (70)	MCV 85 (85)	Alb 37 (3.7)	Uric Acid 595 (10)
CR 610 (6.9)		T Bili 12 (0.7)	Triglycerides 6.32 (560)

Lkc differential: 0.85 (85%) PMN; 0.1 (10%) bands; 0.05 (5%) lymphs

Urinalysis: 1+ proteinuria

Chest x-ray: Mild LVH (left ventricular hypertrophy)

ECG: Normal sinus rhythm; no peaked-T waves

Abdominal ultrasound: CAPD catheter noted; stool impaction noted

Blood cultures × 3: Negative (final result)

Peritoneal dialysate specimen: Cloudy appearance, and white blood cell count of 650 cell/ml (85% PMNs)

Fluid Gram's stain: Many PMNs, no RBCs; many GPC in clusters

Peritoneal fluid culture: *Staphylococcus epidermidis*, positive for β-lactamase (penase)

Sensitivities: penicillin: resistant (MIC >2.0 µg/ml)

nafcillin: sensitive (MIC = 16.0 µg/ml)

rifampin: sensitive (MIC <0.125 µg/ml)

cefazolin: sensitive (MIC = 1.0 µg/ml)

vancomycin: sensitive (MIC = 1.0 µg/ml)

gentamicin: sensitive (MIC = 0.25 µg/ml)

PROBLEM LIST

1. Essential hypertension
2. Open-angle glaucoma
3. Renal failure—on CAPD
4. Osteodystrophy/osteomalacia
5. Chronic constipation
6. Acute bacterial peritonitis

CASE 154

CC: ML is a 6-year-old boy brought to pediatrics clinic by his mother, who states that he has had watery diarrhea, a "tummy ache," and fever of several days duration.

Medical History

ML has a history of multiple episodes of otitis media as a toddler. His last episode occurred 4 months ago. His physician prescribed ampicillin for treatment, and he completed a 10-day course.

He has a history of attention deficit disorder, diagnosed 2 months ago, when school teachers informed his mother that he was inattentive and often disruptive in class—calling out loudly and fidgeting in his seat. His mother states that he has always been "hyperactive," and she thought that it was something he would outgrow. When his school test scores were found to be poor, she thought that something else might be wrong. She states that his new medication has helped his attention span, but he is still very hyperactive and will not go to sleep at night.

He has a history of eczema off and on since infancy. His mother states that he tends to scratch it when it appears because it itches so much.

Family History

Mother: eczema
Sister: asthma

Medication History

Methylphenidate 5 mg po BID
Hydrocortisone cream 0.5% apply QD
Children's vitamins 1 po QD

Allergies

None known

Physical Examination

GEN: Well-developed, well-nourished, fidgety boy

VS: BP 117/68, HR 120, T 38.8°C (axillary), Wt 24 kg

HEENT: Tympanic membranes slightly erythematous with bilateral middle ear effusions; dry, leathery, erythematous excoriated areas on face and neck

COR: Sinus tachycardia, otherwise within normal limits

CHEST: Clear to auscultation

NEURO: Oriented × 3

Results of Laboratory Tests

Na 134 (134)   BUN 5.3 (15)
K 3.4 (3.4)   CR 35.4 (0.4)
Cl 97 (97)   Lkc 5.1 × 10⁹ (5.1 × 10³)
HCO₃ 20 (20)

Stool culture: Gram-negative rods identified as *Shigella sonnei*
Normal GI flora
Sensitivities: Pending

PROBLEM LIST

1. Eczema
2. Chronic otitis media
3. Attention deficit disorder
4. Diarrhea

CASE 155

CC: CR is a 3-year-old boy who was admitted for a 2-day history of lethargy, mental irritability, and confusion.

Medical History

CR was born to a mother who is hepatitis B-positive (HBsAg-positive). He had received hepatitis B immune globulin (HBIG) and the hepatitis B vaccine early during the neonatal period. CR has not demonstrated any episode of symptomatic hepatitis or a serologic diagnosis of hepatitis B infection. Upon reviewing his medical records, no documentation could be found for administration of the usual childhood vaccinations.

Medication History

No medications

Allergies

None known

Physical Examination

      GEN: Ill-appearing boy in moderate distress
       VS: BP 105/68, HR 125, RR 30, T 40.5°C, Wt 15 kg
     SKIN: Pale and dry
    HEENT: PERRLA, no papilledema, ears and nose clear, throat was without inflammation or exudate
     NECK: Without masses or bruits, stiff to movement, positive Brudzinski's sign
      COR: Normal S₁, S₂, (−) S3, (−) S4, normal rhythm
    CHEST: Clear to auscultation
      ABD: Positive bowel sounds, without tenderness
      EXT: Without trauma, full ROM, positive Kernig's sign
    NEURO: Lethargic, irritable, periods of confusion

Results of Laboratory Tests

Na 142 (142)   BUN 4.6 (13)   Plt 242 × 10⁹ (242 × 10³)
K 4.3 (4.3)   Cr 44.2 (0.5)   T Bili 13.7 (0.8)
Cl 102 (102)   HCT 0.44 (44.0)   ALT 0.37 (22)
HCO₃ 22 (22)   Lkcs 19.2 × 10⁹ (19.2 × 10³)   Glu 4.7 (85)

Cerebrospinal fluid: Cloudy appearance
Lkcs 2.3 × 10⁹ (2.3 × 10³), 90% PMN
Pro 1.28 (128)
Glu 1.5 (28)
Gram's stain: Many gram-negative rods

PROBLEM LIST

1. S/P Hepatitis B exposure
2. *Haemophilus influenzae* meningitis
3. Lack of immunizations

CASE 156

CC: GT is a 10-year-old black boy who presented to the emergency room with pain and tenderness in the right lower leg. He also complains of pain in the right knee, but states that the pain in the leg is worse. The pain in his leg had become progressively worse over the past 5 days.

Medical History

GT has a history of sickle-cell anemia and has been admitted to the hospital in the past for supportive treatment and pain management during sickle-cell crisis. GT states that he fell in the playground approximately 2 weeks ago. He attributed his pain to the development of ensuing sickle cell crisis. He had been taking acetaminophen, which seemed to help initially but does not appear to be effective now.

Medication History

Acetaminophen 325 mg q4-6h p.r.n. pain

Allergies

None known

Physical Examination

      GEN: Normal well-developed black boy in obvious pain
       VS: BP 110/75, HR 92, T 38.2°C, Wt 32 kg
    HEENT: WNL
    CHEST: WNL
      COR: WNL, no murmurs
      ABD: Spleen and liver slightly enlarged
       GU: WNL
      EXT: Pain and tenderness in right tibia with a fixed area that is red and swollen, aching pain in the right knee

Results of Laboratory Tests

Na 140 (140)
K 4.4 (4.4)
Cl 101 (101)
HCO₃ 26 (26)
BUN 4.3 (12)
CR 53 (0.6)

Hct 0.248 (24.8)
Hgb 81 (8.1)
Lkcs 20 × 10⁹ (20 × 10³)
Plts 230 × 10⁹ (230 × 10³)
RBC 3.6 × 1012 (3.6 × 106)

Blood cultures: Salmonella species (non-typhi)
X-ray of right tibia suggestive of osteonecroses
Bone scan (four-phase): Consistent with osteomyelitis of the tibia
Blood smear: Normochromic, normocytic cells and sickle cells

PROBLEM LIST

1. Pain in right knee secondary to sickle cell crisis
2. Possible osteomyelitis of the right tibia.

CASE 157

CC: EJ is a 33-year-old man admitted to the hospital because of continued fatigue, shortness of breath (SOB), fevers, and dry, nonproductive cough.

Social History

Tobacco: cigarettes 2 packs/day for 10 years
Alcohol: wine with dinner each evening

Medication History

Dideoxyinosine (DDI; Videx) 200 mg chew tablets po BID (started 4 months ago)
Dapsone 25 mg po QD
Ciprofloxacin 750 mg po QD
Ethambutol 800 mg po q.AM
Rifampin 600 mg po QD
Mylanta 15 ml q4h for upset stomach
Erythropoietin 4000 units s.q. 3 × weekly on M/W/F (12,000 u/week)
Fluconazole 100 mg po QD (ran out 2 weeks ago)

Allergies

Allergy to sulfamethoxazole/trimethoprim (Septra or Bactrim) with total body rash, erythema, and high fevers

Physical Examination

GEN: Ill-appearing cachectic man
VS: BP 150/90, HR 100, RR 25, T 41°C, Wt 50 kg (was 55 kg 1 month ago), Ht 168 cm
HEENT: White plaques on tongue, KOH-positive scraping consistent with thrush; eyes clear
COR: Normal S₁ and S₂; no murmurs, rubs, or gallop
CHEST: Bilateral wheezes and rhonchi
ABD: Bowel sounds present; splenomegaaly; hepatomegaly

GU: WNL
RECT: Guaiac-negative
EXT: Warm, dry skin; pale nail beds; ecchymoses on thighs
NEURO: Transient, intermittent tingling in fingers and toes; no numbness

Results of Laboratory Tests

Na 140 (140)
K 4.0 (4.0)
Cl 102 (102)
HCO₃ 19 (19)
BUN 3.2 (9)
CR 70.7 (0.8)

Hct 0.28 (28)
Hgb 100 (10)
Lkcs 2.4 × 10⁹ (2.4 × 10³)
Plts 90 × 10⁹ (90 × 10³)
MCV 95 (95)

AST 0.83 (50)
ALT 1.5 (90)
LDH 10.6 (634)
Alk Phos 1.83 (110)
T Bili 10.26 (0.6)

Uric Acid 594.8 (10)
Amylase 0.9 (54)

Arterial oxygen 65 mm Hg (on room air)
Serum cryptococcal antigen titer: Positive at 1:128
Glucose-6-phosphate dehydrogenase (G6PD) deficiency screening test—negative (sufficient enzyme present)
Total T cell count = 550; Helper (CD₄)/Suppressor (CD₈) = 50/500
Lkc differential: 0.75 (75%) PMN; 0 (0%) bands; 0.2 (20%) lymphs; 0.05 (5%) monos
Chest x-ray: Diffuse, bilateral interstitial infiltrates
ECG: Normal sinus rhythm; sinus tachycardia—100 rate
PPD skin test (1 month ago): Negative at 72 hr with negative controls
Induced sputum: Positive for *Pneumocystis carinii*

PROBLEM LIST

1. Human immunodeficiency virus infection–AIDS; switched off AZT because of dropping CD₄ count and severe anemia
2. Disseminated infection/ meningitis with *Cryptococcus neoformans*
3. Disseminated *Mycobacterium avium* complex (MAC) infection
4. *Pneumocystis carinii* pneumonia (PCP)

CASE 158

CC: RT is an obese 45-year-old woman who was admitted to the local general hospital for an elective cholecystectomy. She states that she has had recurrent abdominal pain, which radiates to the right upper quadrant of her abdomen. She has had approximately 4 attacks over the past year. The abdominal pain usually resolved within 1 hr or so. However, during her last attack (2 weeks ago), she experienced a low-grade fever, and therefore sought the attention of her primary medical doctor. She underwent several diagnostic studies, including a sonogram that revealed a thickened gallbladder wall, several large stones in the gallbladder, and a gallstone in the common bile duct. Her physician recommended that she undergo an elective cholecystectomy, for which she is admitted today.

Medical History

RT has a history of type II (non-insulin-dependent) diabetes mellitus (NIDDM) for which she was recently (2 months ago) started on glyburide. She also has a history of hypercholesterol-emia and hypertension. She is known to be noncompliant with both her medications and her dietary restrictions (low-salt, low-fat, low-cholesterol, 1200 calories ADA diet).

Medication History

Glyburide 5 mg po q. day
Captopril 25 mg po TID

Allergies

None known

Family History

Mother: diabetes mellitus, CAD, renal failure, myocardial infarction × 2; deceased
Father: hyperlipidemia, died of a stroke

Physical Examination

GEN:	Obese woman in no apparent distress
VS:	BP 132/88, HR 70, T 37.1°C, Wt 100 kg, Ht 150 cm
HEENT:	Retinopathy evidenced by dilated retinal blood vessels
COR:	Regular rhythm, no murmurs
CHEST:	Clear to auscultation and percussion
ABD:	Soft, nondistended, nontender
GU:	Examination deferred
RECT:	No masses, guaiac-negative
EXT:	Warm dry, few xanthomas noted on extremities
NEURO:	Intact

Results of Laboratory Tests

BUN 6.4 (18)	Hct 0.38 (38%)	AST 0.82 (49)
Cr 97.24 (1.1)	Hgb 130 (13)	ALT 0.86 (52)
Glu 12.2 (220)	Lkcs 4.9 × 10⁹ (4.9 × 10³)	LDH 1.67 (100)
LDL 5.17	Plts 165 × 10⁹ (4.9 × 10³)	Alb 50 (5)
HDL 0.91		T. Bili 37.62 (2.2)
PTT 12.2		
PTT 28		

Urine 2% glucose with Clinitest
Cholesterol 8.15 mmol/liter (315 mg/dl) mmol/liter (200 mg/dl) mmol/liter (35 mg/dl)
Triglycerides 4.52 mmol/liter (400 mg/dl)

PROBLEM LIST

1. Hypertension
2. Non-insulin-dependent diabetes mellitus (NIDDM)
3. Hypercholesterolemia
4. Chronic cholecystitis

CASE 159

CC: SH is a 65-year-old retired man who was admitted to the medicine service after suffering a stroke at home. He has left-sided hemiparesis as a result of the stroke. Over the past 3 days, SH has become more confused and lethargic. He also complains of feeling hot, occasional chills and shakes, and shortness of breath relieved by sleeping on a couple of pillows.

Medical History

Angina × 20 years, s/p myocardial infarction (MI) 10 years ago
Hypertension × 25 years, not controlled
Peptic ulcer disease × 30 years

Social History

Tobacco: 45 pack/year history
Alcohol: social drinker

Medication History

Atenolol 100 mg QD.
Hydrochlorothiazide (HCTZ) 100 mg QD
Verapamil SR 240 mg QD
Cimetidine 400 mg BID
Nitroglycerin SL p.r.n.
Mylanta II 30 ml p.r.n.
SH is compliant with his medications

Allergies

None known

Physical Examination

GEN:	Ill-appearing man who looks older than 65 years old
VS:	BP 150/95, HR 95, RR 23, T 39°C, Wt 100 kg (IBW 80 kg), Ht 180 cm
HEENT:	Skin hot to touch, +JVD
COR:	S3 gallop
CHEST:	Bibasilar rales
ABD:	Hepatomegaly
GU:	Foley catheter in place, I/O 2000/ 1500
RECT:	Stool guaiac-negative
EXT:	3+ pedal edema
NEURO:	Oriented to person and place

Results of Laboratory Tests

Na 135 (135)	BUN 7.1 (20)	Glu 6.1 (110)
K 3.1 (3.1)	CR 110 (1.3)	Uric Acid 590 (10)
Cl 110 (110)	Hgb 90 (9)	
HCO₃ 20 (20)	Lkcs 14 × 10⁹ (14 × 10³)	

Lkc differential: Bands 0.12 (12%), PMNs 0.85 (85%), Lymphs 0.005 (0.5%)

Urinalysis: SG 1.020, pH 5.7, Lkcs 500, esterase-positive, nitrite-positive

Urine culture: Gram-negative rods

Blood culture: Gram-negative rods

Echocardiogram: Left ventricular hypertrophy (LVH); 35% ejection fraction

CT scan of head: Infarct in posterior portion of the internal capsule

PROBLEM LIST

1. Peptic ulcer disease
2. Hypertension
3. Angina s/p MI
4. Congestive heart failure (CHF)
5. Hyperuricemia
6. Stroke
7. Sepsis

NEOPLASTIC DISORDERS

CASE 160

CC: RM is a 65-year-old man recently diagnosed with chronic lymphocytic leukemia (CLL) and treated with cyclophosphamide, who presented to the outpatient clinic complaining of weakness, lethargy, confusion, and a cough productive of yellow sputum. Laboratory data included: Scr 88.4 (1.0), Na 115 (115), serum osmolality 250 (250), urine osmolality 600 (600), and urine Na 55 (55). RM was diagnosed with cyclophosphamide-induced syndrome of inappropriate antidiuretic hormone (SIADH), and an acute exacerbation of chronic bronchitis.

Medical History

RM was diagnosed with stage IV chronic lymphocytic leukemia (CLL) 1 week earlier, when he presented to the clinic with fatigue, generalized lymphadenopathy, absolute lymphocyte count 7 (7000), Hct 0.22 (22), and platelets 17×10^9 (17×10^3). He was transfused with PRBCs and platelets and prescribed cyclophosphamide 150 mg po QD. RM has a history of major depression, chronic obstructive pulmonary disease (COPD) with chronic bronchitis, and degenerative joint disease (DJD). RM also has a 20 pack-year history of smoking.

Medication History

Cyclophosphamide 150 mg po QD
Albuterol inhaler 2 puffs q4h p.r.n.
Ipratroprium inhaler 2 puffs QID
Trazodone 150 mg po q.h.s.
Acetaminophen with codeine #3 (30 mg) 2 po q4-6h p.r.n.

Allergies

Penicillin (anaphylaxis)

Physical Examination

GEN: Weak-appearing, confused man
VS: BP 128/88, RR 22, HR 99, T 38°C, Wt 68 kg
HEENT: NC/AT, PERRL, EOMI
COR: Nl S1, S2, no murmurs
CHEST: Breath sounds diminished, coarse rhonchi, wheezes
ABD: Positive bowel sounds, soft NT, splenomegaly
EXT: No clubbing, cyanosis, or edema
NEURO: O × 3 with some mental confusion

Results of Laboratory Tests

Na 115 (115)   CR 88.4 (1.0)   Plts 120×10^9 (120×10^5)
K 3.5 (3.5)   Hct 0.35 (35)   Serum Osm 250 (250)
Cl 99 (99)   Hgb 120 (12)   Urine Osm 800 (800)
HCO₃ 25 (25)   Lkcs 3×10^9 (3×10^3)   Urine Na 55 (55)
BUN 3.6 (10)

PROBLEM LIST

1. COPD
2. Major depression
3. Degenerative joint disease
4. CLL
5. Cyclophosphamide-induced SIADH
6. Acute exacerbation of chronic bronchitis

CASE 160 SOAP NOTES

Problem 4. Chronic Lymphocytic Leukemia

S: RM presented 1 week earlier with fatigue and generalized lymphadenopathy.

O: Increased absolute lymphocyte count, decreased Hct and platelets at time of diagnosis

A: The symptoms of fatigue, generalized lymphadenopathy, lymphocytosis, anemia, and thrombocytopenia indicate that RM is suffering from chronic lymphocytic leukemia. RM will require maintenance therapy to keep his Lkc count down and reverse the anemia and splenomegaly. He was prescribed cyclophosphamide for chronic therapy. Cyclophosphamide may cause bladder cystitis, so patients should be informed to drink plenty of fluids. Chronic therapy with cyclophosphamide can also cause pulmonary fibrosis, so patients should have a baseline and periodic chest x-rays performed.

P: Continue cyclophosphamide 150 mg po QD with plenty of fluids. Check CXR at least yearly. RM will require monitoring of his CBC with differential, platelets, Hgb, Hct, BUN, Scr, and electrolyte, and urinalysis.

Problem 5. Cyclophosphamide-induced SIADH

S: RM presented with weakness, lethargy, and confusion.

O: Hyponatremia, decreased serum osmolality, increased urine osmolality, and increased urinary sodium

A: RM's weakness and confusion with hyponatremia, decreased serum osmolality, increased urine osmolality, and increased urine Na concentration are classic signs of SIADH. Because RM had these symptoms 1 week after beginning cyclophosphamide, the SIADH was most likely induced by cyclophosphamide. Cyclophosphamide has been reported to induce acute SIADH. Fluid restriction is the first-line therapy for SIADH. It is inappropriate to restrict fluids for RM, because he would be at an increased risk for developing cyclophosphamide-induced hemorrhagic cystitis. Because RM will require chronic management of his CLL, the therapeutic options are to choose another agent to treat his CLL or to treat through the SIADH and continue cyclophosphamide. One agent that may be used to reverse SIADH is demeclocycline.

P: Begin demeclocycline 300 mg po BID, and continue cyclophosphamide as prescribed. Demeclocycline may be increased to 1200 mg/day in 2–4 divided doses. If RM's SIADH fails to respond, it may be necessary to discontinue the cyclophosphamide and begin chlorambucil 0.1–0.2 mg/kg/day. RM will require close monitoring of his electrolytes and urinalysis.

Problem 6. Acute Exacerbation of Chronic Bronchitis

S: RM presented with a cough productive of yellow sputum.

O: Diminished breath sounds, coarse rhonchi, wheezes

A: RM has a long history of COPD with chronic bronchitis. His 20 pack/year history of smoking and his COPD increase his risk for recurrent acute exacerbations of his bronchitis. His productive cough and change in the color of sputum indicate the necessity for antibiotic therapy. Because RM has an anaphylactic allergy to PCN, first-line therapy could be either trimethoprim/sulfamethoxazole or erythromycin. However, RM is receiving demeclocycline for SIADH and this may be used to treat his acute exacerbation of his COPD.

P: Continue demeclocycline. If RM's bronchitis does not clear after 14 days, consider changing antibiotics. RM will require monitoring of his cough, sputum production, and breath sounds as well as SOB and other subjective symptoms.

Problem 1. Chronic Obstructive Pulmonary Disease

S: No subjective data

O: Diminished breath sounds, coarse rhonchi, wheezes, slightly increased respiratory rate

A: RM has a long history of COPD, probably secondary to his 20 pack-year history of smoking. He has diminished breath sounds, rhonchi, and wheezes and is slightly tachypneic on physical examination. His COPD is currently managed with a β_2-agonist (albuterol) and ipratroprium. It does not appear severe enough to require systemic steroids.

P: Continue current regimen of albuterol 2 puffs q4h p.r.n. and ipratroprium 2 puffs QID. Monitor RM's pulmonary function tests periodically. RM should be encouraged to stop smoking.

Problem 2. Major Depression

S: None

O: None

A: RM is not exhibiting or complaining of any signs or symptoms of depression. He is without any significant side effects on trazodone. Trazodone is generally well tolerated and can be increased to a maximum dose of 600 mg/day if necessary.

P: Continue trazodone 150 mg po q.h.s. Monitor RM for signs of dry mouth, sedation, orthostatic BP changes, or changes in his mood or affect.

Problem 3. Degenerative Joint Disease

S: None

O: None

A: RM suffers from degenerative joint disease. DJD is a common disorder in the aging population, although the exact cause is unknown. The main goal of therapy is to decrease pain and discomfort. First-line therapy for DJD is an antiinflammatory and analgesic agent. Narcotics should be avoided because patients require chronic therapy, and they may develop tolerance and/or dependency. Narcotics should be avoided in RM because they can also exacerbate depression. Because RM is taking cyclophosphamide (a bone-marrow suppressant), it would be best to avoid aspirin and nonsteroidal antiinflammatory agents because of their antiplatelet activity.

P: Discontinue acetaminophen with codeine. Begin acetaminophen 650 mg po q4-6h p.r.n.

QUESTIONS FOR CASE 160

1. One month later, RM returns to clinic complaining of priapism. What is the most likely cause, and what can be done about it?

2. At the same clinic visit, it is noted that RM's pulse is 140. He admits to increasing his albuterol dose to 4 puffs every 2 hr because his SOB has increased. How should RM's COPD regimen be altered to provide better control without unwanted side effects?

3. The physician is interested in using clonidine to help RM quit smoking. How is this done?

4. A few days after starting co-trimoxazole for another exacerbation of his COPD, RM returns with a rash. What is the most likely cause? What therapeutic intervention (if any) should be used?

CASE 161

CC: ST is a 45-year-old man presented to the emergency room with a 3 day-history of diffuse abdominal pain, fatigue, malaise, pallor, dysphagia, and up to 3–4 episodes of nausea and vomiting per day. The vomitus was usually watery except for this morning, when he had two episodes of bloody emesis. He last ate 5 days ago. Nasogastric (NG) aspirate in the ED was positive for 60 ml of red bloody material. ST was admitted to the Medicine Unit for supportive measure and further GI workup.

History of Present Illness

ST has experienced severe weight loss (40 lb) over the past 2 months and a change in his eating habits. Initially, he experienced early satiety which was unnoticeable until he began to lose weight. Approximately 5 months ago, ST began having upper epigastric pain associated with food, which he thought was secondary to indigestion. He took Maalox, which provided some relief. However, his episodes of pain worsened about 1 week ago; the pain is no longer epigastric but is associated with stomach cramps. The pain occurs throughout the day, had become debilitating to the point where ST is unable to sleep and go to work.

Medical History

Unremarkable except for hypertension diagnosed 7 years ago.

Family History

Father with prostate cancer diagnosed at age 50, and mother with hypertension diagnosed at age 45.

Social History

ST drinks occasionally at parties and smokes about 2 packs of cigarettes per month for 5 years.

Allergies

Penicillin (loss of consciousness at age 5)

Medication History

Procardia XL 30 mg po QD (last taken 3 days ago)
Maalox 30 ml po Q4hrs p.r.n. epigastric pain

Physical Examination

GEN: Thin, pale-looking 45-year-old man in severe distress
VS: Tm 37.0°C, BP 150/95, HR 90, RR 20, Ht 69 in, Wt 62 kg, BSA 1.74 m²
HEENT: (–) head, neck adenopathy, PERRLA, EOMI
COR: Sinus tachycardia, (–) murmurs or gallops
CHEST: Clear to auscultation and percussion
ABD: Diffuse tenderness and distention, (–) bowel sounds
GU: Unremarkable
RECT: (+) guaiac
EXT: Unremarkable
NEURO: Lethargic, oriented × 3, NL gait

Results of Laboratory Tests

Na 133 (133)	WBC 9.5×10^9 (9.5×10^3)	Mg 1.25 (2.5)
Hgb 16 (10.0)	Alb 23 (2.3)	BUN 12.9 (36)
LDH 2.00 (120)	PO₄ 1.59 (4.8)	AST 5.7 (342)
Glu 5.28 (95)	HCO₃ 26 (26)	PT 13.5
K 4.6 (4.6)	Plts 110×10^9 (110×10^3)	Scr 141.4 (1.6)
Hct 0.38 (38)	T Bili 32.7 (1.9)	ALT 7.32 (437)
Alk Phos 18.7 (1120)		Amylase 72 (72)
Ca 39.2 (9.8)		
Cl 104 (104)		

Additional diagnostic findings: (obtained 2 days after admission to the medicine unit)
Abdominal CT scan: (+) multiple liver mass, about 2 × 4 × 3 cm in diameter
Biopsy results: Consistent with adenocarcinoma

Chest CT scan: Normal
Chest x-ray: Clear, (–) infiltrates, (–) metastasis
Colonoscopy: Normal colon, (–) lesions
Barium upper GI series (UGI): Small discrete multiple ulcerative mass 2 cm in diameter with a central necrotic crater confined to the antrum mucosa
Biopsy results: Consistent with adenocarcinoma.
Pathology results: Poorly differentiated adenocarcinoma of signet-ring cell types

PROBLEM LIST

1. Gastrointestinal bleeding secondary to gastric adenocarcinoma
2. Stage IV gastric adenocarcinoma ($T_1N_0M_1$)
3. Prevention of chemotherapy-induced nausea and vomiting

Use SOAP for the above problems.

CASE 161 SOAP NOTES

Problem 1. Gastrointestinal Bleeding (GIB) Secondary to Gastric Adenocarcinoma

S: ST complaints of two episodes of bloody emesis the morning before emergency room presentation.

O: Clinical presentation with malaise, pallor, fatigue, and 60-ml heme-positive NG aspirate in the ER. Rectal examination showed positive guaiac. Workup 2 days after ST admission with barium upper GI series revealed small, discrete multiple ulcerative mass of 2 cm in diameter with a central necrotic crater confined to the antrum mucosa. Biopsy results are consistent with adenocarcinoma.

A: The cause of ST's GIB is attributable to his newly diagnosed stage IV gastric adenocarcinoma with liver metastasis. Gastric malignancies alone can cause bleeding, perforation, obstruction, and pain. The immediate concern for ST is to control the bleeding.

P: Initiate irrigation of the stomach with saline until nasogastric (NG) aspirate is clear. Saline irrigation helps provide an assessment of the rapidity and severity of bleeding, and helps clear the stomach of old blood prior to possible GI workup. Start hydration with IV normal saline 0.9% at 125 ml/hr to restore intravascular volume. The rate of volume infusion should be guided by the patient's condition, the degree of volume loss suspected, and the rate of active bleeding. Continue to observe for evidence of continued blood loss. Monitor recurrent hematemesis, changing vital signs (heart rate, blood pressure), hemodynamics, labs (CBC, platelet, prothrombin time [PT], partial thromboplastin time [PTT], and complete chemistries. Hemoglobin and hematocrit are poor indicators of acute blood loss, because these variables may be normal initially despite significant blood loss and may take hours to reflect the actual degree of hemorrhage.

Problem 2. Stage IV gastric adenocarcinoma ($T_1N_0M_1$)

S: ST complains of diffuse abdominal pain, fatigue, malaise, pallor, dysphagia, N/V up to 3–4 × / day with two episodes of hematemesis, and severe weight loss of 40 lb over the past 2 months. The weight loss is attributed to a change in his eating habits with early satiety.

O: Physical examination of the abdomen showed diffuse tenderness and distention with negative bowel sounds. Laboratory results showed elevation of hepatic enzymes. Abdominal CT scan showed multiple liver mass of about 2 × 4 × 3 cm in diameter. Biopsy results consistent with adenocarcinoma. Barium upper GI series showed the presence of a small, discrete multiple ulcerative mass 2 cm in diameter with a central necrotic crater confined to the antrum mucosa. Biopsy results consistent with adenocarcinoma. Pathology result revealed a poorly differentiated adenocarcinoma of signet-ring cell types. ST was then staged as having a $T_1N_0M_1$, stage IV gastric adenocarcinoma with liver metastasis.

A: Prognosis for ST stage IV gastric adenocarcinoma with liver metastasis is poor. Only 7.7% of patients with stage IV gastric adenocarcinoma survive 5 years. Treatment for primary gastric adenocarcinoma is surgery, with either subtotal gastrectomy or radical total gastrectomy, even in the presence of metastatic disease and adjuvant chemotherapy.

P: ST has elected to undergo subtotal gastrectomy plus adjuvant chemotherapy with methotrexate, 5-fluorouracil, leucovorin, and doxorubicin to begin 3 weeks after surgery. Chemotherapy regimen as follow with cycles repeated every 28 days or as tolerated:

Methotrexate 1.5 gm/m² IV D1
5-fluorouracil 1.5 gm/m² IV D1
Leucovorin 15 mg/m² PO Q 6 hrs × 48 hrs beginning 24 hrs after methotrexate (MTX)
Doxorubicin 30 mg/ m² IV D15

Common toxicities associated with the chemotherapy regimen received by ST are listed in the table below:

CHEMOTHERAPY	ADVERSE REACTIONS
Methotrexate (Rheumatrex) a folate antimetabolite	>10%: myelosuppression, mucositis (dose-limiting, occurs about 5–7 days after therapy, usually resolves within 2 wks), renal failure (common in high dose >3 gm, manifested by an abrupt ⊂ BUN/SCr), nephropathy, hyperuricemia, thrombocytopenia, nausea
1–10%: malaise, fatigue, dizziness, fever, confusion, HA, seizures
5-fluorouracil (Adrucil) a pyrimidine antimetabolite	>10%: heartburn, stomatitis, dermatitis, anorexia, alopecia, diarrhea, N/V (dose-dependent)
1–10%: GI ulceration, dry skin, myelosuppression (granulocytopenia, thrombocytopenia)
Leucovorin (Wellcovorin) methotrexate rescue	<1%: rash, pruritus, erythema, urticaria, wheezing, thrombocytosis
Doxorubicin (Adriamycin) an anthracycline antibiotic *vesicant*	>10%: alopecia, GI (dose-dependent acute N/V, mucositis, ulceration, necrosis of the colon, anorexia, diarrhea), dose-dependent myelosuppression (especially leukopenia)
1–10%: cardiac toxicity (dose-limiting and related to cumulative doses of >550 mg/m²)

Problem 3. Prevention of Chemotherapy-induced Nausea and Vomiting

S: ST is chemotherapy-naive.

O: None

A: Since ST is chemotherapy-naive, prevention of chemotherapy-induced nausea and vomiting with the initial course of chemotherapy is important to prevent the development of anticipatory nausea and vomiting with subsequent courses of chemotherapy. ST is to receive chemotherapy with methotrexate, 5-fluorouracil, leucovorin and doxorubicin beginning 3 weeks after subtotal gastrectomy. The emetogenicity of ST chemotherapy regimen are listed in the table below:

CHEMOTHERAPEUTIC AGENTS	EMETOGENIC POTENTIAL
Methotrexate 1.5 gm/m²	Moderately emetogenic
5-Fluorouracil 1.5 gm/m²	Moderately emetogenic
Doxorubicin 30 mg/m²	Moderately emetogenic

The emetogenicity of chemotherapy increases when combination chemotherapy is administered. ST chemotherapy regimen contained three moderately emetogenic chemotherapy combination which is likely to be highly emetogenic. Consider giving an aggressive antiemetic regimen (i.e., 5HT3 receptor antagonist plus dexamethasone) prior to the initiation of chemotherapy.

P: Start either IV granisetron 10 mcg/kg Q24hrs or Ondansetron 0.15 mg/kg Q4hrs × 3 doses plus dexamethasone 10 mg × 1 about 30 minutes prior to the start of chemotherapy and continue until the end of chemotherapy. Both granisetron and ondansetron are generally well tolerated. Most frequent adverse effects observed are headache and constipation, both of which occur in about 10%–15% of patients. Headache is self-limiting but can be easily treated with acetaminophen if needed. Hot flashes have recently been reported in patients receiving granisetron and dexamethasone; however, it is unclear whether the hot flashes were due to granisetron or dexamethasone. Other adverse effects include somnolence, asthenia, and diarrhea. A clear association with the 5HT3 antagonists has not been established. No extrapyramidal side effects have been reported with the use of 5HT3 antagonists.

QUESTIONS FOR CASE 161

1. What is the current epidemiologic data on gastric adenocarcinoma?
2. What risk factors are associated with gastric adenocarcinoma?
3. Describe the common clinical presentation of patients with gastric adenocarcinoma.
4. How important is screening for early detection of gastric adenocarcinoma?
5. List the common sites of metastases commonly seen in patients with advanced gastric adenocarcinoma.
6. Discuss the different surgical interventions between subtotal gastrectomy and radical total gastrectomy for management of gastric adenocarcinoma.

CASE 162

CC: MF is a 54-year-old postmenopausal woman who was diagnosed 4 months ago with an estrogen-receptor-negative (ER(–)) infiltrating intraductal carcinoma of the right breast. MF is currently undergoing a 6-month course of chemotherapy with cyclophosphamide, doxorubicin, and 5-fluorouracil. During her last course of chemotherapy, she experienced nausea and vomiting up to 2–3 × /day for 2 days after chemotherapy, alopecia, fatigue and a 7-pound weight loss. MF now presents to the Oncology Clinic for her second cycle of chemotherapy and expresses great anxiety about nausea and vomiting, decreasing appetite, weight loss, and further treatment for her breast cancer.

History of Present Illness

MF was in her usual state of health until 4 months ago when on breast self-examination, she found a lump under her arm and sought immediate medical attention from her ob-gyn. Physical examination at the time showed a firm, irregular, fixed nontender nodule in the outer quadrant of the right breast. Mammogram showed a 6 × 3 × 4-cm nodule. Biopsy results were consistent with infiltrating intraductal carcinoma. MF underwent a modified radical mastectomy with axillary node dissection 3 months ago. Pathology revealed a (+) 16/17 lymph-node involvement. The tumor was estrogen-receptor- and progesterone-receptor-negative. MF was then staged as having a $T_3N_1M_0$, stage IIIA, high-risk breast cancer.

Medical History

Cholecystectomy 14 years ago, and a hysterectomy 10 years ago. She has a history of a benign left breast mass. Since her recent diagnosis, MF has been withdrawn and depressed according to family members.

Family History

Grandmother who died of breast cancer at age 65, and a maternal aunt who has had breast cancer since age 40 and is still living.

Social History

Does not smoke or drink alcohol

Allergies

None

Medication History

Conjugated estrogens (Premarin) 0.625 mg po QD
Multivitamin 1 tab po QD
Docusate sodium 100 mg po BID
Chemotherapy regimen: Cycle repeat Q 28 days
Cyclophosphamide 100 mg/m² po D1–14
Doxorubicin 30 mg/m² IV D1,8
5-fluorouracil 500 mg/m² IV D1,8

Physical Examination

GEN: Thin, anxious, withdrawn looking 54-year-old woman
VS: Tm 37.0°C, BP 110/80, HR 80, RR 20, Ht 65 in, Wt 56.7 kg, BSA 1.61m²
HEENT: (–) head, neck adenopathy, alopecia, PEERLA, EOMI
COR: RRR, nl S_1, S_2 CHEST: Clear to auscultation and percussion
ABD: Two well-healed surgical scars; no hepatomegaly
GU: Unremarkable
RECT: Unremarkable, (–) guaiac
EXT: Unremarkable
NEURO: Alert and oriented × 3, NL gait

Results of Laboratory Tests

Na 139 (139)	Ca 43.2 (10.8)	Mg 0.75 (1.5)
Hgb 16 (10.0)	Cl 100 (100)	BUN 7.1 (20)
LDH 3.67 (220)	WBC 3.5 × 10⁹ (3.5 × 10³)	AST 0.58 (35)
Glu 5.28 (95)	Alb 35 (3.5)	PT 13.7
K 4.0 (4.0)	PO₄ 0.83 (2.5)	Scr 97.2 (1.1)
Hct 0.30 (30)	HCO₃ 26 (26)	ALT 0.50 (30)
Alk Phos 1.55 (93)	Plts 100 × 10⁹ (100 × 10³)	
	T Bili 10.3 (0.6)	

Echocardiogram: EF 75%
Abdominal CT scan: Normal
Chest x-ray: Clear, (–) infiltrates, (–) metastasis
Bone scan: Some uptake in the cervical spine
Cervical spine, thoracic spine, pelvis films: Normal, (–) metastasis

PROBLEM LIST

1. Stage IIIA breast cancer
2. Depression
3. Delayed N/V
4. Poor appetite, weight loss

Use SOAP for the above problems.

CASE 162 SOAP NOTES

Problem 1. Stage IIIA Breast Cancer

S: MF on breast self-examination found a lump under her arm 4 months ago

O: Physical examination at the time showed a firm, irregular, fixed nontender nodule in the outer quadrant of the right breast. Mammogram showed a 6 × 3 × 4-cm nodule. Biopsy results were consistent with infiltrating intraductal carcinoma. Pathology results revealed a (+) 16/17 lymph nodes involvement. The tumor was estrogen- and progesterone-receptor-negative. MF was staged as having a $T_3N_1M_0$ stage IIIA breast cancer. MF also has a history of a benign left breast mass, and strong family history of breast cancer.

A: Treatment for stage IIIA breast cancer involves multimodality therapy (surgery, radiation, and chemotherapy) because of the high local-regional recurrence rate (50%–67%). MF had stage IIIA (locally advanced but operable) breast cancer that was at high risk for recurrence because of having greater than 10 involved lymph nodes. MF underwent a modified radical mastectomy with axillary node dissection 3 months ago, and is now receiving a 6-month course of combination chemotherapy. Overall response rates with combination chemotherapy can be up to 90% with 15% complete responses, as well as improved 5-year disease-free survival of 28%–60% and overall survival of 48%–60%.

P: Plan to continue with cycle 2 of induction chemotherapy with cyclophosphamide, doxorubicin, and 5-fluorouracil. Duration of chemotherapy for stage IIIA breast cancer is at least 6 months. Common toxicities associated with the chemotherapy regimen received by MF are listed in the table below:

CHEMOTHERAPY	ADVERSE REACTIONS
Cyclophosphamide (Cytoxan) an alkylating agent	>10%: myelosuppression (especially leukopenia), reversible alopecia, hemorrhagic (bladder) cystitis cardiac dysfunction (CHF, rarely but fatal cardiac necrosis or hemorrhagic myocarditis), N/V 1–10%: thrombocytopenia, anemia, diarrhea, facial flushing
Doxorubicin (Adriamycin) an anthracycline antibiotic *vesicant*	>10%: alopecia, GI (dose-dependent acute N/V, mucositis, ulceration, necrosis of the colon, anorexia, diarrhea), dose-dependent myelosuppression (especially leukopenia) 1–10%: cardiac toxicity (dose-limiting and related to cumulative doses of >550 mg/m²)
5-fluorouracil (Adrucil) a pyrimidine antimetabolite	>10%: heartburn, stomatitis, dermatitis, anorexia, alopecia, diarrhea, N/V (dose-dependent) 1–10%: GI ulceration, dry skin, myelosuppression (granulocytopenia, thrombocytopenia)

Problem 2. Depression

S: None

O: Family members reported MF to be withdrawn and depressed since her recent diagnosis of breast cancer. General appearance on physical examination showed a thin, anxious, withdrawn-looking woman.

A: MF is experiencing common emotional reactions to breast cancer, including anxiety, depression, and social withdrawal. Learning to deal with such feelings is an important task for all patients with cancer. Social support increasingly is recognized as a powerful tool to reduce anxiety and depression, enhance coping, and even possibly to extend life.

P: Refer MF for skilled intervention and counseling with either a psychologist, psychiatrist or clinical social worker with expertise in the treatment of women with breast cancer or other types of life-threatening illness. Also, encourage MF to participate in self-help and support groups for women coping with breast cancer where MF may obtain valuable support and feedback from individuals who share similar experiences and concerns. If MF continues to be depressed after the above attempts, an antidepressant such as TCA or SSRI may be considered as an adjunctive treatment.

Problem 3. Delayed N/V

S: MF complains of N/V 2–3 × /day for 2 days after her last course of chemotherapy

O: None

A: The emetogenicity of MF chemotherapy regimens are listed in the table below:

CHEMOTHERAPEUTIC AGENTS	EMETOGENIC POTENTIAL
Cyclophosphamide 100 mg/m²	Moderately emetogenic
Doxorubicin 30 mg/m²	Moderately emetogenic
5-fluorouracil 500 mg/m²	Mildly emetogenic

The emetogenicity of chemotherapy increases when combination chemotherapy are administered. MF's chemotherapy regimen contain two moderately emetogenic chemotherapy agents which may very well be highly emetogenic when administered in combination. However, the likelihood of delayed N/V from this chemotherapy regimen is not very high. The fact that MF did experience some delayed N/V from this regimen should not be ignored.

P: Plan to start MF on prochlorperazine (Compazine) 10 mg po Q6h p.r.n. N/V. If this regimen fails to control MF's delayed N/V, switch to metoclopramide and low-dose dexamethasone p.r.n. May also educate MF on some nonpharmacologic methods to help decrease N/V such as:
1. Restrict intake to only liquids for several hours preceding chemotherapy
2. For several days after chemotherapy, consume only small, light, bland meals (avoid greasy, spicy, and sweet foods)
3. Advance diet as tolerated
4. Avoid stress and unpleasant environmental stimuli
5. Restriction of activity may help
6. Relaxation techniques

Problem 4. Poor Appetite, Weight Loss

S: MF complains of decreasing appetite, weight loss, and fatigue after her last course of chemotherapy

O: Weight loss of up to 7 pounds over a month in this thin woman who currently weighs 56.7 kg. Ideal body weight is 57 kg for a woman of her height. However, her albumin level is only 35 (3.5), which is little low, indicating decreased body protein stores.

A: Loss of appetite can be a problem for cancer patients. Patients may not feel hungry when they are uncomfortable or tired. Weight loss of up to 7 pounds is unusual with MF's current chemotherapy regimen, although MF's weight loss might be attributable to her poor appetite and N/V after chemotherapy, and her depression over her recent diagnosis of breast cancer. Good nutrition is important. Eating well means getting enough calories and protein to help prevent weight loss, regain strength, and rebuild normal tissues. Patients who eat well often feel better and have more energy, and are better able to withstand the side effects of their treatment.

P: A review of MF's dietary history, including what she is eating and how often, will be important in the assessment of MF's nutritional intake. Advise MF to eat several small meals and snacks during the day rather than trying to have three large meals. May also want to refer MF to a registered dietitian who can design an individual nutritional regimen for MF.

QUESTIONS FOR CASE 162

1. What are the current American Cancer Screening Guidelines for Breast Cancer?
2. What is the rationale for using breast self-examination as an early detector for breast cancer? Describe the steps of how to do a breast self-examination (BSE).
3. How is breast cancer clinically staged and what are some of the sites of metastases?
4. What is the role of tamoxifen in the management of breast cancer?
5. What is Taxol and how should it be administered?

CASE 163

CC: AV is a 52-year-old man who comes to the clinic complaining of blood in the stool, which he has been noticing for 2 weeks. He also reports feeling increasingly fatigued, some vague right upper-abdominal discomfort, and a 10-lb weight loss over the past 5 months.

Medical History
Noncontributory

Medication History
He has been in good health and is not taking any medications.

Social History
Noncontributory.

Physical Examination

GEN: Appears well developed, well nourished
VS: BP 120/80, HR 85, both standing and supine
HEENT: Mild pallor of the conjunctiva
COR: WNL
CHEST: Clear
ABD: The liver is hard, nodular, and palpable at 4 cm below the right costal margin. Total span, 12 cm.
GU: WNL
RECT: No masses felt; stool strongly positive for occult blood

Double-contrast barium enema: A nonobstructing apple-core lesion in the descending colon

CT scan: Multiple 2- to 3-cm mass lesions in both right and left hepatic lobes consistent with metastatic tumor

Biopsy of the colon lesion: Mucinous adenocarcinoma of the colon

Results of Laboratory Tests

Na 140 (140)	Hct 0.31 (31)	AST 1.0 (60)	Glu 4.7 (85)
K 4.0 (4.0)	Hgb 105 (10.5)	ALT 0.92 (55)	Ca 2.3 (9.1)
Cl 98 (98)	Lkcs 7.9 × 10⁹ (7.9 × 10³)	LDH 4.9 (190)	PO₄ 1.5 (4.8)
HCO₃ 20 (20)	Plts 400 × 10⁹ (400 × 10³)	Alk Phos 3.1 (185)	Mg 1.0 (2.0)
BUN 5.4 (15)	MCV 78 (78)	Alb 40 (4.0)	Uric Acid 416 (7)
CR 88.4 (1.0)		T Bili 12 (0.7)	

Lkcs differential: Normal
Peripheral blood smear: Microcytic, hypochromic RBCs with increased number of platelets
Urinalysis: WNL
Chest x-ray: Normal
ECG: Normal

PROBLEM LIST

1. Colon cancer, stage IV, with liver metastasis
2. Iron-deficiency anemia

CASE 163 SOAP NOTES
Problem 1. Adenocarcinoma of the Colon

S: AV complains of a 2-week history of blood loss, increasing fatigability, and vague right upper-abdominal discomfort.

O: AV has enlarged, nodular liver on palpation, positive findings on BE, CT scan, and biopsy of the colon mass, and abnormal SMA-12 of the colon mass and elevated AST, ALT, LDH, and bilirubin levels.

A: AV has colon cancer, stage IV, with liver metastasis; therefore only systemic chemotherapy would be beneficial.

P: Obtain baseline CEA (carcinoembryonic antigen) and recheck in 6 weeks as an indicator of tumor recurrence. Start chemotherapy for systemic disease. Fluorouracil 450 mg/m²/day IV for 5 days and then 450 mg/m² weekly, starting 28 days later. Also begin oral leucovorin, 10 mg/m² every 6 hr for five doses, every other week. Monitor CBC, platelets, LFTs, Cr, and CT scan, liver size, and patient's symptoms. Monitor for side effects of chemotherapy (nausea, vomiting, stomatitis, and diarrhea).

Problem 2. Iron-Deficiency Anemia

S: Recent onset of fatigue; history of recent blood loss

O: Blood in the stool; decreased Hgb and Hct levels; decreased MCV.

A: Iron-deficiency anemia is probably secondary to his blood loss from tumor involvement.

P: Parenteral iron replacement should be considered, because AV is an inappropriate candidate for oral iron at this time because of the unknown extent from gastrointestinal loss. Monitor Hgb and Hct levels, MCV, ferritin concentration, guaiac tests on stools. Advise AV that oral iron therapy may discolor stools (black).

QUESTIONS FOR CASE 163

1. What subjective and objective information does AV have that is consistent with colon cancer?
2. Explain the rationale for obtaining a CEA level.
3. Explain why you agree or disagree to begin prophylactic antibiotic therapy.
4. While receiving his chemotherapy, AV begins to develop stomatitis/mucositis.
   a. What is stomatitis/mucositis?
   b. What are the signs and symptoms?
   c. Which types of organisms is AV susceptible to?
   d. List ways to prevent stomatitis/mucositis.
5. Should AV's elevated platelet count be of concern?

CASE 164

CC: ML is a 72-year-old man diagnosed with pancreatic cancer admitted for pain control, progressive nausea with occasional vomiting, and fatigue. His pain is mainly in the right upper abdomen and epigastric area and can be severe at times. Pain is partially relieved by sitting up, rather than lying. The nausea has prevented him from taking the pain medication as frequently as prescribed, because it worsens the nausea. Despite his poor oral intake, he states that he has to urinate frequently, but only a small amount each time and it burns.

Medical History

Benign prostatic hypertrophy
Ulcer 10 years ago
Hypertension × 10 years

Surgical History

TURP 4 years ago
Appendectomy 40 years ago

Medication History

Hydrochlorothiazide 50 mg + triamterene 75 mg—one every morning
Acetaminophen with codeine 60 mg 1-2 tablets every 4–6 hr
Ibuprofen 600 mg four times daily

Chemotherapy History

Leucovorin 20 mg/M^2/day[7] over 2 hr × 5 days
5-Fluorouracil 400 mg/M^2/day[8] over 15 min × 5 days
Course 2 finished 1 week ago

Allergies

Morphine (hives)
Sulfa (rash)

Physical Examination

VS: BP supine 120/80, HR 82, standing BP 96/60, HR 105, T 38.1°C, Wt 74 kg (80 kg a month ago)
HEENT: Dry mucous membranes, slight oral erythema
COR: WNL
ABD: Tenderness in epigastrium and right upper abdomen
GU: WNL
RECT: Trace guaiac-positive
NEURO: WNL
EXT: Poor skin turgor

Results of Laboratory Tests

Na 148 (148)	Hct 0.44 (44)	AST 1.1 (6.7)	Glu 5.6 (101)
K 4.8 (4.8)	Hgb 139 (13.9)	ALT 0.7 (42)	Ca 1.97 (7.9)
Cl 106 (106)	Lkcs 6.7 × 10^9 (6.7 × 10^3)	LDH 3.2 (190)	PO$_4$ 0.8 (2.4)
HCO$_3$ 25 (25)	Plts 167 × 10^9 (167 × 10^3)	Alk Phos 2.0 (122)	Mg 1.2 (2.4)
BUN 13.6 (38)		Alb 30 (3.0)	
CR 150 (1.7)		T Bili 18.8 (1.1)	

Urinalysis: Many Lkcs, few RBCs, gram-negative rods >10^5 bacteria per ml

Urine culture/sensitivities: *Escherichia coli*
Tetracycline (R) Nitrofurantoin (R)
Cephalothin (S) Sulfamethoxazole (S)
Ampicillin (S) Carbenicillin (S)
Gentamicin (S) Erythromycin (R)
Tobramycin (S) Penicillin G (R)

CT abdomen: 5-cm mass in head of pancreas, enlarged lymph nodes, multiple liver mets, slightly dilated biliary ducts. Impression: disease progression compared with pretreatment scan.

Chest x-ray: WNL

KUB: No evidence of intestinal obstruction

Upper endoscopy: Diffuse erythema, small erosions, no definite ulcers

PROBLEM LIST

1. Hypertension
2. History PUD—inactive
3. BPH-S/P TURP
4. Pancreatic cancer
5. Dehydration
6. Nausea/vomiting/gastritis

7. Pain
8. Urinary tract infection

CASE 164 SOAP NOTES
Problem 4. Pancreatic Cancer Metastatic to Liver (Stage IV)

S: ML is experiencing epigastric and right-sided abdominal pain. He also has nausea, which could be secondary to cancer.

O: CT scan shows mass in pancreas as well as liver mets.[9] LFTs are slightly elevated. Weight loss.

A: ML has stage IV pancreatic cancer, status post two cycles of chemotherapy. He does not appear to be responding to current chemotherapy.

P: Provide supportive care (antiemetics, pain control, nutrition). Consider phase I investigational chemotherapy after symptoms are controlled.

Problem 5. Dehydration

S: ML is experiencing anorexia and fatigue. He admits to poor oral intake.

O: ML has orthostatic hypotension with increased pulse, dry mucous membranes, and poor skin turgor. BUN: Cr ratio >20:1

A: Dehydration (total body salt and water deficit) secondary to poor oral intake and diuretic use; hypovolemic hypernatremia

P: Consider getting urine electrolytes and plasma osmolality to help evaluate dehydration.

   Discontinue hydrochlorothiazide 50 mg + triamterene 75 mg, reevaluate need for antihypertensives after patient is hydrated.

   Replace fluid deficit over 48 hr. Start an intravenous infusion of normal saline at 250 ml/hr. Give 2 liters of normal saline (to replete intravascular volume), then change fluids to D51/4 or D51/2 normal saline at 150 ml/hr for next 36 hr. This should replace salt and water deficits. Once deficits are replaced, maintenance fluids of approximately 1500 ml/m^2/day plus any losses (2–4 liters/ day) will be required until ML resumes adequate oral intake. Replace electrolytes in IV fluids as needed. Monitor serum Na and K, BP, HR, urine output, skin turgor, and mucous membranes. Reassess every 4–6 hr during first 24–48 hr.

Problem 6. Nausea/Vomiting/Gastritis

S: ML is experiencing nausea that appears to be getting worse. He complains of pain in epigastric area and inability to eat or drink secondary to the nausea and vomiting.

O: Nausea, vomiting, poor oral intake, weight loss; gastritis on endoscopy; no evidence of intestinal obstruction; trace guaiac-positive stool

A: ML has pancreatic cancer, received chemotherapy, has been taking oral pain medication (ibuprofen and acetaminophen with codeine), and is dehydrated, all of which can contribute to nausea.

   ML has gastritis secondary to chemotherapy (mucositis), NSAID use, and poor oral intake.

P: Hydrate ML as above. Discontinue ibuprofen because gastric irritation may worsen nausea and gastritis. Discontinue oral acetaminophen with codeine. Use parenteral pain medication until ML can take oral medications. Start prochlorperazine 10 mg IV every 6 hr p.r.n. nausea; can continue prochlorperazine 10 mg po every 6 hr p.r.n. nausea when oral intake is adequate. Start H$_2$-antagonist to decrease gastric irritation and prevent gastrointestinal bleeding. Adjust dosage for renal impairment (estimated CrCl <0.83 ml/sec (50 ml/min)) and switch to oral when ML can tolerate oral medications. Cimetidine 300 mg IV every 8 hr or ranitidine 50 mg IV every 18–24 hr. Can't use antacids or sucralfate because ML is not tolerating oral medications. Monitor: nausea, vomiting, oral intake, guaiac tests of stools, renal function, and side effects from prochlorperazine (sedation, dizziness, extrapyramidal symptoms).

Problem 7. Pain

S: ML complains of pain not relieved by current oral medications, partially relieved by sitting forward.

O: Tumor progressing on CT scan. ML appears to be in pain and has not been able to take oral pain medications.

A: Tumor progression is causing increased pain. There is inadequate pain control with current oral medications. Nausea and vomiting are preventing oral administration temporarily. Pain is exacerbated by gastritis. Need to assess severity of pain.

P: Discontinue APAP with codeine. Treat gastritis as above. Start hydromorphone 2–4 mg IV every 3–4 hr for pain. Do not use morphine because ML had a reaction in the past that was probably due to histamine release and not an allergic reaction. Assess pain medication requirements and adjust accordingly. Schedule pain medication (not p.r.n.) and allow additional medication for breakthrough pain. May switch to oral hydromorphone if desired when ML can tolerate. May consider a slightly longer acting agent such as levorphanol.

   Alternative is to use a patient-controlled analgesic (PCA) device and use hydromorphone with a basal rate of 0.5–1.0 mg/hr and 0.5 mg every 30 min on demand. Assess patient needs and then switch to oral hydromorphone by taking the total 24-hr PCA use and dividing into every-4-hr increments.

   Start a mild laxative to prevent constipation secondary to narcotic use. This will help prevent nausea secondary to constipation. Examples: bisacodyl 5–10 mg per day or senna concentrate 1–3 tablets per day.

   Monitor: pain control, sedation, respiration rate, bowel function (constipation), mental status.

Problem 1. Hypertension/Orthostatic Hypotension

S: History of hypertension

O: BP 120/80, HR 82 supine, BP 96/60, HR 105 standing. Current medications include hydrochlorothiazide 50 mg/triamterene 75 mg.

A: History of hypertension, but currently orthostatic secondary to poor oral intake, nausea, vomiting, and diuretic use resulting in dehydration. May not require drug therapy for hypertension.

P: Discontinue diuretic use. Hydration as in problem 2. Reassess need for antihypertensive therapy after ML is hydrated and taking oral medications.

Problem 8. Urinary Tract Infection and 3. BPH-S/P TURP

S: Urinary frequency and burning with urination

O: Urinalysis: many Lkcs, few RBCs, GNRs, Urine culture: *E. coli.* Temp 38.1°C.

A: *E. coli* urinary tract infection. ML needs parenteral antibiotics, because he is unable to take oral medication. Organism is sensitive to ampicillin, which is probably the cheapest and easiest to give and has minimal toxicity, compared with aminoglycosides. ML is allergic to sulfa, so sulfamethoxazole/trimethoprim cannot be used.

P: Hydrate ML as in problem 2. Start ampicillin 1 g IV every 8 hr. If ML responds to treatment, may consider switching to oral ampicillin after 3–4 days if he can tolerate oral medication.

　　Monitor: urinary symptoms (frequency, burning), temperature, intake/output, repeat urinalysis, and possible nausea or rash from ampicillin.

QUESTIONS FOR CASE 164

1. Approximately 12 hr after the start of the IV hydration, the following laboratory values were reported:

　　Na 145 (145)
　　K 3.2 (3.2)
　　Cl 106 (106)
　　HCO_3 23 (23)
　　BUN 11.4 (32)
　　Cr 141 (1.6)
　　Glu 5.7 (104)

ML is currently receiving $D5_{1/2}NS$ at 150 ml/hr. What adjustments (if any) in his IV fluids are warranted?

2. After 24 hr, ML is still complaining of severe pain. His medication administration record indicates that he has been received hydromorphone via a PCA pump at a basal rate of 0.5 mg/hr and 0.5 mg on demand every 30 min for the last 24 hr. What adjustments in his pain medication regimen would you suggest at this time?

3. What is ML's prognosis?

4. What side effects would you expect from the chemotherapy ML received (leucovorin + 5-fluorouracil)? Which side effects did ML exhibit?

5. If ML's pain cannot be controlled with oral pain medications (once he is taking oral medication), what are the alternatives?

6. On day 3 of hospitalization, ML reports that he has not had a bowel movement in 6 days. On physical examination his abdomen is moderately distended, with faint bowel sounds. He is still not taking any oral medications. A repeat KUB does not show any signs of intestinal obstruction. What options exist for treating ML's constipation?

CASE 165

CC: LL is a 55-year-old woman, last menstrual period >1 year ago, admitted for exploratory laparotomy and debulking of ovarian carcinoma. Fibroids were noted during a routine physical examination 10 months ago. One month PTA, LL noticed distention of abdomen with some abdominal discomfort. Medical examination confirmed presence of larger abdominal mass, and ultrasound revealed complex mass with ascites.

Medical History

Thyroid cancer at age 23 treated with partial thyroidectomy and radiation therapy; now hypothyroid; mitral valve prolapse; gravida 0

Surgical History

Partial thyroidectomy for thyroid cancer at age 23
Cyst removal left jaw 17 years ago
Removal of basal cell cancer from right cheek skin 5 years ago

Medication History

Levothyroxine 0.1 mg
Ferrous sulfate 325 mg po TID
Docusate sodium 250 mg po QD

Allergies

NKDA

Physical Examination (on admission)

　GEN: Well-nourished woman with slight abdominal discomfort
　　VS: BP 110/60, HR 88 regular, RR 18, T 37.2°C, Wt 73 kg, Ht 165 cm
HEENT: Negative except for scar on neck from thyroidectomy
　COR: Clear
CHEST: Lungs clear
　ABD: Distended with ascites and gas; firm irregular mass approximately 15 cm
　　GU: Vagina smooth, narrow; cervix small, smooth; uterus anteverted 5–6 cm; irregular firm right adnexal tumor 15 cm with decreased mobility with tumor extension to the midline
　RECT: Normal
　EXT: Normal

Results of Laboratory Tests (on admission)

Na 143 (143)
K 4.3 (4.3)
Cl 100 (100)
HCO_3 25 (25)
BUN 3.2 (9)
CR 53 (0.6)

Hct 0.37 (37) 0.33 (33) post-op
Hgb 108 (10.8)
Lkcs 6.8×10^9 (6.8×10^3)
Plts 375×10^9 (375×10^3)

TFTs Normal

Lkc differential: P 0.72 (72), L 0.21 (21), M 0.06 (6), B 0.01 (1)

Urinalysis: Yellow, clear; sp. gr. 1.015, negative protein, glucose, bili, Hgb

Chest x-ray: Normal

ECG: Normal

Diagnosis after surgical staging: Stage IIIc epithelial ovarian cancer

PROBLEM LIST

1. Hypothyroidism
2. Chronic constipation
3. Advanced ovarian cancer
4. Malignant ascites
5. Antibiotic prophylaxis for mitral valve prolapse and gynecologic surgery
6. Postoperative anemia

CASE 165 SOAP NOTES

Problem 3. Stage IIIc Epithelial Ovarian Cancer

S: Abdominal discomfort

O: Increase in abdominal size; firm, irregular abdominal mass; positive ultrasound result; surgical confirmation

A: LL has advanced ovarian cancer, which should be treated with chemotherapy in addition to surgery. Therapy should begin after she has recovered from surgery.

P: Begin cisplatin 100 mg/$M^2$10 and cyclophosphamide 600 mg/$M^2$11 on day 1 and repeat every 21 days for 6 cycles. Administer 2 liters of D5W-1/2NS with 50 g of mannitol in first liter over 2 hr as prehydration. If urine output is good, administer cisplatin in 1 liter of NS and infuse over at least 2–6 hr. Follow cisplatin infusion with 1–2 liters of D5W-1/2NS as posthydration, administered over 2 hr. Include 2 g $MgSO_4$ and 20 mEq KCl in first liter of posthydration. LL should be instructed to drink plenty of fluids over the next 24 hr to maintain hydration. Cyclophosphamide can be given by IV push prior to cisplatin therapy.

Problem 4. Malignant Ascites

S: None

O: Ultrasound indicates ascites; abdominal swelling

A: Malignant ascites is due to tumor metastases blocking lymph ducts in the diaphragm, preventing the drainage of peritoneal fluid. Ascites may resolve with debulking surgery and subsequent chemotherapy. If ascites persists, it can cause patient discomfort and put the patient at risk for complications. Mild diuretics and bed rest may help to reduce ascites if it returns after surgery.

P: Monitor fluid collection by monitoring daily weight and abdominal girth.

Problem 5. Antibiotic Prophylaxis

S: None

O: Cor clear on examination; history

A: Mitral valve: Patients with some cardiac abnormalities require antimicrobial prophylaxis to prevent bacterial endocarditis when they undergo certain dental and surgical procedures. LL has mitral valve prolapse but does not have valvular regurgitation and therefore is not at risk.

Surgical: antimicrobial prophylaxis can decrease the incidence of infections after gynecologic operations. Therapy should be directed against *Staphylococcus aureus* and aerobic gram-negative rods. Antibiotics should be administered within 30 min prior to surgery. A single dose of prophylactic antibiotic is sufficient. If surgery is prolonged, the duration of prophylaxis may be increased to 24 hr.

P: Cefazolin 1 g IV immediately prior to surgery.

Problem 2. Chronic Constipation

S: History

O: None

A: Constipation may be aggravated after surgery. LL has been prescribed a stool softener.

P: Continue docusate 250 mg po QD (can increase to BID). Counsel LL on ways to reduce constipation: drink plenty of fluids; increase fiber in diet; and mild exercise (e.g., ambulation) when the surgeon discontinues restriction to bed. A thorough medication history should be taken to determine if LL is taking OTC remedies for constipation.

Problem 6. Anemia

S: None

O: Hct 0.33 (33) postoperative

A: Slight anemia after surgery because of blood loss. LL's Hct was normal on admission. Iron supplementation will help restore Hct to baseline.

P: Ferrous sulfate 325 mg TID po for 1 month

Problem 1. Hypothyroidism

S: None

O: TFTs normal

A: Hypothyroidism is controlled on current dose of levothyroxine.

P: Continue therapy.

QUESTIONS FOR CASE 165

1. Nausea and vomiting due to cisplatin can be expected. What therapy can be given to prevent this?
2. Calculate the dose of cisplatin and cyclophosphamide to be administered.
3. How can the hemorrhagic cystitis associated with cyclophosphamide be monitored and avoided?
4. Under what circumstances should the cisplatin dose be reduced or held?
5. LL has inquired about a new drug, Taxol, that she read about in the paper, and she would like to be given that drug. Is this appropriate in LL's case?

CASE 166

CC: EH is a 50-year-old woman with acute leukemia who presented to the emergency room with progressive fatigue and decreased energy over several weeks, sore throat, nasal congestion, and gum swelling. On admission, EH was noted to have a Lkcs of 15.4 × 10⁹ (15.4 × 10³) and a peripheral smear with leukemic blasts. She was diagnosed through cytogenic testing with acute myelogenous leukemia (AML), and chemotherapy was initiated. EH received an induction course of ARA-C (cytarabine) and daunorubicin. One week after her chemotherapy regimen was initiated, EH complained of intractable nausea and vomiting, rigors, and severe mouth pain. She was noted at this time to have an elevated temperature, a low Lkcs count, decreased fibrinogen, an elevated PT, and decreased platelets.

Medical History

EH has a history of hot flashes secondary to a bilateral salpingo-oopherectomy performed in 1984, and is currently taking conjugated estrogens and medroxyprogesterone.

Medication History

Conjugated estrogens 0.625 mg po QD
Medroxyprogesterone 10 mg po QD

Allergies

No known drug allergies

Physical Examination

GEN: Diaphroretic, weak-appearing woman with alopecia
VS: BP 130/90, HR 88, RR 20, T 39.5°C, Wt 77.5 kg
HEENT: NC/AT, PERRL, EOMI, + prominent gingival hyperplasia, erythematous buccal cavity
COR: N1 S1, S2; no murmurs
CHEST: CTA
ABD: Bowel sounds absent, soft NT, no masses
EXT: No clubbing, cyanosis, or edema
NEURO: A & O × 3, CN II–XII intact

Results of Laboratory Tests

Na 138 (138)	Hct 0.21 (21)	Ca 1.9 (8)
K 3.1 (3.1)	Hgb 80 (8)	PO₄ 0.65 (2)
Cl 115 (115)	Lkcs 0.3 × 10⁹ (300)	PT 24
HCO₃ 28 (28)	Plts 134 × 10⁹ (134 × 10³)	PTT 46.2
BUN 3.2 (9)		Fib (1.06) (106)
CR 88.4 (1.0)		

Bone marrow biopsy: Negative
Peripheral smear: No blasts
Blood cultures: Negative to date
Chest x-ray: No change from baseline

PROBLEM LIST

1. S/P BSO
2. Acute myelogenous leukemia
3. Neutropenia/fevers
4. Intractable nausea and vomiting
5. Disseminated intravascular coagulation
6. Mucositis

QUESTIONS FOR CASE 166

1. Twenty-four hours after her first dose of chemotherapy, EH's laboratory test results are significant for hyperphosphatemia, hypocalcemia, hyperkalemia, and hyperurecemia. A review of the medication administration record indicates that EH never received the allopurinol that was ordered, and she is diagnosed with acute tumor lysis syndrome (TLS). What is the appropriate therapeutic management of TLS?

2. Due to her severe mucositis, EH is unable to take her conjugated estrogens and medroxyprogesterone by mouth. The medical team asks you if these medications can be given intravenously. What is your reply?

3. EH remains febrile on ceftazidime, so the intern adds tobramycin to the regimen. One week later, she is still febrile, and the intern wishes to add amphotericin B. She asks you for an appropriate regimen, including appropriate administration guidelines.

4. One week after amphotericin B was initiated, EH's K level drops to 2.5, and her Mg level drops to 1.0 (2.0). What is the most likely cause of this hypokalemia and hypomagnesemia, and what should be done about it?

5. Three weeks after her chemotherapy induction course, EH remains neutropenic, and the intern wants to start a colony-stimulating factor. What is your advice?

CASE 167

CC: ST is a 40-year-old premenopausal woman with a newly diagnosed 3-cm carcinoma in her right breast, which was discovered during breast self-examination.

Medical History

ST began menstruating at the age of 13. She delivered her first and only child at the age of 38. Prior to this time, she used oral contraceptives for birth control for approximately 15 years.

Social History

ST's mother was diagnosed with breast cancer at the age of 50.
Tobacco: negative.
Alcohol: drinks occasionally socially.

Surgical History

A partial mastectomy and axillary node dissection were performed at the time of diagnosis and have since been followed by local radiation therapy. Pathology studies done at the time of surgery demonstrated 3/15 nodes positive for disease, with estrogen-receptor positivity and negative progesterone receptors. DNA flow cytometry performed on tumor samples indicate that ST's tumor is aneuploid and rapidly dividing. HER-2/neu and cathepsin D levels were not performed on the tumor samples.

Medication History

ST is currently on no medications.

Allergies

Penicillin

Physical Examination

GEN: Well-developed, well-nourished woman in no acute distress

VS: BP 120/70, HR 75, RR 18, T 37°C, Wt 59 kg, Ht 167.6 cm

NEENT: NC/AT, EACs clear, TMs intact, EOMI, PERRL

COR: Normal S_1 and S_2, no murmurs, rubs, or gallop

CHEST: Well-healed 4-cm scar on right breast; clear to auscultation and percussion

ABD: Soft, nontender, no masses or organomegaly

GU: Deferred

RECT: Deferred

EXT: No clubbing, no cyanosis; mild edema noted in right upper extremity; other extremities have no edema present

NEURO: CN II–XII grossly intact

Results of Laboratory Tests

Chem 20 WNL

Hgb 140 (14)

Hct 0.42 (42%)

Lkcs 6.0×10^9 (6.0×10^3)

Plts 300×10^9 (300×10^3)

Lkc differential: Neu 0.537 (53.7%), Lym 0.358 (35.8%), Mono 0.067 (6.7%), Eos 0.023 (2.3%), Baso 0.003 (0.3%)

Urinalysis: Unremarkable

Chest x-ray: Normal; no evidence of breast cancer

Liver, spleen, and bone scan: Negative for metastases

Bone marrow aspirate: Negative for tumor

PROBLEM LIST

1. Breast carcinoma
2. Birth control

QUESTIONS FOR CASE 167

1. Should CMF or CAF be used as initial combination adjuvant chemotherapy in patients with early-stage breast cancer?
2. How long should ST be treated with CMF therapy?
3. Fourteen days after the initiation of her chemotherapy, ST comes to the clinic with a fever of 102°F. The decision is made to admit her to the hospital. Upon admission, ST has some mild mucositis, but her physical examination is otherwise unremarkable. Laboratory results obtained upon admission were the following:

Lkcs 0.1×10^9 (0.1×10^3)

Hgb 120 (12)

Hct 0.40 (40%)

Plts 180×10^9 (180×10^3)

Na 140 (140)

K 4.2 (4.2)

Cl 100 (100)

CO_2 28 (28)

Glu 5.4 (98)

BUN 4.3 (12)

Cr 88.4 (1.0)

Lkc differential: Neutrophils 0.471 (47.1%), Lymphocytes 0.361 (36.1%), Monocytes 0.14 (14.0%), Eosinophils 0.023 (2.3%), Basophils 0.005 (0.5%)

Blood and urine cultures were obtained and the decision was made to start ST on empiric antibiotic coverage. What organisms are likely, and what should be her empiric regimen?

4. Should ST's chemotherapy doses be adjusted on her next treatment course because of the myelosuppression associated with this treatment course?
5. Suggest an appropriate antiemetic regimen for ST while she is receiving her adjuvant systemic chemotherapy with cyclophosphamide, methotrexate, and fluorouracil.

CASE 168

CC: HJ is a 67-year-old woman who presented in 6/95 with a 1-week history of abdominal cramping and bright red blood in her stools. A workup revealed an adenocarcinoma of the sigmoid colon, which was resected and found to be a Dukes B2 lesion. No adjuvant chemotherapy was given. HJ did well until 1 week ago when she presented with right upper quadrant pain unresponsive to ibuprofen, and occasional fevers. On examination, HJ was found to have hepatomegaly and placed on ASA with codeine for pain. Her LFTs and CEA were elevated, and a subsequent CT scan of the abdomen and pelvis revealed multiple bilobar hepatic metastases, but no evident extrahepatic disease. She now returns to clinic to discuss treatment options for her cancer. Additionally, she states that her pain is improved, but she complains of constipation and urinary frequency.

Medical History

UTI 4 months ago

Congestive heart failure (CHF) since age 60

Colonic polyp removed at age 62

Social History

HJ lives with husband who is healthy. Two children are grown and healthy.

1–2 glasses of wine per day

No tobacco

Surgical History
Sigmoid colectomy 6/95
Appendectomy at age 35

Allergies
Penicillin (rash)

Medication History
Digoxin 0.125 mg po QD
ASA with codeine 30 mg one po q4-6h p.r.n.

Physical Examination
GEN: Well-developed, well-nourished distressed woman
VS: BP 120/80, HR 78, RR 15, T 39°C, Wt 65, Ht 177 cm
HEENT: Normal except for IOP (30 rt, 31 lt); goinoscopy revealed open angles in both eyes; no JVD
COR: Normal
CHEST: Normal; no rales
ABD: Liver 6 cm below right costal margin
GU: No CVA tenderness
RECT: Normal
EXT: Normal
NEURO: Normal

Results of Laboratory Tests

Na 140 (140)	Hct 0.41 (41)	AST 0.73 (44)	Glu 5.5 (100)
K 3.5 (140)	Hgb 140 (14)	ALT 0.79 (47)	CA 2.35 (9.4)
Cl 104 (104)	Lkcs 8.0 × 10⁹ (8 × 10³)	LDH 4 (240)	PO₄ 1.1 (3.4)
HCO₃ 26 (26)	Plts 185 × 10⁹ (185 × 10³)	Alk Phos 3 (180)	Mg 1.0 (2)
BUN 5 (14)	MCV 80 (80)	Alb 50 (5.0)	Uric Acid 240 (4.0)
CR 70.7 (0.8)		T bili 10 (0.5)	

CEA 91 mg/liter
Urinalysis: >20 bacteria per HPF, 10–20 Lkcs per HPF
Urine culture: >105 cfu/ml *Escherichia coli* (pansensitive)
Chest x-ray: Normal
Abdominal CT scan: Multiple bilobar liver metastases
KUB: Normal except for large amounts of stool
ECG: Normal
Digoxin level: 1.92 mmol/liter (1.5 mg/ml)

PROBLEM LIST
1. Recurrent urinary tract infection (UTI)
2. Fever
3. Open-angle glaucoma
4. Metastatic colorectal cancer to the liver
5. Pain
6. Constipation
7. Fever

QUESTIONS FOR CASE 168
1. What if HJ responds to hepatic intra-arterial chemotherapy, but develops a small solitary pulmonary metastasis? How should her therapy be changed?

2. What if HJ responds to hepatic intra-arterial chemotherapy, but develops equally significant extrahepatic disease? How should her therapy be changed and what would be the anticipated toxicities?
3. What if HJ responds to hepatic-intra-arterial fluoropyrimidine therapy for several months and then develops progressive hepatic disease, but has no extrahepatic disease? How should she be treated and what are the anticipated toxicities of this therapy?
4. HJ's pain is well controlled during the day, but it wakes her up during the night. What can be done to provide better nocturnal pain relief for HJ?
5. Two months after being treated for her urinary tract infection, HJ develops another urinary tract infection. Is HJ a candidate for antibiotic prophylaxis following successful treatment of this infection?

CASE 169
CC: GC is a 61-year-old, recently widowed woman who was admitted to the hospital eight days ago to begin induction chemotherapy for small cell lung cancer (SCLC). Today she complains of "constant" epigastric pain which has been increasing over the past 3 days.

History of Present Illness
Three weeks ago, GC made an appointment with her primary MD after experiencing an undesired 12-pound weight loss over the previous month. On initial inquiry, her doctor learned that her appetite had been poor and that she had increased smoking from two to three packs per day since the death of her husband 3 months before. GC admitted to frequent episodes of hemoptysis, coughing, and SOB for the past 3 weeks. Suspecting lung cancer, the doctor scheduled GC for a complete workup, including bronchial biopsy, chest and brain CT. After completion of the workup, GC was diagnosed with unresectable, extensive disease with small cell histology. She was scheduled to be admitted for chemotherapy with CAVP-16 (cyclophosphamide, doxorubicin, and etoposide).

Medical History
GC has been in relatively good health all of her life, with the exception of a benign gastric ulcer 2 years ago. She went through menopause 13 years ago, and has been taking estrogen and medroxyprogesterone since that time. GC stopped smoking immediately upon diagnosis 3 weeks ago, and began to use nicotine gum as part of a smoking cessation program.

Medication History
Conjugated estrogens (Premarin) 0.625 mg QD
Medroxyprogesterone (Provera) 5 mg QD (days 16–21 of cycle)
Nicotine gum (was using 25 pieces/day at start of therapy, now using 4 pieces/day)
Bisacodyl 10 mg PR p.r.n. constipation

Cyclophosphamide (CTX) 1000 mg/m^2 Q day 3 weeks
Doxorubicin (DXR) 45 mg/m^2/day Q 3 weeks
Etoposide (VP-16) 50 mg/m^2/day × 5 days Q 3 weeks

Allergies

Sulfa drugs (rash and hives)

Social History

Tobacco: 2 ppd × 30 years
Alcohol: 2 glasses wine per night

Physical Examination

- GEN: Pale, thin woman appearing slightly anxious.
- VS: BP 140/82, HR 82, RR 17, T 38.3°C, Wt 53 kg, Ht 152 cm
- HEENT: PEERLA; oral cavity showing mild mucositis (Stage I)
- COR: RRR; normal S1 and S2
- CHEST: Mild expiratory wheezing R>L; central line shows no redness or erythema
- ABD: Rebound tenderness; no hepatosplenomegaly
- RECT: Guaiac-positive
- EXT: Normal pulses, no bruising, no edema
- NEURO: Oriented to time, place, and person; cranial nerves intact

Results of Laboratory Tests

Na 135 (135)	Cl 98 (98)	T Bili 22.2 (1.3)
Hct 0.31 (31)	WBC 1.5 × 10^9 (1.5)	Plts 70 (70)
LDH 1.65 (99)	Alb 30 (3.0)	BUN 7.5 (21)
Glu 5.55 (100)	PO$_4$ 0.872 (2.7)	AST 0.5 (30)
K 3.5 (3.5)	HCO$_3$ 25 (25)	PT 14
Hgb 4.96 (8.0)	ANC 253	CR 97.2 (1.1)
Alk Phos 1.32 (79)	Mg 0.65 (1.3)	ALT 0.45 (27)
Ca 2.1 (8.5)		

Endoscopy: Positive for two small gastric ulcers

PROBLEM LIST

1. Lung cancer
2. Active peptic ulcer disease
3. Granulocytopenia

Use SOAP for the above problems

CASE 169 SOAP NOTES
Problem 1. SCLC

S: Patient complaining of frequent hemoptysis, coughing, and SOB, as well as poor appetite and an undesired 12-pound weight loss.

O: Patient with SCLC by histology; positive for mild wheezing on examination, as well as a 60 pack year history of smoking.

A: GC has unresectable, extensive disease. Because SCLC progresses rapidly and usually disseminates early in the disease process, surgery is almost never indicated as part of the treatment plan. GC began induction chemotherapy with CAVP-16 because the use of combination chemotherapy regimens has demonstrated a fourfold to fivefold increase in median survival compared to patients who re-

ceived single-drug chemotherapy.

P: Continue with the induction chemotherapy regimen using cyclophosphamide, doxorubicin, and etoposide. Would also consider the addition of chest radiation therapy as well as prophylactic cranial irradiation. The chemotherapy should continue for at least 6–12 months, or until the patient has a relapse of her disease. Common toxicities associated with chemotherapy are usually divided into acute and cumulative toxicities. Cyclophosphamide acutely causes bone-marrow suppression (BMS), and hemorrhagic cystitis. Neurotoxicity in the form of peripheral neuropathy or hearing loss and cystitis are associated with cumulative doses. Doxorubicin acutely causes stomatitis, BMS, and alopecia and may cause vesicant reactions if extravasation occurs. Cumulative doses result in cardiomyopathy. Etoposide acutely causes BMS and alopecia.

Problem 2. Granulocytopenia

S: None.

O: WBC 1.5 × 10^9 (1.5), and ANC 253.

A: Granulocytopenia secondary to the recent chemotherapeutic induction. GC's neutropenia, however, places her at high risk for infection from bacterial, fungal, and viral pathogens. It should be noted that profound BMS is commonly associated with this chemotherapeutic regimen, and that BMS can and should be countered by administration of granulocyte colony stimulating factors.

P: Start filgrastim (G-CSF) 5 mcg/kg/day. For GC, the recommended dose is 265 mcg SQ or IV daily. Plan is to continue to monitor GC's WBC with differential. Also, GC should be monitored for signs and symptoms of infection.

Problem 3. Active Gastric Ulcer

S: Patient with "constant" epigastric pain increasing over the past 3 days.

O: Endoscopy revealed two small gastric ulcers. GC also has epigastric pain, rebound abdominal tenderness, and guaiac-positive stools. Her low Hct may or may not be related to this gastric ulcer.

A: GC has a confirmed diagnosis of active benign gastric ulcer. She is currently not being treated for this condition, but needs to begin treatment immediately to relieve her symptoms and to decrease the risk of serious complications. Her past history of gastric ulcer combined with her history of heavy smoking put her at great risk for ulcer recurrence, especially in the absence of prophylactic treatment. The treatment choices for GC include the histamine (H$_2$) blockers, antacids, sucralfate, and omeprazole. The H$_2$-blockers would be the best choice for GC because antacids and sucralfate require frequent dosing and have poor compliance (also, sucralfate and the aluminum containing antacids may aggravate her periodic constipation), and omeprazole is relatively costly and is usually reserved for refractory cases.

P: Start ranitidine 300 mg QHS for 6–12 weeks. Follow-up UGI series or endoscopy 8 weeks after initiation of therapy should be performed to assess GC's response to therapy.

GC will need to remain on maintenance therapy with ranitidine 150 mg QHS to prevent ulcer recurrence. The patient should be informed that antacids may be used on a p.r.n. basis to relieve pain and that although symptoms may improve, that she must remain on therapy. GC should be monitored periodically for changes in serum CR, CBC, AST, ALT, and CNS status.

QUESTIONS FOR CASE 169

1. In this patient with neutropenia, should prophylactic antibiotics be administered to prevent infection?
2. Calculate the dose of each chemotherapeutic agent for GC.
3. GC's serum calcium is subtherapeutic. What type of calcium supplementation would you recommend?
4. Should GC receive treatment for her malnutrition? What are the options available?
5. Should GC continue to use the nicotine gum in light of the recent reactivation of her gastric ulcer?

CASE 170

CC: RB is a 69-year-old man who presented to the outpatient clinic with complaints of right shoulder pain and urinary retention. On questioning, he also reported fatigue, lethargy, bilateral ankle edema, and the need to use two pillows to sleep comfortably. RB stated that he takes his digoxin daily and never misses a dose.

Medical History

1989: Depression
1990: Congestive heart failure

Medication History

Acetaminophen 2 tablets q6h
Digoxin 0.125 mg po QD
Amitriptyline 50 mg po QD

Allergies

None known

Physical Examination

GEN:	Well-nourished, well-developed adult man in NAD
VS:	BP supine 132/70, HR 76, T 36.5°C, Wt 78 Kg, Ht 183 cm
HEENT:	NCAT
COR:	RR S1S2-MRG
CHEST:	Clear
ABD:	Soft, nontender, positive bowel sounds, -HSM
GU:	WNL
RECT:	Markedly enlarged prostate
EXT:	Painful right shoulder
NEURO:	WNL

Results of Laboratory Tests

Na 136 (136)	Hct 0.41 (41)	AST 0.52 (31)	T Bili 6.84 (0.4)
K 4.5 (4.5)	Hgb 160 (16)	ALT 0.52 (31)	Glu 5.8 (105)
Cl 99 (99)	Lkcs 5.64 × 10⁹ (5.64 × 10³)	LDH 2.32 (139)	Ca 2.69 (10.8)
HCO₃ 27 (27)	Plts 2.68 × 10⁹ (2.68 × 10³)	Alk Phos 18.8 (1125)	POM₄ 0.81 (2.5)
BUN 6.4 (18)	MCV 100 (100)	Alb 44 (4.4)	Mg 1 1 (2 2)
CR 62 (0.7)			Uric Acid 369 (6.2)

Testosterone: 716 ng/ml

PAP: 28.8 ng/ml

PSA: 92 ng/ml

Urinalysis: WNL

Dig: 0.9 nmol/ liter (0.7 ng/ml)

Chest x-ray: Mild cardiomegaly

Pelvic CT scan: Enlarged prostate gland. The prostate gland is in contact with the urinary bladder and rectum. Extension of the neoplasm beyond the capsule of the prostate gland. No abnormal retroperitoneal adenopathy

Bone scan: Extensive skeletal metastases involving primarily the axial skeleton. Appendicular skeletal lesions include the right scapula and the right and left femurs proximally.

Fine-needle aspirate of the prostate: Poorly differentiated adenocarcinoma

PROBLEM LIST

1. Depression
2. Congestive heart failure (CHF)
3. Adenocarcinoma of the prostate (stage D2)
4. Urinary retention
5. Hypercalcemia
6. Right shoulder pain

QUESTIONS FOR CASE 170

1. What symptoms are associated with the various stages of prostate carcinoma?
2. What response rate is expected with the initiation of hormone therapy? How can the response be monitored and what duration of response can be expected?
3. What is the rationale for using leuprolide and flutamide in combination?
4. Is there a role for alternate hormonal therapy if leuprolide and flutamide do not produce a response?
5. What is the role of chemotherapy in the treatment of stage D2 prostate cancer?
6. Define chemoprevention and discuss the rationale for using finasteride as chemoprevention for prostate cancer.

CASE 171

CC: CD is a 58-year-old man who was admitted to the hospital with complaints of anorexia, weight loss, and abdominal pain.

Medical History

Unremarkable until 6 weeks ago when he presented to family physician with symptoms of dyspepsia.

Medication History

Mylanta p.r.n. GI discomfort
Ranitidine 150 mg QD

Allergies

None known

Physical Examination

VS:	BP 150/78, HR 64, T 38°C, Wt 58 kg (down from 64 kg 2 months ago)
HEENT:	WNL
COR:	WNL
CHEST:	Clear to auscultation and percussion
ABD:	Hepatosplenomegaly, enlarged inguinal lymph nodes; 3 × 5-cm mass in the lower right quadrant
GU:	WNL
RECT:	Guaiac-positive
EXT:	WNL
NEURO:	WNL

Results of Laboratory Tests

Na 137 (137)	Hct 0.304 (30.4)	AST 4.45 (267)	Glu 6.1 (110)
K 4.0 (4.0)	Hgb 98 (9.8)	ALT 2.8 (169)	Ca 2.4 (9.8)
Cl 104 (104)	Lkcs 10.7 × 10⁹ (10.7 × 10³)	LDH 4.2 (250)	PO₄ 1.13 (3.5)
HCO₃ 21 (21)	Plts 284 × 10⁹ (284 × 10³)	Alk Phos 6.3 (379)	Mg 1.05 (2.1)
BUN 6.8 (19)	MCV 97 (97)	Alb 30 (3.0)	Uric Acid 249.8 (4.2)
CR 88.4 (1.0)	MCHC 360 (36)	T Bili 20.5 (1.2)	PT 11.7
			PTT 29

Urinalysis: WNL

Abdominal CT scan: Extensive lymphadenopathy, gastric wall thickening; two liver nodules consistent with metastatic disease

Gastric biopsy: Consistent with malignant lymphoma, diffuse large cell

Lymph node biopsy: Malignant lymphoma, diffuse large cell

Bilateral bone marrow biopsies: No evidence of disease

Chest x-ray: WNL

PROBLEM LIST

1. Stage IV malignant lymphoma, diffuse large-cell
2. Risk of tumor cell lysis syndrome
3. Risk of cumulative cardiac toxicities from doxorubicin

CASE 172

CC: SF is a 53-year-old postmenopausal woman who presents 5 years after completion of adjuvant chemotherapy for stage II breast carcinoma with a 2-week history of shortness of breath and mild bone pain in left ribs.

Medical History

Gravida 4, para 4

Menses onset at 14

Hypertension for 13 years, currently treated with enalapril 10 mg BID and furosemide 40 mg QD

Type II (non-insulin-dependent) diabetes mellitus (NIDDM) for 8 years, currently well controlled on glyburide 5 mg po BID

Stage II breast cancer diagnosed 1990; ER+/PR+; 5/19 + nodes. SF received six cycles of adjuvant cyclophosphamide, methotrexate, and 5-fluorouracil and has remained disease-free at follow-up visits to date.

Family History

Breast cancer in mother and sister

Surgical History

Left radical mastectomy in 1990 prior to adjuvant therapy

Medication History

Glyburide 5 mg po BID
Enalapril 10 mg po BID
Furosemide 40 mg QD

Allergies

None known

Physical Examination

GEN:	Well-developed woman in no acute distress
VS:	BP 120/88, HR 80, RR 20, T 37°C, Wt 72.7 kg, Ht 165.1 cm
HEENT:	PERRLA, no JVD, no lymphadenopathy
COR:	Normal S1 and S2, no murmurs, rubs, or gallop
CHEST:	Well-healed scar left breast area; dullness of percussion over left lung bases, decreased breath sounds.
ABD:	Soft, nontender, no masses or organomegaly
GU:	WNL
RECT:	Deferred
EXT:	No clubbing, cyanosis, or edema
NEURO:	Alert and oriented × 3; cranial nerves intact; normal deep tendon reflexes

Results of Laboratory Tests

Na 143 (143)	Hct 0.426 (42.6)	AST 0.62 (37)	Glu 7.7 (138)
K 4.5 (4.5)	Hgb 130 (13)	ALT 0.5 (30)	Ca 2.35 (9.4)
Cl 100 (100)	Lkcs 6.8 × 10⁹ (6.8 × 10³)	LDH 3.4 (204)	PO₄ 1.32 (4.1)
HCO₃ 30 (30)	Plts 372 × 10⁹ (372 × 10³)	Alk Phos 1.5 (90)	Mg 1.1 (2.2)
BUN 3.9 (11)		Alb 40 (4.0)	Uric Acid 286 (4.8)
CR 106 (1.2)		T Prot 68 (6.8)	PT 11.8
		T Bili 5.1 (0.3)	PTT 22.0

Lkc differential: Neut 0.7 (70%), Lym 0.20 (20%), mono 0.065 (6.5%), Baso 0.013 (1.3%), eos 0.022 (2.2%)

Urinalysis: WNL
ECG: Normal sinus rhythm
CXR: Effusion in left lower lobe. Fluid layers out on lateral x-ray.
Bone scan: Multiple metastases to left lower ribs
Pleural fluid thoracentesis: Glucose 5.3 mmol/liter (95 mg/dl), LDH 3.9 mkat/liter (234 u/liter), pH 7.5; Specific gravity 1.025, Protein 50 g/liter (5.0 g/dl), Lkcs 2.6×10^9/liter (2,600/mm^3), RBC 110 $\times 10^{12}$/liter (110×10^6), Cytology adenocarcinoma breast

PROBLEM LIST

1. Hypertension
2. Type II DM
3. S/P adjuvant chemotherapy for breast cancer
4. Shortness of breath
5. Bone pain

CASE 173

CC: JA is a 54-year-old man who is admitted for evaluation of vague epigastric distress that he characterizes as a bloated feeling after meals. There is also early satiety, and he also mentions that he has 2–3 loose stools/day.

Medical History

JA is a construction worker who has noted increased tiredness at the end of each day. He has a several-month history of mild upper abdominal discomfort that is sometimes relieved by antacid therapy. In addition, JA has noticed a small loss of weight.

Medication History

Ranitidine 300 mg po h.s.
Ibuprofen 400 mg po p.r.n. for muscle stiffness
Over-the-counter (OTC) antacid products taken p.r.n. indigestion

Social History

He has smoked one pack/day for 35 years and occasionally consumes a couple of beers after work.

Physical Examination

GEN: Thin, tired-looking man in mild distress
VS: BP 105/70, HR 95, RR 25, T 38.5°C, Wt 75.8 kg, Ht 185.4 cm
HEENT: Normal
COR: WNL
CHEST: Clear
ABD: Epigastric tenderness; bowel sounds present, but diminished

GU: WNL
RECTAL: Guaiac-positive stools

Results of Laboratory Tests

Na 137 (137)	Hct 0.23 (23)	AST 0.25 (15)	Glu 4.6 (83)
K 5.4 (5.4)	Hgb 75 (7.5)	ALT 0.17 (10)	Ca 2.2 (8.9)
Cl 100 (100)	Lkcs 6.5×10^9 (6.5×10^3)	LDH 1.87 (112)	PO$_4$ 1.5 (4.6)
HCO$_3$ 20 (20)	Plts 295×10^9 (295×10^3)	Alk Phos 1.4 (85)	Mg 2.5 (4.9)
BUN 8.9 (25)	MCV 86 (86)	Alb 43 (4.3)	Uric Acid 410 (6.9)
CR 238 (2.7)		T Bili 6.8 (0.4)	

Lkc differential: Normal
Urinalysis: pH 6, SG 1.031, protein-positive (3+), glucose-negative, RBC 0-1/HPF, Lkcs 0-1/HPF, bacteria-negative, hyaline casts and mucus (2+)
Chest x-ray: WNL
ECG: WNL
UGI: Mass in the greater curvature, near fundus
Upper endoscopy and biopsy: Adenocarcinoma, consistent with gastric carcinoma
CT abdomen: No abnormalities noted

PROBLEM LIST

1. Gastric carcinoma
2. Normocytic normochromic anemia
3. Loose stools

CASE 174

RJ is a 72-year-old man with a diagnosis of adenocarcinoma of the lung, admitted to the hospital for evaluation of mental status changes.

History of Present Illness

RJ was in his usual state of health until about 14 months prior to this admission. At that time he noted a productive cough, which had worsened over the preceding months. He also noted the onset of right arm pain, right breast swelling, and hemoptysis. A chest radiograph revealed a mass in both lung fields, and subsequent biopsy revealed adenocarcinoma of the left lung, metastatic to the right lung. Radiation therapy was given to both lung fields, and a complete response was achieved. RJ's disease was then stable until 2 weeks prior to admission, when he began complaining of right-hand numbness and left hip pain. A bone scan and head CT performed at that time revealed metastatic cancer in the left hip and two separate lesions in the brain, presumed to be metastatic disease. At that time RJ was begun on dexamethasone 2 mg po four times daily, and radiation therapy to the brain and left hip was started. Radiation to the hip was completed 1 week PTA; radiation to the brain was completed today. At RJ's clinic visit today, he was observed to exhibit bizarre behavior, with apparent hallucinations. In addition, a CBC revealed pancytopenia. A bone-marrow biopsy was performed; the results are pending.

Medical History

RJ has a history of recurrent gastric ulcer, for which he is followed by a gastroenterologist.

Medication History

Ranitidine 150 mg po BID
Acetaminophen with codeine 30 mg two po q4h p.r.n.
Dexamethasone 2 mg po QID

Allergies

No known medication allergies

Review of Systems

RJ complains of continuous left hip pain, decreased only slightly since radiation therapy. He feels he has been more weak and tired in the past weeks, is aware of his intermittent confusion, and is quite embarrassed about it.

Physical Examination

GEN: Well-developed, slightly cachectic man with somewhat agitated and confused demeanor
VS: BP 180/100, HR 90 reg, RR 16, T 38.5°C, Wt 79 kg, Ht 180 cm
HEENT: Edentulous; tongue stained with nicotine; no acute lesions
COR: Normal S_1, S_2 with occasional systolic click; Gr I/IV systolic ejection murmur at left sternal border; no S_3, S_4
CHEST: Increased AP diameter. Right breast is tender, without discharge. Lungs clear to percussion and auscultation.
ABD: Positive bowel sounds; soft, nontender
GU: Normal man
RECT: External hemorrhoids; no masses; guaiac-negative
EXT: Right arm slightly tender throughout; palmar erythema present; borderline clubbing
NEURO: Oriented × 3 intermittently; at times cannot remember the day or location; no motor deficit; sensory intact

Results of Laboratory Tests

BUN 4.3 (12)   Hgb 72 (7.2)
CR 106 (1.2)   Lkcs 1.4×10^9 (1.4×10^3)
                 Plts 90×10^9 (90×10^3)

Lkc diff: Segs 0.4 (40%), bands 0.03 (3%), lymphs 0.55 (55%), eos 0.02 (2%)
Bone marrow biopsy results pending

PROBLEM LIST

1. Recurrent gastric ulcer
2. Metastatic adenocarcinoma of lung
3. Left hip pain
4. Fever
5. Pancytopenia
6. Mental status changes

CASE 175

CC: JR is a 69-year-old woman who presents to the emergency room complaining of nausea, weakness, fatigue, lethargy, and dizziness. She has had significant nausea in the 24 hr since her cisplatin dose yesterday, with six episodes of vomiting. Her daughter states that JR has lost interest in her usual activities, has trouble sleeping, has lost her appetite, and has lost weight since she was diagnosed with cancer.

Medical History

JR was diagnosed with advanced epithelial ovarian cancer 3 months ago. She successfully completed debulking surgery with residual disease remaining. She has completed two of six cycles of cyclophosphamide and cisplatin chemotherapy, which is being administered in an outpatient infusion center. Her most recent treatment with cisplatin was yesterday.

Medication History

Cisplatin 100 mg/m² IV day 1
Cyclophosphamide 1000 mg/m² IV day 1
Metoclopramide 20 mg IV 1/2 hr before cisplatin infusion
Dexamethasone 5 mg IV 1/2 hr before cisplatin infusion
Lorazepam 1–2 mg s.l. 4–6 hr p.r.n. nausea with chemotherapy
Prochlorperazine 25 mg spansules q. 12 hr p.r.n. × 48 hr
Diazepam 5 mg q.h.s. p.r.n. for sleep and q6h p.r.n. anxiety (prescribed 1 month ago)

Allergies

Penicillin (rash)

Physical Examination

GEN: Elderly woman in moderate distress
VS: BP 110/80 supine, 90/60 standing, HR 105, RR 18, T 37.3°C, Wt 55 kg (56 kg in clinic yesterday), BSA 1.5 m²
HEENT: Mucous membranes dry, otherwise normal
COR: Clear
CHEST: Normal
ABD: Normal; well-healed scar from recent surgery
EXT: Dry to touch, poor skin turgor

Results of Laboratory Tests (Random, non-fasting)

Na 145 (145)	Hct 0.45 (45)	AST 0.4 (24)	Glu 5.6 (100)
K 2.9 (2.9)	Hgb 130 (13)	ALT 0.4 (24)	Ca 2.5 (10)
Cl 140 (140)	Lkcs 6.8 × 10⁹ (6.8 × 10³)	LDH 1.0 (60)	PO₄ 1.5 (4.5)
HCO₃ 25 (25)	Plts 375 × 10⁹ (375 × 10³)	Alk Phos 0.4 (24)	Mg 1.2 (2.4)
BUN 10.7 (30)		Alb 45 (4.5)	Uric Acid 178 (3)
CR 176 (2.0)		T Bili 13.7 (0.8)	

Lkc differential: Not done
Urinalysis: Unable to attain

PROBLEM LIST

1. Advanced ovarian cancer
2. Intractable nausea and vomiting
3. Dehydration
4. Acute renal failure
5. Depression
6. Insomnia

PEDIATRIC AND NEONATAL THERAPY

CASE 176

CC: GJ is a newborn baby girl delivered by cesarean section due to prolonged labor at 38 weeks' gestation, to a 19-year-old unmarried mother with a history of IV drug abuse and seropositivity for hepatitis B surface antigen. The newborn resuscitation team was called for assistance at delivery for high-risk pregnancy. The baby was subsequently admitted to the neonatal intensive care unit.

Birth History, Medical History

Mother's first child, born full-term with no prenatal care with the above described problems. Mother's RPR and FTA-abs are both positive; mother denies having syphilis in the past.

Medication History

None

Allergies

None known

Social History

Mother with known history of IV drug abuse

Review of Systems

Noncontributory

Physical Examination

GEN: Pink, vigorous newborn
VS: BP 61/38, HR 142, RR 36, T 37.4°C, Wt 2.885 kg, Length 48 cm
HEENT: Open anterior fontanelle, EOMI, (+) red reflex, purulent nasal discharge, TM visualized
COR: RRR, no murmur, nl S_1S_2
CHEST: CTA
ABD: (+) BS, soft, NTND, no hepatosplenomegaly
RECT: Patent
EXT: Pulses 2+ DTR patella
NEURO/ DEV: (+) Grasp, good (thumb) suck

Results of Laboratory Tests

Na 137 (137)	Hct 0.50 (50)	AST 1.00 (60)	Glu 4.43 (79)
K 3.8 (3.8)	Hgb 169 (16.9)	ALT 0.08 (5)	Ca 2.4 (9.4)
Cl 102 (102)	Lkcs 13.1 × 10⁹ (13.1 × 10³)	LDH 7.4 (446)	PO₄ 1.74 (5.4)
HCO₃ 22 (22)	Plts 271 × 10⁹ (271 × 10³)	Alk Phos 3.03 (182)	Mg 0.6 (1.1)
BUN 3.9 (11)	MCV 72 (72)	Alb 28 (2.8)	PT 14
Cr 97.2 (1.1)	T Bili 49.6 (2.9)	D Bili 3.42 (0.2)	

WBC differential: Neut 35%, Bands 3%, Lymph 50%, Mono 9%, Eos 3%
Serologic tests for syphilis: RPR (+), FTA-abs (+)
Lumbar puncture: RBC 10, WBC 6, Gluc 51, Prot 163, VDRL pending
EEG: WNL
Tox screen: Negative
Chest x-ray: WNL

PROBLEM LIST

1. Syphilis
2. Hepatitis B exposure
3. Immunization schedule

Use SOAP for the above problems.

CASE 176 SOAP NOTES

Problem 1. Syphilis

S: Mother denies history of syphilis.
O: Baby has some purulent nasal discharge. RPR and FTA-abs are positive in mother and infant.
A: Mother with untreated syphilis exposed neonate in utero. Congenital syphilis is transferred in utero by passage of the *Treponema pallidum* through the placenta. Often, the diagnosis is presumptive and based on serologic titers, such as RPR and FTA-abs. (Definitive diagnosis requires identification of the organism on a darkfield microscope or on a pathologic examination, which occurs only in rare circumstances.) Because most infants are asymptomatic during the first several weeks of life, it is worrisome that GJ presents with purulent nasal discharge. The disease in the newborn is comparable to secondary syphilis in the adult, but is more severe and can be life-threatening. Although GJ has no other symptoms, the LP results show that neurosyphilis cannot be ruled out because the CSF fluid obtained from the lumbar puncture is inconclusive. Therapy with a full 10-day course of penicillin therapy is required.
P: Aqueous crystalline penicillin G (or aqueous procaine penicillin G) 75,000 units IV Q12h (50,000 units/kg/day) × 10 days.

Problem 2. Hepatitis B Exposure

S: None.
O: GJ's mother has documented HBsAg-(+), along with a history of IV drug abuse as a risk factor.
A: Infants can be infected with hepatitis B at the time of delivery, so the standard of practice is to administer the hepatitis B immune globulin (HBIG) as soon as possible after birth to prevent the transfer of seropositivity to the

newborn. However, HBIG will only achieve passive, short-term immunity against the hepatitis B virus. For adequate protection, the three-dose treatment with hepatitis B virus (HBV) vaccine should begin at least by 1 week of age. This allows for active production of antibodies against hepatitis B, and thus long-lasting immunity against the virus.

P: Hepatitis B immune globulin 0.5 ml IM within 12 hours of birth. Hepatitis B virus vaccine 0.5 ml IM at 0–7 days of age, with boosters scheduled at 1 and 6 months of age.

Problem 3. Immunization Schedule

S: None.

O: Newborn infant born to mother with multiple risk factors.

A: Need to emphasize to the mother the importance of immunizations, especially the hepatitis B virus vaccine. Other vaccines should protect against diptheria, tetanus, pertussis, haemophilus type b, polio, measles, mumps, and rubella.

P: The first booster for the hepatitis B virus (HBV) vaccine should be given at 1 month of age. At 2 months of age, the infant should receive the first shots for diptheria, tetanus, pertussis (DTP), haemophilus type b (HbCV) (now available as a single formulation, called Tetrammune), as well as the first dose of oral polio virus (OPV) vaccine. At four months of age, Tetrammune and OPV, boosters should be given. At six months of age, the infant should be given another set of Tetrammune and OPV boosters, as well as the last HBV immunization. At 15 months of age, the child should be given another booster with Tetrammune and OPV, as well as the first measles, mumps, and rubella (MMR) vaccine. At 4 to 6 years of age (before entering school), the child should receive another booster of DTP, OPV, and MMR.

QUESTIONS FOR CASE 176

1. Describe the serologic tests for syphilis, and explain the primary differences between them.
2. What organ systems can be affected by syphilis in a neonate?
3. What is the likelihood that the neonate will develop full-blown hepatitis? What can be done to prevent this?
4. Should GJ receive varicella vaccine? What is the recommended schedule for varicella vaccine?

CASE 177

CC: RS is a 13-month-old girl brought to the pediatrician by her mother because she is still "throwing up all of her special baby formula" 4 days after swallowing some dishwashing liquid. RS's mother is concerned because the physician in the emergency room where she took RS after the ingestion said that the vomiting should stop in 1–2 days. She has tolerated apple juice and oral rehydration fluids. Mother has also noticed a rash developing on RS's face, which RS is frequently scratching.

Medical History

Cow's milk allergy; breast-fed until 4 months of age, when she was placed on Enfamil and subsequently developed diarrhea, vomiting, and atopic eczema. RS has since tolerated Prosobee.

Physical Examination

GEN: Well-developed
VS: BP 95/60, HR 117, RR 45, T 37°C, Wt 10 kg, Ht 76 cm
HEENT: Cheeks are erythematous with exudation
COR: WNL
CHEST: Clear to auscultation
ABD: Protuberant with positive bowel sounds, examination by palpitation WNL
GU: WNL
RECT: WNL
EXT: WNL
NEURO: Alert with a strong cry and normal muscle tone and reflexes

Results of Laboratory Tests

Na 136 (136)	AST 0.45 (27)	Glu 3.3 (60)
K 4.8 (4.8)	ALT 0.3 (18)	Ca 2.5 (10)
Cl 103 (103)	GGT 0.23 (14)	PO$_4$ 1.45 (4.5)
HCO$_3$ 19 (19)	Alb 38 (3.8)	
BUN 2.5 (7)	T Bili 10.7 (0.63)	
CR 53 (0.7)		

PROBLEM LIST

1. S/P Dishwashing liquid ingestion
2. Emesis, cow's milk/soy protein allergy
3. Atopic eczema

CASE 177 SOAP NOTES

Problem 1. Dishwashing Liquid Ingestion

S: Mother states that RS ingested some dishwashing liquid 4 days ago.

O: None

A: Ingestion of nontoxic detergent

P: Dishwashing liquid is a nontoxic detergent that may cause emesis for 1–2 days; therefore RS requires close monitoring at home for dehydration.

Problem 2. Emesis, Cow's Milk/Soy Protein Allergy

S: Mother states that RS has been vomiting for the past 4 days, since the ingestion of dishwashing liquid, but is able to tolerate apple juice and oral rehydration fluids. RS has a history of cow's milk allergy. Prior to the dishwashing liquid ingestion, she was tolerating Prosobee.

O: None

A: Initially, emesis was caused by dishwashing liquid ingestion, but it may now be a soy protein sensitivity. Repeated emesis over the 4-day period may have caused intestinal mucosal damage, allowing increased sensitivity to other protein antigens such as soy protein.

P: Begin feeding with an elemental formula such as Pregestimil to allow intestinal healing. If RS tolerates the elemental formula, continue this formula for 10–14 days. After intestinal regeneration, RS may be able to return to a soy protein formula such as Prosobee, which she was receiving previously.

Problem 3. Atopic Eczema

S: RS's mother has noticed that RS has a rash on her cheeks, which she frequently scratches.

O: RS's cheeks are erythematous and edematous with exudation.

A: Atopic eczema, possibly a manifestation of soy protein allergy

P: Apply sparingly a low-potency topical steroid cream (e.g., triamcinolone cream 0.5%) to affected areas twice daily for 7 days. Supportive care for rash should include avoiding extreme temperatures and humidity and minimizing water contact with rash. Antihistamines may used as needed if RS is irritable and unable to sleep.

QUESTIONS FOR CASE 177

1. Name and describe a computer-generated data base you would search for management information about toxicology.
2. Describe the manifestations of cow's milk allergy. Are cow's milk and soy protein allergies self-limiting, with future development of tolerance to these proteins? What nutritional options are available for each type of protein allergy?
3. Is reversible HPA-axis suppression possible with topical application of corticosteroids in infants and children?
4. Is systemic corticosteroid administration more desirable for treating atopic eczema in infants and children?

CASE 178

CC: JB is an 8-year-old boy brought to the pediatrician by his mother for complaints of a rash that developed shortly after starting an antibiotic for an ear infection.

History of Present Illness

Seven days ago, he visited his uncle in the country for the weekend, where he spent many hours swimming in the lake. During the car ride to the countryside, he started to cough from dust exposure, with increase in frequency and intensity during his stay because his uncle smokes at home. He used his inhaler repeatedly without relief. Upon his return home (5 days ago), the cough and respiratory difficulty persisted but was less severe. He then developed left ear pain, partial hearing loss, and a tactile fever. He was brought to the pediatrician in the morning (4 days ago), and was diagnosed with left otitis media and given a prescription for amoxicillin. This morning, he noticed a rash which began on this abdomen and has since progressed to the rest of his body. He refuses to go to school because he is afraid his classmates will make fun of him.

Medical History

Asthma was diagnosed at 5 years of age, and has been well controlled on albuterol inhalers as needed for wheeze. JB has never been hospitalized for an asthma exacerbation. He has had frequent bouts of otitis media as a young child, but has never had any complications nor required surgical management. His last episode was at 4 years of age. Immunizations are up to date.

Medication History

Albuterol metered-dose inhaler: 2 puffs q6h as needed for wheeze. Normally used once every other week, but this past weekend, patient has used it q4h without relief

Amoxicillin 500 mg po TID × 10 days started 4 days ago.

Allergies

None known

Review of Systems

Noncontributory

Physical Examination

GEN: Comfortable young man with diffuse rash, in NAD

VS: BP 96/58, HR 103, RR 28, T 37.5°C, Wt 32 kg, Ht 114 cm

HEENT: NC/AT, EOMI, PERRL, nl conjunctiva, TMs clear

COR: RRR, no murmur

CHEST: No retractions, breathing comfortably on room air, mild expiratory wheezes bilaterally, no crackles

ABD: Soft, NTND, (+) BS

GU: WNL

RECT: Deferred

EXT: 2+ DTR

SKIN: Diffuse maculopapular rash mainly on the abdomen, with some distribution to all extremities

NEURO: WNL

Results of Laboratory Tests

Na 142 (142)	Hct 0.41 (41)
K 3.6 (3.6)	Hgb 143 (14.3)
Cl 99 (99)	Lkcs 9.2 × 10⁹ (9.2 × 10³)
HCO₃ 19 (19)	Plts 144 × 10⁹ (144 × 10³)
BUN 5.7 (16)	MCV 88 (88)
Cr 53.0 (0.6)	Glu 5.50 (99)

WBC Differential: Neut 65%, Bands 1%, Lymph 23%, Mono 2%, Eos 9%

CXR: RUL bandlike atelectasis, hyperinflated bilaterally consistent with asthma

Sputum: <1 + PMN, no organisms on Gram's stain; culture pending

PROBLEM LIST

1. Drug-induced rash
2. Otitis media

3. Asthma

Use SOAP for the above problems.

CASE 178 SOAP NOTES
Problem 1. Drug-induced Rash

S: JB complains of rash starting on his abdomen, progressing to his whole body.

O: Maculopapular rash developing after 4 days of amoxicillin therapy, with most lesions on the truncal area and some appearing on each limb.

A: The aminopenicillins, ampicillin and amoxicillin, have a higher incidence (5%–10%) of causing a generalized erythematous, maculopapular rash than other penicillins. This rash usually appears 3–14 days into the therapy, and begins on the trunk and spreads to the rest of the body. It is usually mild, and resolves in 6–14 days even if therapy is continued. This is not a dose-related phenomenon, but has a strong association with viral infections (such as mononucleosis and cytomegalovirus) with a 65%–100% incidence. It does not appear to be immunologic in origin because most patients experiencing this rash have a negative skin test for penicillin hypersensitivity, and the same patients have received subsequent ampicillin and other β-lactams without incidents. For this reason, the ampicillin/amoxicillin rash has been deemed to be nonimmunologic, and does not imply hypersensitivity to penicillins, nor is there a contraindication for future use of any penicillins. Although amoxicillin can be continued for the treatment of otitis media, another antibiotic may be chosen to avoid patient discomfort caused by the rash.

P: D/C amoxicillin. Select another antibiotic (see otitis media SOAP). Do not label patient allergic to penicillins.

Problem 2. Otitis Media

S: JB initially complained of ear pain, partial loss of hearing, and fevers.

O: Patient previously diagnosed with otitis media and given 4 days of amoxicillin therapy. Currently has no symptoms of otitis: TMs are clear, patient is afebrile, and WBC is consistent with resolving otitis.

A: This is a case of partially treated otitis media, complicated by development of drug-induced rash. As discussed above, it would be possible to continue amoxicillin for the remaining 6 days of therapy because it is unlikely that the patient is experiencing a true hypersensitivity reaction, and the rash may resolve with continued therapy. However, because JB appears to be bothered cosmetically by the rash, it is acceptable to change the antibiotic. The most common pathogens for otitis media are *S. pneumoniae* and *H. influenzae*, for which amoxicillin (50 mg/kg/day divided into three doses) is the drug of choice. For regions in which β-lactamase-producing organisms are common, trimethoprim/sulfamethoxazole (10 mg/kg/day of TMP in two divided doses) is the first-line agent, primarily because of cost considerations. Other more expensive alternatives (i.e., erythromycin/sulfisoxazole, cefuroxime axetil, cefaclor, and cefixime) have been shown to be similar in efficacy, and may also be selected.

P: Start trimethoprim/sulfamethoxazole double-strength tablet (160 mg TMP/800 mg SMX) po BID × 6 days for the remainder of the 10-day therapy.

Problem 3. Asthma

S: JB has a recent exposure to allergens (i.e., dust and cigarette smoke). His albuterol inhaler has not given him relief as he increased the frequency of use to q4h. He is otherwise normally well controlled with albuterol, with attacks occurring every other week.

O: Patient has persistent cough and respiratory distress. On examination, expiratory wheezes are heard bilaterally. CXR is consistent with asthma. CBC shows eosinophilia (eos = 828 cells/mm^3, versus normal 250–400).

A: JB has extrinsic or allergic asthma, which can be characterized as mild because his attacks occur less than once weekly. Use of a β$_2$-agonist only when symptoms occur is the ideal strategy to control his exacerbations. However, because JB does not use the inhaler daily, he may have forgotten how to use it correctly; this may explain why he was refractory to treatment. The patient and his mother need to have the instructions reinforced periodically. The number of albuterol puffs can also be increased for better efficacy. An AeroChamber may also be added to insure adequate delivery of medication to his lungs. Addition of the cromolyn inhaler may also prove useful, especially for use prior to an anticipated exposure to allergens (i.e., another weekend at his uncle's place).

P: Increase albuterol inhaler to four puffs q6h as needed for wheeze. Add AeroChamber. Add cromolyn inhaler two puffs q6h. Instruct JB and his mother on the correct use of the inhalers and the AeroChamber.

QUESTIONS FOR CASE 178

1. Is it important to note the immunization status of a child with otitis media? Why?
2. Suppose JB still had evidence on examination of otitis media (the tympanic membranes are red, with a purulent discharge) after 4 days of amoxicillin therapy. How would this change the approach in selecting an antibiotic to complete his 10-day therapy?
3. Why is it important to treat otitis media adequately? What are some complications?
4. Why are β$_2$-receptor agonist inhalers now recommended only for p.r.n. usage, and not on the scheduled basis?

CASE 179

CC: JM is a 9-year-old boy whose mother brought him to the clinic today with complaints of stomach aches and cramps, itchy skin, and an 8-day history of intermittent fevers and nausea, with a poor appetite. JM's mom has also noticed that JM's eyes and skin have a yellow discoloration.

Social History

JM attends daycare daily after school. Approximately 2 weeks prior to this visit, he went camping with the Boy Scouts.

Physical Examination

GEN: Well developed and well nourished
VS: BP 90/60, HR 120, RR 20, T 35°C, Wt 26.3 kg (usual weight 28 kg), Ht 132 cm
HEENT: Sunken, icteric eyes with dry mucous membranes
COR: Normal S_1 and S_2, with no murmurs, rubs, or gallops
CHEST: Clear to auscultation
ABD: Soft, hepatomegaly with smooth, tender edge
GU: WNL
RECT: WNL
EXT: Jaundiced skin with pruritis and positive tenting
NEURO: Lethargic, DTR's WNL

Results of Laboratory Tests

Na 138 (138)	Hct 0.49 (49)	AST 8 (480)	Glu 4.8 (87)
K 4.1 (4.1)	Hgb 160 (16)	ALT 6.67 (400)	
Cl 98 (98)	Lkcs 5.1×10^9 (5.1×10^3)	Alk Phos 5.75 (395)	
HCO$_3$ 22 (22)		Alb 44 (4.4)	
BUN 3.6 (10)		T Bili 30 (1.8)	
CR 31 (0.4)			

Hepatitis A antigen: Positive
Hepatitis A antibody: Positive
Urinalysis: pH: 5.6, specific gravity 1.03, urobilin trace, Stool specimen: Clay-colored

PROBLEM LIST

1. Hepatitis A
2. Dehydration
3. Poor appetite

QUESTIONS FOR CASE 179

1. How is hepatitis A transmitted?
2. Is hepatitis A a risk factor for the development of chronic active hepatitis or cirrhosis?
3. Why, in JM's admission laboratory values, would his serum albumin concentration be falsely elevated?
4. Discuss why albumin is used clinically as a nutritional assessment marker and its limitations.

CASE 180

CC: LM is a 7-year-old girl who presents to pulmonary clinic with a several-day history of increase in the frequency of coughing, a slight increase in wheezing, increase in the number of greasy stools per day, and a decrease in her appetite. She also complains of thirst and an increase in frequency of urination at night.

History of Present Illness

LM was diagnosed with cystic fibrosis (CF) at 3 months of age. After birth, she exhibited poor weight gain, chronic diarrhea, and respiratory distress. Several days prior to coming to clinic, LM's mother noticed that LM had developed a productive cough. LM normally has a chronic cough and mild wheezing, but it has been progressing over the past several days. Even though LM is not eating as much as usual, she is experiencing an increase in diarrhea that is characterized by greasy, foul-smelling stool. LM is exhibiting signs of hyperglycemia.

Medical History

LM's CF has been fairly stable; she has never been intubated or required systemic steroids for her respiratory status. She has had several URIs in the past that were treated at home with oral antibiotics. Because of her failure to thrive as an infant, LM was placed on supplemental enteral nutrition as well as enzyme replacements to decrease the amount of diarrhea. LM has mild type I diabetes (IDDM) that has been well controlled with small amounts of insulin.

Medication History

Ferrous Sulfate 25 mg (elemental) po TID
Pancrelipase (Pancrease) two capsules before each meal, one capsule before each snack
Beclomethasone MDI two puffs TID
Regular Insulin 2U SQ before each meal
NPH Insulin 2U SQ at bedtime
Ensure 1 can with each meal
Immunizations up to date

Allergies

Penicillins (facial swelling, urticaria)

Review of Systems

Noncontributory

Physical Examination

GEN: Child small for age, pale skin, noticeably wheezing, in NAD
VS: BP 114/72, HR 87, RR 30, T 38.5°C, Wt 20 kg, Ht 115 cm
HEENT: PERRLA, moist mucous membranes, TM clear
COR: Regular rate and rhythm, no murmur or gallop
CHEST: Coarse BS, bilateral wheezes
ABD: Soft, slightly tender, no masses
RECT: Normal
EXT: Warm, strong pulses
NEURO: Alert and oriented × 3, CN intact

Results of Laboratory Tests

Na 138 (138)	Oxygen saturation 94%
Hct 0.3 (30)	HCO$_3$ 24 (24)
Vit A 0.28 (8)	Plt 300×10^9 (300×10^3)
K 3.6 (3.6)	BUN 3.2 (9)
Hgb 90 (9)	MCV 82 (82)
Vit E 11.6 (0.5)	Cr 60 (0.6)
Cl 101 (101)	Alb 32 (3.2)
WBC 17 (17)	

Chloride sweat test 75 mEq/L

Fasting glucose 07:30 6.9 (125); 11:30 7.2 (130); 17:30 6.6 (120); 02:00 10.5 (190)

UA: No organisms, esterase negative

CXR: No infiltrates, bronchovascular markings consistent with CF

Sputum Gram's stain: Gram-positive cocci in clusters

PROBLEM LIST

1. CF exacerbation
2. Nutritional status
3. IDDM

CASE 180 SOAP NOTES

Problem 1. CF Exacerbation

S: LM complains of a productive cough and increase in wheezing.

O: LM exhibits a low-grade fever, elevated respiratory rate, positive Gram's stain, CXR consistent with CF, coarse breath sounds, and wheezing.

A: The lungs of patients with CF are often colonized with specific organisms. Early in the course of CF, *H. influenzae* and *S. aureus* are the most common organisms isolated from sputum; however, as the disease progresses, most patients become colonized with strains of *P. aeruginosa* and rarely, *P. cepacia*. While a course of antibiotics is indicated, eradication of the organism from the sputum may not always occur. LM is experiencing a mild exacerbation of her CF as evidenced by her symptoms. Because her CXR does not indicate infection and her oxygen saturation is acceptable, she may be treated as an outpatient with oral antibiotics. Furthermore, because LM's wheezing has worsened, she may benefit from increasing the frequency of her steroid inhaler. The use of bronchodilators for treatment in CF is controversial. The responsiveness to bronchodilators varies from 0%–40%; some patients may benefit while others will not.

P: Because LM's Gram's stain indicates *S. aureus*, her therapy should target this organism. Reasonable oral antibiotic selections include cefaclor, cephalexin, cefuroxime axetil, amoxicillin/clavulanic acid, and trimethoprim/sulfamethoxazole. Because LM demonstrates a significant penicillin allergy, trimethoprim/sulfamethoxazole is an appropriate choice dosed at 10 mg/kg/day divided BID for a duration of 14 days. CF patients with lung infections should be treated for a minimum of 2 weeks with antibiotics; experience has shown that shorter courses are inadequate. The goal of the antimicrobial therapy is to eradicate the organism, improve her lung examination, and prevent progression to a severe pneumonia. LM should be monitored for frequency of her cough, wheezing, and temperature. Because LM's wheezing has worsened, she may benefit from increasing the frequency of her beclomethasone inhaler to two puffs QID during her exacerbation. After her exacerbation, she may return to her TID schedule if she is controlled. LM may also benefit from chest physiotherapy (PT). For chest PT, the child is placed in a position in which gravity can drain the lungs, and the chest wall is clapped with a cupped hand followed by supervised coughing. This assists in the drainage of purulent secretions.

Problem 2. Nutritional Status

S: LM has experienced a diminished appetite and an increase in the number of greasy stools daily.

O: LM has frequent diarrhea, is small for her age, has a slightly depressed albumin, and low hemoglobin, hematocrit, and vitamin levels.

A: Pancreatic insufficiency is the main cause of malabsorption in patients with CF. This malabsorption is characterized by greasy stools, an inability to absorb fat-soluble vitamins, and slow growth. Good nutrition and growth are promoted by pancreatic enzyme replacement. Because LM is experiencing gastrointestinal involvement, her current dose of pancreatic enzyme is insufficient, and it should be increased. LM continues to be anemic, so her current dose of ferrous sulfate is insufficient. Furthermore, LM requires external vitamin supplementation with fat-soluble vitamins (A, D, E, K) because her vitamin levels are low.

P: LM's pancreatic enzyme should be increased to three capsules with each meal and two capsules with each snack. The final dose of the pancreatic enzyme will be titrated to the frequency and quality of her bowel movements. The goal is one to four stools daily that are formed and free of fat. LM's stools should be closely monitored as should her abdominal examination (cramping, bloating) and weight. Because LM is slightly anemic, her dose of ferrous sulfate should also be titrated up to 35 mg elemental iron TID. The goal is to elevate her hemoglobin and hematocrit to normal. Finally, LM needs fat-soluble vitamin supplementation. She should receive one tablet daily of a formulation that contains vitamins A, D, E, and K.

Problem 3. IDDM

S: LM complains of thirst and increased urination.

O: LM is displaying polyuria, polydipsia, and an elevated fasting blood glucose during the evening.

A: In patients who have CF, glucose intolerance can occur because of pancreatic destruction, resulting in diminished insulin production. This is rare: only 2%–3% of patients develop IDDM. In patients whom IDDM develops, it is often mild and can be controlled with small daily amounts of insulin; furthermore, CF patients rarely progress to diabetic ketoacidosis (DKA). LM is experiencing only a minor loss of control of her diabetes. Her fasting glucose levels during the day are acceptable, and she does not complain of any symptoms of hyperglycemia during the day. However, LM has an elevated fasting blood glucose and symptoms of hyperglycemia at night. Because her morning, noon, and early evening levels are within the normal limits, it appears that LM's evening dose of regular insulin may be inadequate. Furthermore, increasing the frequency of her inhaled steroids may affect her blood glucose level.

P: Her morning and noon regular insulin and her bedtime

NPH insulin regimen will remain unchanged. Her evening dose of regular insulin (predinner dose) will be increased from two to four units. LM's insulin regimen can be written as follows:

Regular Insulin 2U SQ at 08:00 and 12:00
Regular Insulin 4U SQ at 18:00
NPH Insulin 2U SQ at 22:00

The goal is to return LM's night-time glucose measurement to normal and eliminate her symptoms of hyperglycemia. LM's symptoms and blood glucose levels should be followed closely until each blood glucose level is within the acceptable limit. It is also important to monitor for signs and symptoms of hypoglycemia (such as sweating, shaking, and confusion) whenever an insulin dose is increased.

QUESTIONS FOR CASE 180

1. What other organ systems can be involved in patients with CF?
2. Describe DNase and explain its role in CF therapy.
3. Comment on the use of fluoroquinolones in children.
4. Describe the recent FDA changes in research and approval of medications used in pediatric patients.
5. Counsel LM's mother about appropriate and inappropriate OTC medications for LM.

CASE 181

CC: JD is a 6-month-old boy who presents to the emergency room with a fever, vomiting, decreased urine output, and generalized seizures.

History of Present Illness

Two days ago, JD's mother noticed that he was "not himself." He was not taking as many bottles as usual and was sleeping more than usual. She also commented that JD had only two wet diapers that day. On the day of admission, she noticed that he had a fever of 39°C and began to vomit. Shortly after, he started having seizures, and she brought him to the emergency room.

Medical History

JD had his first case of otitis media (OM) 2 weeks before this visit. His physician prescribed ampicillin for a 10-day course. Because JD had so much diarrhea while taking the ampicillin, and because his symptoms of OM had disappeared, his mother decided to discontinue the medication after only 3 days of treatment.

Social History

JD lives at home with his mom, dad, and two sisters (aged 2 and 3 years) who both attend daycare.

Medication History

Acetaminophen drops for fevers 15 mg/kg/dose Q4-6H

Allergies

None known

Review of Systems

Noncontributory

Physical Examination

GEN: Lethargic infant with generalized seizure activity
VS: BP 93/55, HR 175, RR 35, T 40.0°C, Wt 6 kg (normally 7 kg), Ht 65 cm
HEENT: PERRLA, dry mucous membranes, red, bulging TM bilaterally, bulging fontanel
COR: Normal S_1 and S_2
CHEST: Clear to ascultation and percussion
ABD: Soft, no masses
RECT: Stool guaiac-negative
EXT: Skin tenting noted
NEURO: Generalized seizures, lethargic, nuchal rigidity

Results of Laboratory Tests

Na 135 (135)	Plts 300×10^9 (300×10^3)
Hct 0.35 (35)	BUN 10.5 (30)
Alb 39 (3.9)	Glu 4.4 (80)
K 5.5 (5.5)	
Hgb 105 (10.5)	
Cl 100 (100)	
WBC 21 (21)	
HCO$_3$ 26 (26)	

Cr: 60 (0.7) (Cr was normal at his visit 2 weeks ago)
CSF fluid: Appearance xanthochromic
WBC: 600
Glu: 1.5 (28)
Protein: 0.75 (75)
Gram's stain: Gram-negative bacilli
Blood cultures: Results pending

PROBLEM LIST

1. Septic meningitis
2. Seizure
3. Dehydration
4. Otitis media

CASE 181 SOAP NOTES
Problem 1. Meningitis

S: JD exhibits decreased oral intake, decreased urine output, vomiting, lethargy, and seizure activity.
O: JD has a fever, elevated white blood count, nuchal rigidity, bulging fontanel, and seizures. Examination of CSF fluid parameters (elevated WBC and protein, depressed glucose, and positive gram stain) reveals septic meningitis.
A: JD is suffering from acute meningitis with complications. He was recently diagnosed with acute otitis media for which he was given an incomplete course of antimicrobial ther-

apy. Noncompliance may have resulted in failure to eradicate the organism from the middle ear. Alternatively, because his sisters both attend daycare, they could have transmitted a resistant organism to JD. Daycare centers are associated with a high incidence of resistant organisms. The organism may have then spread either hematogenously or contiguously to the meninges resulting in meningitis. Furthermore, JD's immunizations are not up to date. *H. influenzae* is the most likely pathogen for JD's age group; however, *N. meningitidis* and *S. pneumoniae* are also common in children aged 1 month to 4 years.

P: Treatment for JD's meningitis must be initiated immediately with intravenous antibiotics after CSF and blood cultures are obtained. It is important to obtain the cultures prior to antimicrobial therapy to avoid altering the results of the cultures. Because JD is hypotensive, his renal and hepatic function could be temporarily compromised; therefore, it is wise to avoid treatment with chloramphenicol and aminoglycosides. Approximately 30% of *H. influenzae* is β-lactamase-positive, which renders ampicillin inactive. Initial therapy will be empiric, and therapy will be tailored after the final culture and susceptibilities are available. The initial regimen should be broad enough to cover all of the likely pathogens for JD's age group. Furthermore, it is essential that the antibiotic be able to cross the blood-brain-barrier effectively to ensure adequate CSF drug levels. Doses of antimicrobials should be greater than doses used to treat other systemic infections to ensure adequate CSF penetration. Empirically, a third-generation cephalosporin would be appropriate; for example, cefotaxime 200 mg/kg/day divided Q6H. Other alternatives include ceftriaxone or ceftizoxime both dosed at 200 mg/kg/day divided Q6H. If the culture results indicate that the organism is β-lactamase-negative, ampicillin 200–400 mg/kg/day divided Q4-6H would be adequate. Meningitis due to *H. influenzae* should be treated for a minimum of 10 days. The goals of therapy are to prevent further complications such as cerebral edema, SIADH, deafness, or brain abscesses and to eradicate the organism from the CSF. It is important to monitor CSF (cultures and sensitivities). If JD shows a clinical response to therapy, there is no indication for a repeat LP and CSF examination; however, if he does not improve after 24 to 48 hours of therapy, a second LP should be obtained. Furthermore, it is important to monitor the CBC, renal function, temperature, neurologic status, and vital signs.

Problem 2. Seizures

S: JD is exhibiting seizure activity.

O: JD is experiencing a generalized seizure.

A: JD has developed seizures secondary to his meningitis and this could be compounded by his fever. It is important to stop his seizure activity promptly to avoid permanent damage.

P: For patients who are actively seizing or in status epilepticus as is JD, lorazepam is the drug of choice. Lorazepam is preferred over diazepam for several reasons: lorazepam

stops the seizure within 2 to 3 minutes in approximately 80%–100% of patients and has a longer duration of antiseizure activity (approximately 24–48 hours). Due to the high success with lorazepam, additional anticonvulsants such as phenobarbital often are unnecessary, which helps to avoid drug interactions and additive adverse effects. JD should receive lorazepam 0.1–0.2 mg/kg (0.7–1.4 mg) IV over 2 minutes. A second dose of 0.05 mg/kg may be repeated in 10 to 15 minutes if needed. The goal is to stop seizure activity and prevent neurologic damage. JD should be monitored for any recurrence of seizure activity.

Problem 3. Dehydration

S: JD exhibited decreased oral intake over the past 2 days.

O: JD is hypotensive and tachycardic (normal blood pressure for his age is 106/66; normal heart rate is 130). He has decreased urine output, his BUN and Cr are elevated, and he is demonstrating skin tenting and dry mucous membranes. Furthermore, he has dropped 1 kg in weight.

A: Several factors contribute to JD's dehydration: he has not been taking in as much fluid as he normally does; he has a fever, which increases insensible loss; he has been vomiting; and he has an infection. It is important to determine the severity of JD's dehydration. His percent dehydration can be calculated:

$$\frac{\text{normal body weight} - \text{actual body weight}}{\text{normal body weight}} \times 100 = \% \text{ dehydration}$$

Using JD's weights, his dehydration is calculated at 14%, which is considered severe. JD will need aggressive fluid replacement and maintenance fluids.

P: Fluid replacement is determined by multiplying the weight lost by 1000 ml/kg, so JD will need 1000 ml of replacement fluids. Potassium replacement should be held until his urine output increases and his potassium level decreases to normal; at that point, potassium can be added to the maintenance fluids. The first half of replacement volume (or 500 ml) is given over 8 hours at a rate of 60 ml/hour, and the second half (500 ml) is given over the following 16 hours at a rate of 30 ml/hour. At the same time, his maintenance fluid should be administered. Children weighing less than 10 kg need 120 ml/kg/day (based on normal body weight) for maintenance; for JD this would be 840 ml over 24 hours. However, fever raises the daily maintenance fluid needs in children: 12% for each °C greater than 37°C. JD's fluid requirements will be increased by 36% (or 300 ml) simply due to his fever. JD's total maintenance fluids will be approximately 1200 ml over 24 hours, given at a rate of 50 ml/hour. It is also important to determine the daily sodium requirement. The amount of sodium needed is 2–4 mEq/kg/day; for JD this is 14–28 meq Na+ ≠ day. One-quarter normal saline (0.225%) contains 34 mEq/L; therefore, the fluid that can be used for JD is D51/4NS. In summary, JD's fluid orders could be written as follows: D51/4NS at 110 ml/hour for 8 hours, then at 80 ml/hour for 16 hours. After the first 24 hours, JD's fluid and electrolyte status should be reassessed and adjustments made as needed. The daily requirement for potassium is 2–5 mEq/kg/day, which is 14–35 mEq K+ daily for JD; therefore, when JD's urine output and potassium have normalized, his fluid should be changed to D51/4NS with 20 mEQ K+/L. The goal is to rehydrate JD and reverse his symptoms of dehydration. It is important to monitor his hemodynamic parameters, urine output, weight, electrolytes, and mucous membranes.

Problem 4. Otitis Media

S: JD has exhibited diminished appetite and fever.

O: His TMs are red and bulging and he is febrile.

A: JD's otitis media diagnosed 2 weeks before this visit was inadequately treated, so the organisms were not eradicated. Because this was an acute case of OM, the most likely organisms causing the infection are *S. pneumoniae, H. influenzae,* and *M. catarrhalis.* Resistance rates for *S. pneumoniae* are low, but it is important to consider resistance rates for *H. influenzae* and *M. catarrhalis,* which are 30% and 70%–90% respectively.

P: The antibiotic therapy that JD receives for his meningitis will effectively treat his otitis media, so he does not require any additional therapy. The goals of therapy are to eradicate the organism from the middle ear and prevent further complications such as recurrence or chronic OM. It is important to monitor for resolution of the OM via visual inspection of the ear as well as disappearance of all symptoms.

QUESTIONS FOR CASE 181

1. Explain the role of dexamethasone as adjuvant therapy for children with meningitis.
2. The final culture results of JD's CSF revealed *H. influenzae.* Describe what prophylactic precautions should be taken with JD and his family after his course of septic meningitis.
3. Does JD require ongoing anticonvulsant therapy after discharge from the hospital?
4. If JD develops recurrent bouts of otitis media, how should antimicrobial therapy be approached?
5. Counsel JD's mother about outpatient rehydration principles.

OB-GYN DISORDERS

CASE 182

CC: SK is a 32-year-old woman afflicted with bipolar disorder since age 30. She comes to the ob/gyn clinic today complaining of moderately severe dysmenorrhea, dysuria, and a thick, gray, malodorous vaginal discharge.

Medical History

SK has been having episodes of mania and depression separated by intervals without mood disturbances for the last 2 years. Euphoria, hyperactivity, and flight of ideas often begin suddenly, and these symptoms escalate rapidly in severity over a few days and last for a few days to a few months. Major depressive episodes last for several weeks, during which time SK feels hopeless and depressed. Moderate facial acne has plagued her since age 13. She has had multiple sex partners regularly. She has had a longtime fear of becoming an alcoholic.

Ob/Gyn History

$G_1P_0TAB_1$; last menstrual period was 1 week ago. She has a long history of bothersome heavy periods and had to have her IUD removed because of aggravation of her dysmenorrhea symptoms 3 months ago. She was fitted with a diaphragm, which contributed to two urinary tract infections in the 2 following months, and it was therefore discontinued. She was then given a combination of mestranol and norethindrone (Norinyl) 1 1 + 35, but after taking the first four tablets, she called and said that they triggered a depressive episode and that she was "afraid of birth control pills." Her dysmenorrhea seems to be helped only by acetaminophen with codeine and not by ibuprofen or naproxen. The pelvic cramping lasts for the first 2 days of each menses, when her flow is heaviest. The cramping even occurred when she was diagnosed as having anovulatory cycles for several years.

She had episodes of pelvic inflammatory disease (PID) at ages 19 and 23.

Social History

Single cocktail waitress
Four glasses of wine with dinner for 12 years

Family History

Mother is cyclothymic with a history of substance abuse.

Medication History

Protriptyline 10 mg BID

Acetaminophen 325 mg with codeine 30 mg q3–4h p.r.n. dysmenorrhea
Tetracycline 500 mg BID

Allergies

Clotrimazole vaginal cream

Physical Examination

GEN:	Well developed, well nourished
VS:	BP 126/85 RA (sitting), HR 74, RR 20, T 37°C, Wt 58 kg, Ht 163 cm
HEENT:	Facial skin clear of acne
COR:	WNL
CHEST:	Bilateral fibrocystic breast densities
ABD:	NL
GU:	Thick, gray, malodorus vaginal discharge; "strawberry cervix"; meatal erythema
RECT:	NL
EXT:	NL
NEURO:	WNL

Results of Laboratory Tests

Na 143 (143)	HCO_3 26 (26)	Hct 0.33 (33)	ALT 0.2 (12)
K 4.4 (4.4)	BUN 6.4 (18)	Hgb 120 (12)	T Bili 9 (0.5)
Cl 99 (99)	CR 88 (1.0)	AST 0.17 (10)	Glu (fasting) 5.3 (95)

Protriptyline 380 nmol/liter (100 ng/ml)
Guaiac: Negative
Vaginal fluid: Normal saline slide: highly motile, pear-shaped, unicellular *Trichomonas vaginalis*

PROBLEM LIST

1. Bipolar disorder
2. Facial acne
3. *Trichomonas* vaginitis
4. Dysmenorrhea
5. Contraception

CASE 182 SOAP NOTES

Problem 3. *Trichomonas* Vaginitis

S: Thick, gray, malodorous vaginal discharge and dysuria

O: Normal saline slide: highly motile, pear-shaped, unicellular *Trichomonas vaginalis*; meatal erythema; vaginal malodor; thick, gray vaginal discharge

A: SK has *Trichomonas* vaginitis. Metronidazole is the drug choice; SK probably is not pregnant.

P: Metronidazole 2 g po stat for both patient and her partner(s). Patient education: Warn SK and her partner(s) of the possibility of disulfiram reaction if taken with alcohol, a metallic taste in the mouth, and a brown discoloration of the urine due to metabolites of metronidazole. All those involved should take the metronidazole simultaneously. Monitoring of therapeutic success consists of checking for resolution of symptoms. Follow-up visits are unnecessary if SK and her partner(s) become asymptomatic after treatment. If therapy fails, many practitioners suggest getting liver function tests before repeating therapy, although this is controversial, and SK's were just done and all values were normal. The CDC now recommends that if failure occurs, the patient and her partner(s) should be treated with metronidazole 500 mg twice daily for 7 days. If repeated failure occurs, SK should be treated with a single 2-gm dose of metronidazole once daily for 3–5 days. SK and her partners should be instructed to avoid sex until they are cured.

Problem 4. Dysmenorrhea

S: Moderately severe pelvic cramping for the first 2 days of menses when the flow is heaviest

O: History of dysmenorrhea, even in anovulatory cycles

A: Primary dysmenorrhea occurs in ovulatory cycles and is usually adequately treated with nonsteroidal antiinflammatory drugs (NSAIDs). However, SK failed with both ibuprofen and naproxen, gets relief from acetaminophen and codeine, and has had pelvic inflammatory disease twice. Therefore, adhesions causing secondary dysmenorrhea are probably present.

P: A trial of another class of NSAIDs, mefenamic acid 500 mg po stat, then 250 mg q6h p.r.n. dysmenorrhea, is appropriate, because SK may have both primary and secondary dysmenorrhea. The only way to find out if pelvic adhesions are present, and to avoid long-term use of narcotics in this patient with bipolar disorder, is to do a laparoscopy. Identified adhesions can be lysed at the same time, but they may recur.

Problem 5. Contraception

S: SK has been sexually active with multiple partners since 13 years of age.

O: Currently has sexually transmitted *Trichomonas* vaginitis

A: Her medication history shows that she is not using any form of contraception. Intrauterine devices, diaphragms, and oral contraceptives have been tried and are not acceptable for SK.

P: Because SK has multiple partners and hormonal contraceptives may worsen her bouts of depression, a barrier method of contraception is in order. The most effective barrier method is the use of condoms with contraceptive foam. This will protect her from pregnancy (if used correctly) almost as well as oral contraceptives and will help prevent sexually transmitted diseases. She should be tested for HIV.

Problem 2. Facial Acne

S: History of moderate facial acne since age 13

O: Facial skin is clear at this time.

A: Her current therapy of tetracycline 500 mg po BID appears

adequate.

P: Continue tetracycline 500 mg po BID

Problem 1. Bipolar Disorder

S: SK has been having episodes of mania and depression, separated by intervals without mood disturbances, for the last 2 years. Recently, after taking just the first four birth control pills of her package, a major depressive episode was triggered, and she is now "afraid of birth control pills."

O: Euphoria, hyperactivity, and flight of ideas often begin suddenly, and these symptoms escalate rapidly over a few days and usually last for a few days to a few months. A major depressive episode is manifested in SK as feeling hopeless and depressed, and these symptoms last for several weeks. Her protriptyline level is in the therapeutic range, and she is not complaining of side effects.

P: Continue protriptyline 10 mg po BID. Avoid oral contraceptives and other forms of hormone therapy to avoid aggravation of depression or initiation of depressive episodes.

QUESTIONS FOR CASE 182

1. If metronidazole 500 mg po BID × 7 days fails to cure SK's *Trichomonas* vaginitis, what should be done next?
2. An outside attending physician suggests that SK be given aspirin 650 mg po q4h beginning 2 days before her menstrual flow to treat her dysmenorrhea. Do you agree or disagree with this therapy? Explain.
3. Could SK safely use a Progestasert IUD as a means of contraception?
4. The attending physician suggests that SK be put on disulfiram treatment because she has expressed concern about a drinking problem and is a cocktail waitress. What are your concerns? What other drug is available for alcohol dependence and what would be your concerns about its use in SK?
5. What is a cyclothymic disorder, and why does SK's mother suffer from such a disorder?

CASE 183

CC: HD is a 26-year-old married woman who is seen in the clinic for selection of a contraception method. After intercourse and at certain times of the month she has noted a thin, gray vaginal discharge with a "fishy" odor. In addition, she was instructed to receive follow-up for a urinary tract infection (UTI).

Medical History

HD was diagnosed as having stage IIB Hodgkin's disease 1 year ago. She was treated with radical radiation therapy and did not require chemotherapy at that time. She is in complete remission at this time. Five years ago she took combination oral contraceptives (COC) for 2 years, but has been relying on a diaphragm and spermicide since then. She was treated for an *Escherichia coli* urinary tract infection (UTI) 1 month ago, with a 10-day course of cotrimoxazole. She was previously treated for a UTI 6 months earlier.

Ob/Gyn History

G1P1
LMP 21 days ago, regular 28-day cycle

Surgical History

Appendectomy at age 14 years

Medication History

Vinegar douches after intercourse (self-initiated)
Clotrimoxazole vaginal cream 1 applicatorful QD × 7 days (self-initiated)
Acetaminophen 2 p.r.n. HA

Allergies

None known

Social and Family History

HD is an x-ray technician whose husband is a mechanic. They have a healthy 4-year-old girl. Nonsmoker, drinks no ethanol, vegetarian.

Physical Examination

GEN: Well-developed, well-nourished woman who is a good historian
VS: BP 106/65, HR 50, RR 18, Wt 62 kg, Ht 165 cm
HEENT: WNL
COR: WNL
ABD: Nontender, no masses
GU: Gray, homogeneous vaginal discharge, ovaries were palpable, normal-sized uterus, no tenderness, cervix normal
RECT: Small hemorrhoids
EXT: WNL
NEURO: WNL

Results of Laboratory Tests

Na 140 (140)   Hct 0.34 (34)   Glu 4.4 (80)
K 4.1 (4.1)   Hgb 110 (11)   Chol 4.14 (160)
Cl 100 (100)   Lkcs 7.8 × 10⁹ (7.8 × 10³)   Trig 0.98 (87)
HCO₃ 24 (24)   Plts 220 × 10⁹ (220 × 10³)
BUN 5.36 (15)
CR 61.9 (0.7)

Vaginal discharge: Normal saline wet mount "clue cells"; pH 5, KOH sniff test (+)
Urine culture (–)
Pregnancy test (–)

PROBLEM LIST

1. Stage IIB Hodgkin's disease
2. Contraception
3. Recurrent UTIs
4. Vaginal discharge with "fishy" odor

CASE 183 SOAP NOTES
Problem 2. Contraception

S: Because of the possibility of chemotherapy if her Hodgkin's disease recurs, she is interested in a reliable contraceptive at this time. She and her husband would like to have another child if the Hodgkin's disease does not reappear within 5 years. Although she has been successful with her diaphragm, she admits to noncompliance at times.

O: HD had no problems with COC use previously. Pregnancy test today is negative; no family or personal history of hypertension (HTN), diabetes mellitus (DM), thromboembolic disease, or hyperlipidemia; nonsmoker.

A: HD, a stage II Hodgkin's disease patient, desires a reliable nonpermanent method of birth control. She has no contraindications to use of COC. Douching after intercourse is never recommended and may force sperm around diaphragm and lead to pregnancy.

P: Combination of ethinyl estradiol, mestranol, and norethindrone (Ortho-Novum) 7/7/7 one tablet every day for 21 days, stop 7 days, and repeat × 12 months was prescribed. HD was instructed to begin taking the tablets on the Sunday after her next mensus begins. She should continue to use her diaphragm and spermicide for the first month of COC use. She was instructed to take the COC tablets at the same time each day, use sunscreen when sunbathing to decrease chloasma and other possible dangerous side effects. She will be scheduled for a blood pressure check in 3 months.

Problem 4. Vaginal Discharge

S: HD complains of homogeneous, gray vaginal discharge coating vulva, plus "fishy" odor after intercourse.

O: KOH added to discharge gives off "fishy" odor; normal saline wet mount shows "clue cells"; vaginal pH = 5.

A: Nonspecific vaginosis, also known as *Gardnerella* vaginitis, which is actually a polymicrobial infection. HD's current use of OTC candidal therapy would be expected to have little effect on this bacterial infection and should be discontinued.

P: Begin metronidazole 500 mg BID for 7 days. Instruct HD to avoid alcohol until 24 hr after the last dose, and advise her that a metallic taste in the mouth and brownish discoloration of the urine may occur. No follow-up visit is necessary.

Problem 3. Recurrent UTIs—Follow-up

S: HD's symptoms of burning on urination are gone.

O: Urine culture is negative.

A: Young woman with history of two UTIs in the last 6 months. Both infections were successfully treated with cotrimoxazole. Most likely this is a reinfection rather than a recurrence, and chronic prophylaxis for recurrent urinary tract infections is not warranted at this time. It is most likely related to irritation of the urethra at the time of intercourse.

P: HD should be instructed to urinate shortly after the end of sexual intercourse to flush the urethra of any bacteria.

Problem 1. Stage IIB Hodgkin's Disease

S: No complaints. She is being followed by oncology for this problem every 2 months.

O: No systemic signs or symptoms of recurrent disease. HD was treated with 5000 rads over 4–6 weeks and completed therapy 11 months ago. She understands that the 5-year relapse-free survival rate with subtotal nodal irradiation is 75%–90%. If recurrence occurs, she will be treated with ABVD chemotherapy regimen.

A: A patient with previously diagnosed Hodgkin's disease in complete remission.

P: Oncology to follow.

QUESTIONS FOR CASE 183

1. How much more effective as a contraceptive is a combination oral contraceptive (COC) than a diaphragm and spermicide?

2. If HD misses pill 14 and 15 of her third month of COC use, what advice would you give her?

3. If her BP is 140/90 at her 3-month checkup, what should be done?

4. If HD required chronic treatment for UTIs, what effect would it have on her COC use?

CASE 184

CC: KK is a 45-year-old woman who comes to the gynecology clinic complaining of severe itching of the vulva and vagina and painful burning during urination. She had been treated with metronidazole vaginal gel on a cruise boat last week for a profuse, foul-smelling vaginal discharge with no itching or burning. She is in the luteal phase of her menstrual cycle and is experiencing wide mood swings, forgetfulness, migraine headaches, and a phobia that makes it impossible for her to function at work, thinking that her supervisor has been trying to replace her with a younger, healthier individual for the last several months. She is also asking whether the birth control pill she discontinued several weeks ago may be the cause of her symptoms, migraine headaches, and recently, hairy chin.

Medical History

KK has been experiencing episodic migraine headaches since her menarche at age 13, which usually begin as frontal unilateral dull aches and progress to incapacitating throbbing pain with nausea, vomiting, diarrhea, and vertigo. She also complains of rectal soreness and flatulence intermittently.

Ob/Gyn History

G4P1Mis2Ectopic1; last menstrual period was 2 weeks ago. Recurrent vulvovaginal candidal infections have plagued her

for the last 4 years. Premenstrual syndrome (PMS) was diagnosed 4 years ago; she is only symptom-free for several days after the onset of menses until near ovulation. She had been taking a combination oral contraceptive until 2 weeks ago and is currently using vaginal contraceptive suppositories, which irritate her husband's genitals.

Social History

Smokes 1¾ ppd × 18 years

Family History

Her mother has "common" migraine headaches, hypertension (HTN); her father also has HTN.

Surgical History

She had a left salphingectomy resulting from an ectopic pregnancy at age 23.

Medication History

Progesterone suppositories 200 mg p.r. BID × 4 years
d,l-Norgestrel 0.5 mg with ethinyl estradiol 50 mg, 28 day: 1 daily for 6 months (discontinued 2 weeks ago)
Hydrocodone bitartrate 5 mg/acetaminophen 500 mg p.r.n.
Clotrimazole 500 mg vaginal tablets: 1 p.r.n.
Contraceptive vaginal suppository: p.r.n.

Allergies

Latex

Physical Examination

GEN: Well-developed, well-nourished
VS: BP 124/83 LA (sitting), HR 76, RR 18, T 37.1°C, Wt 61 kg, Ht 168 cm
HEENT: Chin has many short, coarse, dark hair follicles.
COR: WNL
CHEST: Breasts swollen and tender to palpation
ABD: WNL, except for "bikini" scar
GU: Vulvar erythema with white patches; intertrigo with satellite lesions; thick, white, curd-like secretions
RECT: Perianal erythema, flatulence, no hemorrhoids
EXT: WNL
NEURO: WNL

Results of Laboratory Tests

Na 141 (141)	Hct 0.39 liter (39%)
K 4.1 (4.1)	Hgb 130 g/liter (13 g/dl)
Cl 101 (101)	Glu (fasting) 4.9 mmol/liter (89 mg/dl)
HCO₃ 25 (25)	
BUN 5.0 (14)	
Cr 71 (0.8)	

Oral glucose tolerance test: Normal
Guaiac: Positive.
Vaginal fluid: KOH slide: Long threadlike fibers of mycelia with tiny buds of conidia attached

PROBLEM LIST

1. "Common" migraine headaches
2. Premenstrual syndrome
3. Recurrent vulvovaginal candidoasis
4. Hirsutism
5. Desire for contraception
6. Rectal symptoms

QUESTIONS FOR CASE 184

1. Is there a correlation between the etiology and symptoms of PMS?
2. What alternative drug therapies would you suggest if spironolactone failed in the treatment of KK's PMS symptoms?
3. What therapy would you suggest if KK had another recurrence of vulvovaginal candidosis 2 weeks from now?
4. Could depot medroxyprogesterone acetate be used as a contraceptive in KK?
5. Was KK's current vulvovaginal candidosis a recurrence or drug-induced?
6. If KK wishes to become pregnant now, what drug therapies can we safely employ to treat her medical problems?

CASE 185

CC: CC is a 33-year-old woman with a history of epilepsy, type I (insulin-dependent) diabetes mellitus, hypertension, asthma, and impaired renal function. She is 8 weeks pregnant and complains of severe vaginal and vulvar itching, burning, and nonmalodorous vaginal discharge.

Medical History

CC is G2P2 and has had type I (insulin-dependent) diabetes mellitus for 19 years. Her diabetes has been poorly controlled over the last several weeks. CC states that she has decreased the daily amount of insulin because she hasn't been eating "like she should" and is afraid of "overdoing it," but she also states that she has not monitored her blood glucose level in several weeks. She has primary generalized tonic-clonic seizures. Her last seizure was 1 year ago, thought to be due to noncompliance. Mild hypertension has complicated her health for 6 years. She has taken methyldopa during previous pregnancies and has not complained of any problems associated with it. CC was diagnosed with asthma and uses a metoproterenol inhaler on occasion, with relief. During her last asthmatic attack she was given prednisone for control and has continued taking the medication for the last 1½ weeks.

Medication History

Phenytoin 100 mg po q. h.s.
Metaproterenol i-ii puffs QID and p.r.n.
Prednisone 12 mg po q. AM
Methyldopa 250 mg po BID
Insulin ultralente 14 U before breakfast
Insulin reg 7 U before breakfast, lunch, and evening meal

Allergies

NKDA

Social History

Smokes 1 pack/day for 8 years; occasional use of alcohol

Physical Examination

GEN: CC is a 33-year-old woman in acute distress, with complaints of severe vaginal itching and burning and a nonmalodorous vaginal discharge. She recently found out that she is 8 weeks pregnant.

VS: BP 150/100, HR 85, RR 20, T 37°C, Wt 65 kg, Ht 168 cm

HEENT: Pale mucous membranes and skin, no nystagmus, no retinopathy

COR: Normal sinus rhythm, no murmurs, rub, gallop

CHEST: Clear to auscultation

ABD: No pain, tenderness, guarding

GU: Positive vaginal, "cottage cheese"/curd-like discharge, nonmalodorous

EXT: Cool to touch, dry skin; full range of motion of all extremities; no bruises

NEURO: No noticeable neuropathies, peripheral tingling, or numbness; no ataxia, dizziness

Results of Laboratory Tests

BUN 8.9 (25)	Hct 0.38 (38)	Alb 55 (5.5)	Phenytoin 47.6 (12)
CR 123 (1.4)	Hgb 120 (12)	Glu (fasting) 16 (290)	
	MCV 90 (90)	HgbAlC 8%	
	MCHC 330 (33)		

Urinalysis: Protein 1+; glucose ¼%
ABGs pO$_2$ 90, pCO$_2$ 22

PROBLEM LIST

1. Type I (insulin-dependent) diabetes mellitus
2. Epilepsy
3. Hypertension
4. Asthma
5. Impaired renal function
6. *Candida* vaginitis
7. Pregnant (8 weeks)

QUESTIONS FOR CASE 185

1. What alternative drugs could be used to treat CC's *Candida* vaginitis? Give the appropriate drug regimen.
2. If the miconazole therapy fails, what reasons might explain this and what kind of therapy should be initiated?
3. Would oral hypoglycemics be appropriate for CC?
4. Why is folic acid supplementation used for CC?

CASE 186

CC: BB is a 32-year-old woman who comes to the gynecology clinic expressing concern that she can't become pregnant. She also complains of having "bumps" around her rectum for about 6 months.

Medical History

BB has a history of hyperthyroidism 4 years ago, which was successfully treated with propylthiouracil (PTU) for 12 months. Following PTU therapy she has remained chemically euthyroid.

Ob-Gyn History

G0P0

LMP 10 days ago

Regular 31-day cycle except for a decreased menstrual flow during her hyperthyroid state

No history of endometriosis or pelvic inflammatory disease (PID)

Medication History

PTU 100 mg QID × 3 months

100 mg TID × 3 months

100 mg BID × 3 months

100 mg QD × 3 months

This therapy was completed 3 years ago. She takes no medications at this time.

Allergies

Iodine (hypersensitivity following I^{123} scan for assessment of hyperthyroidism)

Social History

BB is an only child. Her husband is a lawyer who has two children by a previous marriage. She has a Master's degree in library science and working at the public library currently. Nonsmoker. Drinks alcohol socially, 1–2 drinks/weekend.

Family History

Her mother had Graves' disease. No family history of other endocrine abnormalities.

Physical Examination

GEN: Well developed, well nourished

VS: BP 110/72, HR 60, T 37°C, Wt 59 kg, Ht 168 cm

HEENT: Mild proptosis that has remained unchanged for 4 years. Thyroid is not enlarged.

COR: WNL

ABD: Nontender, no masses

GU: 5–6 pink-white warts with fine fingerlike fronds on the vulva and perineum. No apparent cervical involvement. Cervix appeared normal; ovaries were palpated. She had a normal-sized uterus. No adnexal tenderness was noted on examination.

RECT: 2–3 small condyloma acuminatum around anus

EXT: No pretibial myxedema

NEURO: No hyperreflexia; no fine resting tremor

Results of Laboratory Tests

Na 138 (138)	Hct 0.41 (41)	AST 0.33 (20)	Glu 5.0 (90)
K 4.5 (4.5)	Hgb 138 (13.8)	ALT 0.27 (16)	Ca 2.37 (9.5)
Cl 100 (100)	Lkcs 6.6 × 10⁹ (6.6 × 10⁵)	LDH 1.92 (115)	PO₄ 0.9 (2.8)
HCO₃ 23 (23)	Plts 298 × 10⁹ (298 × 10⁵)	Alk Phos 0.85 (51)	Chol 4.42 (171)
BUN 4.28 (12)	MCV 91.4 (91.4)	Alb 47 (4.7)	Trig 0.79 (70)
CR 79.56 (0.9)	MCHC 335 (33.5)	T Bili 8.55 (0.5)	

Thyroid function tests: T4: 102.96 (8.0) (RIA); RT3 U: 0.3 (30%); FTI: 30.9 (2.4); Ultrasensitive TSH: 2.1 (2.1)

UA: Glucose (–), ketones (–), protein (–), pH 6.5

PAP: Koilocytosis with mild inflammation

PROBLEM LIST

1. History of hyperthyroidism: Graves' disease
2. "Bumps" around rectum
3. Infertility

CASE 187

CC: JR is a 28-year-old woman who presents to the emergency room complaining of new-onset fever, chills, nausea, and flank pain.

History of Present Illness

JR is a sexually active woman who was seen 5 days ago in the outpatient Ob/gyn clinic for symptoms of severe abdominal cramping associated with her menses and a 3-day history of frequent urination and bladder pain. JR was subsequently diagnosed with a urinary tract infection and sent home with a 10-day supply of trimethoprim-sulfamethoxazole.

Medical History

JR's history is significant for four urinary tract infections over the last 6 months. In each case the infection was successfully treated with a 10-day course of sulfamethoxazole and trimethoprim (Septra). JR also has a history of shortness of breath and wheezing that occur predominately during her aerobic workouts.

Medication History

Septra 1 DS po bid × 10 days (has completed 5 days of 10-day course)

Allergies

Amoxicillin (full body rash)

Social History

Tobacco: 1 pack per week

Alcohol: 2 cocktails/week

Contraception: Diaphragm/condoms for 7 months, previously used condoms only.

Sexual history: Multiple partners in the last year. First pregnancy with abortion 9 months ago.

Physical Examination

GEN: Pale, anxious woman in moderate distress

VS: BP 85/50, HR 120, RR 20, T 39.5°C, Wt 60 kg, Ht 67 in

HEENT: PEERLA, oral cavity and tympanic membranes normal

COR: Normal S_1 and S_2, tachycardic

CHEST: Slight wheezes on expiration

ABD: Liver palpable and non-tender, CVA tenderness

RECTAL: Guaiac-negative

EXT: Normal

NEURO. Oriented to place, time and person; normal deep tendon reflexes and cranial nerves.

Results of Laboratory Tests

Na 137 (137)	WBC 18 × 10⁹ (18 × 10³)	AlPO₄ 1.0 (60)	T Bili 18 (1.0)
Hct 0.32 (32)	LDH 1.7 (101)	PO₄ 1.1 (3.5)	UA 120 (2.0)
K 3.8 (3.8)	Ca 2.3 (9.2)	BUN 3.6 (10)	
Hb 120 (12)	HCO₃ 23 (23)	MCV 90 (90)	
ALT 0.58 (34)	Plts 200 × 10⁹ (200 × 10³)	Alb 40 (4.0)	
Glu 6.1 (110)		Mg 0.80 (1.6)	
Cl 97 (97)		CR 88.4 (1.0)	
		AST 0.58 (35)	

WBC differential: 14PMN/2L/1B/1E

Urinalysis: pH 7.4, SG 1.02; many bacteria, hematuria, WBC casts, 25 WBC/mm³

Urine Gram's stain: GPC in chains.

Blood culture: 1/2 GPC in chains, probable *Enterococcus faecalis*

Chest x-ray: Normal

EKG: Normal

PROBLEM LIST

1. Pyelonephritis with bacteremia
2. Chronic UTI
3. Contraception
4. Asthma

CASE 187 SOAP NOTES

Problem 1. Pyelonephritis with Bacteremia

S: JR is complaining of new-onset fever, chills, nausea, and flank pain.

O: JR has a history of multiple UTIs with the most frequent being 5 days prior to her admission. Her temperature is elevated, her blood pressure is low, and she is exhibiting signs of costovertebral angle tenderness. Additional symptoms include elevated WBC with left shift, UA results, and microbiology findings.

A: JRs recent urinary tract infection has ascended into her kidneys and spread to her blood. JR is exhibiting signs of septic shock as illustrated by her fever and drop in blood pressure. Bacterial growth from her urine and blood cultures suggest systemic infection with *E. faecalis* requiring immediate hospitalization and treatment.

P: IV fluids should be initiated immediately to counteract symptoms of hypotension. *E. faecalis* is typically sensitive to ampicillin and vancomycin. JR's hypersensitivity to amoxicillin precludes the use of ampicillin. Because vancomycin

has bacteriostatic, but not bactericidal activity against enterococcus, an aminoglycoside should be added to produce the bactericidal effect desired in a bacteremic patient such as JR. The aminoglycoside will also provide some gram-negative coverage until final culture results are available. Because JR has adequate renal function, empirically dosed vancomycin 750 mg q 12h and gentamycin 90 mg q 8h may be initiated. Therapy should be continued until JR is afebrile for 48 hours. An additional 10- to 14-day course of oral antibiotics should then be initiated based on culture and sensitivity results. A repeat urinalysis should be conducted 2 to 3 weeks after the completion of therapy to check for eradication of the organism.

Problem 2. Chronic UTI

S: None

O: JR's history is significant for four urinary tract infections during the last 6 months. Symptoms of frequent urination and bladder pain are consistent with an uncomplicated lower UTI.

A: JR has two risk factors for development of a UTI: female gender and diaphragm use. She has experienced a series of UTIs (i.e., four in the last 6 months) which began 1 month after starting to use her diaphragm. The risk of severe infection, such as pyelonephritis, from chronic UTIs is serious. Patients with more than three UTIs in 1 year should be prophylactically treated with antibiotics.

P: The most common organisms associated with community acquired UTIs are *Escherichia coli, Staphlycoccus saprophyticus, Klebsiella pneumoniae, Proteus mirabilis,* and *Enterococcus faecalis.* Prophylactic therapy for JR should include coverage for *Enterococcus,* because this was the cause of her pyelonephritis. Unlike Septra and trimethoprim, nitrofurantoin adequately covers enterococcus in the urine. JR should be started on nitrofurantoin 50 mg po QD for 6 months. Evaluation of other birth control options and proper diaphragm use are discussed under "Contraception."

Problem 3. Contraception

S: None

O: None

A: JR is a sexually active woman who has had multiple partners during the last year. She recently switched her method of contraception from condoms to a diaphragm and condoms after an unwanted pregnancy 9 months ago. JR's sexual history puts her at risk for pregnancy and the development of sexually transmitted diseases. To decrease the risk of both, JR needs adequate contraception. While a diaphragm and condoms can be effective for many patients, JR's frequent UTIs after diaphragm use are cause for concern. Nonintrauterine devices such as birth control pills or contraceptive foam may limit bacterial entry into the uterus. In addition, birth control pills may reduce symptoms of heavy menses. Prior to initiating therapy with birth control pills, JR should be evaluated for a negative history of cerebral vascular accidents, thromboembolic events, coronary artery disease, liver dysfunction, and breast cancer, because these are absolute contraindications. Although JR is not a heavy smoker (e.g., more than 15 cigarettes per day), the risk of CVAs with smoking and increasing age should be weighed against potential benefits of using oral contraceptives.

P: If JR chooses to continue to use her diaphragm, she should be instructed to wash it thoroughly with soap and water after each use and store it in a clean dry container. If JR chooses to switch to oral contraceptives, she should be initiated on a low dose estrogen, triphasic, birth control pill (e.g., Ortho Novum 7/7/7). Triphasic pills mimic the follicular, ovulatory, and luteal phases of the menstrual cycle, minimizing potential side effects. JR should be instructed to take the pill at the same time each day to ensure maximal efficacy. In addition, she should be warned that breakthrough bleeding may occur during the first few cycles of her therapy. Finally, JR should be counseled on the dangers of multiple partners and advised to use condoms to prevent the spread of sexually transmitted diseases.

Problem 4. Asthma

S: JR is complaining of shortness of breath especially during her aerobic workouts.

O: None

A: Shortness of breath and wheezing during exercise occur commonly due to exercise induced asthma (EIA). EIA is thought to be caused by bronchial hyperactivity. A treadmill or bicycle test can confirm the presence of EIA by measuring the FEV1 before and after exercise. A 10% reduction from baseline indicates a positive test. Hyperventilation of cool air can exacerbate EIA. Often the use of a humidifier, which provides warm air, or alternative exercises such as swimming can completely prevent EIA. If JR wishes to continue her aerobic workouts, inhaled, long-acting β_2-agonists have been shown to be superior to anticholinergics, cromolyn, and theophylline.

P: There are many long acting β_2 agonists to choose from. These include albuterol, terbutaline, and salmeterol. The former two drugs provide 2 to 4 hours of relief, while the later can provide up to 8 hours of relief. JR's aerobic workouts probably last up to 1 hour, so albuterol metered-dose inhaler should be sufficient. JR should be instructed to use two to four puffs prior to exercise. Additional puffs can be used for breakthrough asthma.

QUESTIONS FOR CASE 187

1. Why did JR develop pyelonephritis even though she was receiving Septra for her urinary tract infection?

2. Following IV antibiotic therapy, what oral antibiotic would you recommend to complete JR's pyelonephritis treatment?

3. Why are female gender and the use of a diaphragm risk factors for developing a urinary tract infection?

4. Are there any drug interactions the JR should be aware of if she decides to use oral contraceptives?

5. How would the use of birth control pills affect JR's dysmenorrhea and why?

CASE 188

CC: MW is a 20-year-old woman who presents to the clinic with genital pain and newly formed genital vesiculopustules.

Medical History

MW was diagnosed with hepatitis B during her recent pregnancy, for which she has received complete immunization. Recently postpartum, MW has a 6-day-old infant who was born without apparent complications from HSV. MW has genital herpes simplex virus-2, diagnosed at age 18; she has had three recurrences of HSV since diagnosis. Three years ago, MW was assessed for symptoms related to depression. (She was unable to maintain an adequate diet or keep a job. She could not sleep well, woke up early in the morning, and expressed no pleasure in her normal daily activities. MW did not bathe or change clothes regularly.) She was prescribed amitriptyline and responded well. MW did not take her amitriptyline during her pregnancy. MW currently complains of waking up early in the morning and tiredness, and she lacks interest in daily activities. She states that her baby is the only thing "worth it." She wants to breast-feed her infant.

Social History

Unmarried, unemployed; smokes two packs of cigarettes per day for approximately 10 years; "frequent" alcohol use

Allergies

Yeast

Medication History

Docusate sodium 100 mg po q. AM
Acetaminophen w/codeine 15 mg po q4-6h p.r.n.

Physical Examination

GEN: Thin, 20-year-old, depressed, woman 6 days postpartum with painful genital vesicles

VS: BP: 110/85, HR 85, RR 18, T 37°C, Wt 50 kg, Ht 155 cm

HEENT: WNL; no apparent oropharynx or mucosal vesicle formation; normal sclerae

COR: Regular sinus rhythm, no murmurs

CHEST: Clear to auscultation and percussion; tender, full breasts

ABD: No masses or guarding, normal tenderness from recent delivery

GU: Grossly visible vesiculopustules on labia, urethra, and vulva; some with a slight erythematous zone.

RECT: Normal, no vesicles, no hemorrhoids

EXT: Normal-appearing skin color and range of motion

NEURO: Oriented × 3, CN1-12 intact, normal tendon reflexes

Results of Laboratory Tests

BUN 3.2 (9)   Hct 0.33 (33)   Alb 40 (4.0)   Glu 5 (90)
CR 79 (0.9)   Hgb 110 (11)

Antibody to HSV: Positive
Anti-HBs: 7 m IU/ml
Pap smear/Giemsa: Giant cells
Lkc differential: WNL

PROBLEM LIST

1. HBsAg-positive
2. Depression
3. HSV infection
4. Breast-feeding

GERONTOLOGY

CASE 189

CC: EM is an 81-year-old female who has been residing in a nursing home for 3 years. EM is severely demented and has no complaints. She needs assistance in all activities of daily living (dressing, bathing, eating). She spends most of her day in a wheelchair. Because of her dementia and poor eyesight, she cannot participate in activities, read, or watch television. She occasionally gets anxious and repeats ``help me'' over and over again.

Past Medical History

EM had a stroke 4 years ago, and she still suffers from left-sided weakness and unsteady gait. She has a history of atrial fibrillation, is on digoxin 0.125 mg q.d., and has had rheumatoid arthritis for many years for which she receives prednisone 10 mg q.d. She had a right modified mastectomy 5 years ago for breast cancer. Other chronic medical conditions include glaucoma, osteoporosis, and a history of peptic ulcer disease.

History of Present Illness

EM has had a recent decline in her mental status. The nurses note that she seems more disoriented, often slumps over in her wheelchair, and does not respond to commands. She has been unresponsive and very lethargic, sleeping most of the day for the past week. Over the last month, EM lost 6 pounds.

Medication History

Digoxin 0.125 mg q.d. × 20 years
Furosemide 40 mg q.d. × 4 years
KCl 10% 20 mEq q.d. × 4 years
Prednisone 10 mg q.d. (history unknown)
Timolol 0.5% one gtt. O.U. b.i.d. × over 8 years
Ranitidine 150 mg b.i.d. × 4 years
Tamoxifen 10 mg b.i.d. × 4 years
Dipyridamole 25 mg b.i.d.
Tacrine 10 mg po qid × 1 year
Multivitamin with minerals tablet q.d.
Calcium 500 mg b.i.d.
Psyllium 15 ml in fluids b.i.d.

Allergies

Penicillin

Physical Examination

GEN: EM is a very thin, pale female.
VS: BP 110/70, HR 59, T 37, Wt 93.5 lbs. (42.5 kg), Ht 155 cm

HEENT: Cerumen in ear, blocking canal
COR: Irregularly, irregular heart rate
CHEST: WNL, chest clear
ABD: Hypoactive bowel sounds
BACK: Kyphotic
GU: Deferred
RECT: Occult blood—negative
EXT: Skin tear on right forearm; 1+ pitting ankle edema
NEURO: Lethargic, barely arousable when name called; left upper extremity weakness; hyperactive reflexes left elbow and knee; upgoing toe (positive Babinski sign); oriented × 0
SKIN: Dry mucous membranes, poor skin turgor

Results of Laboratory Tests

Na 148 (148)
K 3.3 (3.3)
Cl 115 (115)
HCO$_3$ 28 (28)
BUN 10.5 (30)
CR 120 (1.4)

HCT 0.32 (32)
Hgb 108 (10.8)
Lkcs 10.8 × 10^9 (10.8 × 10^3)
Plts 240 × 10^9 (240 × 10^3)

Glu (fasting) 7.8 (140)
Ca 2.4 (9.6)
Mg 1.0 (2.0)

Lkcs differential: WNL
ESR 25 mm/hr (25 mm/hr)
Rheumatoid factor 1:40
ANA 1:80
Digoxin 3 months prior: 2.3 nmol/liter (1.8 ng/dl)
ECG shows atrial fibrillation, ST-T wave changes
MRI from 2 years ago shows right parietal infarct

PROBLEM LIST

1. Rheumatoid arthritis
2. Atrial fibrillation
3. Status post stroke
4. Glaucoma
5. Osteoporosis
6. History of peptic ulcer disease
7. History of breast cancer
8. Severe dementia, recent decline in mental status
9. Weight loss

CASE 189 SOAP NOTES
Problem 9. Weight Loss

S: EM has lost 6 pounds in the last month. Her status is reported to the physician.
O: Weight 42.5 kg; dry mucous membranes; poor skin turgor, FBS 7.8 (140)
A: Possible causes of weight loss should be evaluated.

Medications: Digoxin can cause anorexia and failure to thrive, especially in the elderly. Prednisone can cause glucose intolerance. Furosemide can cause dehydration and glucose intolerance.

A patient with dementia, especially severe Alzheimer's disease (AD), may be unable to eat unassisted. Food must be provided and fed to patient. Check EM's ability to chew and swallow food. In the terminal stages of AD, patients often stop eating and drinking or cannot maintain enough calories and lose weight. If EM has dentures, need to check that they are in her mouth for meals and the fit needs to be checked during episodes of significant weight loss. EM is dehydrated.

P: Recheck digoxin level. Evaluate the need to continue digoxin; EM is still in atrial fibrillation. EM has a low pulse rate and could be showing other nonspecific toxic reactions to digoxin.

EM is dehydrated because of her diuretic and decreased fluid intake. Consider discontinuing furosemide. EM's edema may be positional edema because she is nonambulatory and in a wheelchair. Need to elevate feet, use Ted hose, and if possible, walk EM with assistance. Order monitoring of input and output and try to increase her fluid intake.

EM has decreased bowel sounds; evaluate for constipation due to decreased muscle tone, dehydration, and malnutrition. Because of dementia, she cannot express GI complaints. Psyllium should be discontinued because of EM's poor fluid intake and its ability to cause impaction in patients with low fluid intake.

Problem 8. Dementia

S: EM is unable to care for herself. She has had recent mental status changes and decreased mental functioning, exhibited by decreased consciousness and inability to follow commands. She cannot participate in many activities.

O: Oriented × 0

A: EM has severe dementia, probably a combination of Alzheimer's disease (AD) and multiinfarct dementia (MID). Her AD has progressed, and there is a possibility of further small infarcts occurring, which would cause decreased functioning.

P: Evaluate any correctable influences on her changed mental status; possible causes are metabolic disturbances such as dehydration, increased or decreased blood sugar, electrolyte imbalance, and thyroid dysfunction. Also need to consider digoxin toxicity, systemic absorption of timolol ophthalmic, bleeding, anemia, and unknown infectious processes. Discontinue Tacrine since the dose is subtherapeutic and it is only indicated in cases of mild to moderate impairment. This patient has severe dementia and no benefit should be expected from Tacrine therapy.

Maximize sensory perception. Need to clean out ear wax to maximize EM's ability to hear. Consider an ophthalmic evaluation; if EM requires glasses, make sure that aides are putting them on her daily.

EM is physically deconditioned. Have her evaluated by occupational and physical therapy to improve her physical functioning and provide mental stimulation and exercise.

Problem 1. Rheumatoid Arthritis (RA)

S: EM has no complaints of pain. She does not exhibit any red, swollen joints. Her fingers are slightly deformed, possibly due to degenerative arthritis, immobility, or lack of use.

O: RF 1:40, ESR 25 (25), ANA 1:80

A: EM has been on chronic steroid therapy for an unknown number of years. All of the above laboratory results, although positive for RA, could be a function of age. Positive titers may not be specific for RA. It is likely that EM would have some degenerative joint disease. If she has RA, she is not experiencing an acute flare and may not need steroids now. Prednisone can cause mental status changes, increase glucose intolerance, and has probably been a factor in the osteoporosis, glaucoma, and ulcer disease.

P: Taper, and if possible, discontinue prednisone. Consider the use of a remissive agent or aspirin or a nonsteroidal antiinflammatory drug (NSAID) if EM becomes symptomatic. EM has a history of ulcers, so NSAIDs should be used judiciously, possibly with sucralfate or misoprostol. Because EM does not seem to have any acute symptoms she may no longer need antiinflammatory treatment. May also suggest the use of an analgesic such as acetaminophen, which can be of benefit in relieving pain and discomfort caused by degenerative joint disease.

Problem 2. Atrial Fibrillation

S: None

O: Pulse 59 apical, irregular
Digoxin level 2.3 (1.8) 3 months prior
K^+ 3.3 (3.3)

A: EM is in atrial fibrillation.

P: Evaluate EM for conduction abnormalities (such as first- or second-degree AV block) due to digoxin. Monitor drug level for increase due to decreased renal function (estimated creatinine clearance 0.35 ml/sec [21 ml/min]). Consider a decreased dose or discontinue digoxin, if it is not maintaining normal sinus rhythm and the last level was on the high side of therapeutic. Increase potassium supplement, to maintain a higher serum potassium concentration to prevent arrhythmias due to low K and digoxin. Would discontinue furosemide because of her dehydration and no current diagnosis apparent for use. Continue potassium and monitor, will discontinue when K^+ concentration is well within normal range.

Problem 3. Status Post Stroke

S: Mental status changes, decreased cognitive function

O: MRI—right parietal infarction

A: Possible small strokes occurring. The efficacy of dipyridamole is controversial, particularly when used alone.

P: It is unlikely that a repeat MRI would be performed; because of EM's dementia, she could not cooperate during the test. Strokes could cause a decompensation in her behavior. Because of her minimal functioning and poor quality of life, minimal treatment is suggested. Start ASA 325 mg q.d. to help in prevention of further small strokes. May evaluate for cardioversion of atrial fibrillation to prevent further stroke activity. Trial of medications is possible, but EM would probably have difficulty coping with electro-cardioconversion.

Problem 4. Glaucoma

S: None, but EM cannot participate in activities due to poor eyesight and dementia.

O: Apical pulse 59

A: Decreased vision combined with dementia limit function and decrease EM's quality of life.

P: Have EM evaluated by an ophthalmologist, monitor ocular pressure. May recommend a change of eye drop because of the remote possibility of CNS effects and decreased pulse from this nonspecific β-blocker. EM is very sensitive to the CNS effects of any medication, and she may be experiencing systemic side effects.

Decreasing dose of steroid may help prevent further eye damage. Need to maximize vision; obtain and use glasses if helpful.

Problem 5. Osteoporosis

S: None

O: Kyphosis

A: Osteoporosis probably secondary to being a postmeno-pausal female on steroid therapy. Due to history of breast cancer, estrogen therapy is contraindicated. No need for calcitonin or etidionate. Both are somewhat controversial and expensive.

P: Questionable benefit from calcium supplement and could exacerbate constipation. May consider discontinuing. Need to try to increase Ca intake in food.

Problem 6. History of Peptic Ulcer Disease

S: None

O: Stool, occult blood—negative

A: EM has been on a therapeutic regimen of ranitidine for many years. Recommended therapy is for only 6–8 weeks. Ulcer disease in the past could have been caused by steroid therapy.

P: EM's renal function is decreased. Ranitidine 150 mg q.d. is a therapeutic dose for her. Would consider a maintenance dose of 75–150 mg q.d. or possibly discontinue therapy. If steroids are continued or NSAIDs are instituted, would suggest the use of misoprostol to prevent ulcer. Sucralfate, the other alternative, would worsen her constipation.

Problem 7. History of Breast Cancer

S: None

A: No masses

P: Patient is 5 years postmastectomy, if no other causes for changes in mental status are found, need to consider the possibility of reoccurrence of breast cancer and metastases to the brain.

Continue tamoxifen at this time. Monitor CBC.

QUESTIONS FOR CASE 189

1. What are the most likely causes of the EM's recent mental status decline?
2. What laboratory tests should be performed to evaluate her change in status?
3. Should medication be prescribed for this patient's dementia?
4. With appropriate medication therapy, what is this patient's prognosis?
5. Would you recommend anticoagulation to prevent further strokes for this patient with atrial fibrillation?
6. What future healthcare decisions can be anticipated?

CASE 190

CC: JM is a 72-year-old female who presents to her local HMO for an annual physical examination and medical clearance for a month cruise to Mexico. Her blood glucose readings at home have been in the range of 180–230 mg/dL. She complains of heartburn, easy fatigueability, some urinary frequency (gets up three times at night) and persistent pains in her hips and knees. At today's appointment she requests a vitamin supplement.

Past Medical History

JM has a history of type II (adult-onset) diabetes mellitus. JM has no family history for cancer. There have been no menopausal vasomotor symptoms for 5 years, and she has denied any vaginal bleeding or discharge in the past. Her lipid profile was normal last year. Her last mammogram was done 5 years ago. JM was clinically euthyroid 12 months ago. She has a 40 pack-year history of smoking, but has not smoked for 10 years; she reports moderate alcohol use.

Past Surgical History

She had thyroidectomy surgery in 1978 to treat her hyperthyroidism.

Medication History

Levothyroxine 0.05 mg q. AM (1985)
Conjugated estrogens 1.25 mg q.d. (1976)
Medroxyprogesterone 10 mg ut dict. (1976)
Glyburide .5 mg bid (1991)
Piroxicam 20 mg q. AM (started 3 months ago)
Naproxen 200 mg 2 tabs q 8h p.r.n. (recent OTC)

Allergies

Codeine, sulfa

Physical Examination

GEN: Pale, overweight woman with no acute distress or symptoms

VS: BP 160/80 (lying), HR 60, RR 16, T 38.2, Wt 70 kg (increased from 65 kg on last visit), Ht 162.5 cm (164 cm on prior visit)

HEENT: Hair coarse, arteriole-venule nicking in the eye, thyroid slightly enlarged, mild lid lag

COR: WNL

CHEST: Lungs clear, breast examination normal

ABD: WNL

GU: Atrophic changes present on pelvic examination

RECTAL: No hemorrhoids present

EXT: Skin warm and dry to touch, grooved nails and decrease in deep tendon reflexes, with no edema present, bilateral varicose veins

NEURO: WNL

Results of Laboratory Tests

K 4.7 (4.7)	RBC 3.7×10^{12} (3.7×10^6)	T3 uptake .39 (39)
CR 120 (1.4)	Glu (fasting) 13 (234)	Iron 9.2 (51.4)
Hct 0.34 (34)	T4 54 (4.2)	HgbA$_k$ 12%
Hgb 117 (11.7)	TSH 5.2 (5.2)	

Urinalysis: negative for Lkcs, bacteria, ketones, 1+ protein, glucose negative

Pap smear: Atypical cells present (normal 2 years ago)

Occult blood: Guaiac-positive

PROBLEM LIST

1. Postmenopausal hormone replacement therapy
2. Hypothyroidism
3. Type II diabetes mellitus (DM)
4. Degenerative joint disease (DJD)
5. Traveler's diarrhea prophylaxis

CASE 190 SOAP NOTES

Problem 1. Postmenopausal Hormone Replacement Therapy

S: JM has not experienced "hot flashes" for 5 years while on conjugated estrogen therapy, but continues to have hip and knee pain. She denies any recent onset of vaginal bleeding or unusual discharge.

O: Atrophic changes on pelvic examination; annual Pap smear reveals atypical cells not present 2 years ago. Negative family history for cancer. Breast examination showed no lumps. Some loss of height since last visit.

A: The growth of precancerous cells may be enhanced with hormonal therapy. JM is asymptomatic, but the risk of endometrial cancer may now outweigh the benefit of preventing osteoporosis in this patient. Except for the diabetes, the risk of coronary heart disease appears minimal. The dose of estrogen may be unnecessarily high.

P: Refer to GYN for colposcopy based on abnormal pap and the age of the patient. Even if it is normal, consider tapering and discontinue the estrogens. Consider placing the patient on a calcium supplement such as Tus and a multivitamin (with Vitamin D) with minerals, especially if her diet is deficient. Encourage mild aerobic exercise such as walking. Monitor pap smear every six months. A mammogram should be ordered. Provide brochures to instruct JM to self-examine breasts on a routine basis and report any lumps immediately to her physician.

Problem 2. Hypothyroidism

S: JM complains of lack of energy since her last visit, 6 months ago. Compliant (takes every morning with her coffee) on levothyroxine 0.15 mg q.d. (switched to generic 6 months ago because of cost savings). Needs annual check of thyroid function tests.

O: Thyroidectomy in 1978; 5-kg increase in weight without edema. Skin dry to touch and hair coarse in texture. Thyroid gland slightly enlarged. Blood pressure is 170/80 mm Hg and pulse is 60 beats/min. No arrhythmias or overt heart disease present. Thyroid tests include T4 54 (4.2) (low), TSH 5.2 (5.2) (high), and T3 uptake 0.39 (39) (high). Decrease in deep tendon reflexes.

A: JM is clinically hypothyroid despite levothyroxine replacement therapy. Lack of energy may be due to inadequate diabetes control or iron loss, however vital sign changes are classic for hypothyroidism. Conjugated estrogen therapy may be interfering with the T4 result. The recent switch to a generic product may not be a factor in loss of control; the disease may be progressing. Dose is low on a µg/kg basis.

P: Counsel JM on the need to stay on one brand for proper control. Either discontinue the generic levothyroxine product and initiate treatment with the branded product and titrate dose. Repeat thyroid laboratory test profile in 1 month. If values remain low and/or JM is symptomatic, consider dosage increase to 0.175 mg. Counsel JM on expected side effects of the higher doses. Monitor weight, blood pressure, pulse, and blood sugar response with thyroid control.

Problem 3. Type II Diabetes Mellitus

S: JM complains of lack of energy and urinary frequency (she says she gets up three times a night); she self-reports (when she remembers) that her blood sugars have been "high" using Accu-Chek III.

O: Urinalysis is negative for glucose and ketones. Fasting blood sugar is reported by the laboratory to be 13 (234). The results of a glycosylated hemoglobin (Hgb A$_{1c}$) were reported to be 12%. Weight has increased from 65 kg to 70 kg in last 6 months. Levothyroxine dose is maintained at 0.15 mg. Serum creatinine is 120 (1.4) and JM is spilling protein in the urine. A-V nicking is evident on fundoscopic examination.

A: JM's diabetes is not tightly controlled as evidenced by her symptoms, blood sugar level, and weight gain. She has evidence of early microvascular complications, as evidenced by changes in the eye and kidney and diminution of tendon reflexes. With the patient planning a cruise, major counseling on importance of diet, exercise, and disease monitoring is needed.

P: Increase glyburide dose to 5 mg po bid. Have the patient return to the clinic in two weeks for dosage adjustment with the goal of asymptomatic control before the cruise leaves in four weeks. Continue testing or ordering liver function tests. The patient needs counseling on: 1) side effects of increased dose of glyburide, 2) correct use of Accu-Chek III blood glucose monitoring kit, 3) importance of diet control, 4) signs and symptoms of hyper and hypoglycemia. Attempts to initiate a 1500 calorie ADA diet for one month should be made with recommendations for light exercise such as swimming several times a weeks.

Problem 4. DJD

S: JM complains of increased hip and knee pain and has recently started naproxen OTC to help ease the pain. She also complains of "not having as much energy as I used to have" and requests vitamins.

O: The RBCs, hematocrit, hemoglobin, and serum iron test results are low or low-normal, and a stool guaiac test shows blood. She appears somewhat pale in the face to her family physician. She does not have hemorrhoids or a family history for cancer.

A: Pain is not controlled on current therapy. JM appears to be experiencing blood loss from regular use of the NSAID piroxicam, exacerbated by the recent OTC purchase of ibuprofen. The uncontrolled diabetes and hypothyroidism may be contributing to her loss of energy.

P: Discontinue the piroxicam and the naproxen, which may be precipitating factors in the GI blood loss. Since the patient is still having pain in the weight-bearing joints, recommend a switch to acetaminophen 650 mg po qid on a prn basis. The acetaminophen is a cost-effective, relatively safe and efficacious analgesic for a majority of cases of osteoarthritis, most cases of which do not have an inflammatory component.

Problem 5. Traveler's Diarrhea Prophylaxis

S: Not applicable

O: JM is traveling for an extended length of time to a tropical area with poor hygiene with "high risk" for developing diarrhea. JM is allergic by history to sulfa drugs.

A: Prophylaxis against traveler's diarrhea may be indicated, due to risk factors and possible complications (dehydration) with diabetes mellitus control. The benefit of preventive therapy appears to outweigh the risk of side effects to the patient.

P: Patient education on precautions such as avoid water (including ice), uncooked foods, unpeeled fruits and vegetables. For rehydration use bottled or canned beverages or fruit juices, or water that has been boiled (hot tea or coffee). A single daily dose of doxycycline 100 mg is prescribed; JM is counseled on sunscreen precautions to avoid a photosensitivity reaction. Treatment is started on the first day of travel and continued until the second day home. Patient recommended to purchase loperamide OTC for any self-limited diarrheal episodes.

QUESTIONS FOR CASE 190

1. How long should hormonal estrogen treatment be continued in a postmenopausal patient? What are the patient risk factors to long term estrogen therapy?

2. How should levothyroxine be dosed in the elderly? How fast can dosage be increased? What are the precautions and expected side effects?

3. How strictly should the blood sugar level be controlled in an elderly patient with type II diabetes mellitus? Can long-term complications be prevented or delayed?

4. Why is JM's urine glucose level normal? Why should the daily checking of urine sugars be discontinued? Why are blood sugar determinations better for the elderly diabetic?

5. Recommend treatment with an NSAID in this elderly patient who has compromised renal function. Are any of the NSAIDs more "renal-sparing" than others? What parameters would a pharmacist monitor for renal toxicity?

6. When is prophylaxis for traveler's diarrhea indicated?

CASE 191

CC: LB is a 79-year-old male who lives at home with his wife of 52 years. He is a retired manager of a clothing manufacturing firm. He has no aphysical complaints and states, "I'm tired, getting old is no fun." LB seems unable to find the words he wants to express himself during the interview. He knew his name and the year, but he could not tell the interviewer what month it was or where he was, nor could he recall if he had eaten breakfast.

Much of the medical and social history is provided by LB's wife and daughter. LB's wife states that he has been well except for "that heart attack last year, that's when all this started." LB has been forgetful and nervous; he has had a 12-pound weight loss in the past 3 months. He spends most of his time around the house with his wife. LB used to go outside for hours tending his garden but has not shown interest this past year. He has gotten more irritable with Mrs. B and has recently begun to have trouble dressing and sometimes refuses to take a bath. In the last few weeks there have been two episodes of agitation, where he has been very unreasonable and angry. He has been verbally abusive, calling his wife names and accusing her and others of stealing his tools. He naps during the day and goes to bed at 8 PM, often awakening at 2 AM. He is unable to return to sleep and goes through drawers searching for misplaced items. He feels someone is taking his things and hiding them. LB still drives short distances such as to the grocery store. In the last year he has had one minor traffic accident where "someone hit him and it wasn't my fault." He denies getting lost, but his wife remembers a trip to his daughter's last month where he got confused and made several wrong turns before getting to her house. LB's daughter adds that she has seen a decline in her father's memory over the last 4–5 years, but the last few years he seems to have gotten much worse. She has concerns about her mother, who she feels is "stressed out," and she believes her father's alcohol intake makes matters worse. She feels that her mother has taken over the entire burden of maintaining the household. Her mother cannot rest because her father constantly awakens her early in the morning and makes demands on her throughout the day.

Past Medical History

LB had a nontransmural myocardial infarction (MI) 13 months ago. He had complained of severe indigestion and was taken to the emergency room. He was hospitalized for 5 days, during which time he got very confused and agitated, had visual hallucinations, and had to be given "tranquilizers" to calm him down. He is being treated for arrhythmias and has had angina and congestive heart failure (CHF).

Medication History

Digoxin 0.25 mg q.d. × 1 year
Furosemide 40 mg q.d. × 1 year
KCl 10% 15 ml (20 mEq) q.d. × 1 year
Verapamil 80 mg q8h × 6 months
Diphenhydramine 50 mg q. h.s. × 1 month
Nitroglycerin 0.4 mg 1 tablet s.l. p.r.n. chest pain

Allergies

No known allergies

Social History

Tobacco: 75 pack-year history, quit about 3 years ago
Ethanol: History of chronic alcohol use (heavy in the past, averaging 2–5 scotch and sodas a day). Currently drinks 2–3 drinks per day (per daughter).

Physical Examination

GEN: LB is a well-developed, well-nourished male. He is clean and his clothes are neat and well matched.
VS: BP 150/90, HR 71, T 37, Wt 71.4 kg, Ht 172 cm
HEENT: WNL
COR: Regular rate and rhythm with frequent extrasystoles
CHEST: Inspiratory crackles at both bases
ABD: Mild left lower quadrant tenderness
GU: WNL
RECT: Slightly enlarged prostate
EXT: 2+ pitting edema of feet and ankles
NEURO: Oriented × 1. Minimental status examination: 11/30

Results of Laboratory Tests

Na 140 (140)	HCO₃ 25 (25)	AST 0.65 (39)
K 4.0 (4.0)	BUN 7.5 (21)	ALT 0.58 (35)
Cl 102 (102)	CR 105 (1.2)	Glu 5.3 (95)

Digoxin: 2.2 nmol/liter (1.7 ng/ml)

ECG: NSR with frequent (greater than 30/hr), multifocal PVCs; left axis deviation.
Echocardiogram: Normal chamber size; mild aortic stenosis, normal systolic function

PROBLEM LIST

1. S/P MI with arrhythmias
2. Angina
3. CHF
4. Mental status changes
5. Alcohol abuse
6. Weight loss

QUESTIONS FOR CASE 191

1. What signs and symptoms of dementia does LB exhibit?
2. What are the main differential diagnoses that need to be considered for LB's dementia?
3. What medication recommendations could be made to treat LB's symptoms of dementia?
4. LB's family is asking for help to maintain him at home. His wife wants to continue to care for him. What can you offer?

CASE 192

CC: SP is a 72-year-old male who is reported to have a mental status decline over the last 2 weeks. He has become disoriented in his home and is not able to recognize familiar people. He is also reported to be drowsy most of the day, with periods of severe agitation.

Past Medical History

SP has a history of Parkinson's disease (1991); SP suffers from gout (1985) controlled with medication; hypertension (1983) controlled with medication; gastric resection for PUD in 1976, and now has pernicious anemia and chronic constipation with frequent impactions. Recently, SP has been diagnosed with "sundowning" and has been prescribed medications.

Medication History

Levodopa/carbidopa 25/250 2 tabs p.o. t.i.d.
Benztropine 2 mg p.o. t.i.d.
Allopurinol 300 mg p.o. q.d.
Hydrochlorothiazide (HCTZ) 50 mg p.o. q.d.
KCl 20 mEq p.o. b.i.d.
Cyanocolbalamine 6 μg p.o. q. AM
Thioridazine 50 mg at dinner
Phenolphthalein 60 mg ii tabs p.o. of AM p.r.n.
Alprazolam 1 mg p.o. q.i.d. p.r.n. agitation
Flurazepam 15 mg p.o. h.s. p.r.n. sleep, may repeat

Social History

Tobacco—negative
Alcohol—occasional social drinker

Physical Examination

GEN: Well-developed, overweight, confused male in no acute distress who appears extremely drowsy.

VS: BP 130/90, HR 85, RR 20, T 38.4, Wt 72 kg, Ht 185.42 cm

HEENT: WNL; wears corrective lenses

COR: Normal S1 and S2, no murmurs, rubs, or gallops

CHEST: Clear, no rales present

ABD: Flat, nontender

GU: Prostatic hypertrophy

RECT: Hard stool in rectum

EXT: No skin tears or lesions; slightly pale

NEURO: Bilateral rigidity; slight tremor present, oriented to person only

Results of Laboratory Tests

Na 137 (137)	AST 0.40 (24)	Glu 7.1 (128)
K 4.8 (4.8)	ALT 0.47 (28)	Ca 2.3 (9.2)
Cl 102 (102)	LDH 2.5 (150)	PO₄ 1.4 (4.2)
HCO₃ 28 (28)	Alk Phos 1.75 (1105)	Uric Acid 420 (7.0)
BUN 8.6 (24)	Alb 41 (4.1)	Chol 6.47 (250)
CR 97 (1.1)	T. Protein 72 (7.2)	Iron 15 (85)
	T Bili 14 (0.82)	

Urinalysis: Negative for glucose and microorganisms
Chest x-ray: WNL
ECG: WNL

PROBLEM LIST

1. Hypertension
2. Gout
3. Pernicious anemia
4. Parkinson's disease
5. Constipation
6. Agitation (sundowning)

CRITICAL CARE

CASE 193

CC: FF is a 36-year-old male brought to the hospital by the paramedics after he collapsed at home. His family states that FF was acting normally throughout the day and was working in his yard when he complained of severe headache and collapsed. The family did not observe any seizure activity. A paramedic unit was called, and FF was transported to the ER.

Past Medical History

Unremarkable

Social History

No alcohol, tobacco, or recreational drug use

Medication History

Currently taking no medication. Occasionally takes aspirin for headache. Last known intake of aspirin was 1 week ago.

Allergies

No known allergies to medication, no food intolerance

Review of Symptoms

Negative per family members

Physical Examination

GEN: Well-developed, well-nourished male, unresponsive to verbal stimuli
VS: BP 190/140, HR 95, RR 18, T 37 (rectal), Wt 80 kg, Ht 185 cm
HEENT: Rigid neck; funduscopic examination reveals bilateral retinal hemorrhages; right pupil dilated and unresponsive to light
COR: S1, S2 normal, no murmurs or gallops
CHEST: Clear to ascultation
ABD: Soft, no masses or rigidity
GU: Normal male genitalia
RECT: Deferred
EXT: Normal, no clubbing, cyanosis, or edema
NEURO: Patient unresponsive to verbal and painful stimuli; reflexes symmetrical and increased; (+) Babinski, sucking, and grasp reflexes.

Results of Laboratory Tests

Na 139 (139)	Hct 0.40 (40%)	AST WNL	Glu 6.4 (115)
K 3.9 (3.9)	Hgb 155 (15.5)	ALT WNL	Ca 2.6 (10.0)
Cl 100 (100)	Lkcs 7.0 × 10⁹ (7.8 × 10⁹)	LDH WNL	PO₄ 1.1 (3.4)
CO₂ 24 (24)	Plts 220 × 10⁹ (220 × 10⁵)	Alk Phos WNL	Mg 1.05 (2.1)
BUN 4.3 (12)	MCV 82 (82)	Alb WNL	Uric Acid WNL
CR 70.7 (0.8)		T bili 94 (5.5)	

Lkc differential: Normal
Urinalysis: Normal
Chest x-ray: Clear
ECG: Normal

Hospital Course

After admission to the ER, FF was given 100 mg thiamine and 25 ml of 50% dextrose intravenously. A CT scan of the head revealed a large subarachnoid hemorrhage. While being transported to the ICU, FF sustained two tonic-clonic seizures, each lasting 20 sec. The seizures were approximately 5 min apart. Upon arrival to the ICU, FF sustained a third seizure, lasting 15 sec.

PROBLEM LIST

1. Subarachnoid hemorrhage
2. Status epilepticus
3. Hypertension

CASE 193 SOAP NOTES
Problem 2. Status Epilepticus

S: None

O: FF had three seizures without regaining consciousness. There is no history of a seizure disorder or head trauma.

A: FF is experiencing status epileticus due to a subarachnoid hemorrhage. FF has sustained multiple seizures without regaining consciousness. Aggressive therapy is indicated because seizure activity may increase intracranial pressure and worsen neurologic function. Therefore FF should receive intravenous anticonvulsants.

P: Diazepam 5 mg IVP should be administered at a rate of 2 mg/min. This dose may be repeated at 10-min intervals until seizures stop or a total of 20 mg is administered. The intravenous fluid should be changed to 0.9% sodium chloride and FF should receive 1500 mg of phenytoin infused over 30 min. The therapeutic end point is cessation of seizure activity. FF should be monitored closely for hypotension and the development of respiratory depression. Hypotension is treated by decreasing the phenytoin infusion rate and/or administering a fluid bolus. Respiratory depression caused by diazepam may be controlled with intubation and mechanical ventilation.

Problem 1. Subarachnoid Hemorrhage

S: FF complained of acute onset of severe headache.

O: Acute onset of coma, rigid neck, presence of bilateral retinal hemorrhages on funduscopic examination. Positive Babinski, grasp, and sucking reflexes are neurologic signs that do not help to localize the lesion.

A: FF has sustained a subarachnoid hemorrhage. The clinical presentation of abrupt onset of headache, loss of consciousness without incidence of previous symptoms, and absence of lateralizing signs is consistent with a subarachnoid hemorrhage caused by a ruptured aneurysm. Most commonly, vascular aneurysms are located at bifurcations of the cerebral vasculature. The increase in extravascular blood due to the intracranial hemorrhage increases the intracranial pressure (ICP). Progressive increases in the ICP should be prevented, to avoid additional neuronal death. Patients with acute neurologic events are also at high risk for developing stress ulcers.

P: Change intravenous fluids from dextrose in water to a balanced salt solution. The level of the head should be elevated to 15–30 degrees. FF should be intubated and hyperventilated to achieve an arterial PCO_2 of 20–25 torr. Mannitol should be administered in a dose of 500 ml of a 20% solution (1.25 g/kg). This dose should be repeated every 4–6 hr. Monitoring parameters should include hourly neurologic assessment, arterial blood gas determination, and hourly assessment of fluid intake and urine output. Serum sodium, potassium, chloride, bicarbonate, blood urea nitrogen, and creatinine should also be closely monitored. Serum osmolarity should be measured at least twice daily. The hemoglobin and hematocrit should be monitored to detect further bleeding. Placement of a nasogastric tube would be useful for intragastric pH monitoring when there is a risk of markedly increasing ICP. Histamine-2 receptor antagonist infusion of cimetidine 900 mg/24 hr or ranitidine 150 mg/24 hr should be initiated.

Problem 3. Severe Hypertension

S: None

O: BP 190/140 on admission

A: Severe hypertension may result from an intracranial hemorrhage. Left untreated, the hypertension may worsen the subarachnoid bleeding.

P: Treatment should be initiated with intravenous nitroprusside at a rate of 0.25 µg/kg/min and the dose titrated to the patient's response. The blood pressure should initially be decreased to a mean arterial pressure (MAP) of 120 mm Hg. The neurologic examination should be followed closely to identify deterioration with lowering of the blood pressure. If FF remains stable at a MAP of 120 mm Hg, the blood pressure may be slowly decreased to a MAP of 80–90 mm Hg.

QUESTIONS FOR CASE 193

1. What should be done to FF if phenytoin loading fails to control the status epilepticus?

2. What may be done to FF to prevent neurologic sequelae from his subarachnoid hemorrhage?

3. What drug interactions are present in FF's case?

4. Can corticosteroids be used to treat the increased ICP in FF?

5. What complications would result from tube feedings in FF?

CASE 194

CC: DK is a 58-year-old male who has undergone three-vessel coronary artery bypass graft surgery. As he was being taken off the bypass machine, it was noted that he was hypotensive. DK was transferred to the intensive care unit postoperatively with a blood pressure of 90/50 mm Hg.

Past Medical History

Unstable angina × 10 years
Myocardial infarction 5 years prior to admission
Hypertension × 15 years
Insulin-dependent diabetes mellitus since age 35

Social History

Smoked 1 1/2 ppd × 30 years—quit 5 years ago
No alcohol or recreational drug use

Medication History

Hydrochlorothiazide 25 mg p.o. q.AM
ASA 325 mg p.o. q.AM
Isosorbide dinitrate 30 mg p.o. t.i.d.
Verapamil 120 mg p.o. t.i.d.
Nitroglycerin 0.4 mg s.l. p.r.n. chest pain
Insulin NPH (human) 26 units s.q. q.AM/12 units s.q. q.PM

Allergies

None known

Review of Systems

Noncontributory

Physical Examination (upon admission to ICU postoperatively)

GEN: Well-developed, well-nourished male intubated and appearing drowsy post CABG

VS: BP 90/50/63, HR 110, RR 18 (controlled ventilation), T 37 (rectal), Wt 85 kg, Ht 183 cm

HEENT: WNL

COR: Tachycardic with nl S1, S2; grade III/VI SEM at LLSB

CHEST: Bibasilar rales

ABD: Soft, no masses or rigidity

GU: WNL

RECT: Deferred

EXT: Slightly cool

NEURO: Responsive to verbal stimuli, reflexes normal

Results of Laboratory Tests

Na 136 (136)	Hct 0.38 (38%)	AST WNL	Glu 6.7 (120)
K 4.0 (3.5)	Hgb 140 (14.0)	ALT WNL	Ca 2.6 (10.0)
Cl 105 (105)	Lkcs 8.2 × 10⁹ (8.2 × 10³)	LDH WNL	PO₄ 1.29 (4.0)
CO₂ 24 (24)	Plts 220 × 10⁹ (220 × 10³)	Alk Phos WNL	Mg 1.0 (2.0)
BUN 7.14 (20)	MCV 82 (82)	Alb WNL	Uric Acid WNL
CR 150 (1.7)		T bili WNL	

Lkc differential: Normal
Urinalysis: Normal
Chest x-ray: Cardiomegaly; mild pulmonary edema
ECG: NSR, rate 120, evidence of LVH

Hospital Course

After admission to the intensive care unit, the following hemodynamic parameters were obtained. In addition to these findings, DK had a urine output of 20 ml/hr.

Hemodynamic Parameters

BP	90/50/63 mm Hg (S/D/M)
HR	110 beats/min
Right atrial pressure (RAP)	10 mm Hg (mean)
Pulmonary artery pressure (PAP)	38/24/29 mm Hg (S/D/M)
Pulmonary capillary wedge pressure (PCWP)	21 mm Hg
Cardiac index (CI)	1.2 liter/min/m²
Systemic vascular resistance (SVR)	2080 dynes sec cm-5

PROBLEM LIST

1. Type I (insulin-dependent) diabetes mellitus
2. Acute heart failure—s/p CABG

CASE 194 SOAP NOTES
Problem 2. Acute Heart Failure

S: None
O: BP 90/50 with a mean of 63 mm Hg
   HR 110 beats/min
   PCWP 21 mm Hg
   CI 1.2 liter/min/m²
   SVR 2080 dynes sec cm-5
   Chest x-ray: Mild pulmonary edema
   Urine output: 20 ml/hr
A: DK has acute heart failure following bypass surgery. Objective parameters that are consistent with heart failure are hypotension, tachycardia, low cardiac index, and high systemic vascular resistance. DK also has reduced urine output and cool extremities, reflecting tissue hypoperfusion. The elevated pulmonary capillary wedge pressure (preload) and the chest x-ray results suggest that DK has mild pulmonary edema caused by heart failure. DK requires inotropic support. Dopamine possesses dose-dependent inotropic, chronotropic, and vasoactive properties. At doses of 0.5–2 μ/kg/min, dopamine stimulates dopaminergic receptors in the renal vascular beds, producing an increase in renal blood flow, glomerular filtration rate, and urine output. With infusion rates of 2–5 μg/kg/min, dopamine increases cardiac output and contractility, with little change in heart

rate, blood pressure, or systemic vascular resistance. Doses up to 10 μg/kg/min result in a further increase in cardiac output, with small increases in heart rate and blood pressure. Infusion rates in excess of 10 μ/kg/min produce an increase in mean arterial pressure and vasoconstriction of the renal vasculature, and may increase pulmonary capillary wedge pressure.
P: DK requires immediate blood pressure and inotropic support. When a patient is hypotensive, one therapeutic option is fluid therapy with crystalloids (normal saline) or colloids (albumin or hetastarch). DK already has an elevated pulmonary capillary wedge pressure and evidence of pulmonary edema. Thus the administration of a fluid challenge would probably not result in a beneficial effect. DK requires a vasoactive drug, such as dopamine, to support his blood pressure and cardiac output. Dopamine should be initiated at a dose of 5 μ/kg/min and titrated to response. All hemodynamic parameters should be monitored closely in this patient. Specific end points are: mean arterial pressure 70 mm Hg, cardiac index >2.2 liter/min/m², heart rate below 120 beats/min, a reduction in pulmonary capillary wedge pressure (to 16–18 mm Hg) with resolution of pulmonary edema, and a urine output of 0.5 ml/kg/hr. Warm, perfused extremities are also desirable. The clinician should strive to use the lowest possible dose of dopamine to achieve these end points.

Problem 1. Type I (Insulin-dependent) Diabetes Mellitus

S: None
O: DK has a history of Type I (insulin-dependent) diabetes mellitus since age 35. DK was receiving 26 units of NPH insulin every morning and 12 units of NPH insulin every evening. His blood glucose is now normal.
A: DK has type I (insulin-dependent) diabetes mellitus; he does not exhibit hyperglycemia presently. If DK does not receive insulin, hepatic glycogenolysis, gluconeogenesis, and lipolysis will occur. Hyperglycemia will cause an osmotic diuresis and intravascular volume contraction. The resultant increased catecholamine levels will increase free fatty acid mobilization. Stress-related release of cortisol and growth hormone augments this process by their anti-insulin activities. Hyperglycemia and ketone body accumulation cause large losses of water, sodium, potassium, calcium, and phosphate. Additionally, DK could develop diabetic ketoacidosis if insulin is withheld for a long enough period of time. A number of factors will alter the amount of insulin ICU patients require. Glucose tolerance varies greatly in response to glucagon, cortisol, growth hormone, and catecholamine levels. Additionally, the administration of intravenous fluids containing dextrose or parenteral or enteral nutrition will alter insulin requirements.
P: DK will require insulin coverage during his ICU admission. DK should have his blood glucose level checked every 6 hr, and he should receive intermittent doses of regular insulin. Elevations in the blood glucose level may be treated with a sliding-scale insulin regimen as follows:

Blood glucose <8.3 mmol/liter (150 mg/dl)	0 units
Blood glucose 8.3–11.1 mmol/liter (150–200 mg/dl)	3 units
Blood glucose 11.1–13.9 mmol/liter (200–250 mg/dl)	6 units
Blood glucose >13.9 mmol/liter (250 mg/dl)	10 units

The insulin dose may be adjusted to the patient's response. DK should be monitored for clinical evidence of hypoglycemia throughout the period of insulin administration. Unexplained agitation, tachycardia, or CNS depression require assessment of the blood glucose concentration and prompt treatment with 25 ml of 50% dextrose administered IVP if hypoglycemia is present. The development of seizures would require empiric administration of 25–50 ml of 50% dextrose solution IVP.

QUESTIONS FOR CASE 194

1. If DK's blood pressure is stabilized with dopamine but the cardiac index remains inadequate, should vasodilator therapy be initiated?
2. What potential problems exist if nitroprusside is used in DK?
3. What is the role of dobutamine in DK?
4. What should be done if DK becomes agitated?

CASE 195

CC: CL is a 49-year-old male being admitted to the hospital for normalization of his blood sugar levels, which have been progressively increasing over several months. His fasting blood sugar level from this morning was 23.3 mmol/liter (420 mg/dl), and 2 hr after breakfast his blood glucose concentration was 26.4 mmol/liter (475 mg/dl). CL has been experiencing significant nocturia, polyuria, and polydipsia for several weeks. His urine has been negative for ketones.

Past Medical History

CL received an orthotopic heart transplantation (OHT) 7 months before admission for treatment of severe dilated cardiomyopathy. Over the last 3 months, CL has developed hypertension. Treatment with diltiazem was initiated 1 month ago.

Medication History

Cyclosporine liquid 200 mg b.i.d.
Prednisone 5 mg b.i.d.
Azathioprine 200 mg q.d.
Trimethoprim 80 mg/sulfamethoxazole 400 mg q.o.d.
Digoxin 0.125 mg q.d.
Ethacrynic acid 25 mg q.o.d.
Diltiazem, sustained-release capsules 90 mg q.d.
Magnesium complex 600 mg b.i.d.
Multivitamins 1 q.AM
Aspirin, enteric-coated 80 mg q.d.

Review of Systems

CL states that he is unable to sleep through the night because he is frequently getting up to urinate. CL complains that he is experiencing bothersome headaches. CL has developed a hand tremor, tingling sensation in his hands and feet, and tender and sore gums.

Physical Examination

GEN: Thin-appearing male with painful, macular, weeping rash that follows the T10 dermatome
VS: BP 130/100, HR 80 reg, RR 22, T 37.4, Wt 77 (was 68 kg 7 months ago, IBW 81 kg)
HEENT: PEERL, red swollen gums
COR: JVP normal, +S4
CHEST: Lungs clear
GU: WNL
EXT: No edema

Results of Laboratory Tests

Na 132 (132)	Hct 0.43 (43.2)	AST 0.55 (33)	Glu 23.3 (420)
K 4.9 (4.9)	Hgb 131 (13.1)	ALT 0.3 (18)	Ca 2.3 (9.3)
Cl 104 (104)	Lkcs 4.8 × 10⁹ (4.8 × 10³)	Alk Phos 1.1 (68)	Mg 0.75 (1.5)
HCO₃ 22 (22)	Plts 251 × 10⁹ (251 × 10³)	Alb 32 (3.2)	Chol 7.3 (275)
BUN 9.6 (27)	MCV 98 (98)	T Bili 17 (1.0)	LDL 5.8 (225)
Cr 115 (1.3)			TG 1.9 (168)

Cyclosporine: 660 ng/ml, whole blood HPLC (375 ng/ml 1 month ago)
Digoxin: 1.2 nmol/liter (0.9 μ/liter)

PROBLEM LIST

1. S/P heart transplant on immunosuppressive therapy
2. Hypertension
3. Cyclosporine (CSA) toxicity
4. Steroid-induced diabetes
5. Herpes zoster
6. Hypercholesterolemia
7. Gingival hyperplasia

CASE 195 SOAP NOTES
Problem 1. S/P OHT on Immunosuppressive Therapy

S: None
O: CSA 660
A: CL received his OHT 7 months ago and is on CSA, AZA, and prednisone for immunosuppressive therapy. There are no signs of rejection. He is currently experiencing problems related to his immunosuppressive therapy: CSA toxicity, prednisone-induced diabetes, CSA and prednisone exacerbation of hypertension and activation of herpes zoster; the CSA toxicity and hyperglycemia need acute management (see problems 4 and 5). There are no signs of CSA nephrotoxicity, although this requires continued monitoring. CL's weight has increased 9 kg toward his IBW of 81 kg. CL is receiving TMP/SMX for PCP prophylaxis and magnesium complex for replacement of Mg due to CSA-induced Mg wasting.

P: Hold CSA for now, restart when levels are 250 ng/ml. Continue prednisone, AZA, TMP/SMX, and magnesium complex. Continue to monitor for signs of rejection.

Problem 4. Steroid-induced Diabetes

S: Nocturia, polyuria, polydipsia

O: FBG 23.3 mmol/liter (420 mg/dl), Glu 26.4 mmol/liter (475 mg/dl)

A: Steroids can cause significant resistance to the action of insulin and also increase glucose production by the liver. Although the current prednisone dose is approaching physiologic levels, it is still sufficient to induce diabetes. CL needs to have his blood sugar normalized.

P: Initiate therapy with s.q. insulin. Start insulin dose at 0.6 units/kg/day, divide the dose 2/3 in the morning and 1/3 in the evening. An initial insulin regimen for CL would be NPH 20 u/Reg 10 u in the morning and NPH 17 u in the evening. Check blood sugar levels before meals and at bedtime. The goal is to achieve FBS 6–10 mmol/liter (100–180 mg/dl). Monitor for signs of hyperglycemia, polyuria, nocturia, and polydipsia. For long-term management of CL's diabetes, give glipizide 10 mg p.o. b.i.d., 30 min before breakfast and dinner. CL should be taught how to monitor his blood sugar levels at home.

Problem 5. Herpes Zoster

S: Painful rash

O: Macular weeping rash that follows the T10 dermatome.

A: CL's rash is consistent with herpes zoster (varicella-zoster virus, VZV) virus. Intravenous acyclovir has been shown to be effective in preventing dissemination of infections, promoting cutaneous healing, and relieving pain. The dose of acyclovir to treat VZV is 10 mg/kg IV every 8 hr. The dose should be infused over at least 1 hr to prevent renal damage due to drug precipitation and crystallization in the distal tubules. The dose of acyclovir for CL is 800 mg IV q8h. Aspirin 650 mg alone or with codeine 15–30 mg, p.o. q4-6h p.r.n. may relieve the pain.

P: Acyclovir 800 mg via slow IV infusion every 8 hr for 10 days, then switch to p.o. 200 mg 5 × per day for 5 months. Monitor SCr, BUN and the number and severity of herpetic lesions. Give aspirin 650 mg alone or with codeine 15–30 mg, p.o. q. 4-6 hr p.r.n. pain.

Problem 3. Cyclosporine Toxicity

S: Tremor, tingling of hand and feet, headache

O: CSA level 660 ng/ml

A: CL is exhibiting symptoms of CSA toxicity, most likely caused by his elevated CSA level. The current CSA level is significantly elevated, as compared with 1 month ago on the same CSA dose. Diltiazem, which had recently been added to his regimen, decreases CSA metabolism, thereby causing an increase in CSA levels. CL has been using the CSA liquid, and it is possible that he is drawing up an inaccurate dose; his technique for drawing up his CSA dose should be checked. The dose of CSA should be held until the level falls to 250 ng/ml. The CSA should then be restarted at a lower dose, and the dose adjusted based on CSA levels. Consider switching CL to an alternative antihypertensive agent, since the diltiazem is not controlling his blood pressure and is interfering with his CSA levels. If the decision is made to discontinue the diltiazem, then it will be unnecessary to restart the cyclosporine at a lower dose.

P: Hold CSA for now. Check CSA levels. When levels are 250 ng/ml, restart CSA. Switch to CSA gel caps 200 mg p.o. b.i.d. (since diltiazem is to be discontinued). Continue to monitor CSA levels.

Problem 2. Hypertension

S: None

O: History, elevated BP measurements

A: CL's blood pressure remains elevated in spite of treatment with diltiazem. The increase in the CSA concentration secondary to diltiazem inhibition of CSA metabolism may also be contributing to CL's hypertension. An alternative antihypertensive agent should be selected. Avoid the use of β-adrenergic blockers, since these can worsen CL's lipid profile and mask symptoms of hypoglycemia. Angiotensin converting enzyme (ACE)-inhibitors, clonidine tablets or patches, and prazosin are suitable alternative agents.

P: Discontinue diltiazem. Start captopril 12.5 mg p.o. t.i.d. Monitor BP, BUN, SCr, and K

Problem 6. Hypercholesterolemia

S: None

O: Chol 7.3 (275), LDL 5.8 (225), TG 1.9 (168)

A: CL's hyperlipidemia should be treated. He is at increased risk for the development of coronary disease in his newly transplanted heart. Dietary measures should be instituted with drug therapy. The use of niacin should be avoided, since it can worsen CL's glucose control. Bile acid-binding resins may lead to decreased absorption of prednisone and digoxin in CL. The bulky powders may prove unpalatable, and in view of the numerous other drugs CL must take each day, he may be noncompliant with his regimen. The combined use of lovastatin and immunosuppressive agents has been shown to have an increased incidence of myopathy. If used in transplant recipients, close monitoring is required. Gemfibrozol would be a satisfactory choice, especially considering CL's lipid profile. Suggest gemfibrozol 600 mg p.o. b.i.d., 30 min before the morning and evening meals.

P: Start gemfibrozol 600 mg p.o. b.i.d., 30 min before the morning and evening meals. Instruct CL about appropriate dietary measures he should be following.

Problem 7. Gingival Hyperplasia Therapy

S: Gums are swollen, red, tender, and sore.

O: None

A: CL's sore gums may lead to poor nutritional intake. They are also a potential source of systemic infection if CL's gums should become infected or bleed. Cyclosporine and calcium-channel blockers can cause gingival hyperplasia.

P: Instruct CL to practice good oral hygiene. He should brush his teeth with a soft toothbrush and floss regularly. CL should visit his dentist on a regular basis.

QUESTIONS FOR CASE 195

1. CL states that since his heart transplant he seems to become short of breath whenever he begins his daily exercise program, but this resolves before the end of his routine. Explain what is happening.
2. What other types of opportunistic infections is CL at risk for developing?
3. On a routine visit to the transplant clinic 2 weeks after being discharged from the hospital, CL was noted to be in atrial fibrillation with heart rates up to 118 beats/min. His digoxin level was 0.9 nmol/liter (0.7 μ/liter). The clinic physician increased CL's digoxin dose to 0.25 mg per day.
   a. Give the possible explanations for the decrease in CL's digoxin concentration.
   b. Calculate the new expected digoxin steady-state concentration.
4. CL is going to the dentist next week to have two teeth extracted. His physician would like to give him prophylactic antibiotic therapy. What do you recommend?

CASE 196

CC: DD is a 45-year-old male transferred to the ICU with a rectal temperature of 39.4°C, abdominal pain, and a change in mental status.

Hospital Course

Gastrointestinal Bleeding. DD was admitted 4 days ago after vomiting bright red blood. He failed to stop bleeding after nasogastric tube lavage. He has a history of gastrointestinal bleeding due to esophageal varices, with 4 GI hemorrhages in the past year. A vasopressin infusion was begun at 0.4 units/min and increased to 0.8 units/min to control the bleeding. An esophagogastroduodenoscopy (EGD) revealed large esophagal varices that were actively bleeding. The varices were sclerosed. DD's hematocrit fell from 0.30 (30) on admission to 0.22 (22) after hydration. DD required transfusion of 8 units of packed red blood cells and 4 units of fresh frozen plasma. The vasopressin infusion was discontinued 12 hr ago.

Ethanol Withdrawal. DD has a long history of ethanol abuse, with his last drink 4 hr prior to admission. DD was begun on lorazepam 2 mg every 8 hr i.m. He became agitated and experienced visual and auditory hallucinations. Additionally, he developed tachycardia and developed a temperature elevation to 100°F. DD required restraints and a total of 12 mg of intravenous lorazepam to control the agitation.

Past Medical History

As above

Cirrhosis of the liver was confirmed by liver biopsy; cause is probably long-term alcohol abuse. DD has had multiple

episodes of alcoholic hepatitis. He has no history of hepatic encephalopathy.

Chronic obstructive pulmonary disease (COPD): FEV_1 65% predicted; FEF_{25-75} 55% predicted, and FVC 72% predicted. DD has a cough producing a small amount of sputum.

Social History

Ethanol abuse for 20 years
Has smoked 2 packs/day for 22 years
No recreational drug use

Medication History

DD was not taking any prescription medications. He uses aspirin occasionally to relieve headaches.

Allergies

None known

Physical Examination

GEN: Thin male, arousable to voice, oriented to person only
VS: BP 120/85, HR 110, RR 20 unlabored, T 39.4 (rectal), Wt 64 kg, Ht 170 cm
HEENT: Icteric sclera, EOM intact, PERRLA, throat clear, poor dentition, no nuchal rigidity
CHEST: Clear to auscultation and percussion, spider angiomas seen on chest
COR: S_1, S_2 normal, no murmurs or gallops
ABD: Protuberant abdomen, diffuse tenderness, no rebound, could not palpate liver or spleen, hypoactive bowel sounds, fluid wave present, shifting dullness present
EXT: No clubbing, cyanosis, or edema; palmar erythema, no asterixis, IV catheter insertion sites are clean
GU: Bilateral testicular atrophy, no penile or scrotal lesions
RECT: No stool in rectal vault, no masses, normal prostate
NEURO: Drowsy but answers to name, no focal neurologic signs, all reflexes present and equal, cranial nerves II-XII intact.

Results of Laboratory Tests

Na 136 (136)	Hct 0.30 (30%)	AST 4.5 (270)	Glu 4.4 (80)
K 3.5 (3.5)	Hgb 102 (10.2)	ALT 3.7 (220)	Ca 2.00 (8.0)
Cl 98 (98)	Lkcs 17×10^9 (17×10^3)	LDH 3.33 (200)	PO_4 1.29 (4.0)
CO_2 22 (22)	Plts 220×10^9 (220×10^3)	Alk Phos 2.0 (118)	Mg 1.0 (2.0)
BUN 4.3 (12)	MCV 82 (82)	Alb 20 (2.0)	Uric Acid 387 (6.5)
CR 70.7 (0.8)		T Bili 94 (5.5)	

Lkcs differential: 0.79 (79%) polys, 0.14 (14%) bands, 0.04 (4%) lymphocytes, 0.02 (2%) monocytes
Urinalysis: Bilirubin-positive
Chest x-ray: Clear
ECG: Normal

Prothrombin time: 14.0 sec/12.4 sec (control)

Arterial blood gas: pH 7.41 pCO_2 42 mm Hg, pO_2 92 mm Hg, room air

Paracentesis: Cloudy fluid; Lkcs 500/mm^3 with 96% polys; Gram stain reveals many Lkcs and Gram-negative rods; culture pending

Medication List

Sucralfate 1.0 g every 6 hr since admission

Cefoxitin 1.0 g every 6 hr since admission

Lactulose 30 ml every 6 hr since admission

Diazepam 5.0 mg every 6 hr begun day 2 of admission

Multivitamin 1 every morning begun day 3 of admission

Folic acid 1 mg every morning begun day 3 of admission

Thiamine 100 mg every morning since admission

PROBLEM LIST

1. Alcoholic liver disease—cirrhosis of the liver, h/o alcoholic hepatitis
2. H/O COPD
3. GI bleeding—secondary to esophageal varices
4. H/O ethanol withdrawal
5. Sepsis—subacute bacterial peritonitis
6. Coagulopathy
7. Change in mental status

QUESTIONS FOR CASE 196

1. Defend your rationale for altering his antibiotic therapy.
2. What could be done to prevent further recurrence of variceal bleeding?
3. What are the adverse effects of vasopressin administration?
4. What types of intravenous fluid should be administered to DD?

CASE 197

CC: AM is a 40-year-old man who is admitted to the hospital with a 2-day history of fevers to 37.9°C, chills, malaise, decreased appetite, abdominal pain, loose stools, pus from his orthotopic liver transplant abdominal wound, and headache.

Past Medical History

AM received an orthotopic liver transplant (OLT) 2 months ago for treatment of chronic active hepatitis secondary to IV drug abuse and alcoholic cirrhosis. His postoperative course was complicated by an ascites leak, *Staphylococcus aureus* wound infection and bacteremia. AM was treated for an episode of acute rejection 1 week prior to admission. AM also has a history of peptic ulcer disease and upper GI bleeding with encephalopathy.

Social History

AM quit drinking alcohol and smoking cigarettes about 1 year ago; he smokes cigars occasionally and denies recreational drug use.

Medication History

Cyclosporine (CSA) capsules 400 mg b.i.d.

Prednisone 7.5 mg q.d.

Azathioprine (AZA) 50 mg q.h.s.

Trimethoprim 80 mg/sulfamethoxazole (TMP/SMX) 400 mg q.o.d.

Magnesium complex 300 mg q.d.

Acyclovir 800 mg q.i.d.

Multivitamins 1 q.AM

Physical Examination

GEN: Thin, ill-appearing male in no apparent distress.

VS: BP 130/70, HR 100 regular, RR 16, T 37.7, Wt 54.3

HEENT: Normocephalic; no JVD, thyromegaly, or nodes noted

COR: Nl. S1, S2, soft I/IV systolic murmur

CHEST: Lungs clear to auscultation

ABD: Soft, thin, positive bowel sounds; liver and spleen not appreciated, abdominal scar with multiple areas of pinkish material and raised areas of skin

GU: WNL

RECT: Guaiac-negative

EXT: WNL

NEURO: Alert and oriented × 3

Results of Laboratory Tests

Na 134 (134)	Hct 0.24 (24.4)	AST 0.95 (57)	Glu 5.3 (96)
K 4.5 (4.5)	Hgb 73 (7.3)	ALT 1.15 (69)	Mg 0.6 (1.2)
Cl 109 (109)	Lkcs 2.7 × 10^9 (2.7 × 10^3)		Alk Phos 1.18 (71)
HCO$_3$ 26 (26)	Plts 164 × 10^9 (164 × 10^3)		Alb 18 (1.8)
BUN 11.1 (31)	MCV 102 (102)		T Bili 39.3 (2.3)
Cr 150 (1.7)			

Lkcs differential: 0.62 (62%) N, 0.3 (30%) L, 0.05 (5%) M, 0.02 (2%) E, 0.01 (1%B)

Urinalysis: WNL

Blood culture: CMV-positive

Liver biopsy: Areas of focal cellular necrosis consistent with CMV hepatitis with viral inclusions

Cyclosporine: 295 ng/ml, whole blood HPLC

PROBLEM LIST

1. S/P liver transplant on immunosuppressive therapy
2. CMV infection
3. Infected surgical abdominal wound
4. Diarrhea
5. Peptic ulcer disease
6. Renal insufficiency
7. Anemia
8. Hypomagnesemia

QUESTIONS FOR CASE 197

1. How should AM's fever and headache be managed?
2. The cultures are positive for *Staphylococcus epidermidis* and *Pseudomonas aeruginosa*. What alterations in AM's antibiotic regimen should be made?
3. A follow-up liver biopsy is positive for mononuclear cell infiltrates consistent with mild rejection. How should this be treated?
4. Five days later, AM develops a fever of 39°C. Blood cultures are obtained and come back 1 of 4 positive for Aspergillus. Treatment with intravenous amphotericin is to be started. Give an appropriate dose and administration guidelines for its use.
5. Discuss the use of ketoconazole for antifungal prophylaxis.

CASE 198

CC: MP is a 30-year-old, 75-kg male who is recently S/P pancreas-renal transplant and is currently being managed posttransplantation. Fourteen days following transplantation he is experiencing a sudden decrease in renal and pancreas function.

History of Present Illness

MP underwent combined cadaveric pancreas-renal transplantation 14 days ago. He is currently managed with cyclosporine, azathioprine, and prednisone. His postoperative course has been uneventful, with Cr decreasing to 97.2 μmol/liter (1.1) by day 6 postoperative, his serum and urine amylase levels stabilizing at 0.90 μkat/liter (54) and 2247 μkat/liter (134.800), respectively, and his fasting blood sugars averaging 5.6 mmol/liter (102). Since his surgery, he has not required insulin. Unfortunately, MP is experiencing a sudden change in renal and pancreatic function with increasing serum Cr and amylase levels as above. Decreased renal function may be due to rejection, CMV infection, or CSA toxicity (most recent level 398). Pancreas rejection may also be a possibility. Renal biopsy reveals 1+ vasculitis and 1+ interstitial rejection.

Past Medical History

His past medical history includes type I (insulin-dependent) diabetes mellitus since age 2 resulting in the development of diabetic nephropathy and peripheral neuropathy as an adult. His renal insufficiency has worsened from 10/86 to the time of transplant [Cr increased from 336 μmol/liter (3.8) to 1185 μmol/liter (13.4)]. Hemodialysis was initiated in 1989. Other PMH is significant for hypertension, prostatitis, and anemia.

Medication History

Cyclosporine 300 mg b.i.d.
Prednisone 40 mg q.d.
Azathioprine 50 mg q.d.
Nifedipine XL 30 mg q.AM

Clonidine 0.1 mg b.i.d.
Clonidine patch #2 q. week
Ranitidine 150 mg b.i.d.
Acyclovir 800 mg q.i.d.
Clotrimazole troches 10 mg q.i.d.

Allergies

None known

Physical Examination

GEN: Well-developed male in no acute distress
VS: BP 142/96, HR 82, RR 18, T 37.8, Wt 65 kg, Ht 162 cm
HEENT: Normocephalic, fundal examination shows laser scarring
COR: WNL
CHEST: Lungs clear
ABD: WNL except for allograft incision scar
GU: WNL
RECT: Guaiac-negative, firm prostate
EXT: No clubbing, cyanosis, or edema
NEURO: Oriented × 3

Results of Laboratory Tests

Na 131 (131)	Hct 0.3 (30)	AST 0.17 (10)	Glu 6.1 (111)
K 5.0 (5.0)	Hgb 94 (9.4)	ALT 0.25 (15)	Ca 2.5 (10.1)
Cl 100 (100)	Lkcs 18 × 10⁹ (18 × 10³)	LDH 1.7 (100)	PO₄ 1.1 (3.4)
HCO₃ 25 (25)	Plts 431 × 10⁹ (431 × 10⁵)	Alk Phos 0.9 (53)	Mg 1.05 (2.1)
BUN 12.5 (35)	MCV 88 (88)	Alb 33 (3.3)	Uric Acid 188 (3.1)
CR 239 (2.7)		T Bili 34.2 (2)	

Serum amylase: 2.7 μkat/liter (162)
Urine amylase: 1095 μkat/liter (65,700)
CSA level: 398 (whole blood HPLC)
Anti-OKT3 antibodies: negative
Urinalysis: pH 6.2, specific gravity 1.0, color yellow, appearance cloudy, Lkcs esterase positive, protein-neg, glucose-neg, ketones-neg, occult blood-neg.
CMV blood culture: negative
Renal biopsy: 1+ Vasculitis, 1+ interstitial changes

PROBLEM LIST

1. S/P renal-pancreatic transplant
2. Cyclosporine toxicity
3. Hypertension
4. Prostatitis
5. Anemia
6. Allograft rejection

QUESTIONS FOR CASE 198

1. MP should be informed of drugs that may interact with cyclosporine and cause substantial changes in his cyclosporine levels. List six examples.
2. Immediately following his renal-pancreas transplant, MP was managed with antilymphocyte globulin (ALG), azathioprine, and prednisone. Cyclosporine therapy was started

approximately 10 days after transplantation. Why was his therapy with CSA delayed?

3. MP shows signs of both kidney and pancreas rejection. Results of a renal biopsy confirm that MP's alterations in renal function are at least partially due to rejection. How is pancreas rejection best diagnosed?

4. MP is managed with acyclovir (800 mg q.i.d.) as prophylaxis for CMV infection and ranitidine (150 mg b.i.d.) for prevention of gastrointestinal complications associated with steroid use. Considering his decline in renal function, should these doses be adjusted?

5. The CSA level for MP is 398 ng/ml, measured by HPLC. What are some of the different tests available for measuring CSA?

CASE 199

CC: TT is a 45-year-old male admitted to the ICU with a fever of 39.4°C, a change in mental status, blood pressure of 80/50, and a urine output of 100 ml over the last 8 hr.

Hospital Course

TT presented with a 1-week history of fatigue and sore throat. Count was 43 10^9/liter with (43 × 10^3/ml), 0.4 (40%) blasts. A bone marrow biopsy revealed acute myelocytic leukemia (AML). TT received an induction regimen of daunorubicin 45 mg/m² on days 1–3 and cytarabine 100 mg/m² on days 1–7. Chemotherapy was completed 8 days ago. Lkc count has fallen since chemotherapy.

Social History

Noncontributory

Review of Systems

As above

Medication History

As above for hospital course. TT was taking no medications prior to admission.

Allergies

TT has no allergies or history of food intolerance

Physical Examination

GEN: Well-developed, well-nourished male, obtunded but arousable

VS: BP 80/50, HR 136, RR 40, T 39.4 (rectal), Wt 80 kg, Ht 183 cm

HEENT: Mouth ulcerations, no evidence of oral thrush, EOM intact, PERRLA, funduscopic examination is normal

CHEST: Diffuse rales throughout both lung fields

CV: S_1, S_2 normal, no murmurs or gallops heard

ABD: Soft, liver and spleen enlarged and palpable, no tenderness to palpation, active bowel sounds, no rebound tenderness

GU: Normal male genitalia

RECT: Guaiac-negative

EXT: Extremities warm bilaterally, no petechiae, IV sites clean and without tenderness

NEURO: Reflexes normal and symmetrical, no nuchal rigidity, CN II-XII intact.

Results of Laboratory Tests

Na 136 (136)	Hct 0.31 (31%)	AST 0.58 (35)	Glu 6.1 (120)
K 4.7 (4.7)	Hgb 100 (10.0)	ALT 0.50 (30)	Ca 2.27 (9.1)
Cl 101 (101)	Lkcs 0.2 × 10^9 (0.2 × 10^3)	Alk Phos 1.8 (110)	PO$_4$ 1.58 (4.9)
CO$_2$ 12 (12)	Plts 20 × 10^9 (20 × 10^3)		Mg 1.05 (2.1)
BUN 21 (60)	MCV 82 (82)		Uric Acid WNL
Cr 185 (2.1)			

Lkcs differential: Cannot be done due to low Lkcs count

Prothrombin time: 13.0 sec/12.5 sec (control)

Fibrinogen: 3.3 (330)

FSP: negative

Urinalysis: Specific gravity 1.033; (+) granular casts; 0 RBC; 0 Lkcs; Gram stain: no organisms seen

Chest x-ray: Diffuse infiltrates throughout both lung fields

Arterial blood gases: pH 7.24, pCO$_2$ 25 mm Hg, pO$_2$ 55 mm Hg; 82% hemoglobin saturation on 50% oxygen via facemask

Sputum Gram stain: Few Lkcs, many Gram-negative rods; culture pending

Blood cultures: Pending

PROBLEM LIST

1. AML: s/p induction with daunorubicin and cytarabine; chemotherapy-induced leukopenia, thrombocytopenia, mucosal ulceration
2. Septic shock
3. Acute respiratory failure: adult respiratory distress syndrome (ARDS) and gram-negative pneumonia
4. Renal insufficiency

CASE 200

CC: RH is a 36-year-old male with a history of renal transplantation, who presents to the kidney transplant clinic with complaints of low-grade fever over the last few days accompanied by pain around the allograft transplant site.

History of Present Illness

RH is admitted to the hospital to rule out allograft rejection. Differential diagnosis besides rejection includes CMV infection, cyclosporine toxicity, and an increase in Cr secondary to drugs such as cimetidine, cotrimoxazole (trimethoprin component). CMV infection may also result in decreased allograft function; CMV cultures are currently negative. Cyclosporine trough level is 78 ng/ml, within the normal therapeutic range. Biopsy results include 2+ vascular and 2+ interstitial changes consistent with acute rejection. High-dose prednisolone was implemented at a dose of 7 mg/kg IV with no response.

Past Medical History

RH's past medical history includes end-stage renal disease (ESRD) secondary to glomerulonephritis. He underwent a cadaver renal transplant on 3/26, which was managed postoperatively with sequential immunosuppression including prednisone, azathioprine, and antilymphocyte globulin (ALG) followed by cyclosporine (CSA). HLA tissue typing for donor and recipient revealed 4/6 HLA antigen match. RH experienced one episode of mild allograft rejection on 5/5, which responded to high-dose prednisolone (7 mg/kg q.d. for 3 days). Baseline Cr level since this episode has been 123.8 μmol/liter (1.4). Other medical problems include hypertension, currently controlled with nifedipine and a clonidine patch. RH also complains of pain on urination, suggesting a possible urinary tract infection.

Medication History

Cyclosporine 200 mg b.i.d.
Prednisone 200 mg q.d.
Azathioprine 50 mg q.d.
Nifedipine 10 mg p.o. q6h
Clonidine patch #1 q. week
Cotrimoxazole DS 1 tab 3 times weekly (PCP prophylaxis)

Allergies

None known

Physical Examination

GEN: Well-developed male in mild distress; cushingoid appearance secondary to prednisone use
VS: BP 126/86, HR 92, RR 16, T 38.5, Wt 71 kg, Ht 176 cm
HEENT: Normocephalic, cushingoid facial features
COR: WNL
CHEST: Lungs clear
ABD: Pain at allograft site upon palpitation
GU: WNL
RECT: Guaiac-negative
EXT: Some muscle wasting; no clubbing, cyanosis, or edema

Results of Laboratory Tests

Na 136 (136)	Hct 0.36 (36)	AST 0.3 (18)	Glu 6.1 (110)
K 4.2 (4.2)	Hgb 132 (13.2)	ALT 0.27 (16)	Ca 2.5 (10.1)
Cl 101 (101)	Lkcs 1.5×10^9 (1.5×10^3)	LDH 1.3 (78)	PO$_4$ 0.84 (2.6)
HCO$_3$ 26 (26)	Plts 155×10^9 (155×10^3)	Alk Phos 1.0 (62)	Mg 1.0 (2.0)
BUN 12.5 (35)	MCV 88 (88)	Alb 35 (3.5)	Uric Acid 184 (3.1)
CR 221 (2.5)		T Bili 10.3 (0.6)	

Urinalysis: pH 6.2, specific gravity 1.0, color yellow, appearance cloudy, Lkcs esterase positive, protein neg., glucose neg., ketones neg., occult blood neg., bacterial smear positive

Culture: 100,000 colonies *Escherichia coli*

Sensitivity: resistance to amp but sensitive to cefazolin, gentamicin, tobramycin, ceftizoxime, and ciprofloxacin.

CMV culture: Negative

Renal biopsy: 2+ vasculitis, 2+ interstitial rejection

PROBLEM LIST

1. Renal transplant managed with immunosuppression
2. Possible allograft rejection
3. Hypertension
4. Urinary tract infection (UTI)

ANSWERS TO QUESTIONS

SECTION 1

GENERAL

CASE 1

1. Furosemide inhibits free water reabsorption to a greater extent than it increases sodium, potassium, and chloride excretion. This effect in combination with the electrolyte replacement provided by the saline, can facilitate the correction of the hypoosmolality resulting from SIADH.

2. Sulfonamides are found in a number of drug classes including the previously mentioned antimicrobial class, diuretics, oral hypoglycemics (i.e., sulfonylureas), and carbonic anhydrase inhibitors. However, the incidence of cross sensitivity among these agents has not been determined. Although they may cause immediate hypersensitivity reactions, the sulfonamides have been associated more frequently with delayed reactions which are cutaneous in nature. Gastrointestinal, hepatic, renal, and hematologic complications have also been noted to occur secondary to sulfonamides.

CASE 2

1. The rationale for using the combination of penicillin and gentamicin in *Streptococcus viridans* is the synergy achieved with this combination. Animal studies have demonstrated more rapid sterilization of vegetations and clinical experience supports a high response rate secondary to this synergy. However, the use of combination therapy for such a relatively susceptible organism has been questioned. The combination appears to provide for shorter treatment regimens with apparently comparable success to penicillin therapy alone.

2. In the non-penicillin allergic patient, the options for therapy include 4 weeks of penicillin alone, 2 weeks of combination penicillin and gentamicin, or 2 weeks of combination therapy followed by 2 weeks of penicillin alone. The combination of penicillin and gentamicin for two weeks is the standard regimen for patients without complicated infection (e.g., shock). Therapy with four weeks of penicillin alone has been shown to be equally effective. The choice between the two regimens is dependent on the risk/benefit of using an aminoglycoside in the particular patient versus the convenience and lower cost associated with the de-creased length of therapy with the combination. When patients present with complicated infection, combination therapy with penicillin and gentamicin for two weeks followed by 2 weeks of penicillin is recommended.

3. Rash has been reported more frequently with ampicillin and amoxicillin than with other penicillins. A high incidence of rash occurs with the use of aminopenicillins in patients with viral diseases. Rash has been reported in 65–100% of patients with mononucleosis treated with ampicillin and in a large percentage of those treated with amoxicillin. The rash reported with the aminopenicillins appears to be non-immunogenic and skin testing for penicillin hypersensitivity in the majority of these patients has been negative. Because the published experience with penicillins in endocarditis is more extensive than with other agents, it is important to confirm a reported penicillin allergy before choosing an alternative agent.

4. Echocardiography is considered to be important in the diagnosis of infective endocarditis. It is second only to blood cultures in diagnostic importance. However, the sensitivity of transthoracic echo for the detection of vegetations is 50–75% but can reach 95% with the transesophageal method. A negative result, however, does not exclude the diagnosis of endocarditis and a positive result may actually report the existence of a vegetation which does not exist. Sequential echocardiograms provide information on the need for, and timing of, surgical intervention.

CASE 3

1. The most likely reason that CS developed anaphylaxis after IM penicillin but not after PO penicillin is that the PO penicillin was her initial, sensitizing exposure. It is likely that her five day course of penicillin three months ago stimulated the production of an IgE penicillin antibody. Once produced, this antibody would bind to mast cells and basophils with very high affinity.

2. Anaphylaxis can be divided into three different phases: sensitization, activation, and effector phases. The sensitization phase involves production of IgE and its binding to mast cells

and basophils. The activation phase involves re-exposure to the antigen (penicillin in this case), triggering mast cells and basophils to respond by releasing their contents, including histamine, serotonin, heparin, slow-reacting substance of anaphylaxis (SRS-A), and eosinophilic chemotactic factor of anaphylaxis (ECF-A). The effector phase occurs when substances released from mast cells and basophils exert their pharmacologic effect on the body. Histamine and serotonin have been shown to be responsible for increasing vascular permeability (which may cause a decrease in blood pressure due to extravasation of fluid into tissue spaces) and smooth muscle constriction (which may cause bronchoconstriction). ECF-A has been shown to attract eosinophils to the site of its release. SRS-A has been shown to cause prolonged constriction of smooth muscle.

3. Other types of drug-induced hypersensitivity reactions include Type II cytotoxic reactions, Type III immune reactions, and anaphylactoid reactions. Type II cytotoxic reactions occur as a result of antibodies binding to target cells, activating either the complement cascade (causing cell lysis) or phagocytic cells (resulting in cell death). Examples of this type of hypersensitivity reaction include agranulocytosis and thrombocytopenia. Type III immune reactions involve the formation of antigen-antibody complexes that activate the complement cascade. Local cell damage results wherever the complexes are located. Finally, anaphylactoid reactions clinically resemble Type I hypersensitivity reactions, but the causative agent directly stimulates release of mediators from mast cells and basophils without IgE.

4. Common agents associated with anaphylaxis include: venom from insects and snakes, penicillins, cephalosporins, sulfonamides, insulin, and tetanus anti-toxin.

5. Recently, it has been estimated that 100 to 500 penicillin deaths occur each year in the United States, and that the rate of penicillin-induced anaphylaxis is 10 to 40 cases per 100,000 injections.

CASE 4

1. Enzymatic patterns for acetaminophen hepatotoxicity are greatly elevated transaminase values, usually above 50 μkat/liter, 3000 units/liter, with ALT > AST. These transaminase levels are usually elevated more than all other enzymes. Alcoholic hepatitis has only mild elevations in transaminase levels (usually <17 μkat/liter, 1020 units/liter), with AST > ALT and GGTP elevated above all others. Choledocholithiasis and cholestastic jaundice cause elevations in ALP and GGTP levels above all other liver enzymes, and only when there is significant hepatic damage do transaminase levels rise to any significant degree. Alcoholic patients are predisposed to the hepatotoxicity of acetaminophen by induction of the cytochrome P-450 system and depletion of glutathione. Alcoholics exposed to acetaminophen at doses slightly above therapeutic (approximately 6 g/d) have hepatotoxicity that has an unusual enzymatic pattern. Transaminase levels are elevated, with AST >50 (3000), but AST > ALT.

2. There are two major isoenzymes of amylase that are clinically relevant, S-type isoamylase and P-type isoamylase. Several tissues release both types of isoamylases, but S-type

isoamylase is released predominantly from salivary glands, while P-type isoamylase is released predominantly from the pancreas. This patient has a normal lipase level, which is a much more specific indicator of acute pancreatitis than amylase level and probably eliminates acute pancreatitis as a possibility. In chronic alcoholics, the S-type isoamylase level is increased due to simple carbohydrate stimulation of salivary glands by alcohol. This patient's amylase level is probably due to increased salivary amylase.

3. ALP and GGTP are eliminated in the bile. Obstruction of the biliary tract will increase levels of these enzymes in the serum faster and higher than hepatocellular enzymes.

4. Alcoholic hepatitis should now be considered, since the patient has a history of alcohol abuse and AST > ALT with GGTP having the highest elevation.

5. Acute pancreatitis should now be considered because the patient again has a history of alcohol abuse, but now both her lipase and amylase levels are elevated, with relatively normal hepatic enzyme levels.

CASE 5

1. The risk factors TT has for CAD include advanced age (>50), male sex, and a family history of CAD, all of which cannot be altered. Risk factors that can be altered include hypertension, weight, hypercholesteremia, and sedentary lifestyle.

2. Isosorbide dinitrate and isosorbide mononitrate are potent vasodilators. The new isosorbide mononitrates appear to be as effective as, but not superior to, isosorbide dinitrate. Some of the isosorbide mononitrates can be taken once or twice daily. Tolerance has been seen with some of the mononitrates, and a nitrate-free period is still essential in preventing nitrate tolerance even with a twice-daily regimen. Isosorbide mononitrates are more expensive than isosorbide dinitrate but currently do not offer any significant advantage. Isosorbide dinitrate remains to be an effective and economical nitrate for use in patients with CAD, and TT should continue to take it.

3. ACE inhibitor–induced cough occurs in approximately 5–20% of patients treated with ACE inhibitors. ACE inhibitor–induced cough, which is more annoying than disabling, occurs more frequently in women than in men. It typically occurs within a week to 6 months after initiation of therapy, and often recurs with rechallenge of the same or another ACE inhibitor. The cough is usually not dose related, but in some cases it may diminish with a dose reduction. After discontinuation of the ACE inhibitor, it often subsides in 1 to 4 days, but may take up to 4 weeks to resolve. There are a number of proposed mechanisms for ACE inhibitor–induced cough. The cough is thought to be mediated by vagal C fibers and an increase in prostaglandins, kinins (i.e., bradykinin), or substance P (a neurotransmitter in C fibers of the respiratory tract) levels.

4. TT should keep the tablets with him at all times. He should keep them in the original glass container, remove the cotton filler after it is opened, and write the date when he opened it on the bottle. He should obtain a new bottle every six months, even if the tablets are not completely used, to ensure

potency. The tablets should be stored in a cool, dry place, but not refrigerated. When TT has an angina attack, he should stop his activity immediately, sit down, and place one tablet under his tongue; he should not swallow it. He should take the nitroglycerin when the pain first starts; he should not wait for the pain to worsen. The onset of action is within 1 to 2 minutes and pain is usually relieved within 3 to 5 minutes. If the chest pain persists after 5 minutes, TT should take another tablet, and if he has the pain after 5 more minutes, he should take one more tablet. TT should not take more than three tablets in 15 minutes. If TT still has pain after three tablets, he should call his doctor, or dial 911, or go to the nearest emergency room for evaluation.

TT may have a stinging or burning sensation under the tongue after taking a sublingual nitroglycerin tablet. He may also experience warmth, flushing, lightheadedness, faintness, tachycardia, headache, and a feeling of fullness in his head after use. Sitting when taking the tablets may help minimize the dizziness and lightheadedness. TT should keep his nitroglycerin SL tablets out of reach of children.

CASE 6

1. Thiazide and other non-potassium-sparing diuretics would not be a good choice to treat RH's hypertension since they cause glucose intolerance. The exact mechanism of this effect is unknown, but it may be related to diuretic-induced hypokalemia. The effect is most important in patients with diabetes, such as RH. Since other drugs are available to treat his hypertension, these diuretics should not be used.

2. Certain cephalosporins, especially cefoperazone, cefamandole, cefotetan, and amoxalactam, furazolidone, metronidazole, and perhaps procarbazine, can produce a disulfiram-like reaction.

3. Yes, the copper reductase method (Clinitest) does not interact with vitamin C, although this is a cumbersome method for testing urine glucose concentration.

4. There are no known drug interactions between ibuprofen and oral hypoglycemic agents. RH should be cautioned against taking large doses of aspirin (3 g/day) because aspirin will increase the hypoglycemic effect of oral sulfonylureas. Acetaminophen may be a better choice than ibuprofen because NSAIDs may antagonize the effects of antihypertensive medications such as propranolol in some patients.

5. Glycosylated hemoglobin helps determine the extent of hyperglycemia over time. Normal levels indicate that a diabetic patient has been well controlled, and they may be more useful than single measurements such as a fasting blood glucose level.

CASE 7

1. Knowing the postdose time of SDCs is crucial to the proper interpretation of a patient's drug therapy. Digoxin has a relatively long alpha phase that dictates that SDCs not be drawn any sooner than 6 hr postdose. The concentrations in the alpha phase are ignored, because they do not correlate with the clinical efficacy or toxicity of digoxin. If JK's digoxin SDC had been collected 1 hr postdose, then the SDC could not be used to recommend a dose change. The proper recommendation would be to draw another SDC after the next dose with a postdose time of at least 6 hr.

2. Digoxin slows the ventricular response rate to atrial fibrillation, but it does not have efficacy in converting the patient back to normal sinus rhythm. Thus, the therapeutic end point of digoxin therapy in atrial fibrillation is the ventricular response rate.

3. The estimated C_{SS} would be 3.20 nmol/liter (2.5 ng/ml) (using equation (1.42)). The clinician must be careful in the evaluation of SDCs for drugs that have long half-lives. A prematurely drawn sample level interpreted without respect to the length of time the patient has been taking the drug is inappropriate. For digoxin this problem is compounded in patients who have significant renal insufficiency, as digoxin is 75% renally eliminated.

4. Common symptoms of digoxin intoxication include bradycardia, nausea, vomiting, cardiac arrhythmias, and mental confusion. Bradycardia is the most easily identified symptom of digoxin toxicity, though a slow ventricular rate may be due to other causes such as verapamil or sick sinus syndrome. Nausea, vomiting, and mental confusion are very nonspecific, and a temporal relationship between digoxin SDCs and symptoms would be required to establish the probability of a symptom of digoxin toxicity. Cardiac arrhythmias caused by digoxin cannot be distinguished from cardiac arrhythmias secondary to various pathologic conditions of the heart. This example is typical of adverse reactions from drug therapy, in that the symptoms of drug intoxication are difficult to attribute conclusively to drug therapy, and this ambiguity has led to the underreporting of adverse drug reactions in general.

CASE 8

1. Samples for serum iron level determinations should be drawn 2–4 hr after ingestion of an immediate-release iron product. If the product is sustained-release, another sample for iron level determination should be drawn approximately 6 hr after ingestion. After absorption from the GI tract, iron is normally transported in the blood bound to transferrin. In an overdose, transferrin becomes saturated, and free iron is present. The free iron is cleared rapidly from the plasma and distributes intracellularly. Therefore, the serum iron level will drop rapidly. This drop reflects the distribution of the iron out of the plasma, not clearance from the body. It is more difficult to interpret a serum iron level at this point, since the level may not reflect the potential severity of the intoxication. Therefore, if the timing of the serum iron level sampling is delayed, it is more important to follow the progression of clinical manifestations to assess the seriousness of intoxication rather than the serum iron levels.

2. A strong correlation has been shown between leukocytosis and serum iron levels. Blood glucose levels <8.3 mmol/liter (150 mg/100 ml) and/or a white blood cell count 15 × 10^9 (15,000) correlate with a serum iron concentration of 53.7 μmol/liter (300 μg/100 ml) or more. This patient

has leukocytosis and hyperglycemia, both of which are consistent with an elevated serum iron level.

3. The clinical manifestations of iron poisoning are often described as consisting of five phases. The initial phase usually occurs within 2 hr of the ingestion and consists primarily of GI symptoms including vomiting, hematemesis, abdominal pain, and diarrhea. Depending on the severity of the fluid and blood loss from the GI tract, hypotension and shock may develop. Lethargy and coma can also occur. During the second phase the patient's symptoms improve. This apparent improvement can then be followed by shock and acidosis, which appear 2–12 hr after the first phase. Iron is toxic to the liver, and the peak hepatotoxic effects occur 2–4 days after ingestion. While relatively uncommon, pyloric scarring and obstruction may become evident 2–4 weeks later.

4. The primary methods of emptying the stomach in an iron overdose are ipecac syrup–induced emesis and lavage. Activated charcoal is ineffective, since it does not adsorb iron. Whole bowel irrigation can be considered when an abdominal radiograph demonstrates iron tablets in the stomach and/or intestines following gastric emptying. Whole bowel irrigation involves instilling a large volume of a polyethylene glycol electrolyte lavage solution into the GI tract, with the subsequent development of diarrhea that evacuates the GI tract. Several case series and case reports have demonstrated that whole bowel irrigation successfully removes iron tablets from the GI tract without complications. In cases where ipecac and/or lavage were unsuccessful, it is conceivable that the iron tablets had adhered to the GI mucosa or formed tablet bezoars that could be removed with whole bowel irrigation. In some cases, gastrotomy has been performed to surgically remove iron tablets embedded in the gastric mucosa.

5. The presence of ferrioxamine in the urine generally changes the color to pink or orange. Whether a color change occurs, and its intensity, depends upon the concentration of ferrioxamine and other factors such as urine pH. Particularly at low concentrations, there is a great deal of subjectivity in determining whether a color change is present. In some cases the urine does not appear to change color, despite very high serum iron levels. If a color change is present, ferrioxamine is present, and this is evidence that iron chelation is occurring. Lack of a color change is not a sensitive indicator that significant iron poisoning is not present.

CASE 10

1. The most common side effect of alpha-interferon is its flu-like syndrome. Warn CF about the possibility of fever, chills, HA, malaise, and myalgia. If the symptoms are intolerable, he can take Tylenol 650 mg every 6 hours. Also warn CF about the possibility of developing nausea/vomiting and/or diarrhea. If he develops nausea/vomiting and/or diarrhea, he should call his doctor. Alpha-interferon may also cause fatigue. If CF experiences worsening fatigue, he should call his doctor.

2. The factors contributing to his anemia include:
   CML
   Chronic Disease Status
   Busulfan
   Due to the fact that CF has a normocytic anemia and is symptomatic with low endogenous erythropoietin levels, it is appropriate to treat CF with erythropoietin. CF should be started on erythropoietin at a dose of 100 U/kg sq TIW. Also, begin ferrous sulfate 325 mg oral BID-TID. CF should return in 4 weeks to check a Hgb level at which time if he has not achieved at least a 1 gm/dl rise in Hgb, his dose should be increased to 150–200 U/kg sq TIW. Hemoglobin should be checked in another 4 weeks at which time if he has not achieved at least a 1 gm/dl rise in hemoglobin, a ferritin level should be checked; if that is normal, increase erythropoietin again to 300 U/kg sq TIW. Repeat Hgb level in 4 weeks. If CF has not achieved a 1 gm/dl rise in Hgb, discontinue erythropoietin and consider RBC transfusion.

3. Candidates for abciximab include patients with a high-risk of vessel reclosure after angioplasty. In general, high-risk patients include those with unstable angina, non-Q-wave myocardial infarction, acute Q-wave MI, or existing lesions in the artery to be dilated. CF has none of these risks. Additionally, abciximab is associated with an increased frequency of major bleeding. CF is already anemic and has been on an anti-platelet drug-aspirin since 1981. Due to these factors, CF does not appear to be an appropriate candidate for abciximab.

SECTION 2

FLUIDS AND ELECTROLYTES AND NUTRITION

CASE 17

1. The half-life of phenobarbital is approximately 5 days, so it can be given once daily without unacceptable variations in serum concentration. HR had not been taking his Pb (blood level was zero when he was admitted to the hospital), so a simplified dosing regimen combined with patient education about the importance of taking his phenobarbital as prescribed is indicated.

2. At 60 kg, HR's maintenance fluid requirement is 2300 ml/day. He has impressive signs and symptoms of dehydration, but the only indication of hypovolemia is a low urine output; this is consistent with a total body volume deficit of 3–4 liters. Fluid replacement at 250 ml/hr will provide 6 liters in 24 hr; this infusion rate should meet HR's total fluid need without causing volume overload.

3. It would seem, with an 18-kg (40 lb) weight loss over the past 3 months, that HR has been eating very little and that most of his calories have probably been coming from alcohol. The half-life of red blood cells is 120 days, so even if HR's smear is normal, he may have depleted body stores of iron and folic acid. B_{12} deficiency takes years to develop, so it is probably not an important issue in this patient. Water-soluble vitamins are not stored in the body to any appreciable degree, and alcoholics, with their high carbohydrate (alcohol) diet, are particularly at risk for thiamine deficiency. A vitamin preparation containing the recommended daily allowance (RDA) will meet HR's maintenance and repletion needs for vitamins. He would also benefit from $FeSO_4$ 325 mg q.d.–t.i.d. if his anemia workup indicates depletion of iron stores.

4. While HR's serum albumin level is below normal, it indicates only that he probably has a modest deficit in his visceral protein mass. The rate at which any individual will repair a nutritional deficit is most dependent on the maximal synthetic rate of the portion of the body cell mass that makes protein. In the case of albumin, this is the liver. Giving calories and protein beyond the amounts needed to support the maximal protein synthetic rate will cause complications related to a high rate of fat synthesis, without accelerating nutritional repletion. If 1800–2000 kcal/day does not result in a 1-kg (2 lb) weekly gain in weight, HR's nutrition prescription should be reevaluated.

5. HR's total serum calcium concentration is normal, and displacement of it from albumin binding sites during acidosis is no longer an issue, but his serum albumin is now 31 g/liter (3.1 g/dl). The total serum calcium concentration is 0.2 mmol/liter (0.8 mg/dl) lower for every 10 g/liter (1 g/dl) albumin below the normal value (because of the smaller number of albumin binding sites), but the ionized level is unaffected. Using 40 g/liter (4 g/dl) as the normal albumin value, HR's total serum calcium level "corrects" to 2.7 mmol/liter (10.9 mg/dl). It can be inferred from this that HR's ionized calcium level is above the upper limit of the normal range; HR should be treated for hypercalcemia to see if his mental status will improve. The quickest and least invasive way to lower serum calcium is to give a loop diuretic to increase calcium excretion, along with normal saline and potassium replacement to prevent fluid and electrolyte abnormalities. Give furosemide 40 mg IV and begin an infusion of normal saline with KCl 20 mmol/liter (20 mEq/liter). The goal is to reach a urine output of 200–500 ml/hr; furosemide is repeated in a dose and at a dosing interval to achieve this goal. The rate of infusion of the normal saline is titrated to replace the urine output. Serum potassium concentration should be checked every 4–6 hr, and the amount of potassium given adjusted as indicated to keep the value in the normal range.

CASE 18

1. 59.7 g protein × 2.64 liter = 158 g protein/day
   158/6.25 = 25.3 g nitrogen/24 hr [in]
   8.2 × 2.6 = 21.3 + 4 = 25.3 g nitrogen/24 hr [out]
   Nitrogen balance = 25.3 − 25.3 = zero nitrogen balance
   JR is in nitrogen balance on his current regimen. No changes are needed.

2. JR may be changed to a concentrated enteral formula, such as TwoCal (2 kcal/ml). His new goal rate would be 55 ml/hr.

3. Since JR's gastrointestinal tract is functional, it is better for him to receive nutrition by the enteral route. Some benefits of enteral nutrition, compared with parenteral nutrition, include a decreased chance of septic morbidity, decreased likelihood of gut atrophy, cost savings, and a decreased chance of serious complications.

SECTION 3

DISEASES OF THE BLOOD

CASE 24

1. Monotherapy with agents such as ceftazidime or imipenem have been shown in special populations to be an effective alternative to combination therapy in treating initial febrile episodes in neutropenic patients. However, monotherapy should be limited to those patients who have been neutropenic for only a brief period of time and who have an ANC > 500. Patients who are clinically unstable, septic or are experiencing an extended period of neutropenia should receive more aggressive therapy with a combination of an aminoglycoside and anti-pseudomonal beta-lactam, or an aminoglycoside and imipenem. Aztreonam may be substituted for the beta-lactam or imipenem in penicillin-allergic patients.

2. The decision of when to initiate anti-fungal therapy is still controversial. Some institutions institute amphotericin B at the onset of nonfebrile neutropenia and others institute amphotericin B at the first onset of febrile neutropenia. Most practitioners agree that if febrile neutropenia persists despite antimicrobial therapy in adequate doses, amphotericin B therapy should be initiated.

3. A test dose of 1mg should be administered when initiating amphotericin therapy to assess tolerability. If the patient tolerates the test dose, then the daily amphotericin dose should be escalated to reach 0.5–1 mg/kg/day. If fungal infection is documented, the patient should receive a cumulative dose >1 gram. If no fungal infection can be found, therapy should be continued until the ANC>500 and the clinical picture improves. Patients should be premedicated to prevent fever, chills, and rigors associated with administration of amphoteracin B. Premedication includes diphenhydramine, hydrocortisone, and sometimes an NSAID such as ibuprofen. Heparin may be placed in the bag to help minimize infusion-related phlebitis. Monitor electrolytes (especially potassium and magnesium) and serum creatinine daily. Dosage adjustments of other agents may be required as serum creatinine increases. Daily supplements of potassium and magnesium may also be required.

4. The use of growth factors in this setting is still controversial due to the potential for stimulating any remaining leukemic cells. SB will undergo bone marrow biopsy at day 14 to determine if all leukemic cells have been eradicated. Although not supported by any particular data, the general clinical consensus is if there are no remaining leukemic cells at day 14, growth factors such as G-CSF may be administered to shorten the duration of neutropenia with little risk of causing a relapse of AML.

CASE 25

1. Since RB is taking a sustained-release formulation, assume that plasma procainamide concentrations will fluctuate minimally during the dosing interval. Therefore, 3.4 mg/liter is approximately equal to the patient's current steady-state procainamide level. The following equation can be used to calculate procainamide clearance:

$$Cl = \frac{(S)(F)(D/\tau)}{Cpss_{ave}}$$

$$= \frac{(0.87)(0.85)(500 \text{ mg}/6 \text{ hr})}{(3.4 \text{ mg/liter})}$$

$$= 18.1 \text{ liter/hr}$$

With RB's actual procainamide clearance and the desired steady-state plasma concentration known, the above equation can be rearranged to solve for dose. Since it is usually necessary to dose sustained-release procainamide every 6 hr in patients with normal renal function, the dosing interval will not be changed.

$$Dose = \frac{(Cl)(Cpss_{desired})(\tau)}{(S)(F)}$$

$$= \frac{(18.1 \text{ liter/hr})(6 \text{ mg/liter})(6 \text{ hr})}{(0.87)(0.85)}$$

$$= 880 \text{ mg}$$

Sustained-release procainamide is available as 250-mg, 500-mg, 750-mg, and 1000-mg tablets. Therefore, an appropriate dose may be 750 mg or 1000 mg every 6 hr. If 1000 mg every 6 hr was chosen as the dose, the resulting steady-state procainamide plasma concentration could be estimated by rearranging the same equation to solve for Cpss.

$$Cpss_{ave} = \frac{(S)(F)(D/\tau)}{(Cl)}$$

$$= \frac{(0.87)(0.85)(1000 \text{ mg}/6 \text{ hr})}{(18.1 \text{ liter/hr})}$$

$$= 6.8 \text{ mg/liter}$$

2. Procainamide-induced hemolysis is a warm-antibody immunohemolytic process. The proposed mechanism for this

event is the autoimmune or "methyldopa" type reaction, where the offending agent stimulates antibody production against altered (antigenic) sites on the red blood cell membrane. The inhibition of suppressor T cells may also be involved. When the red cells become coated with IgG, they undergo phagocytic destruction in the reticuloendothelial system.

3. The incidence of positive direct antiglobulin (Coombs') tests in patients receiving agents such as procainamide or methyldopa is as high as 10–20%. However, the prevalence of actual immunohemolytic anemia is much lower. The incidence of actual hemolysis in patients receiving procainamide is reported to be 3% overall, and 14% in patients who develop a positive direct Coombs' test.

4. During moderate-to-severe hemolysis, the liver's capacity to conjugate bilirubin may be exceeded. If this occurs, indirect (unconjugated) bilirubin serum levels will increase disproportionately, relative to those of direct (conjugated) bilirubin. For this reason, an elevated indirect bilirubin serum level is a useful laboratory marker of red blood cell lysis.

5. When hemolysis is clinically significant (i.e., hemodynamic instability or other severe symptoms), corticosteroid therapy is the initial treatment of choice and produces a beneficial response in most patients. A common steroid regimen is prednisone 1 mg/kg/day given until hemoglobin levels have normalized. Therapy may then be slowly tapered over a period of several months.

CASE 26

1. Some potential side effects of glucocorticoids are sodium retention, hypertension, diabetes mellitus, and behavioral disturbances. More long-term use is associated with ocular cataracts, glaucoma, osteoporosis, Cushing's syndrome, and suppression of pituitary function. Corticosteroids may also cause cutaneous atrophy and impairment of wound healing. These are particularly important in UC patients who are already predisposed to intestinal perforation. Glucocorticoids may also mask the symptoms of peritonitis, which is one of the major symptoms of intestinal perforation. Patients must be monitored very closely for the development of these side effects and also counseled about them.

2. Sulfasalazine structure is a sulfapyridine moiety linked to 5-aminosalicylic acid (5-ASA) by a diazo bond. The diazo bond is cleaved in the colon by enteric bacterial azoreductase, releasing the active component, 5-ASA (mesalamine). The 5-ASA inhibits natural killer activity, auto-antibody synthesis, and the cyclooxygenase (inhibition of prostaglandins) and lipooxygenase (inhibition of neutrophilic production of chemotactic substances) pathways, and also acts as an oxygen-derived free radical scavenger. It is proposed that 5-ASA's beneficial activity is primarily due to local effects.

3. Oral mesalamine is indicated for patients with involvement of the duodenum, ileum, or proximal large bowel. Asacol is an enteric-coated tablet that releases 5-ASA at a pH greater than 7 (in the terminal ileum/colon). The recommended daily dose of 2.4gm provides 2.4gm of 5-ASA, which is comparable to 1gm of sulfasalazine. Pentasa, which contains enteric-coated microgranules compressed into tablets, is both time and pH dependent. The recommended daily dose is 4gm, which provides 4gm of 5-ASA or the equivalent of 10gm of sulfasalazine. It releases 5-ASA in the duodenum, jejunum, ileum, and colon. In comparison, a 4gm daily dose of sulfasalazine provides only 1.6gm of 5-ASA. Since AM's extent of disease is not to the ileum, these agents would not yet be necessary to use if olsalazine is effective.

4. Toxic megacolon is a very serious complication of UC, involving an acute dilation of the colon and systemic toxemia. Signs and symptoms include those of an infection, such as a high temperature, increased heart rate and WBC. Also, the patient may complain of a sudden increase in frequency of bowel movements and significant abdominal pain. Toxic megacolon is life-threatening and has an overall mortality rate of up to 30%. Some predisposing factors are use of antispasmodics and irritant cathartics and hypokalemia. The major complications of toxic megacolon are colonic perforation, peritonitis, and hemorrhage. Treatment includes bowel rest, correction of fluid and electrolyte imbalances, high-dose steroids, and initiation of empiric antibiotics.

5. The adverse effects of parenteral iron therapy may be divided into hypersensitivity reactions and local reactions. The hypersensitivity reactions may be further broken down into immediate and delayed reactions. The immediate acute hypersensitivity reactions include anaphylaxis (0.3%), urticaria, rashes, dyspnea, fever, arthralgias, sweating, and dizziness. There is no difference in the incidence of anaphylaxis with IV vs. IM administration. Delayed reactions (24–48 hours) are usually associated with larger IV doses. Delayed reactions from IM administrations usually occur 3–7 days after the dose. They include chills, fever, backache, headache, myalgias, arthralgias, malaise, and N/V. Local reactions associated include pain at the injection site (specifically IM), inflammation, sterile abscesses, necrosis, atrophy, and fibrosis. Phlebitis associated with IV administration can be minimized by infusing over 2–6 hours and diluting the iron in 0.9% NaCl.

CASE 30

1. Oral dosing is not recommended for vitamin B_{12} for several reasons. The percent of vitamin B_{12} absorbed decreases with increasing doses. Erratic dose absorption may occur with larger doses. There is potential for decreased compliance if multiple daily doses are administered. This can put the patient at risk of neurological damage from low vitamin B_{12} levels; most physicians will avoid oral dosing unless patients have a contraindication to IM injections.

2. The preferred time of administration of H_2-receptor antagonists is at night. This is because acid secretion follows a circadian rhythm and peaks at night. Also, food can buffer much of the lower amounts of acid secretions produced throughout the day.

3. There are three different salt formations of iron available: ferrous sulfate, ferrous gluconate, and ferrous fumarate.

All three of these salts are readily absorbed; however, there is a different amount of elemental iron in each form: ferrous sulfate contains 64mg/325mg tablet, ferrous fumarate contains 66mg/200mg tablet, and ferrous gluconate contains 37mg/325mg tablet. Ferrous sulfate and ferrous fumarate contain approximately the same amount of Fe^{++} per tablet, while ferrous gluconate contains about half the Fe^{++} of the other two salt forms. Thus, twice as many ferrous gluconate tablets would need to be taken to equal the dose of elemental iron provided by a given number of ferrous sulfate or ferrous fumarate tablets.

4. *Helicobacter pylori* is a pathogen that has been associated with peptic ulcer disease. It is still controversial as to when practitioners will use antibiotic therapy for their patients to eradicate the pathogen. Some physicians feel that therapy should be started for any patient who has a positive culture to prevent peptic ulcer disease from occurring. Others feel that patients should be started on antibiotic therapy once an ulcer has occurred and a positive culture is found, while others will wait for a recurrence of the ulcer to initiate antibiotic therapy. It has been shown in several studies that triple therapy (including bismuth subsalicylate, metronidazole, and amoxicillin or tetracycline) decreases the recurrence of peptic ulcer disease by 20–100%. Also, a combination of omeprazole and one antibiotic such as amoxicillin has been shown to be effective. The length of these treatments is at least two weeks; patient compliance with multiple drug therapy is always an issue to consider.

SECTION 4

ENDOCRINE AND METABOLIC DISEASES

CASE 31

1. Ophthalmic, neuropathic, nephrotoxic complications are the most common adverse events associated with long-term diabetes. Ophthalmic complications include diabetic retinopathy, which may progress into visual disturbances and eventually blindness. Annual ophthalmology exams should begin 5 years after onset of type I diabetes, or at the time of diagnosis of type II diabetes. Diabetic neuropathy may involve pain, sensory deficit, motor deficit, or autonomic neuropathy (including postural hypotension, neurogenic bladder, and incontinence). Physical exams should include an extensive neurologic exam. Diabetic nephropathy may be preceded by hypertension and proteinuria, both of which may easily be monitored at home as well as in the clinic. Symptoms of both neuropathy and nephropathy are present in JG.

2. Angiotensin-converting enzyme inhibitors (ACEI) are useful in preventing microalbuminuria from developing into overt diabetic nephropathy when therapy is instituted early. Due to the elevated serum glucose in patients with diabetes mellitus, the kidneys become hyperperfused as free water is drawn osmotically to suger, which has exceeded the renal threshold (approximately 180 mg/dL in normal patients). This results in glomerular hypertension, and leads to microalbuminuria as glomerular cell damage occurs. Clinical proteinuria precedes azotemia and end-stage renal disease. ACEI lower systemic blood pressure via inhibition of angiotensin II–mediated vasoconstriction (resulting in vasodilation). This decreased systemic blood pressure results in decreased afferent arteriolar pressure. At the same time, the efferent arteriolar pressure is also decreased, by the primary action of ACEI on angiotensin II. Since both inflow and outflow are alleviated, the renal damage due to excessive pressures can be prevented. Obviously, once damage has already occurred, little can be done to reverse the events. Thus, therapy must be initiated as soon as proteins are detected on urinalysis.

3. Metformin is the second biguanide antihyperglycemic agent approved by the FDA (the first one, phenformin, was withdrawn in 1977 due to its association with fatal lactic acidosis). The exact mechanism is unknown; it is believed to decrease hepatic glucose production, decrease intestinal absorption of glucose, and improve insulin sensitivity. Sulfonylureas, on the other hand, act by stimulating the release of insulin from beta cells and increase beta cell sensitivity to glucose. Sulfonylureas also act outside of the pancreas by increasing and sensitizing insulin receptors in tissues. Since the mechanisms of action of biguanides and sulfonylureas are dissimilar, it is reasonable to use them together for additive effects in patients whose blood glucose is not controlled by a single agent.

4. One method of bacterial resistance against beta-lactams is the production of beta-lactamase enzymes, either plasmid or chromosomally mediated, that inactivate beta-lactams. The presence of beta-lactamase inhibitors counteracts the inactivating enzymes, thereby broadening the spectrum of coverage of the parent beta-lactams. Beta-lactam/beta-lactamase inhibitor combinations cover the same bacterial

spectrum as the parent beta-lactams except for enhancement in the following areas: improved *Bacteroides* coverage (similar to metronidazole), improved coverage for *Staphylococcus aureus* (similar to nafcillin), and improved coverage for *Hemophilis influenzae* (from 70–85% to almost 100%). For JG, switching from amoxicillin to amoxicillin/clavulanate is appropriate.

CASE 32

1. Long-term complications of diabetes mellitus include diabetic nephropathy, retinopathy, peripheral neuropathy, peripheral vascular disease and cardiovascular complications such as coronary artery disease, hypertension, and stroke. The results of the Diabetes Control and Complications Trial (DCCT) Research Group suggested that intensive therapy effectively delays the onset and slows the progression of diabetic nephropathy, retinopathy, and neuropathy. Intensive therapy means three or more daily insulin injections as guided by frequent blood glucose monitoring. The occurrence of retinopathy and nephropathy were found to be reduced by 47% and 39%, respectively. The major adverse event of intensive therapy is a two-fold increased risk of severe hypoglycemia.

2. Since TT has insulin-dependent diabetes mellitus, beta-blockers should be avoided because they can mask the signs and symptoms of and prolong hypoglycemia. Diuretics may worsen TT's hypercholesterolemia because they can increase serum cholesterol and triglycerides. TT has no contraindications for calcium-channel blockers and angiotensin-converting enzyme inhibitors.

3. Risk factors for coronary artery disease in TT include: a positive family history for premature coronary heart disease, diabetes mellitus, hypertension, high low-density lipoprotein levels, and low high-density lipoprotein levels.

4. According to the report of the National Cholesterol Education Program (NCEP) Expert Panel on Detection, Evaluation, and Treatment of high blood cholesterol in adults, the desired total cholesterol is < 200 mg/dL and LDL is < 130 mg/dL. Cholesterol levels of 200–239 mg/dL and LDL of 130–159 mg/dL put her at borderline risk.

5. No. NSAID are less effective than tricyclic antidepressants for the treatment of neuropathic pain. NSAID are most effective for inflammatory pain. Moreover, NSAID may result in sodium and water retention, and thus may antagonize the antihypertensive effect of TT's benazepril. Furthermore, NSAID should be avoided in TT to prevent worsening of her renal function.

CASE 33

1. (*a*) Moon facies, (*b*) truncal obesity, (*c*) thin extremities, (*d*) proximal muscle weakness, (*e*) striae on abdomen.
   (*a*) Bruises, (*b*) acne, (*c*) hirsutism, (*d*) osteoporosis, (*e*) hypertension, (*f*) stunted growth, (*g*) poor wound healing, (*h*) buffalo hump, (*i*) thin, transparent skin, (*j*) facial plethora, (*k*) skin hyperpigmentation, (*l*) psychiatric disturbances, (*m*) opportunistic skin infections.

2. (*a*) Blood pressure, (*b*) confusion, (*c*) nausea and vomiting, (*d*) abdominal pain and tenderness, (*e*) fatigue.
   Laboratory monitoring parameters: (*a*) serum sodium, (*b*) serum potassium, (*c*) eosinophils, (*d*) lymphocytes, (*e*) serum glucose, (*f*) blood urea nitrogen.

3. There are two ACTH-stimulation tests:
   1) Rapid ACTH-stimulation test: Administer 25 units of ACTH or 0.25 mg of cosyntropin IV or i.m. Obtain serum cortisol levels before ACTH is administered (baseline), 30 min after ACTH is administered, and 2 hr after ACTH is administered. EM has secondary adrenal insufficiency, which would not show a response to this ACTH-stimulation test. The serum cortisol levels would not be expected to increase up to 690 nmol/liter (25 μg/dl) or increase 193–276 nmol/liter (7–10 μg/dl) over the baseline serum cortisol level.

   2) The 3-day ACTH-stimulation test: Administer 25 units of Acthar-gel i.m. or 0.25 mg of cosyntropin in 500–1000 ml normal saline to run in over 6–8 hr. Either of these is administered daily for 3 days. During this time, collect 24-hr urine specimens to measure for the 24-hr urinary free cortisol level. Since EM has secondary adrenal insufficiency, the 24-hr urinary cortisol level would be expected to show a gradual increase over the 3 days.

4. Acute gastrointestinal bleeding could lead to severe blood loss and hypovolemia. This could result in worsening confusion, tachycardia, azotemia, hypoxia, hypotension, and shock. Treatment is supportive—administer plasma expanders (crystalloids or colloids) and administer oxygen. A medication to inhibit gastric acidity (e.g., histamine-2 blocking agents, antacids, or omeprazole) should be administered to prevent further gastric erosion.

5. Patient education should include:
   1) Do not stop taking prednisone without consulting your doctor.
   2) Carry an identification card that lists your current medications and dosages, and your doctor's name, address, and telephone number.
   3) Take the steroid with food or milk to reduce gastric irritation. Do not take other medications that irritate the stomach, such as aspirin, ibuprofen, and alcohol.
   4) Always make sure to have enough of the steroid medication on hand so that no doses are missed.

CASE 34

1. Agranulocytosis is a reduction of the infection-fighting neutrophils to fewer than 500 cells. It is the most dangerous but infrequent adverse reaction to the thioamides. The onset of fever, malaise, gingivitis, and sore throat is so abrupt that routine monitoring of the white blood cell count and differential is not helpful. Instead, all patients should be told to immediately report fever associated with flu-like symptoms to a pharmacist or a physician. Older patients (age >40 years) and those receiving high-dose methimazole (>40 mg/day) are at greater risk for developing this toxic reaction. Low doses (<30 mg daily) of methimazole appear safer than any dosage of PTU. This reaction may occur at any time during the course of therapy but is

more likely during the first 3 months of therapy. Fortunately, complete reversal of symptoms and return of granulocytes is seen after discontinuation of the thioamide. Rechallenge with the same drug or the alternative thioamide is not recommended because the risk of recurrent agranulocytosis is great.

2. The autoregulatory effect of the thyroid gland to prevent excessive hormone production, if a large iodide load is present, is known as the Wolff-Chaikoff block. This hormone block is not overcome by TSH stimulation and occurs when a critical intrathyroid iodide concentration is established in the gland. Iodide-induced thyrotoxicosis or Jod-Basedow disease occurs in abnormal thyroid glands that have lost the protective Wolff-Chaikoff block. Most cases of Jod-Basedow disease occur in patients with multinodular goiters who have autonomous functioning nodules that are activated by the increased iodide substrate. Agents that contain large amounts of iodide (e.g., amiodarone, which contains 37.2% iodine by weight) have also been implicated.

3. Pregnancy and hyperthyroidism create special management problems because the fetal thyroid, which begins functioning during the 12–14th week, will be at risk. Pregnancy appears to ameliorate the symptoms of thyrotoxicosis during the pregnancy; management difficulties arise during delivery, when the thyrotoxicosis typically reactivates. Therefore, it is preferable that the hyperthyroidism be definitely treated with either surgery or radioactive iodine prior to pregnancy. During pregnancy, radioactive iodine is absolutely contraindicated because the transplacental passage of I^{131} will destroy the fetal thyroid. Chronic iodide administration should also be avoided during pregnancy because fetal goiter and asphyxiation can occur. Thioamides, which cross the placenta, can be used throughout pregnancy if certain precautions are followed. PTU (rather than methimazole) is the drug of choice in pregnancy because methimazole has been (rarely) associated with congenital skin defects. The dosage of PTU should be maintained below 300 mg daily to reduce the risks of fetal goiter and hypothyroidism. In patients with mild or moderate allergic reactions to PTU, methimazole should still be entertained because untreated maternal thyrotoxicosis results in abortion and perinatal death. Clinically, the mother should be maintained in a comfortable "mildly hyperthyroid" state with her FT_4D or FT_4I in the upper ranges to prevent fetal thyroid suppression. The appearance of an enlarged maternal goiter is alarming because it implies the development of maternal and fetal hypothyroidism. The concomitant use of thyroid hormone is not recommended because thyroid does not cross the placenta, the fetus makes its own thyroid hormone, and exogenous thyroid administration may make maternal control more difficult. Once euthyroid, surgery can be safely performed in the second trimester, after suitable preparation with thioamides. During the last trimester, surgery increases the risk of precipitating spontaneous abortion.

4. Surgery is an effective method of therapy for patients who desire surgery; patients for whom radioactive iodine or thioamides are contraindicated; patients with large goiters causing respiratory, cosmetic, or swallowing difficulties; and selected pregnant and pediatric patients. Surgery is as safe as other nonsurgical hyperthyroid treatments if it is performed by an experienced surgeon in a patient who has been adequately prepared prior to surgery. If possible, surgery should not be done unless the patient has been rendered euthyroid by thioamides or properly pretreated with a combination of iodides or ipodate and β-blockers to prevent thyroid storm. Lugol's solution or saturated potassium iodide is frequently given for 10–14 days preoperatively to decrease gland vascularity, increase gland firmness, and thereby, facilitate surgical removal. The major complication of surgery is hypothyroidism. In experienced hands, vocal cord paralysis, permanent hypothyroidism, risks of anesthesia, and other postoperative complications (i.e., infection) occur rarely. Disadvantages of surgery include expense, hospitalization, and the patient's fear of surgery.

5. The most common side effects associated with the thioamides include rash and gastrointestinal effects of nausea, bitter taste, and diarrhea. A pruritic maculopapular rash, without other systemic reactions, is the most frequent adverse effect. In mild cases, the rash may disappear spontaneously despite continued thioamide therapy or respond successfully to antihistamines. If the rash persists, another thioamide can be substituted because little cross-sensitivity exists. However, if the rash is associated with concomitant systemic symptoms (i.e., fever, arthralgias, angioneurotic edema, and anaphylactoid reactions), the thioamides should be discontinued and substitution with another thiooamide deferred. Less common but serious reactions include agranulocytosis, hepatocellular or obstructive hepatitis, hypoprothrombinema, rheumatologic abnormalities such as lupus, and severe hypoglycemia secondary to an autoimmune disorder.

6. Radioactive iodine therapy appears to be safe, quick, painless, and effective. It is indicated in patients past adolescence, in patients with a history of prior thyroid surgery, in patients who are poor surgical risks, in patients with Graves' ophthalmopathy, and in patients who fail or are unable to tolerate thioamide therapy. It is the treatment of choice in the elderly patient with cardiac disease and in patients with autonomous toxic multinodular goiters. RAI is absolutely contraindicated in pregnancy because RAI destroys the fetal thyroid. The dose of RAI administered is estimated from the gland size and the 24-hr RAIU. Prior to RAI therapy, patients should be pretreated with thioamides to deplete glandular hormone stores and prevent the risk of thyroid storm. Iodides should not be used for several months prior to RAI therapy because they will impair the uptake of the RAI therapy. Thioamides should be discontinued at least 1 week prior to and after RAI therapy to encourage optimal RAI uptake. The major complication of RAI therapy is hypothyroidism. Fears of carcinogenesis, leukemia, and genetic damage have not been substantiated. Immediate side effects of RAI are minimal and may include mild thyroid pain and tenderness. Ophthalmopathy may occur or worsen. A course of systemic corticosteroids may be required to decrease ocular inflammation and conjunctivitis.

CASE 35

1. Lipoatrophy is an immunologically mediated process that results in the wasting away of fat tissue. This atrophy more commonly occurs adjacent to the injection site, but it may (rarely) occur at a site distant from the injection site. Lipoatrophy is more common in females than in males. The treatment for lipoatrophy is doses of purified pork insulin or human insulin injected directly into the atrophied area. Use of these less immunogenic insulins usually causes resolution of the atrophied area within a few weeks. After the atrophy has resolved, the patient should continue to inject at that site once or twice a week. Discontinuation may result in reappearance of the problem.

2. A decrease in the dose of thyroid replacement medication may reduce the metabolic clearance of insulin, thereby decreasing insulin requirements.

3. The appropriate dose of regular insulin should be drawn into the syringe. The NPH vial should be gently rolled between the palms to resuspend the insulin particles. (Shaking the vial may result in foaming and flocculation.) The appropriate dose of NPH insulin should then be drawn into the syringe. (Injecting air into the vial is no longer recommended.)

4. Yes, this patient should possess at least one glucagon kit for the treatment of hypoglycemia (if the patient is unconscious).

5. Glucagon once resuspended (with diluent provided in the glucagon emergency kit) should be administered subcutaneously. The adult dose ranges from 0.5 to 1.0 mg. Glucagon may cause nausea and vomiting; therefore the patient should be positioned so as to avoid aspiration. Once the patient regains consciousness, oral glucose should be administered immediately.

CASE 36

1. Adrenal suppression, evidenced by decreased endogenous cortisol levels, hyperglycemia, fluid retention, behavioral disturbances, poor wound healing, cataracts, and Cushing's syndrome (buffalo hump, moon face, central obesity, easy bruising, acne, hirsutism, and striae).

2. Acetaminophen can be used to relieve pain, but it will have no effect on inflammation.

3. Possibly, but at increased expense with equivocal benefit. In addition, sustained-release niacin can elevate liver function test results and cause possible liver toxicity; it should be avoided if possible.

4. Niacin is not a reasonable option because of the patient's history of stomach distress and diabetes. Gemfibrozil is effective at lowering both triglyceride and cholesterol levels and is a good first- or second-line drug in mixed hyperlipidemias. Long-term studies have also documented its effectiveness in reducing the risk of CHD. In JN, a reasonable starting dose would be 600 mg b.i.d. given 30 min before the morning and evening meals.

5. Physical therapy helps preserve muscle strength and range of motion. Cooling or warming inflamed joints may be helpful.

SECTION 5

RENAL DISEASES

CASE 43

1. HJ's renal dysfunction and/or heart failure could have been better than expected, leading to a faster clearance and a lower observed drug level. Secondly, HJ could have been noncompliant, which would also lead to a decreased level.

2. Would hold digoxin for approximately 3 days (1 $t_{1/2}$) and recheck level. If 2.1 represents an average steady-state level, restarting at 0.125 mg q.d. will achieve a level of approximately 1.28 nmol/liter (1 µg/ml), which is in the desired therapeutic range.

3.

   $$IBW = 50 + 2.3 \ (Ht(in) - 60)$$
   $$50 + 2.3 \ (68 - 60) = 68.4 \ kg$$
   $$CrCl = \frac{(140 - 67) \ (68.4)}{3.5 \ (72)} = 19.8 \ ml/min = 1.2 \ liter/hr$$
   $$Cl_{AMG} = CrCl = 1.2 \ liter/hr$$
   $$Vd = 0.25 \ (68.4) = 17.1 \ liter$$
   $$Kel = \frac{Cl}{V} = \frac{1.2}{17.1} = 0.0695 \ hr^{-1}$$
   $$T_{1/2} = \frac{.693}{\tau} = 9.97 \ hr$$

   2 $t_{1/2}$'s ≈ 20 hr. Could dose q24h to achieve levels of ~6 and 1.5 mg/liter (6 → 3 → 1.5).

   $$Cpeak = \frac{\dfrac{SFD}{V}}{1 - e^{-k\tau}} = \frac{\dfrac{90}{17.1}}{e^{-kt} \ (1 - e^{-.07(24)})} \ e^{-.07(1)} = 6.03 \ \mu g/liter$$
   $$trough = Cpeak \ e^{-k(\tau - t)} = 6.03 \ e^{-.07(23)} = 1.21 \ \mu g/liter$$

   90 mg q24h = Dose. Steady-state will be achieved in approximately 33 hr; check peak and trough levels around or after 3rd dose.

4.

   $$Vd = 2 \ liters/kg \ (73) = 144 \ liters$$
   $$Cl = Cl \ acetylation + Cl \ renal + Cl \ other$$
   $$= 0.134 \ kg \ (wt) + 3(CrCl) + 0.1 \ liter/kg \ (wt)$$
   $$= 0.13 \ (73) + 3(1.2) + 0.1(73) = 20.4 \ liters/hr$$

   *Cl decreased by 25% due to CHF

   $$Cl = 20.4(0.75) = 15.3 \ liters/hr$$

   $$Kel = \frac{Cl}{V} = \frac{15.3}{144} = 0.1063 \ hr^{-1}$$

   $$T_{1/2} = \frac{0.693}{K} = 6.52 \ hr$$

   $$Css = \frac{SFD/\tau}{Cl}$$

   To achieve a Css of 6 mg/liter

   $$6 = \frac{(0.85) \ (0.87) \ Dose/6}{15.3}$$

   Dose = 744.8 ≈ 750 mg p.o. SR q6h

5. Quinidine decreases the clearance of digoxin by about 50% and increases the volume of distribution by about 30%. The change in volume is thought to be due to a rapid (<24 hr) tissue displacement. Because of these changes, many people recommend holding one dose of digoxin and restarting with one-half the previous maintenance dose. This assumes that you wish to maintain the current steady-state level.

CASE 44

1. Diabetic ketoacidosis occurs commonly in IDDM patients who have an infection. Infection influences the development of DKA by stimulating the release of insulin counter-regulatory hormones such as glucagon. CL presents to the ED with a 1-week history of chills, fever, and nausea, which could be secondary to a viral or bacterial infection. She also has a history of noncompliance with insulin, which predisposes her to develop DKA.

2. Treatment of DKA consists of correcting hyperglycemia (insulin), dehydration (fluid therapy), and electrolyte imbalances (electrolyte replacement).
   Hyperglycemia/dehydration: A bolus dose of insulin (0.1–0.2 unit/kg) followed by a continous infusion of 0.1 unit/kg/hr is administered concomitantly with normal saline at a rate of 0.5 to 1 liter/hr. Once the BP and pulse have been stabilized, sodium chloride 0.45% may be substituted. When blood glucose approaches normal limits, D5 0.45% sodium chloride may be used.
   Electrolyte imbalances: Na: Sodium is usually adequately replaced by sodium chloride. K: Serum K levels could be high, normal, or low depending on the degree of DKA. If K levels are high, no potassium should be administered until the levels reach normal limits. Then, 10–20 meq/hr of potassium may be administered. Hypokalemic patients may be given higher doses. PO_4: Phosphate use in patients

---

*Would not expect much fluctuation in levels using the sustained-release dosage form.

with DKA is controversial. If PO_4 replacement is indicated, it should be administered at a rate of 5–10 mmol/hr. HCO_3: Bicarbonate should only be administered to patients with arterial PH levels < 7.1. If HCO_3 replacement is indicated, it should be administered in doses of 44 meq/hr.

3. Chronic complications of diabetes can be divided into several categories such as neuropathy, macrovascular, microvascular, and podiatric. *Neuropathy:* May be divided into two major categories: autonomic (gastroparesis, sexual dysfunction, orthostatic hypotension, etc.) and peripheral (bilateral symmetrical, cranial neuropathies, truncal neuropathies, etc.). Bilateral symmetrical neuropathy is the most commonly encountered neuropathy. Patients present with burning pain, tingling, and/or numbness in the feet or hands. Non-narcotic analgesics, narcotic analgesics, anticonvulsants, tricyclic antidepressants (TCAs), and capsaicin can be used for symptomatic treatment of peripheral neuropathies. In general, TCAs are considered the drugs of choice. *Macrovascular disease:* Includes peripheral vascular disease, coronary heart disease, and cerebrovascular disease. The treatment of macrovascular disease is preventive therapy which may include weight reduction, blood glucose control, cessation of cigarette smoking, treatment of hypertension, and treatment of hyperlipidemia. *Microvascular disease:* Includes retinopathy and nephropathy. The treatment of microvascular disease is also preventive. Diabetic patients should receive annual ophthalmologic exams. Laser therapy may be used to treat active retinopathy. Currently, captopril is the only medication with an FDA approval to decrease mortality and morbidity due to diabetic nephropathy. *Podiatric:* When neuropathy develops, patients with diabetes may be less aware of foot trauma when it occurs. Trauma may result in infections which resolve slowly due to poor peripheral circulation. Prevention of podiatric problems may be avoided by maintenance of good foot hygiene, including daily self-examination of the feet for cuts or other trauma, keeping toenails cut neatly, and daily cleaning of the feet.

4. Diabetic nephropathy, hypovolemia, use of ACE inhibitors (captopril), and the use of large doses of an NSAID (ibuprofen).

5. It is recommended that patients with diabetes check their blood glucose concentrations before meals, one to two hours after meals, at bedtime, and occasionally around 3 am. Most patients do not follow this rigorous schedule. Since CL has frequent DKA episodes, the importance of frequent blood glucose testing should be emphasized with her and with her husband.

CASE 48

1. Total iron dose (mg) = (0.66)(50 kg) {(100 – (100)(8.5)/ (14.8)} = 1404 mg
   Volume of iron dextran = 1404 mg × 1 ml/50mg elemental iron = 28 ml iron dextran
   TR is a small elderly woman with likely limited muscle mass; therefore, IV therapy may be preferred over the IM route. TR should be premedicated with diphenhydramine 30 minutes prior to administration of the iron dextran. The iron dextran should be diluted in 0.9% NaCl or D5W. A 25 mg test dose should be given over 5–10 minutes to observe for acute hypersensitivity reactions. After an hour, if no reaction occurs, the remaining dose should be administered over 2 to 6 hours.

2. In choosing an antihypertensive regimen for TR, K-sparing diuretics should be avoided due to the potential for hyperkalemia. ACE inhibitors should also be used with caution due to the potential for hyperkalemia. Thiazides should be avoided with TR's low CL_{cr}. Felodipine is a reasonable choice; however, 5 mg is a low dose. The dose can gradually be increased up to 20 mg/day. If a 2nd agent is needed, a centrally acting adrenergic agonist (e.g. clonidine) may be tried.

3. In patients with chronic renal failure, it would be preferable to avoid agents with antiplatelet activity due to the increased tendency for bleeding. (Aspirin irreversibly inhibits platelet aggregation). Therefore, suggest starting acetaminophen rather than aspirin.

4. Vitamin C does increase iron absorption (by maintaining iron in the ferrous state) but only by about 10% with 500–1000 mg of vitamin C; therefore, the low doses of vitamin C in the available preparations are unlikely to significantly increase absorption and do not justify their cost.

5. Long-term aluminum ingestion in patients with chronic renal failure can lead to increased serum aluminum. Neurotoxicity can result, including encephalopathy and dementia. Aluminum may also accumulate in the bone and osteomalacia may develop.

SECTION 6

GASTROINTESTINAL DISEASES

CASE 49

1. PTU is the drug of choice for Graves' disease during pregnancy and should be continued. PTU crosses the placenta and may cause goiter and hypothyroidism in the fetus. Using the lowest possible dose to control hyperthyroidism would be prudent. Many women require lower PTU doses during pregnancy. The risks of the effects of thyrotoxicosis on the baby outweigh the potential benefit of discontinuing the PTU.

2. Propylthiouracil: PTU is primarily metabolized with only 1–3% of the parent compound being eliminated unchanged. Although hemodialysis has not been studied for this agent specifically, based on the intrinsic clearance of the drug, volume of distribution, and protein binding, hemodialysis will not contribute significantly to the overall clearance of this agent. The dose should not be reduced in renal failure.

   Ranitidine: Ranitidine is 70% renally eliminated. When the CrCl falls below 0.83 ml/sec (50 ml/min), the oral ranitidine dose should be decreased to 150 mg p.o. q24h. Hemodialysis removes a significant amount of ranitidine; therefore, the daily dose should be given after dialysis.

3. First assess whether AJ has been compliant. Assuming compliance, a further workup to determine the cause of the anemia is in order. The workup should include MCV, MCHC, guaiac test, reticulocyte count, folate and B_{12} levels, peripheral blood smear, and erythropoietin level. AJ has two fairly obvious reasons to have persistent anemia. Chronic renal failure causes anemia secondary to a low erythropoietin level. PUD can cause a blood-loss anemia.

4. Combination therapy with histamine type-2 receptor antagonists and sucralfate has not been shown to be of more benefit than either agent alone. If AJ fails ranitidine, she should be switched to sucralfate.

5. This is AJ's first diagnosis of PUD. Since not all patients will have recurrent PUD, long-term prophylaxis is reserved for patients with recurrent disease.

CASE 50

1. Azathioprine is metabolized by the liver to 6-mercaptopurine (6-MP), which interferes with nucleic acid synthesis. Immunosuppressive agents are not first-line therapy in Crohn's disease. Trials support the use of immunosuppressive(s) as steroid-sparing agents in chronic steroid-dependent disease and in the treatment of refractory fistulas. However, these effects are usually seen after several months of continual therapy.

   Adverse effects associated with immunosuppressive agents include bone marrow suppression and infection, pancreatitis, drug-induced hepatitis, and allergic-type reactions. Neoplasms have also been reported. These adverse effects may limit the long-term use of immunosuppressive agents.

   The indications for immunosuppressive therapy in IBD include treatment of severe, steroid-dependent Crohn's disease, Crohn's patients with fistulas unresponsive to metronidazole and/or steroids, and unresponsive ulcerative colitis when surgery is not a viable option.

2. Cyclosporine (CSA) appears to have a beneficial therapeutic effect in active chronic severe Crohn's disease. Continual oral therapy at dosages ranging from 5 to 10 mg/kg/day results in a rapid improvement in disease symptoms, which is an advantage of CSA therapy over azathioprine and 6-mercaptopurine. However, relapse usually occurs upon discontinuation of the drug. (Long-term, low-dose CSA therapy (2 mg/kg/day) does not appear to maintain remission, although further study is required.)

   Nephrotoxicity is a major concern with CSA therapy. Reversible renal impairment may result in a decrease in GFR and an increase in BUN, potassium, and uric acid. These renal effects usually occur with higher dosages and reverse within several months of discontinuing the drug. Mild-to-moderate hypertertension requiring pharmacologic intervention is associated with the nephrotoxicity. Other adverse effects include parathesias, tremor, hirsutism, hyperplasia of the gums, headache, GI effects, and abnormal liver function test results.

   A potential role for CSA may be in the rapid control of severe Crohn's disease symptoms, thus allowing time for slower-acting, long-term agents to take effect. Further controlled trials are necessary to fully delineate the role of CSA in Crohn's disease.

3. Sulfasalazine is used in Crohn's disease with varying degrees of success. Although evidence does support some therapeutic benefit of sulfasalazine in the treatment of mild-to-moderate Crohn's disease, it has not been shown to be effective in severe disease. Variables that affect sulfasalazine therapy in Crohn's disease include disease severity (mild-to-moderate versus severe) and the location of disease involvement (small versus large bowel).

   Colonic bacteria cleave the diazo bond of sulfasalazine to sulfapyridine and 5-ASA, the active moiety. Because 5-ASA is released in the colon, sulfasalazine is most effective in Crohn's disease with colonic involvement. This fact may explain the decreased efficacy of sulfasalazine in Crohn's disease of the small bowel. However, a trial of sulfasalazine in these patients may be attempted since backwash of colonic bacteria into the terminal ileum may cleave sulfasalazine and liberate active 5-ASA.

Clinical trials have failed to provide adequate evidence supporting the use of sulfasalazine as maintenance therapy in Crohn's disease.

GK's Crohn's disease involves the colon as well as the ileum. His disease has been controlled in the past with oral steroids and sulfasalazine. The recent resection of his terminal ileum may increase his response to sulfasalazine. Following surgery, sulfasalazine may be reintroduced at a dose of 2 g/day.

4. Toxic megacolon is characterized by an acute dilation of all or a portion of the colon to more than 6 cm. Toxic megacolon is considered to be a medical emergency, with a mortality of approximately 15–35%. Clinical manifestations include a high fever, profound weakness, tachycardia, leukocytosis, abdominal pain, distention and tenderness, volume depletion, and electrolyte imbalances.

The use of antimotility agents to control diarrhea, and narcotics to manage abdominal pain in mild-to-moderate Crohn's disease is appropriate. However, controversy surrounds the use of these agents in more severe Crohn's disease. The ability of these agents to induce toxic megacolon, although not well substantiated within the literature, is a major concern.

Since GK is postoperative and under medical supervision, the necessity of pain control probably outweighs the risk of developing toxic megacolon.

5. The efficacy of metronidazole in active colonic Crohn's disease, fistulas, and perianal disease is substantiated by case reports and several clinical trials. Patients with colonic disease who are unresponsive to sulfasalazine may respond to metronidazole therapy, which may be considered an alternative to sulfasalazine therapy.

The dose of metronidazole ranges from 500 mg/day to >1 g/day. Several months of continual metronidazole therapy are necessary to elicit a therapeutic response, but recurrence of active disease usually follows dosage reductions or discontinuation of therapy. It appears that long-term, high-dose therapy is necessary to maintain disease remission. Thus, the use of metronidazole in Crohn's disease must be weighed against the potential long-term adverse effects of the drug.

High-dose metronidazole (>1 g/day) and/or therapy lasting longer than 6 months may be associated with peripheral neuropathy, hematologic manifestations, and the development of malignancies. Other adverse effects of metronidazole include metallic taste, GI upset, glossitis, urticaria, and darkening of the urine. These effects are reported frequently, but they are generally considered to be mild. Metronidazole may also induce a disulfiram-like reaction with concurrent alcohol administration.

6. Corticotropin (ACTH) may be a possible therapeutic option in steroid-naive IBD patients requiring steroid therapy for control of their disease. A recent study suggests the superiority of ACTH over parenteral hydrocortisone in ulcerative co-

litis patients who are steroid-free for 30 days prior to receiving ACTH. Patients who had received recent steroid therapy showed no difference between the two drugs. Corticosteroids, such as parenteral prednisolone and methylprednisolone, are preferred because they induce a more predictable effect, possess less mineralocorticoid activity, and do not depend upon adrenal responsiveness.

GK has been on long-term steroid therapy, so ACTH would not be an appropriate therapeutic choice.

7. Nonsteroidal antiinflammatory drugs (NSAIDs) inhibit the synthesis of prostaglandins, which are known mediators of inflammation. By virtue of this action and the proposed inflammatory component of IBD, it would seem that NSAID therapy would be beneficial. However, NSAIDs have been reported to induce or exacerbate Crohn's disease. Because of this potential, patients should be monitored for exacerbation of their disease during NSAID therapy.

CASE 51

1. Bisacodyl is a stimulant laxative that should be used infrequently (less than once every few weeks); daily usage should be discouraged. Since DH has prolonged therapy beyond 1 week, he should be advised to discontinue its use. He should be informed that use of stimulant laxatives in outpatients beyond 1 week is not recommended.

2. Tap water or saline enemas may be used for short-term management of fecal impaction. Phosphate-containing enemas cause evacuation of the bowel within 2–15 min and may be inappropriate for DH because of his renal failure. To administer the enema, DH should be instructed to lie on his left side with one knee bent or to assume the knee-to-chest position. The nozzle should be inserted in the rectum and the solution slowly introduced. DH should be informed that he may experience an urge to defecate shortly after administering the enema. Single doses should be administered per treatment. Recommend to DH that he should not use saline enemas because he may be at risk for hyperphosphatemia.

DH should be informed of nonpharmacologic interventions to prevent constipation:

a. Increase fiber in diet with bran and whole grain cereals and breads, fruits, and green vegetables
b. Increase fluid intake to 6–8 full glasses of liquid (water, juice, milk)
c. Incorporate regular exercise in daily living (e.g., walking)

3. Two androgens are available for use to increase erythropoiesis: nandrolone decanoate and fluoxymesterone. Nandrolone decanoate has the higher anabolic:androgenic ratio, which results in fewer masculinizing side effects. Side effects commonly reported with androgens include virilization, weight gain, muscle soreness, hirsutism, priapism, acne, swelling, and hematoma at the injection site. Since DH is male, either agent may be appropriate in terms of side effects. However, since DH is already taking i.m. injections of iron dextran, it may be prudent to recommend fluoxymesterone, which is available orally. Recommendation: fluoxymesterone 30 mg/day p.o. up to 6 months. Therapy

should be discontinued after 6 months regardless of response, to avoid the risk of hepatotoxicity.

4. Recombinant human erythropoietin is now available for the treatment of anemia of chronic renal failure either dialysis- or non-dialysis-dependent. Starting doses of 50–100 units/kg three times a week are appropriate (DH requires 3500–7100 units three times weekly). After DH's Hct reaches 0.3–0.33 (30–33%) or increases more than 4 points in any 2-week period, then the dose should be decreased by 10–25 units/kg three times a week. If the Hct exceeds 0.36 (36%), therapy should be withheld until it falls to 0.3–0.33 (30–33%). After therapy is reinitiated, the dose should be reduced by 25 units/kg three times a week. The maintenance dose of erythropoietin should be individualized to maintain a Hct in the target range 0.3–0.33 (30–33%), using dose adjustments (increases or decreases) in 25-unit/kg increments. Increases should occur no more than once per month. Monitoring parameters necessary during therapy include: Hct, CBC with differential, platelets, BUN, creatinine, and potassium levels, iron stores, and blood pressure (see Chapter 13, "Other Anemias" for monitoring intervals).

5. Allopurinol is metabolized to an active metabolite (oxypurinol), which may accumulate in patients with chronic renal failure. Patients with ClCr <1.3 ml/sec (80 ml/min) should receive dosages below 300 mg/day. DH has a ClCr=0.45 ml/sec (27 ml/min). He is on 100 mg daily, with good control of his urate concentration. Recommend to resume allopurinol 100 mg p.o. q.d.

SECTION 7

HEPATIC AND PANCREATIC DISORDERS

CASE 57

1. Several factors affect the immediate nutrition decisions: the semicomatose state, the GI upset, and the acute liver problem. Oral ingestion of anything should be avoided in an unconscious patient, who should be maintained on adequate intravenous calories without protein until the acute problem is under control. Then TPN may be started. An enteral diet, oral or via n/g tube, may be considered when the patient is fully conscious.

2. The amount of protein supplied by the feeding product is of concern in patients with liver problems. The total daily protein intake should be kept at 20–30 g. TPN and enteral products with a high content of branched-chain amino acids should be used. This is thought to help decrease ammonia production.

3. Ascites is an accumulation of fluid in the abdomen. It is better treated conservatively with salt restrictions and a mild diuretic. The goal of therapy is to produce a moderate rate of diuresis—not more than 1 kg/day. Spironolactone, in doses ranging from 50 to 200 mg/day, is usually used. In more severe ascites or in cases resistant to spironolactone, furosemide may be added to the regimen.

4. In addition to the decreased RBC indices, serum iron concentration is expected to be decreased and total iron-binding capacity (TIBC) is expected to be elevated. Also, a decreased serum folic acid level is found consistently in chronic alcoholics. Once the acute problem has resolved, a regimen of folic acid 1 mg/day p.o. for 1 month and ferrous gluconate 300 mg t.i.d. p.o. for 3 months should replete the liver stores. A good multiple vitamin and well-balanced diet should eliminate the need for iron and folic acid after liver stores are repleted.

5. Glycosylated hemoglobin levels are often used to assess compliance by the diabetic. In the nondiabetic, 3–8% of hemoglobin becomes attached to glucose. If the diabetic is maintaining good control, the glycosylated hemoglobin concentration should be less than 8%. This parameter gives a good indication of control during the preceding 2 months.

CASE 58

1. Vitamins that are absorbed through the small intestine by active transport or stored in the liver may be deficient in patients with a history of chronic alcohol use. Specifically, LF may be deficient in folate, pyridoxine (vitamin B_6), thiamine (vitamin B_1), niacin (vitamin B_3), and vitamin A. Folate deficiency can cause anemia, and thiamine deficiency can cause Wernicke's and Korsakoff's syndromes. LF's anemia is addressed in the next question. Wernicke's and Korsakoff's syndromes are serious neurological sequelae of thiamine deficiency, and LF should receive thiamine 100 mg orally each day for 10 to 14 days. LF may also benefit from a multivitamin daily. Liver disease can impair the production of vitamin K–dependent clotting factors and result in an impaired clotting system and prolonged serum prothrombin time. LF should receive vitamin K 10 mg subcutaneously for three days to help prevent bleeding.

2. Megaloblastic anemia caused by folate deficiency is usually the cause of anemia in patients with chronic alcohol use; however, these patients are also at risk for microcytic anemia caused by iron deficiency secondary to blood loss. It is important to first identify the underlying cause of the anemia and then replace the deficient factor, otherwise neurologic abnormalities caused by vitamin B_{12} deficiency may progress if the megaloblastic anemia is treated empirically with folic acid. Check LF's serum iron, vitamin B_{12}, and folate levels, and then treat with the appropriate agent(s).

3. Routine use of anticonvulsant medications to prevent alcohol-withdrawal seizures has not been well documented in the medical literature. The seizures associated with acute alcohol withdrawal are usually brief, self-limiting, and rarely focal in nature. Electroencephalographic abnormalities are mild and usually return to normal within several days. Also, the risk of seizures during acute alcohol withdrawal has generally passed by the time adequate drug levels of anticonvulsants have been achieved. In addition, LF is receiving benzodiazepines, which have antiseizure activity.

4. Patients with ascites are at risk for developing primary or spontaneous bacterial peritonitis (SBP), for which there is no obvious source for the infection. The classic presenting symptoms are fever, chills, abdominal pain, diffuse abdominal tenderness, and rebound tenderness. Some infected patients may not exhibit the classic symptoms of SBP, but may present with worsening jaundice or encephalopathy. A paracentesis diagnostic of SBP will be cloudy in appearance, have a white cell count greater than 500 cells/m³, and usually positive bacterial cultures. Enteric gram-negative rods are implicated about 70 percent of the time; however, empiric antibiotic treatment should include coverage for gram-positive cocci (primarily non-enterococcal streptococci species). Empiric antibiotic therapy with an aminoglycoside and ampicillin or a third-generation cephalosporin should be initiated, and then specific antibiotic therapy can be selected after bacterial culture results are available. Many patients show clinical improvement after 24 to 48 hours of therapy, and they may complete their treatment course as an outpatient with appropriate oral antibiotics. The duration of antibiotic therapy is usually 10 to 14 days.

5. The risk of rebleeding from esophageal varices is very high. Given the high mortality and morbidity associated with bleeding esophageal varices, prophylaxis of gastrointestinal ulceration is a reasonable precaution in these patients. Prophylaxis with antacids, histamine-2 antagonists, and/or sucralfate may be initiated with the same regimens as those recommended for the treatment of peptic ulcer disease or reflux esophagitis.

6. The preferred method of treating ascites is to gradually reduce the ascites with bed rest, salt restriction, and diuretics to avoid abrupt plasma volume changes that may lead to shock, renal failure, and encephalopathy. However, some patients may develop ascites refractory to intensive medical therapy which become tense, painful, and can cause respiratory distress as the ascites progresses. These patients may require therapeutic paracentesis (aspiration of peritoneal fluid) to remove the ascitic fluid. During the paracentesis, albumin is infused intravenously in amounts proportional to the albumin removed by paracentesis to minimize fluid and electrolyte imbalance. The patient's renal function and serum electrolytes should be monitored.

CASE 61

1. The proposed mechanism of action of lactulose is by decreasing the pH of colonic contents to 5.5 or lower, and altering the ratio of ammonia to ammonium ion. By increasing the amount of ammonium ion, less ammonia is available to be absorbed, thereby lowering the serum level of ammonia. Neomycin destroys colonic bacteria by preventing the degradation of protein to ammonia, thereby reducing the serum level of ammonia.

2. The usual dose of vasopressin is 0.2–0.4 units per minute by continuous IV infusion. Infusions may be continued up to 72 hours, with slow tapering of the dose over time. The vasoconstrictor activity of vasopressin may decrease cardiac output and cause coronary ischemia. Bradycardia is frequently observed. GI cramping, bowel ischemia, and dilutional hyponatremia are other possible complications.

3. Phytonadione is the preferred agent. Its onset of action is quicker than oral vitamin K. Intravenous administration is the most effective, but there is a small risk of anaphylactic reactions due to the colloid suspension of the preparation. Intramuscular administration should not be used in this patient due to the risk of bleeding.

4. Theoretically bowel sterilization by neomycin may limit the efficacy of lactulose as lactulose must be degraded by colonic flora in order to acidify the lumen of the bowel. However, clinical evidence suggests that both agents work synergistically and can be used together.

SECTION 8

RHEUMATIC DISEASES

CASE 62

1. Osteoarthritis is characterized by progressive degeneration of cartilage with secondary bone changes. Secondary synovial inflammation may occur occasionally but is not necessarily a characteristic of the disease. Thus, systemic steroids do not have a role in the treatment of osteoarthritis. Intraarticular administration of hydrocortisone, betamethasone, methylprednisolone, triamcinolone, and dexamethasone may be beneficial for temporary pain relief and associated local inflammation. Long-term use of intraarticular corticosteroids is controversial because of the potential for serious adverse effects.

2. Nonpharmacologic therapy is extremely important for the management of osteoarthritis and may be sufficient for managing mild-to-moderate osteoarthritis. A proper balance between exercise and rest may improve range of motion, relieve joint stiffness, decrease joint stress, and strengthen periarticular muscles. Patients should be taught gentle range-of-motion exercises during periods of inactivity. Patient such as VB should also be educated on the need to limit excessive stress to the joints by decreasing weight bearing exercise and on the usefulness of walking aids (e.g., canes, crutches) to relieve joint pain and stress. Moderate application of heat may aid muscle relaxation, and ice packs may aid acute inflammation.

3. The causes of VB's insomnia include psychosocial stressors (i.e., relatively recent death of her husband and worry about her DJD and potential upcoming surgery), ingestion of caffeine and alcohol in the afternoon and evening, and physical pain from her DJD.

4. Disagree. Flurazepam has two short-acting metabolites and a long-acting metabolite, N-desalkylflurazepam, which accumulates with nightly doses. The half-life of N-desalkylflurazepam is 40 to 150 hours. Elderly patients are more susceptible to suffering adverse experiences from a dose of 30 mg flurazepam than younger patients. Studies have shown an association between the use of long-acting benzodiazepines and increased incidence of hip fracture in elderly individuals. The efficacy of flurazepam 15 mg is comparable to flurazepam 30 mg; the lower dose is more appropriate for elderly patients, such as VB.

CASE 63

1. This patient has mild renal insufficiency, which is probably secondary to prostaglandin inhibition by high-dose ibuprofen therapy because of temporal relationship and lack of signs of allergic or autoimmune renal disease. The main predisposing factor for prostaglandin-induced decreased renal blood flow is the high dose of ibuprofen. Sulindac is relatively renally sparing compared to other nonsteroidal antiinflammatory drugs and therefore may be a reasonable choice in this patient. However, ibuprofen is one of the least expensive nonsteroidal antiinflammatory drugs.

Aspirin, indomethacin, meclofenamate and phenylbutazone may have a higher incidence of adverse effects. Aspirin causes more gastrointestinal microbleeding and inhibits platelet aggregation for a longer time than other nonsteroidal antiinflammatory drugs. Aspirin may be associated with more drug interactions, and may even increase the hepatotoxicity of methotrexate (see the Textbook). Nonacetylated salicylates have little effect on platelet function or renal blood flow. Meclofenamate has a much higher incidence of diarrhea. Nabumetone has been reported to cause less GI ulceration, but this remains somewhat speculative at this time. Otherwise, there are few differences in the incidence of gastrointestinal bleeding or ulceration in general. Indomethacin is much more commonly associated with central nervous system effects. Phenylbutazone may be more commonly associated with agranulocytosis. Many other differences among these agents are unproven—particularly effectiveness in treating RA.

2. Corticosteroids would ideally not be needed in any patient with rheumatoid arthritis because of potential adverse effects. However, corticosteroids provide relatively rapid, dramatic antiinflammatory effects. This patient has immediate needs—to continue to work and to take care of herself and her family—and will be considered to be a candidate for corticosteroid therapy.

The choice of route and nature of corticosteroid administration are based on the patient's joint and extraarticular involvement. Intraarticular injections of corticosteroids are very beneficial, but only in patients with a limited number of severely inflamed joints. This patient has many joints involved. Intravenous high-dose pulse corticosteroid therapy is beneficial, but this effect is only temporary, patients must come into the hospital for a few days, and severe toxicities such as arrhythmias and death rarely occur. In some clinics, this may be a preferred choice.

Oral low-dose corticosteroids given chronically are used in many such patients, particularly when a rapid generalized response is needed. Although the initial intent may be to taper and discontinue this therapy as soon as possible due to the many adverse effects associated with chronic therapy, many patients continue on chronic low-dose corticosteroids for years. Most patients respond well to a fixed schedule of prednisone 5 to 15 mg per day, but some investigators have begun to allow patients some flexibility in determining their daily doses similar to the concept of patient-controlled analgesia using opioid analgesics. A major factor in using oral low-dose corticosteroids in this patient is an economic need for continued employment by the patient.

3. The major reasons for discontinuation of methotrexate or other second-line agents are lack of effect and development of adverse effects, but other reasons also arise. A second-line agent should not be labelled ineffective in a patient until used 4 to 6 months, or possibly even longer if some response is seen.

The toxicity seen is dependent on the agent used. Mucositis, rash, gastrointestinal intolerance, and pulmonary, hematologic, and hepatotoxic effects are common reasons for discontinuing methotrexate. Select patients will have an increase in the formation of rheumatoid nodules while on methotrexate. Some of these toxicities can be diminished by properly screening and educating patients. Hepatotoxicity, for example, may be more common in patients who are obese, diabetics, alcoholics, or receiving aspirin. The use of folic acid may diminish certain toxicities (anemia and stomatitis), but not others. Lower doses are always a consideration, but may not be effective.

Patients stop taking second-line agents for other reasons such as inability to pay for the drug and its associated monitoring, inconvenience of routine monitoring visits, lack of rapid response, and just giving up hope of response. Social services and patient education help diminish these types of withdrawals.

4. It is not necessary to stop the methotrexate, depending upon the activity of the disease and other factors. Discontinuation of methotrexate may result in a severe flare in the arthritis. This differs from discontinuation of other second-line agents that result in a more gradual increase in disease activity.

If the methotrexate is still considered to be working somewhat, then another second-line agent or a change in the NSAID may be considered. Combinations of methotrexate with hydroxychloroquine or azathioprine may be helpful, whereas combinations with auranofin are probably not helpful.

However, if the methotrexate is not considered to be working or if it is not desirable to use combination therapy, then another second-line agent should be considered.

CASE 64

1. The etiology of OA appears to be multifactorial. Although not the sole cause, trauma may lead to joint destruction and changes consistent with OA.

2. If septic arthritis is ruled out, MJ's disease has probably progressed to include an inflammatory component. Simple analgesia will no longer suffice; an agent with antiinflammatory properties is indicated. In light of her gastrointestinal complaints, the nonacetylated salicylates (e.g., salsalate) would be a good choice. The nonacetylated salicylates have

been associated with less GI discomfort than any other NSAIDs. Enteric-coated aspirin is another option, if cost is an important concern for MJ.

3. Drug-induced lupus syndrome is typically characterized by (a) a delayed onset between 1 month to 5 years (MJ's onset was after 2 years), (b) an 80–90% incidence of symmetrical, nondeforming polyarthritis frequently in the small joints of the hands and wrists (MJ had recent onset of pain in hands, wrists, and feet), (c) fever and myalgia in up to 50% of cases (MJ's T = 38^2), and (d) pleuropulmonary features in up to 50% of patients with procainamide-induced lupus syndrome (MJ did not have these manifestations). Central nervous system and renal involvement do not occur. Rashes, alopecia, discoid lesions, and mucosal ulcers characteristic of idiopathic SLE occur in less than 25% of drug-induced lupus syndromes. Antinuclear antibodies (ANA) appear in 100% of symptomatic procainamide-induced lupus syndromes. Other common serologic findings include elevated ESR (46%), presence of LE cells (77%), positive RF (35%), and false-positive test results for syphilis (28%). A normocytic, normochromic anemia secondary to hemolysis may also occur in 9–21% of procainamide-induced lupus syndrome cases.

4. Several drugs have been associated with lupus-like syndromes and are divided into three categories according to occurrences. The first group is drugs that demonstrate a definite association with lupus syndromes, such as hydralazine, procainamide, isoniazid, methyldopa, quinidine, and chlorpromazine. The second group contains drugs less frequently associated with lupus syndromes, such as anticonvulsants, β-blockers, sulfasalazine, penicillamine, lithium, and antithyroid drugs. The third group includes drugs only rarely associated with lupus syndromes, such as estrogen, gold salts, penicillin, griseofulvin, reserpine, captopril, phenylbutazone, and tetracycline. Many of the implicated agents have a chemical moiety in common, such as the amino or hydrazino group on procainamide, hydralazine, and isoniazid compounds, or the sulfhydryl group on captopril, penicillamine, and antithyroid compounds. These chemical moieties may exist in the environment, in foods and natural products such as herbicides, pesticides, alfalfa sprouts, mushrooms, and tobacco, which may induce lupus-like syndromes. Finally, a few case reports of agents possibly exacerbating idiopathic SLE include estrogen, ibuprofen, sulindac, and tolmentin.

5. No. MJ's symptoms are consistent with osteoarthritis (i.e., the characterization of her pain and the absence of systemic manifestations). The positive rheumatoid factor probably results from MJ's procainamide-induced lupus syndrome, since it occurs in up to 35% of these cases. This question emphasizes the importance of an accurate and detailed patient history.

CASE 65

1. Clinical S/S of drug-induced lupus (DIL): Overall, the clinical presentation is considered to be mild with little organ involvement. Most patients have migratory arthralgias that affect the small joints of the hands, elbows, knees, shoul-

ders, and feet. Patients also complain of myalgias, weight loss, and malaise. Up to 50% of patients also complain of dyspnea/pleurisy and rashes, which are described as malar and photosensitive. Renal, central nervous system, and hematologic involvement is not common in DIL. Symptoms usually occur within 3 months to 2 years after initiation of drug therapy. Patients with some of these signs and symptoms should have their medication regimen evaluated for possible drug-related lupus. Several laboratory values can be used to confirm the diagnosis.

2. Laboratory results used to diagnosis SLE and DIL: The fluorescent antinuclear antibody (ANA) test is used most frequently to confirm any type of lupus. The ANA test results vary with each laboratory and include whether the result is positive or negative, the titer levels, and the pattern reported. The ANA result will be positive in 95% of patients with any type of lupus (including DIL); however, the ANA test is not specific: it is positive in 50% of patients with other connective tissue diseases such as rheumatoid arthritis and scleroderma. The titers will vary, but most laboratories consider a dilution above 1:40 to be positive, with higher titers (e.g., 1:1280) being more important. Despite the titers, many patients will have their ANA tested two or three times if a diagnosis is questionable. A positive ANA result may be diagnostic for any type of SLE or other connective tissue disease, but it will not help differentiate between lupus, scleroderma, and rheumatoid arthritis. One way to help differentiate between them is to look at the four ANA patterns that may be reported: homogeneous, speckled, peripheral, and nucleolar. The speckled and nucleolar patterns are considered to be specific for scleroderma, but the speckled pattern can be found in SLE or rheumatoid arthritis. The homogeneous pattern can be found in scleroderma, rheumatoid arthritis, and SLE (including drug-related type). Therefore the ANA pattern is of some usefulness, but its lack of complete specificity makes it a less powerful tool than a specific antigen-antibody reaction test. The presence of specific antibodies to certain cellular components will enable a clinician to differentiate between SLE and other connective tissue diseases. The most widely used is the anti-dsDNA test.

A positive anti-dsDNA (antibodies to double-stranded DNA) result is highly specific for SLE. Antibodies made to RNA, which are often found in SLE patients, include anti-Sm and anti-nRNP. Another laboratory result diagnostic for idiopathic SLE is decreased complement (C3) levels. Drug-induced lupus usually does not involve increased anti-dsDNA or anti-Sm antibodies or decreased complement levels. However, antihistone antibodies are found in 90% of patients with DIL.

If a clinician suspects DIL from a patient's clinical manifestations, a positive ANA result usually warrants discontinuation of the suspected medication. If no medication is the obvious culprit, specific antigen-antibody tests will help confirm the diagnosis of DIL.

3. DIL versus idiopathic SLE: Patients who develop DIL are usually older (50s to 60s) than SLE patients (20s to 30s). Women account for approximately 50% of DIL and 90%

of SLE patients. Caucasian patients account for 90–95% of those with DIL, 65% of those with SLE.

Clinical presentations: Patients with DIL usually have a much milder disease than SLE, with arthralgias, myalgias, weight loss, chest pain, and rashes as the most prevalent symptoms. SLE patients present with all of the above plus episodic fevers, dyspepsia, neurologic manifestations (headaches, seizures, psychoses, dementia), cardiac signs (pericarditis, myocarditis, hypertension), hematologic problems (anemia, thrombocytopenia), and most importantly, various stages of lupus nephritis.

Prognosis: Since DIL does not involve the major organ systems (in most patients), the prognosis is considered to be much better than idiopathic SLE. Most cases of DIL will resolve in time without intense therapeutic intervention.

4. Many patients (25–50%) diagnosed with SLE suffer from depression or other psychiatric disturbances, such as anxiety, dementia, or psychoses. Depression usually occurs soon after diagnosis of SLE, and it is not known whether the actual depression is endogenous (from the effect of SLE on the brain tissue) or exogenous (reactive depression), following the diagnosis of a disease that cannot be cured and which has the potential to alter the quality of life and shorten the patient's life-span. Counseling by a clinical psychologist or a support group to help the patient learn to deal with SLE and its manifestations is recommended. Many areas have special SLE support groups for this specific purpose. If medication is needed to help the patient recover from the initial stages of depression, several factors must be considered when choosing an antidepressant. Since most antidepressants are considered equally efficacious, the selection of an agent should be based upon the adverse-effect profile and the cost to the patient. Of the tricyclic agents, the tertiary amines (e.g., amitriptyline) tend to cause a great deal of sedation, orthostatic hypotension, and anticholinergic effects, making them undesirable for elderly patients (who often suffer from urinary retention, glaucoma, hypertension) if used in large doses. These agents also have long half-lives and active metabolites that can accumulate, making the previously mentioned adverse effects worse in the elderly. If they are used, they should be started in low doses (e.g., amitriptyline 25 mg q.h.s., which is 1/3–1/2 the starting dose for a younger patient). In general, the secondary amines (e.g., desipramine) or nontricyclics (e.g., fluoxetine, trazodone, bupropion) may have a better adverse-effect profile for elderly patients, but they may be more expensive. Some of the newer agents (e.g., SSRIs, venlafaxine, bupropion) produce little sedation and can actually have a stimulatory effect, which many patients find desirable.

Patients with a history of seizure disorders should probably not receive bupropion or maprotiline (>225 mg/day), since these drugs can alter seizure control. The tricyclic agents are usually not recommended for patients with cardiac conduction abnormalities; however, many patients with cardiac abnormalities will not experience arrhythmias unless they receive very large doses or an overdose of the medication. After weighing the patient's medical history with the adverse-effect profile of each antidepressant, the cost of therapy must be considered.

5. Drugs associated with DIL: The two medications most often associated with DIL are hydralazine and procainamide. Less commonly associated with DIL are isoniazid, chlorpromazine, and methyldopa.

    Theory: The most popular theory links DIL to HLA-DR4, specifying patients with genetically slow acetylation rates as more susceptible to DIL. Slow acetylation results in an accumulation of drug, allowing it to complex with nuclear proteins (DNA or histones). Antinuclear antibodies are then formed against the complexes, resulting in further stimulation of the immune system (T and B cells), which can ultimately result in an inflammatory response and clinical symptoms.

    Dose and DIL relationship: There appears to be a dose-dependent relationship in the number of patients on procainamide or hydralazine who develop DIL. Patients who have received >14 g total or >1600 mg daily of procainamide or >200 mg daily of hydralazine have a greater chance of developing DIL.

    Percentage of patients developing (+) ANA: Approximately 50–100% of patients on procainamide develop a positive ANA titer within 2 months after initiating therapy. Up to 30% of these patients will develop clinical manifestations of DIL within 2 years. Between 50 and 100% of patients on hydralazine will develop a positive ANA titer within the first 6 months of therapy, with up to 10% of patients becoming symptomatic within 2 years.

CASE 67

1. The two drugs most commonly associated with lupus erythematosus are procainamide and hydralazine. Drug-induced lupus (DIL) patients present clinically with arthralagias, myalgias, weight loss and malaise, joint pain, and rash. DIL occurs within 3 months to 2 years after initiating drug therapy. However, DIL is reversible and symptoms typically resolve within days to months after discontinuation of the drug.

2. A positive antinuclear antibody (ANA) test is specific for SLE. The ANA titer is usually greater than 1:160 in SLE patients. There are four fluorescent ANA patterns (rims, homogeneous, speckled, and nucleolar). An ANA titer greater than 1:160 with rim immunofluorescent pattern is most specific for SLE.

3. Hydroxychloroquine and chloroquine have ocular side effects. Corneal deposits can develop within a few months of therapy and are usually benign. However, retinopathy can also develop with anti-malarial therapy. The risk for retinopathy appears to be dose related. Symptoms of antimalarial retinopathy include peripheral and central vision loss, color disturbance, blurred vision, night blindness, light flashes and streaks, and photophobia. Patients should have regularly scheduled ophthalmologic examinations.

4. Hyperkalemia treatment depends on the patient's serum levels and if the patient is experiencing any ECG changes (cardiac effects). PS's potassium level is at the higher range of normal. She is asymptomatic and does not need any intervention at this time. However, her serum potassium levels should be monitored. If symptoms are seen or her serum potassium levels increase, sodium polystyrene sulfonate should be started. To actually reduce potassium from the body, sodium polystyrene sulfonate (Kayexalate) is given, which exchanges sodium for potassium in the intestinal tract. The usual dose is fifteen to thirty grams orally or given rectally as an enema.

5. Calcium may be given if hyperkalemia results in EKG abnormalities. Calcium does not change the total body potassium level, but counteracts the myocardial effects of excess potassium. Other options include sodium bicarbonate administration, which lowers extracellular potassium levels but does not change the total body potassium. Administration of glucose with regular insulin will also shift extracellular potassium back into cells. Sodium polystyrene or hemodialysis are required to actually remove potassium from the body.

CASE 70

1. Since noncompliance has been ruled out as an etiology, other alternatives need to be investigated. Reinfection with a different strain of *P. aeruginosa* than the one previously treated may be an explanation. The most likely etiology, however, is related to this patient's antacid and multivitamin with mineral use. Antacids and minerals (as well as dairy products) will bind ciprofloxacin (via chelation) thereby preventing drug absorption. This patient, who was taking antacids around the clock, should have been counseled to take ciprofloxacin 1 hour before or 2 hours after her antacids (dairy products and minerals).

2. In patients with cellulitis, the most common group of infecting organisms is the Gm+ cocci (i.e., *Staph* or *Strep*). Ciprofloxacin has poor activity against these pathogens and would therefore be a poor choice for cellulitis even in this patient with a history of diabetes. Trimethoprim/ sulfamethoxazole (TMP/SMX) would have been an appropriate agent to treat the initial episode of cellulitis in this penicillin-allergic patient. TMP/SMX covers *Staph/Strep* and a large number of Gm– pathogens (except *P. aeruginosa*). It does not cover Gm– anaerobes (i.e., *Bacteroides* species); however, at her initial presentation for cellulitis 3 months ago, this was not part of the differential since there was no drainage.

3. EK's wound cultures reveal 3 distinct pathogens: *S. aureus*, *P. aeruginosa*, *B. fragilis*. Therapy should be focused on treating these organisms. Monotherapy will not cover all of these pathogens, and it appears that 2 antibiotics will be needed to complete therapy. Clindamycin or metronidazole will adequately cover *B. fragilis*. However, clindamycin will also cover *S. aureus*. Clindamycin IV/PO are equivalent doses and subsequently the patient can be converted directly to the same regimen orally. It should be noted that diarrhea occurs in approximately 30% of patients on clindamycin and *C. difficile*-associated pseudomembranous colitis has also been reported to occur with its use. Abdominal pain, cramping with fevers, and loose stools are signs of pseudomembranous colitis. Ciprofloxacin is an appropriate choice for this patient's *P. aeruginosa*, especially since

the isolate is sensitive to ciprofloxacin. The patient should be advised to avoid antacids and dairy products as above in answer #1. Clindamycin 900mg po TID and ciprofloxacin 750mg po BID for 2–4 weeks would be appropriate to complete therapy.

4. Sucralfate has been shown to decrease ciprofloxacin's absorption. Sucralfate is a nonabsorbable aluminum sulfated polysaccharide which dissociates into aluminum and a highly polar anion in an acidic environment. This polar anion is the active moiety that binds to the ulceration. Aluminum is now free to bind (chelate) with ciprofloxacin and prevent drug absorption. It is therefore recommended that ciprofloxacin be taken 1 hr before or 2 hrs after sucralfate.

5. Naproxen and ibuprofen are both NSAIDs from the same chemical class (the proprionic acids). Both agents have had an adequate trial (>2 weeks) at maximal doses and have failed to produce a clinical benefit. A trial of an NSAID from a different chemical class (i.e., the indoles, oxicams, or fenamates) may provide an adequate response and would be worthwhile prior to the initiation of gold therapy. In this patient, however, the severity of disease progression (i.e., swan-neck deformities of both hands) suggests that more aggressive therapy with a SAARD, in addition to NSAIDs, may be required.

CASE 72

1. The therapy most often used to eradicate *H. pylori* is as described previously for TF. Other antibacterial drugs which may be used are amoxicillin, clarithromycin, metronidazole, and tetracycline. Any two or three of these antibiotics together with an anti-secretary agent (acid-reducing agent) should be efficacious. Other options found to be effective include concurrent amoxicillin 500mg po qid with omeprazole 20mg po bid for 2 weeks. Clarithromycin with omeprazole has also been shown to be effective.

2. Drugs for treatment of peptic ulcers have been used now for many years. Antibacterial treatment as described previously works well in cases where *H. pylori* is responsible. Histamine-receptor antagonists are effective for acute treatment and long-term maintenance for decreasing the incidence of relapse. Histamine-receptor blockers (ranitidine, cimetidine, famotidine, nizatidine) decrease acid secretion, and are relatively safe agents. Omeprazole is a proton pump inhibitor which inhibits more than 90% of a 24-hour acid secretion. Omeprazole relieves pain and usually is given once daily. Sucralfate is an aluminum hydroxide complex of sucrose which protects ulcers from exposure to acid. Sucralfate is effective for acute treatment and prevention of relapse. Sucralfate is also not systemically absorbed and usually does not interact with many drugs. Misoprostol is a prostaglandin analog effective for prevention of gastric ulcers in patients on chronic NSAID therapy. However, misoprostol is not as effective as histamine-receptor antagonists for acute treatment. Antacids can be effective in promoting healing of ulcers; however, the need for multiple daily doses increases the likelihood of noncompliance.

3. Several risk factors for osteoporosis are known that pinpoint individuals. These include female gender, Caucasian or Asian ethnicity, positive family history, early menopause or oophorectomy in women, hypogonadism in males, reduced ovarian function prior to menopause, nutritional deficiencies, and social habits including alcohol abuse or cigarette smoking.

Clinicians should consider any endocrine abnormalities including hypogonadism, hyperparathyroidism, or hyperthyroidism, drug-induced osteoporosis, bone marrow malignancy especially myeloma, osteomalacia, and other disorders that may represent secondary causes of osteopenia.

4. Estrogen replacement therapy is contraindicated in women who have had breast cancer in the past or presently have breast cancer. Estrogen replacement therapy may increase the risk of breast cancer after 10 or more years. Patients with endometrial cancer within the past 3 to 5 years should not receive estrogen replacement therapy. Estrogen replacement therapy has been shown to increase the risk of endometrial cancer. Patients with undiagnosed abnormal genital bleeding, active thrombophlebitis or thromboembolic disorders, and transient ischemic attacks (TIAs) should not receive estrogen replacement therapy also.

Relative contraindications include active liver disease, past history of thrombophlebitis and breast cancer in first-degree relatives.

SECTION 9

RESPIRATORY DISEASES

CASE 73

1. $V_d = (65 \text{ kg})(0.48 \text{ liter/kg}) = 31.2 \text{ liter}$

$Cl = (F)(S)Dose/(Cp_{ss})(T)$

$= (1)(1)400 \text{ mg}/(25 \text{ mg/liter})(12 \text{ hr})$

$= 1.3 \text{ liter/hr}$

$k = Cl/V_d$

$= (1.3 \text{ liter/hr})/(31.2 \text{ liter})$

$= 0.042 \text{ hr}^{-1}$

$t_{1/2} = 0.693/k$

$= 16.5 \text{ hr}$

Assumptions:
a) Patient is at steady-state.
b) Volume of distribution is constant and within population values.
c) Sustained-release product used: F = 1, little fluctuation in peaks and troughs since half-life is close to τ (continuous release).

2. $Cp_{desired} = 10\text{--}20 \text{ mg/liter}$ (55.5--111 μmol/liter)

$S_{aminophylline} = 0.86$

$F_{aminophylline} = 1.0$

$Dose = (Cl)(Cp_{ss})(\tau)/(F)(S)$

$= (1.3 \text{ liter/hr})(15 \text{ mg/liter})/(1)(0.86)$

$= 23 \text{ mg/hr}$

a) Loading dose is not required since BJ is already at steady-state.
b) If aminophylline is required, hold until levels fall into therapeutic range.

3. Although the use of prophylactic antibiotics in asthma patients is controversial, certain benefits are apparent in specific patient populations. Patients who experience multiple pulmonary infections with subsequent clinic visits or hospitalizations may benefit from prophylactic antibiotics. However, daily use of oral antibiotics usually results in bacterial resistance and adverse reactions. Some practitioners advocate the use of "p.r.n." antibiotics. Many patients familiar with their disease can recognize the onset of respiratory infection. These patients are supplied with antibiotics that are initiated by the patient when symptoms of infection are apparent (i.e., change in sputum color or amount of sputum production). This may help prevent acute exacerbation of asthma and subsequent hospitalization in this patient population. This practice is more common in patients with COPD. Since the history of BJ's previous hospitalizations is not given, prophylactic antibiotics are not necessary. Also, erythromycin should be discontinued because daily antibiotics can foster bacterial resistance. Theophylline levels should be monitored; since erythromycin can inhibit theophylline metabolism, discontinuing the drug may lead to decreased theophylline levels.

4. If BJ does not respond to current inhaled therapy, an anticholinergic agent such as ipratropium is a logical addition to the regimen. Anticholinergic agents are additive with B_2-agonist therapy. Pulmonary function indicators (FVC) improve with addition of an anticholinergic agent to a B_2-agonist-containing regimen. Should BJ not respond to the change in her regimen, ipratropium 2 puffs q.i.d. can be initiated.

5. Patient education:
a) Correctly place cap on canister and shake gently.
b) Hold mouthpiece 1--1.5 inches from mouth, between lips, and be sure tongue is out of the way.
c) Breathe in slowly and depress during slow, deep inhalation.
d) Hold breath for 10 sec. Wait 1--5 min between inhalations if possible. (Recommend spacer if needed.)
e) Try to use the metoproterenol inhaler before the beclomethasone inhaler.
f) Rinse mouth with water after using the beclomethasone inhaler, to prevent thrush.

CASE 74

1. Place 1 tablet under the tongue at the onset of chest pain. May repeat the dose every 5 minutes for a maximum of three doses as needed. If chest pain is not relieved with the third dose, call 911. Keep nitroglycerin tablets in the original container and store in a cool dry place. Do not store in the refrigerator as this is a moist environment. After opening a new bottle, immediately remove the cotton and discard, as the cotton may absorb moisture and degrade the tablets. Once open, the tablets have an expiration of 6 months.

2. Not all calcium-channel blockers have the same hemodynamic profile. Diltiazem and verapamil are generally considered to have substantial myocardial depressant actions as well as mediating vasodilation. Nifedipine is generally considered to have primarily a vasodilatory effect and much less of an effect on the myocardium. The other dihydropyridine calcium-channel blockers such as amlodipine, isradipine, and felodipine are believed to have even less negative inotropic effect on the myocardium and are potent vasodilators. Objectives in the treatment of angina involve either improving oxygen supply or decreasing myocardial oxygen demand. Diltiazem and verapamil may improve both supply and demand via their myocardial depressant effects and potentially mediating coronary vasodilatation. Nifedipine and the other dihydropyridine calcium-channel blockers may worsen angina due to reflex tachycardia, which occurs secondary to the primary vasodilating effect of these agents, thereby increasing oxygen demand.

3. If SB's hyperuricemia persisted and he continued to experience frequent gouty attacks despite the interventions, pharmacologic therapy may be indicated. Choice of pharmacologic agent depends on whether SB's uric acid is increased from overproduction or underexcretion. A 24-hour uric acid collection is needed to determine the cause. A uric acid collection of >800 mg/dl indicates overproduction. Overproducers should be treated with allopurinol since it decreases the production of uric acid by blocking xanthine oxidase. A uric acid collection of <750 mg/dl indicates underexcretion. Underexcretors of uric acid should be treated with probenecid as this drug enhances uric acid excretion in the kidneys.

SECTION 10

CARDIOVASCULAR DISORDERS

CASE 79

1. There are a large number of drug interactions with warfarin that should be avoided when caring for patients that need anticoagulation. Amiodarone, clofibrate, metronidazole, and TMP/SMX have been shown to increase the anticoagulant effect of warfarin in clinical studies. Erythromycin is thought to have a similar interaction but has not been documented in the medical literature. These medications have major effects that typically occur days after the medication is started.

2. Cholestyramine, rifampin, and carbamazepine are thought to decrease the anticoagulant effect of warfarin. Cholestyramine can have a rapid effect due to a decreased absorption of warfarin.

3. For most conditions treated with anticoagulation, warfarin doses should be adjusted to maintain an INR between 2.0 to 3.0. Two indications that require more aggressive warfarin therapy are mechanical prosthetic heart valves and recurrent systemic embolism despite therapeutic anticoagulation; INR should be maintained between 2.5 and 3.5. All other indications such as venous thrombosis and atrial fibrillation, should be treated with anticoagulation at an INR between 2.0 to 3.0.

4. Drugs that aggravate gastroesophageal reflux disorder do so by decreasing lower esophageal sphincter pressure, allowing acid to travel back into the esophagus and cause symptoms of heartburn. Drugs known to have this effect are calcium-channel blockers, progesterone, alcohol, methylxanthines (including caffeine), estrogens, and nicotine.

5. There are at least four compensatory mechanisms that the body develops to maintain normal cardiac output as a result of congestive heart failure. These include cardiac dilation, activation of the sympathetic nervous system, sodium and water retention, and cardiac hypertrophy. Cardiac dilation occurs when the amount of blood pumped out of the heart is less than the amount of blood returning to the heart. Congestive heart failure results in decreased perfusion of the body's tissues, leading to activation of the sympathetic nervous system. In addition, decreased perfusion to the kidneys causes an increase in sodium and water retention. All of these factors increase workload on the heart, resulting in proliferation of cardiac muscle.

CASE 80

1. $ClCr_{estimated}$ = 36.7 ml/min (0.6 ml/sec)

$CLDIG_{CHF}$ = 0.88(CLCR) + 23 ml/min = 55.3 ml/min = 3.3 liter/hr

$Cpss_{estimated}$ = F S Dose/Cl τ = (0.65)(125 µg)/(0.9 µg/liter)(72 hr) = 0.34 ng/ml

$Cpss_{actual}$ = 0.9 ng/ml

$CLDIG_{actual}$ = (0.65)(125 µg)/(0.9 µg/liter)(72 hr) = 1.25 liter/hr

The digoxin clearance calculated (from the steady-state level of 0.9 ng/ml (1.15 nmol/liter) of 1.25 liter/hr is approximately 1/3 of the expected clearance, which would give a steady-state level of approximately 0.3 ng/ml (0.38

nmol/liter) with the dose of 0.125 mg q. 3 days. This decreased digoxin clearance in ED is most probably caused by an interaction with amiodarone, which has been shown to increase digoxin levels by up to 70%. Other factors, including renal insufficiency and severe congestive heart failure, also affect digoxin clearance, but they are accounted for in the calculations.

2. Although ED is taking 120 mg of furosemide daily, her potassium level is within normal limits. ED is receiving two other medications that conserve potassium, both Maxzide (triamterene/HCTZ) and lisinopril. In addition, patients with CHF are encouraged to avoid salt in their diet, and ED may be using a salt-substitute that contains potassium.

3. Metolazone is a quinazoline-derivative diuretic structurally and pharmacologically similar to the thiazides. Metolazone may be more effective than thiazides in the treatment of edema in patients with impaired renal function. Therefore, since ED's estimated creatinine clearance is 0.6 ml/sec (36 ml/min), metolazone may be a useful alternative if her edema is uncontrolled with Maxzide (triamterene/HCTZ).

4. Drug-induced SLE usually subsides once the offending agent is discontinued. Since ED is experiencing only mild SLE symptoms, no treatment is necessary now. For patients with more severe symptoms, prednisone in doses of 0.5–1 mg/kg/day may be beneficial.

5. If ED's CHF continued to worsen despite increasing the doses of her lisinopril and furosemide, other medications may be added. Nitrates, such as isosorbide dinitrate or topical nitroglycerin, may be added to enhance vasodilation. Another medication to consider would be an α-blocker such as prazosin, terazosin, or doxazosin. Some patients with severe CHF have been treated with intermittent home dobutamine infusions. However, this regimen has not been shown to decrease morbidity or mortality in these patients.

CASE 82

1. Acidosis decreases the sensitivity of receptors to catecholamine stimulation, so higher doses may be needed until the acidosis is alleviated. Correction of acidosis by the use of bicarbonate has not proved to be very effective, because it does not treat the underlying cause. Treatment of BL's hypoxemia with intubation and 100% oxygen will increase O_2 delivery to the tissues and stop anaerobic metabolism and the production of acid.

2. BL has a high SVR, which indicates vasoconstriction, probably secondary to high levels of circulating endogenous catecholamines. Additional vasoconstriction with agents such as norepinephrine will only increase afterload and most likely decrease cardiac output further. His primary need is enhanced perfusion, not pressure; the only effective way to increase perfusion is to increase cardiac output.

3. Stimulation of contractility increases the work of the heart, which always carries with it the need for increased myocardial oxygen delivery and the risk of deleterious effects on already jeopardized ischemic tissue.

4. The cardiovascular effects of dopamine are dose-dependent. Generally, positive inotropic (β_1) activity is seen at doses from 5–10 μg/kg/min. Above this level a strong vasoconstricting (α_1) component is added to its activity. Dobutamine, in addition to positive inotropic (β_1) effects, also causes vasodilation (β_2), which may decrease BL's blood pressure and compromise perfusion further. The combination of dopamine and dobutamine allows greater β_1 stimulation at lower doses of each. Additionally, the conflicting secondary effects allow the use of higher doses of both drugs, if necessary. This requires very delicate titration and close monitoring.

5. BL is at high risk for embolization and subsequent CVA because he is in cardiogenic shock (a high-risk group) and has had a large transmural anterior MI (see Chapter 39, "Acute Myocardial Infarction"). Approximately 60% of patients with this type of MI develop left ventricular thrombi (LVT). Early anticoagulation with heparin reduces the incidence to about 24%. Anticoagulation with oral agents is justified if BL develops LVT or has large akinetic regions; a 2-dimensional echocardiogram before heparin is discontinued will help assess the risk of delayed embolization. If indicated, anticoagulation should be continued for 3–6 months with warfarin.

6. Metoprolol is usually given as prophylaxis against reperfusion arrhythmias. BL is receiving anticoagulation therapy for prevention of embolization of a ventricular thrombus, not for reperfusion; therefore β-blocker therapy is not indicated. However, addition of a cardioselective β-blocker may be useful, if BL continues to be tachycardic.

7. Diazepam and other benzodiazepines are very useful in treating anxiety. Most MI patients have anxiety, which causes tachycardia, which in turn increases myocardial oxygen demand and hence the work the heart must do. All benzodiazepines given IV decrease blood pressure, and BL is already hypotensive. This effect can be minimized by decreasing the rate of injection. Diazepam is metabolized in the liver, and BL has hepatic cirrhosis and congestion. While this is an important consideration in severe cirrhosis, prolonged congestion, and liver failure, BL's congestion is being treated and he has mild cirrhosis, which should not cause significant alterations in metabolic function. Diazepam has many active metabolites; most are renally eliminated. One metabolite, desmethyldiazepam, has a half-life about 5 times that of diazepam and is known to have negative effects on mental status. BL has impaired renal function secondary to cardiogenic shock and heart failure. A clouded sensorium is not desirable, because it will make evaluation of AWS difficult. Caution should be exercised in using diazepam in BL for prolonged periods of time. If BL's hepatic and renal function does not improve, changing to another benzodiazepine (e.g., lorazepam) may be warranted.

8. Caution should be used in the presence of hepatic cirrhosis because all of the agents currently available to treat hypertriglyceridemia can elevate liver enzyme levels. Aggressive therapy in treating hypercholesterolemia may help reduce triglyceride levels as well. BL should be monitored closely.

CASE 83

1. The duration of anticoagulant therapy for patients with atrial fibrillation depends upon a number of factors. The duration of the atrial fibrillation is the most important. A patient with a recent onset of atrial fibrillation, who is likely to be successfully converted either electrically or pharmacologically, will only need to be anticoagulated for 6–8 weeks. These patients should be therapeutically anticoagulated for 3–4 weeks prior to cardioversion and for 2–3 weeks following successful conversion. If the patient remains in atrial fibrillation, the therapy should be continued indefinitely. Patients who have evidence of systemic embolization while in atrial fibrillation should be anticoagulated indefinitely.

2. The recommended intensity of warfarin therapy is to an INR 2.0–3.0. The published studies vary with respect to the intensity, but experience adequately documents anticoagulating to this range.

3. β-Blocker therapy for MB is appropriate if the therapeutic goal is rate control and not conversion to normal sinus rhythm and it is demonstrated that her left ventricular function is well preserved. Assuming this is the case, the question of selecting a β-blocker with intrinsic sympathomimetic activity (ISA) should be considered. MB has several problems that must be considered in the selection of a β-blocker: mild renal insufficiency, elderly age group, relative hypotension, possible altered mental function follow-ing her stroke, and her present hyperthyroid state. β-Blockers with ISA are proposed to provide β-blocking effects without excessive bradycardia and are thought to decrease systemic vascular resistance and so be helpful in treating hypertension. One of the therapeutic goals in MB is to slow the ventricular rate and not to decrease the blood pressure further. In this case, the selection of a drug such as pindolol or acebutolol, both of which have ISA, would be inappropriate. Based on this, either of the agents discussed in the case would be better.

4. Estrogens have been implicated in interacting with warfarin by two mechanisms, both of which have been suggested to lead to antagonism of warfarin effect and therefore more clotting. Estrogens have been thought to increase clotting factor synthesis and increase antithrombin III (ATIII) levels. While both of these have been documented in the laboratory, not every patient receiving estrogens and warfarin demonstrates antagonism of warfarin effect or development of thromboembolism. The influence of estrogens must be considered (as discussed) as well as the potential risk and benefits.

5. Additional risk factors that may place MB in jeopardy of bleeding include any residual motor function disturbances, any residual dizziness, any seizure problems that might develop and require antiseizure therapy, and confusion, which might alter her ability to take the medication on a reliable basis.

SECTION 11

SKIN DISEASES

CASE 92

1. BF is still complaining of withdrawal symptoms. Because blood levels of nicotine vary among individuals using the same strength nicotine patch, the nicotine level in BF may be suboptimal. Nicotine gum (polacrilex) can be added on top of the patch at this time to increase nicotine levels. (This will also give BF something to do with her mouth.) If this does not help, the dose of transderm nicotine dose can be increased. Recent studies have suggested that a 35 mg patch (21 mg + 14 mg) may be useful.

2. The nicotine gum is usually started at 2 mg taken every 1–2 hours or whenever there is the urge to smoke. A maximum of 30 pieces/day has been recommended. The gum should be chewed slowly, until the taste of nicotine or a slight tingling sensation is felt. This will promote a slow absorption. Continue chewing until this tingling is gone. Each piece should last ~30 minutes. The gum should be continued until the craving to smoke is satisfied by 1–2 pieces of gum daily. A gradual decrease in number of pieces/day is recommended. BF needs to be counseled to chew only one piece at a time and to avoid smoking cigarettes while using the gum. Local adverse effects include mouth, throat, and tongue irritation and ulceration; however, most of these local effects are transient.

3. Signs of nicotine excess include nausea, abdominal pain, vomiting, dizziness, headache, diarrhea, cold sweats, blurred vision, difficulty hearing, weakness, and confusion.

4. It is in patients with extensive psoriatic plaques who use steroids on large areas of their body in whom there is the greatest concern for systemic side effects. When high-potency agents are applied to large areas of diseased skin, systemic side effects, including HPA-axis suppression and glucose intolerance, have been reported. Caution should be taken to avoid applying topical steroids on or near mu-

cous membranes. BF's psoriasis is fairly localized on the elbows and knees. A short course of moderate- to high-potency steroids is unlikely to produce systemic side effects.

5. Initially, to treat the scalp involvement, a coal tar shampoo should be used. Lathering the shampoo into the scalp for five to ten minutes and then rinsing seems to help decrease the scaling and itching. For more resistant scalp involvement, a steroid gel can be applied. For even more severe involvement, a formulation containing salicylic acid in propylene glycol may be tried. Anthralin is another option; however, it is quite irritating, and should be reserved for more severe, thick scales.

CASE 93

1. The extent of the rash may appear atypical in that areas of the skin normally protected by clothing are involved. The oleoresin, urushiol oil, is responsible for AM's contact dermatitis. Direct contact with the plant is not always necessary. In this case, AM probably had direct contact with the plant with her hands and arms as she cleaned out weeds and brush. Because AM wore the same clothes (unwashed) the next day, further contact with oleoresin that remained on the clothing caused involvement on her abdomen and legs. This is supported by the fact that the rash in these areas appears to be at an earlier stage than that on the hands and arms.

2. Drugs should be considered as a possible cause since she is on several medications. Dermatologic reactions can occur with all of the agents that she is receiving. Eczema, pruritus, erythema, and various eruptions can occur with glyburide. Various skin manifestations have been reported with both enalapril and cimetidine, but these are generally rare. The key factor in this case is the recent history of exposure to an area where there was likely to be poison ivy. Also, while she has no history of prior allergics, she reported that she was "finishing" the task. Therefore, prior exposure for sensitization is possible.

3. Glucocorticoids increase gluconeogenesis, and glucose tolerance and sensitivity to insulin are both decreased. The glucose level should be monitored by AM as planned. If the level increases, the magnitude of the elevation must be evaluated because AM may be able to tolerate some elevation until the completion of steroid therapy, which will be short-term. When steroids are discontinued, the glucose should return to previous levels. If the elevation is considered significant, AM's dose of glyburide might be increased until the steroid is discontinued.

4. The potential exists for involvement of further areas of the skin (e.g., genitalia) or possibly the eyes, as AM's rash is still developing because of the further contact with the clothing that still had the oleoresin on it. If the eyes/eyelids become involved, cold compresses may be helpful. An ophthalmic steroid ointment may be indicated. The use of systemic steroids in this case should help minimize the development of further problems.

5. If areas of the poison ivy became infected, several factors are considered. If the area is small and confined, either erythromycin or bacitracin could be applied topically. Neomycin is best avoided because of potential sensitization. The secondary infection would be likely caused by *Staphylococcus aureus*. If the area of infection involved is more extensive or has the potential to spread, then systemic antibiotics should be used. A penicillinase-resistant penicillin or a first-generation cephalasporin should be used.

CASE 94

1. No. Although prophylactic penicillin was useful in preventing death from β-hemolytic streptococcal infections during the 1950s and 1960s, recent blinded evaluations demonstrate no benefit from routine administration of systemic prophylactic antibiotics to burn patients.

2. Yes. The guidelines from the American College of Surgeons call for i.m. administration of 250 units tetanus immune globulin.

3. Because burn patients demonstrate impaired phase I hepatic metabolism (diazepam and chlordiazepoxide), the preferred parenteral benzodiazepine is lorazepam (phase II hepatic metabolism). Because severe and potentially fatal hyperkalemia is associated with succinylcholine administration in burn patients, its use should be avoided. Decreased potency of nondepolarizing neuromuscular blocking agents such as pancuronium and atracurium is observed after the first postburn week, and increased dosage is required. This is not a problem because dosing can be guided by assessment of the degree of muscle relaxation by a peripheral nerve stimulator.

4. No. Early enteral nutrition can be accomplished even in the absence of bowel sounds. Because of gastric ileus, successful insertion of a nasoduodenal feeding tube may require use of an endoscope.

5. No. A transient leukopenia is commonly observed following burn injury and is probably due to margination and movement of Lkcs from the systemic circulation.

SECTION 12

DISEASES OF THE EYE AND EAR

CASE 99

1. *Staphylococcus aureus, Streptococcus pneumoniae, Pseudomonas aeruginosa, Neisseria gonorrhoeae, Moraxella liquefacins,* and α streptococci are the organisms most likely to cause corneal infiltrations. The occurrence of Gram-negative infections is increasing, possibly as a result of extended-wear contact lenses.

   If bacterial keratitis is suspected, a stat corneal culture must be obtained and broad-spectrum topical antibiotic therapy should be applied immediately while the results of these cultures are pending. The progression of *Pseudomonas* infections is very rapid, and tobramycin or polymyxin B should be included in initial local therapy. Topical bacitracin, erythromycin, or tetracycline will cover the possible Gram-positive organisms. Systemic antibiotics are generally not indicated unless one is dealing with highly pathogenic organisms such as *Pseudomonas* spp. or if the conjunctivitis or keratitis is only one manifestation of a more generalized condition.

2. Bacterial conjunctivitis causes a profuse discharge with moderate tearing. The eye itches minimally, and nodal involvement is uncommon. Bacteria and PMNs can be seen on a stained smear. Unlike bacterial conjunctivitis, viral, fungal, and allergic conjunctivitis cause a minimal discharge. Tearing is profuse with viral, but minimal and moderate for fungal and allergic conjunctivitis. Nodal involvement is common for viral and fungal infections. The allergens cause profound itching. Monocytes and eosinophils can be seen on stained smears of viral and allergic conjunctivitis, respectively, while the smear is usually negative for fungal infections.

3. No, never patch an infected eye; this enhances the bacterial growth. Corticosteroid ophthalmic preparations are used for a variety of inflammatory eye conditions that may cause permanent tissue damage and blindness if not treated correctly. The use of corticosteroids in combination with antimicrobial agents is controversial because corticosteroids reduce the local immune reaction and mask the signs and symptoms of the infection.

   The complications of topical ophthalmic steroids are well-described and include acute glaucoma, corneal ulceration, fungal keratitis, and progressive herpes simplex virus keratitis. Considering these risks, it seems warranted to avoid steroids unless the patient is under the observation of an ophthalmologist.

4. Elderly patients are usually more sensitive to volume depletion and sympathetic inhibition than are younger patients. Therefore a diuretic is the drug of choice to initiate therapy.

The higher dosage of hydrochlorothiazide did control GT's blood pressure, but unfortunately it caused some electrolyte disturbances. A decrease in dose did correct the electrolyte problem, but an increase in blood pressure occurred. A sympathetic inhibitor like clonidine can be added. Start with a low dose of 0.1 mg at bedtime and gradually increase at 1- to 2-week intervals. Inform GT about the sedation and dry mouth that may occur with oral clonidine. These symptoms often disappear after the first few weeks.

After the therapeutic dose has been found, GT can be switched over to the transdermal therapeutic system (TTS), which is a once-a-week dosage form. Seventy-five percent of patients with mild hypertension can be controlled on this dosage form. An acute withdrawal rebound hypertension is unlikely to occur.

CASE 100

1. Omperazole works by inhibiting the H^+/K^+ ATPase enzyme system at the secretory surface of the gastric parietal cells, thereby suppressing gastric acid secretion. Omeprazole is FDA-approved for the treatment of poorly responsive gastroesophageal reflux disease. An appropriate starting dose would be 20 mg p.o. q.d. × 4–8 weeks. The capsule should be taken on an empty stomach, and it should not be opened, crushed, or chewed. Omeprazole should not be used for maintenance therapy since the long-term side-effects have not yet been established in humans, although gastric carcinoid tumors have been observed in rats. The patient should be monitored for side-effects such as diarrhea, nausea, vomiting, abdominal pain, numbness in extremities, weakness, dizziness, and HA.

2. Long-acting nitrate compounds have been associated with nitrate tolerance. This may result from sulfhydryl depletion at the nitrate receptor which in turn leads to decreased production in cyclic GMP and decreased vasodilation. Nitrate schedules should be arranged to ensure that the patient has a nitrate-free period of approximately 10–12 hr/day. This allows time for the receptors to replete their sulfhydryl stores and limits the amount of tolerance seen.

3. Pindolol is a β-blocker that exhibits intrinsic sympathomimetic activity (ISA). This type of activity is favorable in patients who develop symptomatic bradycardia on β-blockers. The partial agonist activity produces a small amount of β-stimulation, which helps alleviate some of the symptoms of bradycardia, such as dizziness. Although ISA may be beneficial in hypertension patients who develop symptomatic bradycardia, it is unfavorable in CAD patients, because it may lead to anginal pain.

SECTION 13

NEUROLOGIC DISORDERS

CASE 105

1. If after loading MJ with phenytoin he is still seizing, another smaller load of phenytoin should be administered. The dose should be 7mg/kg IV (420mg) at 50mg/minute. Should the seizures still persist after this load, phenobarbital should be administered at 18mg/kg IV (~1100mg) at 50–75mg/minute. An additional load of 7mg/kg IV (420mg) of phenobarbital can be given at 50–75mg/min should the seizures still persist. If these measures fail to halt the seizures, the patient should be admitted to the ICU and pentobarbital 15mg/kg IV over 1 hour should be administered and a maintenance infusion of 0.5mg/ kg/ hr should be started. Alternatively, midazolam 200ug/ kg IV load followed by a continous infusion of 0.75-10ug/ kg/min can be administered. These infusions should be titrated to clinical and EEG response.

2. Risk factors that contribute to antiepileptic-induced osteomalacia include chronic anticonvulsant use (> 6months), multiple antiepileptic agents, inadequate vitamin D intake, decreased exposure to ultraviolet light (i.e., sunlight) and lack of physical activity. Dose-dependent osteomalacia does not appear to occur and reports of osteomalacia have occurred with doses as small as 200mg/day of phenytoin. Duration of therapy and number of anticonvulsant agents appear to play a more significant role than dose. MJ's history of institutionalization may contribute to his osteomalacia since he has decreased exposure to ultraviolet light and lack of physical activity. His history is also positive for antiepileptic use greater than 6 months; however, he has not been on multiple anticonvulsants.

3. The exact mechanism of antiepileptic-induced osteomalacia is unknown; however, it is believed that these agents affect vitamin D metabolism by the induction of hepatic enzymes, thereby producing a deficiency in active vitamin D. This decrease in active vitamin D subsequently leads to a decreased serum Ca, secondary hyperparathyoidism with subsequent bone resorption and osteomalacia. Other proposed effects include the inhibition of bone resorption, inhibition of intestinal calcium absorption, inhibition of calcitonin secretion, and inhibition of phosphate excretion.

4. Phenytoin-induced gingival hyperplasia is a dose-related effect with an unknown mechanism of action. Risk factors include poor oral hygiene and possibly increased saliva phenytoin concentrations. MJ's phenytoin needs to be at 300mg po HS in order to control his seizures as indicated by his past medical history; however, there are some changes that may help his gingival hyperplasia. MJ's nursing staff should be counseled on good oral hygiene such as the proper brushing and flossing of his teeth and regular dentist appointments. MJ should also be changed from chewable tablets to capsules if possible, since saliva concentrations may play a role in the etiology of this adverse drug reaction. Should these measures not help to control and improve MJ's gums, gum resection may be required or a change to another antiepileptic may be warranted.

CASE 106

1. Only diazepam, lorazepam, phenytoin, and phenobarbital are available for intravenous use. Benzodiazepine agents are useful for the acute termination of seizures, but they are not routinely used for maintaining an anticonvulsant effect after termination of status epilepticus. Lorazepam has been anecdotally reported to be effective in this setting, but it has not been extensively evaluated. Either phenytoin or phenobarbital may be used for JZ; however, since JZ responded well to the initial loading dose of phenytoin, it is reasonable to continue maintenance therapy with this drug.

2. The hematologic adverse effects of carbamazepine therapy include leukopenia, thrombocytopenia, and aplastic anemia. Before initiation of carbamazepine, a baseline complete blood count with differential and platelets should be ordered. The complete blood count should be repeated at 2, 4, 6, and 8 weeks of carbamazepine therapy. JZ should be told to return to clinic immediately if she develops abrupt onset of fever, infection, petechiae, or fatigue. Carbamazepine should be discontinued if the white blood cell count drops below 1.5×10^9/liter (1,500/mm^3) or if bleeding or infection occurs. After the first 2 months of carbamazepine therapy, laboratory monitoring for hematologic adverse effects should be repeated at 3-month intervals.

3. Carbamazepine, phenytoin, and valproate are approximately equally effective and well-tolerated for the treatment of generalized tonic-clonic seizures. JZ was noncompliant with phenytoin therapy because of gingival hyperplasia, which would probably recur if the drug were restarted. Carbamazepine is the apparent cause of JZ's current rash, and this drug should be discontinued as soon as possible, to prevent worsening of the rash or other organ involvement. Although likely to be effective for JZ's seizures, valproate should be avoided because it has been associated with pancreatitis and may worsen her chronic pancreatic dysfunction. Phenobarbital would be a reasonable choice for treatment of JZ, although she should be monitored closely for

adverse effects. Some patients who develop a rash on carbamazepine demonstrate similar hypersensitivity symptoms on phenobarbital. Thus, JZ should be monitored for rash, hepatitis, lymphadenopathy, and other signs or symptoms of phenobarbital hypersensitivity. JZ should also be monitored for the central nervous system adverse effects associated with phenobarbital including sedation, decreased mentation, and impairment of motor skills. Phenobarbital can be initiated at a dose of approximately 90 mg daily and increased according to the clinical status of the patient.

4. JZ's exacerbation of SLE should be treated with prednisone at an initial dose of 30–60 mg p.o. q.d. A response should be seen within 2–4 weeks. Higher doses of prednisone or intravenous methylprednisolone may be effective if the initial response to prednisone is inadequate. Once JZ's condition has improved, the dose of prednisone should be slowly tapered to the lowest amount that is effective for suppressing the debilitating symptoms of the disease.

5. JZ's symptoms suggest exocrine insufficiency of the pancreas with resultant malabsorption of fat. Supplementation with pancreatic enzymes is usually effective for improving fat absorption and should be initiated with 3–4 capsules with each meal. The choice of specific product (e.g., Pancrease EC, Viokase, Cotazyme) is guided by cost, availability, and patient preference. The dose of pancreatic enzymes should be titrated according to relief of JZ's symptoms (bloating, anorexia, and fat in the stools). Concurrent treatment with cimetidine may improve the absorption of pancreatic enzymes by reducing enzyme degradation by gastric acid. JZ should be educated about the need for continued enzyme supplementation and the goals of treatment.

CASE 107

1. Dermatologic reactions are common with sulfasalazine and are best treated by discontinuation of the medication. A mild antihistamine such as diphenhydramine may be given p.r.n. for itching, and corticosteroids used to induce remission of her Crohn's disease should help.

2. DW would respond to an appropriate tricyclic antidepressant or an anticonvulsant. However, before initiating antidepressant therapy, her MAOI should be discontinued for a 2-week period to avoid potential serious drug interactions. Secondary amines such as nortriptyline or desipramine provide adequate relief of neuropathic pain and are better tolerated than amitriptyline or other tertiary amines. Since she did not respond to amitriptyline in the past, DW should be started on 25 mg of desipramine, with the dose titrated upward by 25 mg per week until a therapeutic dose of 150–300 mg per day is attained. Anticonvulsants are an alternative choice, but they should be reserved for failure of antidepressants, as they have a more extensive side-effect profile, and DW will require concomitant treatment of her depression.

3. Before beginning desipramine, an ECG is advisable to rule out cardiac disease. Once she has begun taking the drug, she should have serum desipramine levels monitored as her dose reaches 150 mg per day. These levels will indicate

if further increases are necessary. If she develops intolerable side effects, such as rapid heart rate or urinary retention, an earlier drug level should be obtained.

4. Because DW is currently experiencing significant pain that is supported by demonstrable pathology, she should not undergo abrupt withdrawal of her opiates. Clonidine alone will not provide adequate relief of her pain and may intensify her depression. However, after symptoms of her Crohn's disease subside and her pain levels have receded, clonidine may be useful in weaning her from opiates and preventing myalgias, agitation, and diarrhea commonly observed with opiate withdrawal. A transdermal clonidine patch releasing 0.1 mg/hr should be applied to the skin. Since approximately 2 days are required to reach steady-state, oral clonidine, 0.1 mg t.i.d., should be given for the first 48 hr that the patch is worn. Each patch must be replaced after 5–7 days, and DW should be evaluated for increased depression and orthostasis while receiving the clonidine. After 7–10 days, the clonidine may be discontinued.

5. DW's increased blood pressure is a likely result of sodium and water retention noted with chronic glucocorticoid use. A natriuretic/diuretic may be used to counter this effect, but it should be combined with a potassium-sparing agent to avert increased potassium-wasting. She may be given a trial of hydrochlorothiazide/triamterene and monitored for changes in her blood pressure.

CASE 108

1. A non-modifiable risk factor is her race. Broderick et al reported that blacks had a 2.1 times the risk of SAH of whites and 2.3 times the risk of intracerebral hemorrhage in those under the age of 75. There is an increased frequency of aneurysms with hypertension and smoking (also with age, lean body mass, and atherosclerosis). This supports the degenerative theory for the pathogenesis of aneurysms, which suggests an acquired defect in the vessel wall versus the congenital or medial defect theory, which suggests there is a weakness of the arterial wall due to maldevelopment.

2. The exact mechanism of action of calcium-channel blocker for prevention of cerebral vasospasm and delayed ischemic changes is unclear. The proposed mechanism is multifold. The primary action of the dihydropyridine calcium-channel blockers nimodipine, nicardipine, and nifedipine is the inhibition of Ca^{2+} influx through voltage-dependent calcium channels in the plasma membrane, leading to relaxation and vasodilation of vascular smooth muscle as well as to negative inotropic, chronotropic, and dromotropic responses in the myocardium. They also interfere with erythrocyte lysis, prevent platelet aggregation, and decrease endothelial degeneration caused by catecholamines. The agents most studied, nimodipine and nicardipine, have high selectivity in cerebral blood vessels, which in addition to their effect on vasculature (including improvement of collateral circulation to ischemic areas), appears to increase cerebral blood flow. However, calcium-channel blockers probably do not reverse vasospasm, but reduce the incidence of symptoms due to vasospasm and delayed ischemic

deficits by cell membrane stabilization, minimizing secondary cell injury effected by calcium disequilibrium. They have been shown to significantly reduce severe neurological deficits from cerebral vasospasm. The most commonly observed side effects are hypotension (5–8%), tachycardia/bradycardia, rash, and headache.

3. Prophylactic antiepileptic therapy is generally accepted as a wise practice for prevention of seizures in patients with SAH. Phenytoin is the most commonly used agent as it is less sedating than phenobarbital and is available in an injectable dosage form. Carbamazepine is an alternative but is not available in parenteral form. A loading dose of phenytoin 15–20mg/kg should be given (typically 1 gm). The dose should be divided (for example, 500mg q3h × 2) to avoid excessive sedation and should not be administered at a rate greater than 50mg/min. A maintenance dose of 5–7 mg/kg/day (typically 100mg i.v. q8h) should be started immediately, and dosage adjusted to maintain a serum phenytoin concentration of 10–20 μg/ml, usually closer to >15μg/ml. Duration of therapy is variable and may range from 1–2 years, unless the patient experiences a seizure. Patients should be monitored for toxicity, such as nystagmus, lethargy, hepatoxicity, hemolytic anemia, rash, neutropenia, and thrombocytopenia. Patients need to be counseled about these potential side effects as well as good dental hygiene.

4. Selection of antiemetic medication should be made considering the risk of seizures in patients S/P SAH. Phenothiazines should be avoided due to their potential for lowering the seizure threshold. Droperidol is a commonly used agent (0.625 mg i.v. q4–6h prn); metoclopramide and lorazepam are also commonly given. Hydroxyzine may be used; however, it is associated with a rare incidence of involuntary motor activity, including seizures, trembling, and shaking, especially when higher than recommended doses are administered.

5. Hunt and Hess developed a clinical grading scale for intracranial aneurysms which correlates the patient's clinical status with prognosis. Their classifications are graded according to surgical risk based on the presence or absence of neurologic deficits and significant associated disease. Treatment protocols are recommended based on grade in order to reduce the morbidity of rebleeding in good grade patients and surgery in poor grade patients. Patients who meet Grade I criteria are asymptomatic or have minimal headache and slight nuchal rigidity. Grade II criteria include moderate to severe headache, nuchal rigidity, no neurological deficit other than cranial nerve palsy. Grade III criteria are drowsiness, confusion, or mild focal deficit. Grade IV criteria include stupor, moderate to severe hemiparesis, possibly early decerebrate rigidity and vegetative disturbances. Finally, grade V criteria are deep coma, decerebrate rigidity, and moribund appearance. Serious systemic diseases such as hypertension, diabetes, severe arteriosclerosis, COPD, and severe vasospasm result in placement of the patient in the next less favorable category. Patients who are grade I or II at presentation have a relatively good prognosis, grade III patients have intermediate prognosis, and grade IV and V patients have a poorer prognosis. In terms of timing of surgery, patients with grade I to III presentation should undergo surgery in most instances, early (0–3 days post SAH) if patient is alert, and late (11–14 days post SAH) if patient is lethargic. Patients with grade IV or V presentation are rarely candidates for early surgery; however, some believe patients may be candidates if they are radiographically free of vasospasm.

CASE 110

1. Chlorpromazine given parenterally is effective in aborting an acute migraine headache which is unresponsive to ergotamine or to oral analgesics. It may be given by intramuscular or intravenous injection. Intravenous injection should be used with caution since hypotension may occur. Prednisone 40–60 mg daily for 3 to 5 days has also been used to abort intractable migraine headache pain. Corticosteroids such as prednisone and dexamethasone presumably work by suppressing the sterile perivascular inflammation of resistant headache.

2. Heartburn or GERD is often described as retrosternal burning chest pain that may radiate to the neck. Other symptoms of GERD include regurgitation, dysphagia, and bleeding. Elevating the head of the bed 6 to 8 inches may help to minimize the reflux symptoms. Patients should avoid eating 3 hours before bedtime and avoid eating food that may irritate the esophageal mucosa and lower esophageal sphincter tone. Eating three small meals per day may also help. Obesity and smoking also seem to aggravate reflux symptoms.

3. Foods that have been known to precipitate migraines include monosodium glutamate (MSG), found in Chinese food and canned soups. Tyramine may also trigger migraine attacks and is found in red wine and ripened cheeses. Cured meats may also aggravate migraine headaches due to their nitrite content. Finally, chocolate and cheese with phenylethylamine may also trigger migraine attacks. If a migraine attack is triggered by any of these foods, the patient should be instructed to avoid the component responsible.

4. Many antimigraine medications cause vasospasm, which should be avoided in SA due to her history of thrombophlebitis. These medications include ergotamine derivatives and isometheptene, a component found in Midrin®. In addition, sumatriptan, which may also work by vasoconstriction, should be reserved for migraine attacks not responsive to narcotic analgesics.

SECTION 14

PSYCHIATRIC DISORDERS

CASE 114

1. Buspirone, a chemically unique agent used in the treatment of anxiety disorders, differs from benzodiazepines in that it has a low abuse potential and low potential for causing physiologic dependence, causes little sedation and minimal psychomotor or cognitive impairment, and is not cross-tolerant with alcohol or other CNS depressants. Buspirone is equally effective with benzodiazepines in the treatment of GAD. This is an attractive agent for patients unable to tolerate the sedative and cognitive impairment of benzodiazepines, those with a substance abuse history, and those who require long-term therapy.

2. Buspirone treatment is associated with a lag time of 1–2 weeks before the onset of antianxiety activity. Patients who have been treated previously with benzodiazepines may expect immediate anxiety relief, based on their past experience. These patients may be dissatisfied with buspirone treatment and elect not to comply with a regimen that does not meet their immediate expectations. Careful counseling should be given to the patient, explaining the slow onset of antianxiety effects and the advantages of buspirone over benzodiazepines. This education may improve patient acceptance of buspirone and prevent early discontinuation of the medication before an adequate therapeutic trial.

   At higher doses, buspirone can cause dysphoria and irritability. Buspirone theoretically has antidopaminergic activity, but extrapyramidal symptoms and tardive dyskinesia have not been reported.

3. Antihistamines such as hydroxyzine and diphenhydramine do produce sedation and slight relief of anxiety, but are well known to cause anticholinergic side effects. TB's symptoms justify an agent with better documented efficacy. As TB has no substance abuse history, initial therapy with a benzodiazepine is warranted.

4. Nonpharmacologic treatment plays an important role in the treatment of GAD. In certain cases, pharmacotherapy may be warranted initially to quickly reduce distressing anxious symptoms, but long-term management of GAD should include nondrug psychotherapeutic approaches. In many cases of GAD, a few sessions of supportive therapy or relaxation therapy may significantly lessen anxiety complaints and may even eliminate the need for pharmacotherapy. In some cases of GAD, cognitive therapy is used. In this treatment approach it is assumed that anxious symptoms are caused by cognitions (thoughts or images) or schemata (silent assumptions). Cognitive therapy is directed at reducing anxious symptoms that are derived from these cognitions.

The patient is assisted in developing new cognitions that do not produce anxious symptoms. The patient is also directed toward modifying the schemata. Hopefully these approaches will enable the patient to reduce or eliminate anxiety without the long-term need for medication.

5. The initial goal of therapy was to relieve inflammation and itching. Administration of a medium-strength topical corticosteroid 3 times daily is an appropriate initial therapy, as this will probably produce rapid control of her symptoms. After initial control, maintenance therapy should include use of the weakest strength corticosteroid preparation that will control the problem. This will avoid systemic toxicity that can be associated with using medium-to-high potency products for long periods of time. Counsel TB to use the low potency product sparingly as maintenance therapy by rubbing in the product thoroughly once or twice daily while the skin is moist. The stronger corticosteroids can be kept on hand should a flare-up occur, but they should not be used on a regular maintenance basis. Hopefully, as TB's GAD is controlled and she learns appropriate stress management techniques, this will help to lessen the severity of her eczema. Maintenance therapy should gradually be tapered off to reduce the chance of rebound flares of the topical lesions.

CASE 115

1. There is a 75 to 80% correlation between the pathogens found in bacteruria and those cultured from a rectal swab. The most common pathogens in UTI are the enteric bacteria. *Escherichia coli, Proteus, Klebsiella,* and *Pseudomonas* are responsible for the majority of UTIs. *E. coli* is responsible for 80% of initial infections. *Enterococcus faecalis* and *Staphylococcus saprophyticus* are also common.

2. Women who develop three or more UTIs per year may benefit from prophylaxis. Since RF has had four UTIs this year, she is a candidate for prophylactic therapy. Trimethoprim-sulfamethoxazole (TMP/SMX) and nitrofurantoin are commonly used as prophylactic agents. Nitrofurantoin at doses of 50–100 mg at bedtime and TMP/SMX at doses of 1/2 DS tablet at bedtime have been used for prophylaxis. Some recent studies have shown that doses of TMP/SMX as low as 1/2 tablet three times weekly are as effective as traditional daily dosing.

3. Patient counseling is an important part of therapy for genital herpes. For patients like RF with frequent recurrences, extra effort should be made to provide adequate education about the disease and its treatment. In addition to empha-

sizing the importance of compliance with medications, the following points should be discussed with RF:

5. Patient education:
   a) During the periods of infectivity, sexual activity should be avoided because there is no proven way to prevent the transmission.
   b) Both partners should be tested for herpes and be treated if needed.
   c) Women with herpes should obtain yearly pap smears.
4. Benzoyl peroxide, Retin-A, and antibiotics are commonly used to treat acne.

   Benzoyl peroxide: A safe and effective agent that is used topically. It is a bactericidal agent that reduces the production of fatty acids in sebum. Retin-A: It is a topical vitamin A acid that increases the turnover rate of skin cells and decreases the cohesiveness of skin cells. As a result, it removes comedones and inhibits the formation of new comedones. Antibiotics: Tetracycline is commonly used to treat acne. Besides its antibacterial action, it has other mechanisms of action that reduce acne.

5. Anorexia nervosa and bulimia are the two common eating disorders (EDs). Anorexia is characterized by self-starvation, extreme weight loss, body image disturbances, and a fear of becoming obese. Bulimia is characterized by binge eating followed by some form of purging. To date, there is no satisfactory treatment for anorexia and bulimia. Psychotherapy is the major treatment modality used in EDs. Recent studies have suggested that patients with eating disorders also have a major depressive component. Imipramine, desipramine, and phenelzine have been shown to reduce binging behavior in bulimic patients.

CASE 116

1. Patients have experienced nausea and vomiting, as well as increased agitation, restlessness, and aggressiveness, when fluoxetine and L-tryptophan were given together. The mechanism for this drug interaction is unknown, but it may involve the inhibition of serotonin reuptake by fluoxetine. Note that this interaction differs from that observed when fluoxetine is taken together with a monoamine oxidase inhibitor (MAOI). In the latter situation, a "serotonin syndrome" may result, which refers to the CNS irritability, shivering, altered consciousness, and myoclonus that may develop from a drug interaction between fluoxetine and the MAOIs.

2. MK should be free of symptoms of depression for at least 4–5 months on fluoxetine before the drug is discontinued. If this is done, watch for symptoms of relapse and withdrawal. The risk of relapse is highest during the first 2 months after discontinuation of the drug. To prevent withdrawal, decrease his fluoxetine dose by 25% every 1–2 weeks.

3. If MK is not responding to the maximum recommended dose of fluoxetine (after a minimum of 1–2 months), consider changing to another antidepressant such as a tricyclic antidepressant (TCA) or an MAOI. Given MK's preoccupation with suicide, neither class of agent is ideal. Therefore, starting MK on trazodone may be a better option, since overdoses from trazodone often result in less severe consequences than the TCAs or the MAOIs. The initial dose of trazodone is 150 mg p.o. q.d. Increase the dose by 50 mg/day every 3–4 days, not to exceed a daily dose of 400–600 mg.

4. MK is experiencing signs and symptoms of acetaminophen (APAP) overdose. Note that the sample for MK's acetaminophen level was drawn only 2 hr postingestion of the Darvocet-N, which gives a false reading (sample should be taken 4 hr postingestion). The initial 24–48 hr of an APAP overdose is usually characterized by mild GI symptoms. Hepatic manifestations of an overdose become evident approximately 3–4 days postingestion.

5. Ingestion of >150 mg/kg of acetaminophen can result in early signs and symptoms of acetaminophen toxicity. MK weighs 68 kg, so he would have had to ingest a minimum of 16 Darvocet-N tablets to experience signs of APAP toxicity [i.e., (68 kg × 150 mg/kg)/650 mg APAP per Darvocet-N tablet]. MK would have had to ingest at least 20–30 tablets to see the symptoms that he is experiencing.

CASE 117

1. The clinical symptoms of tardive dyskinesia (TD) and withdrawal dyskinesia (WD) are very similar. The symptoms of WD usually appear within 2 weeks of discontinuation of neuroleptic therapy. These effects dissipate and disappear within 3 months. By comparison, the symptoms of TD persist beyond 3 months after the discontinuation of a neuroleptic agent. MJ's condition may be due to a recent decrease in her haloperidol dose (i.e., withdrawal dyskinesia). However, it is also entirely possible that MJ is experiencing TD, since this can occur independent of neuroleptic therapy, especially in the elderly.

2. It is premature to start MJ on an antidepressant simply because she "looks depressed." If MJ's depression is real and progresses, it may be appropriate to start her on an antidepressant. Antidepressants high in sedative and anticholinergic effects (such as amitriptyline, doxepin, imipramine, nortriptyline) should be avoided because MJ is lethargic and is experiencing anticholinergic effects. Bupropion and maprotiline, although relatively low in sedative and anticholinergic activity, are contraindicated by MJ's seizure history, since these drugs have been associated with seizures. The best antidepressant for MJ would be desipramine or fluoxetine. Initiate either of these agents only if clinically indicated, and note that the addition of an antidepressant to a neuroleptic agent may actually worsen psychosis.

3. MJ experienced rash in the past with chlorpromazine. This reaction is not uncommon with neuroleptic agents and can occur between 14–60 days after starting the neuroleptic drug. These allergic reactions can be treated symptomatically with antihistamines, without having to discontinue the neuroleptic agent. Therefore, the use of haloperidol is safe in MJ. In general, the incidence of cross-sensitivity between the neuroleptics is low, but if a patient has an anaphylactic reaction to a particular neuroleptic agent, it is crucial to avoid agents with similar chemical structures.

4. Many drug interactions are associated with haloperidol. However, clinically significant interactions have been seen only with anticholinergics (increased psychosis, decreased

serum haloperidol, and development of TD); with lithium (altered consciousness, EPS effects, leukocytosis); and with carbamazepine (decreased therapeutic effects of haloperidol).

5. MJ is not a good candidate for clozapine because her psychosis had been in control in the past with haloperidol. Furthermore, MJ would be at risk for toxicity since the drug's adverse effect profile includes sedation, anticholinergic effects, and dose-related seizures.

CASE 118

1. Most children with ADHD will outgrow this disorder. In all probability, Kevin will be able to discontinue his medication sometime during the ages of 12–15 years old. In the meantime, the concept of "medication-free" periods during school vacations and summers should be emphasized to the parents. They must be reassured that, once Kevin reaches 13 years of age, he will receive a trial without medication in an effort to wean him from the psychostimulant medication. If this is successful, which it is in over 70% of children with this disorder, he will no longer need to use medication.

2. During therapy with the psychostimulant agents, it is important to monitor Kevin's weight and height. While these may not keep up with Kevin's peers during his medicated periods, growth spurts will occur commonly during non-medicated periods to compensate. A close watch should also be kept on his sleep patterns to insure that he is not experiencing excessive interruption associated with the potential central nervous system stimulant properties of pemoline. It is most important that blood pressure and pulse rate be recorded, since the possibility of irreversible damage to the cardiovascular system is present. Myocardial hypertrophy has been reported in association with chronic use of agents of this type. If significant increases are noted in blood pressure or heart rate, dosage should be reduced or an alternative agent should be considered. If stomach upset is mentioned by Kevin or his parents, it may be due to pemoline; however, in a child this age, a number of other causes must be ruled out before therapy should be modified. It is of particular importance to perform liver function tests because of the possibility of hypersensitivity reactions; these should be done every 3–6 months, depending upon the dosing schedule. If Kevin is maintained drug-free during the summer, these tests would best be done at the midpoint of each school semester. It is also best to evaluate liver function approximately 4–6 weeks after the initiation of dosage, so if medication is initiated at the beginning of the fall semester, a 6-week liver evaluation is consistent with good therapeutic practice.

3. Since Kevin is receiving 75 mg/day of pemoline, the dose may be increased. The recommended rate would be to increase the dose to 93.75 mg/day for a week, and then evaluate Kevin's performance for the subsequent week. If this does not have an effect, another dose increase to 112.5 mg/day could be done and evaluated for a further 1-week period. If this is unsuccessful, alternate therapy should be considered.

4. Although there is no direct pharmacokinetic drug interaction in this situation, the possibility of central nervous system excitation from triprolidine, a component in this hay fever medication, should not be overlooked. If CNS excitation were to occur, an alternative antihistamine should be selected. However, central nervous depression is just as likely to occur in a child this age, so careful monitoring for excessive drowsiness is also essential.

5. Assuming that Kevin's liver function test results have not changed with pemoline therapy, there should be no problem with use of theophylline in this asthmatic patient. The dose of the drug should be very carefully titrated to achieve an optimal bronchodilator effect. The monitoring procedures (refer to answer 2) should be closely watched. In addition, any central nervous system excitation from theophylline must be screened, so that there will not be pharmacodynamic antagonism of the therapeutic effects of pemoline.

6. A lack of response to pemoline does not rule out the possibility of response to one of the other centrally acting sympathomimetics, such as methylphenidate or dextroamphetamine. If Kevin fails to respond to pemoline, a trial with methylphenidate (Ritalin) would be appropriate. Therapy should be initiated with a dose of 20 mg/day, with subsequent increases dependent upon the patient's response. The monitoring parameters described for pemoline should also be observed during the use of methylphenidate. In addition, because of the reported inhibition of hepatic drug metabolism with methylphenidate, a close watch should be kept on theophylline serum concentrations even though a drug interaction has never been reported between these two agents. It is possible that theophylline levels could increase in conjunction with this CNS stimulant.

CASE 119

1. Clonidine, a centrally acting α-agonist, has been used to reduce the withdrawal symptoms of narcotic(s) in methadone detoxification. Clonidine has also been used as adjunctive therapy in alcohol withdrawal. Clonidine inhibits the sympathetic outflow of the locus ceruleus. Clonidine decreases the symptoms caused by excessive activity of the sympathetic nervous system when it is used for either narcotic or alcohol withdrawal. Two limiting effects are hypotension and sedation. Most patients experiencing alcohol or narcotic withdrawal have increased sympathetic nervous system activity and may benefit from the sedation caused by clonidine. A typical clonidine regimen for use in this setting is oral clonidine 0.4–1.2 mg for two days (in divided doses) followed by the application of two Catapres (transdermal clonidine) TTS-2 patches. The rationale for this recommendation is that clonidine release should be constant for 7 days. The patches may be replaced (one at a time to decrease the potential for an increase in side effects and to facilitate a taper of the clonidine) one time, for a total treatment time of 14 days.

2. Caffeine is the most socially accepted stimulant drug in the world in the form of coffee and cola-containing soft drinks. Over the counter (OTC) diet pills and some cough

syrups contain phenylpropanolamine, a CNS stimulant. Amphetamines are the prototype CNS prescription stimulant and are Schedule II Controlled Substances. Many other drugs and look-alike drugs of abuse have CNS stimulant properties. Some of these include pseudoephedrine, ephedrine, cocaine, methamphetamine, and caffeine. Use and/or abuse of CNS stimulants is currently very prevalent in our society.

3. The signs and symptoms observed with cocaine overdose are central nervous stimulant–type effects. Because cocaine blocks the reuptake of catecholamines at adrenergic nerve endings, excitatory and inhibitory stimulant responses are stimulated. Heart rate, blood pressure, and respiratory rate increase. The initial increase in respiratory rate may be followed by a rapid but shallow breathing pattern. In addition, cocaine can have cardiotoxic effects and may cause an arrhythmia (especially in those who have compromised cardiac function). Other sympathomimetic actions that may be observed in cocaine abuse include talkativeness, euphoria, and restlessness. Physiologic effects include mydriasis, vasoconstriction, hyperthermia, dry mouth, sweating, tics, increased muscle activity, and myoclonic jerking. Seizures may develop, especially if the dose taken is excessive, and the "abuser" with a history of seizures may be at increased risk. The initial euphoria experienced with cocaine use eventually progresses to a dysphoric stage (possibly including a component of depression) and may even progress to hallucinations or psychosis. Chronic cocaine users tend to exhibit hostility, impulsiveness, aggressive behavior, and wide swings in mood and behavior. Because many cocaine abusers typically go on "binges," their personal hygiene, sleep patterns, and mood changes may indicate that they are abusing a CNS stimulant.

Treatment of cocaine overdose may include use of a short-acting β-blocker (such as esmolol), fluid replacement (if sweating or dehydration is apparent), and use of an antiarrhythmic drug if a cocaine-induced arrhythmia develops (e.g., ventricular tachycardia—lidocaine). If cocaine-induced seizures develop, phenytoin, diazepam, or phenobarbital may be used for treatment.

4. Cocaine acts on the sympathetic nervous system by blocking the reuptake of catecholamines at adrenergic nerve endings. By blocking catecholamine reuptake, cocaine potentiates both inhibitory and excitatory responses of sympathetically innervated structures. In addition, cocaine has a local anesthetic action that is due to a direct effect on nerve cell membranes. Cocaine prevents the generation and transmission of nerve impulses at cell membranes and thus has an anesthetic action in addition to a CNS stimulant action.

5. If RS were to develop signs and symptoms of alcohol withdrawal it would be best to consider a shorter-acting benzodiazepine. RS came into the emergency room with signs and symptoms of having taken two CNS depressants (alcohol and diazepam). Because RS has some signs and symptoms of decreased liver function (increased liver function test results: ALT, AST, alkaline phosphatase, and an increased PT), her ability to metabolize a longer-acting benzodiazepine medication may be compromised. Therefore, it would be best to use a shorter-acting benzodiazepine. The use of clonidine orally (in conjunction with clonidine patches) could also be considered, depending on RS's blood pressure when the signs and symptoms of alcohol withdrawal become apparent. Caution must be exercised in starting both clonidine and a benzodiazepine because both can lower the blood pressure. It is important to begin thiamine 100 mg IV (and then oral) q.d. to prevent the development/or progression of Wernicke-Korsakoff psychosis.

CASE 120

1. Phenothiazines are not recommended therapy for the management of alcohol detoxification because they may result in increased seizures, impaired thermoregulation, extrapyramidal effects, postural hypotension, syncope, and arrhythmias. As phenothiazines have not been shown to be any more effective than benzodiazepines, their increased risk of adverse effects prevents them from being used.

2. Due to the advent of the flexible fiberoptic esophagoscope in the 1970s, direct injection of a sclerosing agent into the bleeding varix has become much safer and is gaining popularity in the treatment of bleeding varices. The most commonly used sclerosant in the United States is sodium tetradecyl sulfate, although sodium morrhuate and ethanolamine oleate have been used. It appears that sclerotherapy is more effective in stopping acute bleeding and preventing rebleeding than more conventional therapy.

3. If vasopressin is to be used, continuous intravenous infusion is the recommended route, thus avoiding the toxicity of intermittent large doses of vasopressin. The drug is diluted in D5W or NS to a concentration of 0.1–1.0 unit/ml. The initial infusion rate is 0.2–0.4 u/min and may be increased to 0.9 u/min if necessary. Attempts should be made to taper the drug after 24–72 hr of treatment, based on patient response.

4. Although disulfiram has been available for 30 years, a consensus on its therapeutic use has not been reached for several reasons. One is the methodologic problems involved in study design for assessment of compliance and efficacy of the drug. The disulfiram reaction can be produced with a small amount of alcohol, and although the course of the reaction is usually short-lived and benign, in rare cases and with higher doses, it may proceed to cardiac arrhythmias, heart failure, and death. The safest use of the drug is in a close counseling and rehabilitation relationship where doses and behavior can be closely monitored.

5. The United States Public Health Service Immunization Practices Advisory Committee currently recommends the use of polyvalent pneumococcal vaccine in immunocompetent adults who are at increased risk of pneumococcal disease or its complications. This includes patients who are suffering from chronic diseases, including alcoholism and liver cirrhosis. The recommendation is also made for immunocompromised adults with splenic dysfunction (among other diseases). It is wise to recommend that TR receive one dose of 0.5 ml pneumococcal vaccine, either i.m. or s.c., before he is discharged.

CASE 129 ANSWERS

1.

Characteristic	Anorexia nervosa	Bulimia
Method of weight control	reduced intake	vomiting
Binge-eating	uncommon	common
Body weight	emaciated	normal/increased
Exercise	vigorous	rare
Amenorrhea	frequent	50% of time
Anti-social	rare	frequent
Bradycardia & hypotension	common	uncommon
Complications	hypokalemia	hypokalemia aspiration pneumonia esophageal tear

2. The majority of bulimics can be successfully treated on an outpatient basis as long as thorough follow-up monitoring is possible. Hospitalization of bulimic patients is necessary only in situations when life-threatening hypokalemia associated arrhythmias, esophageal or gastric tears, severe depression and other serious complications are present.

3. The effectiveness of a number of drugs have been evaluated in the management of bulimia:

Tricyclic Antidepressants
—imipramine
—desipramine
—amitriptyline (+/−)
Monoamine Oxidase Inhibitors
—phenelzine
Miscellaneous Agents
—bupropion (+/−)
—lithium (+/−)
—naloxone (+/−)

Serotonergic Agents
—fluoxetine
—trazodone
—sertraline
—fenfluramine
Anticonvulsants
—phenytoin (+/−)
—carbamazepine (+/−)
—valproic acid (+/−)

4. Although antidepressants appear to be effective in managing bulimia, especially in those patients with depressive signs and symptoms, pharmacologic intervention as the sole therapy is not curative. Often times in studies where antidepressants alone appear to successfully manage bulimia, most patients relapse upon discontinuation of the drug. Optimal therapy should include a combination of both behavioral and drug therapies.

SECTION 15

INFECTIOUS DISEASES

CASE 131

1. Without treatment 90% of patients with retinitis will show disease progression leading to retinal necrosis, scarring, and eventually detachment of the retina. There are presently 2 available agents used in the treatment of CMV retinitis: ganciclovir and foscarnet. A greater survival benefit has been noted with the use of foscarnet. Both agents are equally efficacious in arresting or improving CMV retinitis; however, many providers begin with ganciclovir unless the patient's platelet is less than 30,000. Ganciclovir is renally eliminated, so the dose must be adjusted for renal insufficiency. Its main toxicity is hematologic (neutropenia and thrombocytopenia), so CBCs must be monitored. Foscarnet's toxicity is mainly renal and patients must be prehydrated with normal saline prior to infusion. This drug must be given via a central line using a special continuous infusion pump over at least 2 hours daily for life. Maintenance ganciclovir therapy given 6mg/kg IV q24h is administered five times a week as a 1-hour infusion without prehydration. These quality-of-life issues are important factors affecting choice of agents. In addition, foscarnet has a higher cost to the patient. Oral ganciclovir recently approved by the FDA is in capsule form and may be preferred by patients stabilized on ganciclovir injection.

2. Education points are as follows:

a) DDI are large tablets and 2 tablets must be taken to provide adequate buffer to enhance absorption of the drug.

b) DDI can be crushed, chewed, or dissolved in an 8-oz glass of water. Fruit juices should be avoided as they are acidic and will react with the buffer in the tablet, impairing absorption of the drug.

c) Patients should avoid antacids and should be told to check with the pharmacist or physician prior to starting new medications (OTC and prescription). Some medications may impair absorption of ddI or be impaired by ddI's buffers. Staggering the dose by 2 hours is generally sufficient.

d) Avoid drinking alcohol as this is another risk factor for pancreatitis. Pancreatitis is a significant adverse effect associated with ddI.

e) Patients must report any tingling, needle point sensations in extremities since peripheral neuropathy is a possible side effect of ddI therapy.

3. Patients should be counseled on self-administration of G-CSF; the main instructions include:

a) The patient must be instructed on appropriate SQ sterile aseptic technique, and must also be educated on the risk involved if this technique is not adhered to.

b) The vial should not be shaken.

c) G-CSF should be refrigerated.

d) The product should not be frozen.

e) The colony stimulating factor can be stored in the refrigerator in a syringe; therefore it can be drawn up in two syringes (one used and the balance stored).

4. Health care assessment and maintenance issues for all HIV (+) patients are important because they allow successful management of disease progression and their pharmacologic therapy (treatment and prophylaxis). The average HIV patient is usually on a number of pharmacologic agents (6–12 medications) and requires appropriate baseline health care maintenance to effectively monitor therapeutic efficacy and toxicity of these drugs. As CD4 cell count declines, the risk for opportunistic infections increases. Therefore baseline laboratory values and serology tests must be conducted to monitor progression of disease (lymphocyte count, electrolyte status, hematologic profile, and hepatic and renal function). Respiratory infections (TB, PCP, pneumonia, sinusitis, etc.) develop frequently, and baseline chest x-rays are necessary. Baseline PPD with controls must also be done. HIV-positive patients, because of their immune status, are susceptible to the common cold and the "flu" virus, and should be encouraged to receive appropriate vaccinations to prevent tremendous increase in viral burden. The fifth most important assessment is a drug/allergy history from the patient, to allow the provider to select optimum therapy for the patient

5. Currently the following agents are used in the treatment of disseminated MAC.

Drug	Dose	Common Toxicity
Clarithromycin (Biaxin®)	500mg po qd	Macrolides cause GI upset (N/V), rash, hearing loss, aminotransferase elevation
Azithromycin (Zithromax®)	500mg po qd	
Ethambutol (Myambutol®)	15 mg/kg po qd (1g po max) dose modification in renal failure	GI, optic neuritis (>25mg/kg/d)
Rifabutin/Rifampin (Mycobutin®/Rifadin®)	300–600 mg po qd	Elevated LFTs, GI, red-orange discoloration of body secretions
Clofazamine (Lamprene®)	100mg po qd	N/V and pink → brown → black discoloration of skin
Ciprofloxacin (Cipro®)	500–750mg po bid	N/V, anxiety, abd pain, seizures
Amikacin	15mg/kg IV bid	Nephrotoxicity, ototoxicity

CASE 132

1. There is no risk for transmission of HIV with hepatitis B immunization. All products are manufactured using recombinant DNA technology.

2. If TC is prescribed a medication containing sulfa, she should be counseled about the likelihood of developing a rash and the need to discontinue the medication should a rash appear. If this happens, she should be evaluated by a physician, since there is the possibility for development of Stevens-Johnson syndrome. TC should also be counseled about the photosensitization that may occur with use of the sulfonamides.

3. Because the oral typhoid vaccine contains viable organisms, the concurrent administration of antibiotics may inactivate the vaccine and not provide the desired immunologic response.

4. While IgG is prepared from pooled plasma, each unit is screened to exclude the virus and the antibody. In addition, purification steps known to inactivate HIV are used in the preparation of IgG. No cases of HIV transmission have been attributed to IgG.

5. An IgG dose of 0.02 ml/kg is recommended for stays of up to 3 months. If TC were going to travel for longer than 3 months, the recommended dose is 0.06 ml/kg given every 5 months or until immunity to hepatitis A develops.

CASE 133

1. Cephalosporins are effective alternate agents in patients with mild (nonanaphylactic) reactions to penicillins. Obviously, JS should not receive a cephalosporin, even though there is only an 8–15% cross-sensitivity pattern between the agents. When patients experience anaphylactic reactions, it is best to avoid drugs in the same class if possible. In this case, erythromycin would be an effective agent for treatment of *Streptococcus pneumoniae*. The drug can be given intravenously initially (5–7 days) and then changed to the oral route if JS is responding to therapy. Erythromycin 500 mg IV every 6 hr should be initiated. Some side effects of erythromycin to monitor include GI disturbances (nausea/vomiting), rash, and ototoxicity.

2. Theophylline kinetics:

$$Vd = 0.48 \text{ liter/kg} \times 65 \text{ kg} = 31.2 \text{ liter}$$

(Vd is normally based on total body weight. If this patient had been obese, total body weight would still be used.)

$$\text{Loading dose} = \frac{(Vd) \times (Cp)}{(S) \times (F)}$$

$$= \frac{(31.2 \text{ liter}) \times (15 \text{ mg/liter})}{(1) \times (1)}$$

$$= 468 \text{ mg} \approx 500 \text{ mg}$$

The loading dose for JS would be 500 mg of sustained-release theophylline orally. In order to calculate a maintenance dose for JS, we need to calculate his expected clearance:

$$Cl = (0.04 \text{ liter/hr/kg}) \times (65 \text{ kg}) = 2.6 \text{ liter/hr}$$

(However, JS is a smoker with COPD, so the expected clearance must be multiplied by the associated factors):

Cl = 2.6 liter/hr × 1.6 (smoking) × 0.8 (COPD)
    = 3.3 liter/hr

Other expected parameters:

$$k = Cl/Vd = 3.3 \text{ liter/hr}/31.2 \text{ liter} = 0.11 \text{ hr}^{-1}$$

$$T_{1/2} = 0.693/k = 0.693/0.11 = 6.3 \text{ hr}$$

$$MD = \frac{(Cl) \times (C_{pss}) \times (\tau)}{(S) \times (F)}$$

(where τ = dosing interval) [as18]

Since we will be administering sustained-release theophylline, the dosing interval will be 24 hr, with the total dose divided into 3 doses (every 8 hr):

$$MD = \frac{(3.3 \text{ liter/hr}) \times (15 \text{ mg/liter}) \times (24 \text{ hr})}{(1) \times (1)}$$
$$= 1188 \text{ mg} \approx 1200 \text{ mg}$$
$$= 400 \text{ mg p.o. q8h}$$

Since this dose is based on expected parameters and appears high, levels should be checked to ensure that JS is within the therapeutic window.

3. Phenytoin adverse reactions:

Dose-related:
Drowsiness
Nystagmus
Diplopia
Dizziness/ataxia
Extrapyramidal movements
Exacerbation of seizure
    disorder

Non-dose-related:
Gingival hyperplasia
GI upset
Hypersensitivity reactions
Systemic lupus erythema-
    tosus
Stevens-Johnson
    syndrome
Hair loss
Megaloblastic anemia
Hypocalcemia
Osteomalacia
Peripheral neuropathy

4. a. Shake the canister thoroughly.
   b. Place the mouthpiece between the lips, making sure the teeth and tongue are out of the way.
   c. Actuate the canister during a slow, deep inhalation.
   d. Hold the breath at full inspiration for 10 sec.
   e. Pause at least 1 min, preferably 5 min, before the next inhalation from the canister.
5. Acute poisoning may be manifested by nausea, vomiting, drowsiness, confusion, liver tenderness, hypotension, cardiac arrhythmias, jaundice, and acute hepatic and renal failure. Generally, acetaminophen overdoses can be classified into 4 stages (time measured from time of ingestion):

Stage 1 (12–24 hr): Nausea, vomiting, diaphoresis, an-
    orexia
Stage 2 (24–48 hr): Clinically improved; AST, ALT, biliru-
    bin and prothrombin levels begin
    to rise.
Stage 3 (72–96 hr): Peak hepatotoxicity; AST can be 333
    (20,000)
Stage 4 (7–8 days): Recovery

Acetaminophen is rapidly absorbed; therefore, activated charcoal, forced emesis, or gastric lavage are helpful only if given during the first 1–2 hr of ingestion. Acetylcysteine is given orally or intravenously and is effective if given during the first 24 hr of ingestion. A loading dose of 140 mg/kg should be given immediately. A maintenance dose of 70 mg/kg every 4–8 hr should be continued for 3 days. Since JS had a level of 118 (13 hr after ingestion), we can expect the hepatic damage to be minimal.

CASE 134

1. In general, patients with primary generalized seizures, an EEG without abnormalities, and a seizure-free period of two or more years are good candidates for withdrawal of anticonvulsant therapy. Other factors to consider are the etiology of seizures and age of onset. The potential benefits of drug withdrawal include elimination of the chronic dosing, adverse effects, and potential drug interactions associated with the anticonvulsant drug therapy. Other potential benefits include elimination of the costs associated with the medications, laboratory monitoring, and clinic visits. The risk for the patient is seizure recurrence, status epilepticus, physical injury, and difficulties with the social issues associated with recurrence of seizures (loss of employment, driving privileges, social stigma). The decision is a medically and socially complex one that should be discussed with the patient over a series of clinic visits. If MS's phenytoin is discontinued, it should be tapered gradually over several months.
2. MS needs to be aware he is at risk for bleeding and he should avoid situations that increase the risk of bleeding. MS should avoid trauma, rectal suppositories or enemas, hard toothbrushes, dental floss, metal razors, aspirin, and nonsteroidal antiinflammatory drugs. If he does start to hemorrhage, he needs to know to seek early medical treatment.
3. Hepatitis C (HCV) is an RNA virus that is generally transmitted via intravenous drug use or blood transfusion. Sexual transmission may occur, but at a lower rate compared to hepatitis B. The incubation period is 2 weeks to 6 months. The diagnosis is made by detection of anti-HCV antibody. Prophylaxis for hepatitis C is not available at this time. About 50 percent of acute cases of hepatitis C result in chronic infection.
4. Lactulose, a nonabsorbable disaccharide that acts as an osmotic laxative, decreases ammonia absorption and reverses the symptoms of hepatic encephalopathy. Lactulose should be administered in doses of 30 mL every hour until diarrhea occurs, and then titrated to a dose that results in 2 to 4 loose stools per day. If the patient is unconscious or unable to take oral medications, lactulose may be given as a retention enema. Adverse effects of lactulose include nausea, abdominal distension, and diarrhea. In addition, the patient should be monitored for fluid and electrolyte losses secondary to diarrhea.
5. The term "liver function tests" (LFTs) commonly refers to bilirubin, alkaline phosphatase, aspartate aminotransferase (AST, formerly SGOT), and alanine aminotransferase (ALT, formerly SGPT). However, these tests actually reflect

cell damage as opposed to "function." Bilirubin is a metabolic byproduct of the lysis of erythrocytes by the reticuloendothelial system. Hepatocellular injury from viral hepatitis, alcoholic hepatitis, or cirrhosis may impair bilirubin metabolism and elevate serum bilirubin concentrations. Alkaline phosphatase, AST, and ALT are serum enzymes that have a certain specificity for hepatocellular injury and biliary tract dysfunction or obstruction. Elevated alkaline phosphatase levels usually reflect impaired biliary tract function, although this enzyme is also found in high concentrations in skeletal, intestinal, and placental tissue. In contrast to ALT, which is found primarily in hepatic tissue, AST is also found in cardiac, skeletal, and renal tissue.

Laboratory values such as albumin and prothrombin time actually represent the synthetic "function" of the liver rather than just cell injury because albumin and prothrombin are proteins synthesized exclusively by the hepatocytes. In addition, the prothrombin time is dependent on hepatic synthesis of vitamin K–dependent clotting factors and sufficient uptake of vitamin K, both of which may be impaired in liver or biliary disease. While albumin levels and prothrombin times represent liver synthetic function, they are not early or sensitive indicators of liver disease, and decreases in their levels are not specific for liver disease.

A single test is not a reliable indicator of, and may not be specific to, liver disease. A set of appropriate laboratory values that assess different parameters of liver damage and function should be monitored serially and used in conjunction with the clinical findings to guide the therapy of the individual patient.

CASE 135

1. Intravenous drug users develop endocarditis more frequently than the general population because they commonly use nonsterile syringes and needles. This allows introduction of skin organisms, such as *Staphylococcus aureus*, into the blood stream. The organism then reaches the cardiac tissue and subsequently adheres to the cardiac valve. One factor necessary for adherence of the organism is a previously damaged heart valve. Intravenous drug abusers commonly inject contaminated preparations that travel through the venous system and may produce endocardial damage. Thrombi develop on the damaged endocardial surface and serve as foci for bacterial implantation. The tricuspid valve is located in the right side of the heart, and therefore is the first valve to be exposed to the contaminants injected by the intravenous drug abuser. Bacterial implantation therefore occurs more commonly on the tricuspid valve.

2. Infective endocarditis leads to the deposition of fibrin and platelets (thrombus) around the site of infection, resulting in a vegetation. These vegetations can become quite large and friable and may be released into the arterial circulation or pulmonary vasculature, depending on which side of the heart is infected. These emboli may vary in size and most often affect the brain, spleen, kidneys, gastrointestinal tract, heart, or extremities. Pulmonary infarction may occur in right-sided endocarditis. Petechial skin lesions, known as splinter hemorrhages, are characterized by acute vasculitis. These lesions were once thought to be embolic, but may instead be an immunologic reaction. Other skin lesions associated with pain, tenderness, and cellulitis may be embolic. Renal lesions may result from emboli to the kidneys, which may be manifested by hematuria. Roth spots are petechial hemorrhages that are occasionally found in the retina. Janeway lesions are nontender, subcutaneous, erythematous maculopapular lesions. Osler's nodes are painful tender nodules that may develop on the palms of the hands or soles of the feet. These are most likely the result of embolization.

3. The transthoracic echocardiogram has a sensitivity between 60 and 80%; therefore, vegetations are commonly missed. However, with clinical symptoms, the patient's history, a positive blood culture, and a cardiac murmur, a clinical diagnosis of endocarditis can be made with a negative transthoracic echocardiogram result. To help prevent a misdiagnosis that may result in the unnecessary long-term use of antibiotics, the transesophageal echocardiogram has been developed. This test is much more sensitive in finding cardiac vegetations, and thus, some practitioners feel comfortable ruling out the diagnosis of endocarditis in the presence of positive clinical symptoms but a negative transesophageal echocardiogram result. However, more experience is needed with this diagnostic test to assess its reliability.

4. As stated previously, intravenous drug abusers commonly use nonsterile needles and syringes for injection. These paraphernalia are colonized with bacteria such as *Staphylococcus aureus*, so this organism is much more likely to be the cause of endocarditis in intravenous drug users than is any other organism. *Staphylococcus aureus* is the cause of endocarditis in more than 85% of the patients. *Streptococcus* spp. and Gram-negative organisms such as *Pseudomonas aeruginosa* may also cause endocarditis in this patient population. Outbreaks of endocarditis caused by different bacteria (e.g., *Serratia, Pseudomonas*) have been traced to contaminated water used to inject the illicit substance intravenously.

5. β-Lactamase-stable penicillins (BLSPs) are the drugs of choice for empirically treating endocarditis in an intravenous drug user. Commonly, penicillin is added as initial therapy to cover streptococcal infections, as failures have occurred with streptococcal infections when treated with BLSPs. Vancomycin is an alternative for patients who have a serious penicillin allergy. Vancomycin has the advantage that when used empirically it will cover streptococcal and staphylococcal species, including methicillin-resistant *S. aureus*. The disadvantage of vancomycin is that it may not be as effective as the penicillins for treating staphylococcal infections, as failures have been reported. If vancomycin must be used, minimal bactericidal concentrations and serum bactericidal titers should be determined to demonstrate that killing of the organism is occurring. An aminoglycoside such as gentamicin may be necessary in combination with vancomycin for the entire treatment course. Alternatively, rifampin may be added to vancomycin to enhance bactericidal effects. Vancomycin should be reserved for situations in which there are no other alternatives. The

first-generation cephalosporins, such as cefazolin, have been used for endocarditis; however, their routine use is not recommended. Cefazolin is highly susceptible to inoculum effects. Such an environment exists with endocarditis, allowing degradation of β-lactamase-labile antibiotics, such as cefazolin.

CASE 136

1. Alternatives to erythromycin for the treatment of *Campylobacter* infection include tetracycline and ciprofloxacin and norfloxacin. However, both of these agents may cause photosensitivity, which may be a concern while FT is on a cruise.
2. Questions include:

Any recent travel?	Recent diet changes?
Recent antibiotic use?	Any ill contacts?
Underlying diseases?	Appearance of stools?
Number of bowel movements?	Volume of stools?
Medications being taken?	

3. Alka-Seltzer is not a good choice of antacid for FT, since it contains a large amount of sodium, which may cause fluid overload. Mylanta and Maalox have been reformulated to minimize the sodium content and therefore would be acceptable agents to treat his heartburn. In general, antacid suspensions no longer contain significant amounts of sodium. Those that still do would have to be taken many times each day to negatively affect CHF. Calcium carbonate–containing products such as Tums are safe to use in CHF patients, provided they are not hypercalcemic.
4. The only medication that FT is taking that may be photosensitizing is the furosemide. He should limit his sunlight exposure or use a topical sunblock or protectant.
5. Factors that predispose to digoxin toxicity include age, renal insufficiency, metabolic alkalosis, hypokalemia, hypothyroidism, hypomagnesemia, and hypercalcemia.

CASE 137

1. Recent evidence has demonstrated that patients with low CD_4 counts who are diagnosed with syphilis have a higher occurrence of neurosyphilis. The reason for this has not been completely elucidated; however, it is thought to be due to the low CSF levels obtained with benzathine penicillin. In patients with intact cellular immunity, the levels obtained with benzathine penicillin are sufficient to eradicate the infection. Since AIDS patients do not have an intact immune system, they are thought to be predisposed to infection of the central nervous system. Case reports suggest that unusual clinical manifestations of syphilis may be more common and the clinical course more rapid in HIV-infected patients. Some clinicians offer their patients treatment for neurosyphilis if the CSF is abnormal (elevated protein, leukocytosis, +/– VDRL); however, small studies have shown that both normal and HIV-infected patients can have abnormal CSF findings during primary or secondary syphilis infections but do not demonstrate neurological findings. Other clinicians empirically treat all of their HIV-infected patients with serologic documented syphilis as neurosyphilis. This is not currently recommended by the CDC and is not supported by reports found in the literature. Others do not believe that the few case reports justify routine CSF examination in all HIV-infected patients. CSF abnormalities are common in HIV-infected patients with primary and secondary syphilis and are of unknown prognostic significance. Currently the CDC recommends CSF examination in any HIV-infected patient diagnosed with latent syphilis, regardless of the duration of infection. Any HIV-infected patient with unexplained neurological symptoms should include neurosyphilis as part of the differential. Additionally, patients treated for primary or secondary syphilis should have follow-up titers to ensure treatment success (fourfold decrease by 3 months). A lumbar puncture can also provide baseline CSF titers, which may be useful for a later diagnosis. Treatment schedules recommended by the CDC differ slightly for HIV-infected patients. Patients with primary or secondary syphilis should receive benzathine penicillin 2.4 million units IM as a single dose. Patients with non-neurologic latent syphilis should have their CSF examined and, if negative, should be treated as latent syphilis regardless of the duration (2.4 MU I q week for 3 weeks). Some clinicians will treat primary and secondary syphilis as latent; however, no studies have examined the ability of this regimen to prevent neurosyphilis in HIV-infected patients.
2. Generally, a VDRL titer greater than 1:32 indicates neurosyphilis. However, neurosyphilis cannot be diagnosed by CSF VDRL titers alone. On CSF examination, high levels of protein, an elevated white count, and an elevated VDRL are consistent with neurosyphilis. If the VDRL is negative, neurosyphilis cannot be ruled out; however, a negative FTA-ABS will provide evidence against the diagnosis of syphilis. Unfortunately, the diagnosis of neurosyphilis in HIV-infected patients is complicated by high false-negative and high false-positive rates. Non-treponemal tests detect antibodies against cardiolipin-lecithins; therefore cross-reactivity occurs with *T. pallidum* antigens and subsequently a false-positive VDRL or RPR test. Since HIV-infected patients often have polygammopathy and abnormally high levels of anti-cardiolipin antibodies, they have a high occurrence of false-positive tests. Additionally, HIV-infected patients may not demonstrate positive findings on CSF examination due to impaired immune responses; therefore, negative CSF findings do not always rule out neurosyphilis. The treatment for neurosyphilis is high-dose intravenous penicillin. The normal dose for neurosyphilis is 2–4 million units every 4 hr intravenously for a duration of 14 days, unless renal function or other factors preclude the use of high penicillin doses.
3. A descriptive history of an allergic reaction should always be elicited from patients who report a penicillin allergy. If a patient describes the allergy as anaphylactoid (respiratory distress, any symptoms of edema or swelling), the patient should receive an alternative agent for the treatment of syphilis. However, patients who report reactions that occurred after the treatment of a prior syphilis infection could be describing the Jarisch-Herxheimer reaction. The symptoms of this reaction include rash, fever, chills, diffuse

myalgias, and headache. It is a self-limiting reaction that begins approximately 4–6 hr after the initial treatment and usually resolves within 24 hr. Patients reporting a penicillin allergy, or patients who have never received penicillin previously, may have a skin test placed to detect an allergic reaction. The CDC currently recommends a tetracycline to treat penicillin-allergic patients. Erythromycin is not recommended because an unacceptable number of treatment failures have occurred. Doxycycline 100 mg b.i.d. p.o. should be given for 14 days. Follow-up is important in patients receiving this regimen, to determine compliance and treatment failure, which is not uncommon in patients treated with agents other than penicillin. The CDC does not recommend the use of doxycycline, cephalosporins, or erythromycin to treat syphilis in HIV-infected patients due to high failure rates. Desensitization is recommended for those patients with a true penicillin allergy.

4. Currently, the point at which antiretroviral therapy should be initiated is under debate. Several studies have indicated viral resistance in patients with progressive disease who received long-term antiretroviral therapy. Initiation of antiretroviral therapy especially in asymptomatic patients should be discussed with the patient to determine if the risk/benefit ratio is acceptable. Initiation of zidovudine would be appropriate for RC since her CD4 counts are less than 500 mm³. Zidovudine may slow progression to the development of AIDS. Current dosing recommendations are 200 mg p.o. t.i.d. Patients should be monitored monthly initially and every few months thereafter. The most common adverse effects are anemia and headache, but other effects include thrombocytopenia, hepatitis, and myositis. Appropriate clinical laboratory monitoring should be performed as well as a physical examination and patient history during subsequent clinic visits.

5. RC should begin *Pneumocystis* prophylaxis with cotrimoxazole (TMP-SMX) or aerosolized pentamidine. Studies have documented a higher incidence of opportunistic infections in patients with CD4 counts below 200/mm³, particularly *Pneumocystis carinii* pneumonia (PCP). The usual dose of cotrimoxazole is one double-strength tablet twice daily three times per week. Many AIDS patients cannot tolerate cotrimoxazole because of its adverse effects, in which case aerosolized pentamidine can be used. Cotrimoxazole is the drug of choice for PCP prophylaxis, since several reports have documented extrapulmonary PCP with the aerosolized pentamidine. TMP/SMX can also be used as primary prophylaxis against *Toxoplasma gondii*. Primary prophylaxis for esophageal or vaginal candidiasis or cryptococcal infection is not recommended at this time. Primary prophylaxis for *Mycobacterium avium* intracellular may be initiated when the CD4 count is below 100 mm³. Addition of rifabutin at this stage of disease has shown a protective effect against systemic MAI infection.

CASE 138

1. The macrolides clarithromycin 500 mg po bid and azithromycin 500 mg po qd are drugs awaiting FDA approval of an indication for MAC prophylaxis. However, rapid resistance has been observed with clarithromycin. It is unknown whether single or combination therapy should be used for prophylaxis. Data on rifabutin prophylaxis as monotherapy against MAC disease indicates a reduction in mycobacteremia but offers no survival benefits and appears to be unable to prevent disseminated MAC.

2. The benefits of antiretroviral therapy wane with time. There are instances, however, when switching from zidovudine to ddI is appropriate:
   a) The duration of zidovudine's benefit is controversial. If a patient is on zidovudine for one year or more and demonstrates progression of disease (indicated by fall in CD4 cell count or increase in opportunistic infection), this may be evidence of failure secondary to resistance.
   b) If a patient develops toxic myopathy (with elevated creatinine kinase CPK) with long-term use, zidovudine should be changed to ddI.
   c) If a patient has hepatomegaly and significant aminotransferase elevations ALT and AST, zidovudine should be discontinued.
   d) If a patient on zidovudine develops anemia, granulocytopenia, and thrombocytopenia, therapy should be changed to ddI.

3. Studies of multidrug antiretroviral therapy remain inconclusive. Many providers have various opinions about combination therapy. Currently, combination therapy is used in patients who demonstrate intolerance to zidovudine or have a decline in CD4 count. The usual treatment algorithm utilized by most practitioners is to start ddC and zidovudine after the patient has failed monotherapy with zidovudine and monotherapy with ddI. There is a growing belief that multiple therapies may be necessary to effectively slow the virus, because different agents work at different sites in the replication cycle of the virus. Preliminary data on combination treatment with zidovudine plus 3TC (Lamivudine, an investigational antiretroviral agent) suggest that this combination produces the most pronounced and prolonged effect of any anti-HIV drug regimen yet studied in suppressing HIV replication and increasing CD4 count. The future of HIV eradication may rest with combination therapy, triple- or four-drug combination use.

4. Wasting is defined as an unexplained loss of 10% or more of normal lean body mass. This can occur at any CD4 cell count. However, the risk of wasting and serious malnutrition increases dramatically when the CD4 cell count falls below 100 cells/mm³ in AIDS patients.

5. Weight loss and malnutrition are common problems associated with HIV. The timing of death has been correlated with two indicators of malnutrition: weight loss and albumin levels. The first indicator, weight loss (20% or more of body weight), correlates with a median survival of less than two months. The second indicator, albumin levels less than 2.5 g/dl, has been correlated with a median survival of less than three weeks.

CASE 139

1. The three most common pathogens of community-acquired pneumonia are *Streptococcus pneumoniae*, *Hemophilus influenzae*, and *Legionella pneumophila*.
2. The incidence of cross-reactivity between penicillins and cephalosporins is approximately 6%. Studies have shown that a penicillin-allergic patient is about three times more likely to develop an allergic reaction to cephalosporin than a non-penicillin-allergic patient.
3. Only angiotensin-converting enzyme inhibitors and combinations of hydralazine and isosorbide dinitrate have been shown to reduce mortality in patients with congestive heart failure. Conventional diuretics and digitalis therapy have not been shown to reduce mortality, although they may help control undesirable symptoms associated with CHF.
4. Although patients with elevated uric acid levels are more likely to develop gouty attacks, the treatment of asymptomatic hyperuricemia is not recommended since the risk of adverse drug reactions and the costs of treatment outweigh the benefits of therapy.
5. Causes of chronic insomnia include sleep apnea, nocturnal myoclonus, psychiatric disorders such as depression, and medical disorders such as angina, asthma, congestive heart failure, hyperthyroidism, peptic ulcer disease, and renal insufficiency. Chronic insomnia may be induced by serotonin-specific reuptake inhibitors, antihypertensives such as beta-blockers and clonidine, sympathomimetic amines such as amphetamines, caffeine and cocaine, and other drugs such as oral contraceptives, phenytoin, and thyroid preparations. Withdrawal of alcohol, benzodiazepines, tricyclic antidepressants and sympathomimetics can also induce insomnia.

CASE 140

1. Monotherapy with ceftazidime, cefoperazone, and imipenem/cilastatin has been shown in selected populations to be an effective alternative to combination therapy for treatment of the initial febrile episode in neutropenic patients. While the more established regimens consisting of an aminoglycoside in combination with an antipseudomonal β-lactam drug are preferred for profoundly neutropenic or "shocky"/septic-appearing patients, monotherapy does have a role in special situations. Patients with preexisting renal insufficiency or those receiving nephrotoxic drugs such as cisplatin, cyclosporine, or amphotericin B are candidates for nonaminoglycoside regimens. Monotherapy should be limited to those patients who have been neutropenic for only a brief period of time and have an ANC >500. Patients who seem clinically unstable or are septic-appearing should receive more aggressive combination therapy regimens containing an aminoglycoside and an antipseudomonal β-lactam agent.
2. The decision to initiate antifungal therapy in febrile neutropenia is a highly controversial one. It has been reported that up to one-third of neutropenic patients persistently febrile after a week of antibacterial therapy will have systemic fungal infections. Given these data, the consensus among experts in the field is that patients who remain febrile and profoundly neutropenic for 1 week, despite broad-spectrum antibiotics in adequate dosages, should receive amphotericin B therapy.
3. The single most important determinant for the duration of antimicrobial therapy in febrile neutropenia is the patient's ANC. Once the ANC is <500, the risks of infectious complications are much lower. In general, febrile neutropenic patients will require a minimum of 1 week of systemic antibiotics. If a patient is afebrile for 48–72 hr with an ANC <500 and negative cultures, the patient should complete a 7-day course of therapy. For those patients afebrile with ANC >500 who appear clinically stable, most experts would continue antibiotics for an additional 5–7 afebrile days before considering discontinuation of therapy. If at that time the patient shows no signs of infection and appears clinically well, it is reasonable to stop antibiotic therapy. Many clinicians, however, recommend continuation of antibiotics until the ANC is <500. Profoundly neutropenic (ANC <100) patients who are afebrile but appear unstable should continue antibiotics until the ANC is <500. In all cases, when antibiotics are discontinued during neutropenia, the patient must be followed carefully, and systemic antibiotics reinstituted immediately for fever or signs of infection.
4. Patients receiving chemotherapy for acute leukemia are at risk for opportunistic infections, including infection with *Pneumocystis carinii*. The risk of *Pneumocystis carinii* pneumonia can be dramatically reduced by the prophylactic administration of TMP-SMX (trimethoprim/sulfamethoxazole). Various regimens including daily and thrice-weekly administration have been used. Thrice-weekly administration of TMP-SMX (one double-strength TMP-SMX b.i.d. on three consecutive days) has been shown to be as effective as daily administration (one single-strength b.i.d.) and may be the preferred schedule, to minimize TMP-SMX-induced bone marrow suppression. BF should continue to receive prophylactic TMP-SMX throughout the maintenance therapy period for his ALL.
5. The colony-stimulating factors (CSFs) are hematopoietic growth factors that regulate the differentiation and proliferation of hematopoietic precursor cells. Currently there are two products available through recombinant DNA technology. The primary pharmacologic effect of these agents is to increase the production of neutrophils by the bone marrow. G-CSF (filgrastim) is lineage-specific and preferentially stimulates the neutrophil cell line. GM-CSF (sargramostim/molgramostim) acts predominantly on pluripotent stem cells and immature progenitor cells. It is not lineage-specific and promotes the differentiation of neutrophil, eosinophil, thrombocyte, monocyte, and macrophage cell lines.

   Prolonged neutropenia (ANC <1000) is the primary risk factor for the development of infectious complications and mortality in patients receiving cytotoxic chemotherapy. The CSFs, which reduce both the severity and the duration of neutropenia, should therefore reduce the infectious complications associated with myelosuppressive chemotherapy. To date, there has been one controlled prospective trial using G-CSF in patients with relapsed or refractory leukemias. Patients receiving the CSF experienced a shorter duration of neutropenia and had fewer documented infections than the control group. Additionally, there was no evidence that G-CSF accelerated the regrowth of leukemic blasts in bone marrow. This finding is important, as many clinicians believe CSFs should not be used in patients with myeloid leukemias because of the potential for stimulation of leukemic subclones. BF is receiving induction chemotherapy for ALL with daunorubicin and vincristine, both of which are potent bone marrow suppressive agents. BF will be profoundly neutropenic (ANC <500) for >7 days, and although there are limited data in this patient population, it is reasonable to consider the addition of a CSF to his regimen.

SECTION 16

NEOPLASTIC DISORDERS

CASE 160

1. Priapism is an unfortunate side effect of trazodone. It should resolve upon discontinuation of trazodone. RM's depression must be managed with another antidepressant. Tricyclics should be avoided in older patients, as they may be more sensitive to the anticholinergic, orthostatic, and potential arrythmogenic properties of the tricyclics. Fluoxetine would be an appropriate alternative, and should be started at 20 mg p.o. q.d. and titrated according to RM's signs and symptoms of depression, or RM may no longer require treatment for his depression if he has been treated for 6 months or longer.

2. RM's COPD regimen is no longer controlling his symptoms. The next logical step in the therapeutic management of RM's COPD is to add an inhaled steroid to the regimen. Beclomethasone 4 puffs q.i.d. should be initiated, and RM should be instructed to decrease the use of his albuterol to 2 puffs q4–6h as needed. He should be instructed to use the albuterol before inhaling the beclomethasone and to rinse his mouth thoroughly after each administration.

3. Clonidine has been used to help control the withdrawal symptoms associated with the cessation of smoking. RM should be given clonidine 0.1 mg s.l. and have his BP rechecked about 45 min later, to ensure that his BP will not decrease markedly after administration of clonidine. If his BP can tolerate the drug, clonidine patches can be started. The patches are applied to the upper torso once weekly. However, clonidine may aggravate his depression, so nicotine chewing gum or patch may be a better alternative for RM.

4. Trimethoprim/sulfamethoxazole may frequently cause a rash in certain individuals. The rash should resolve upon discontinuation of the drug. RM should be started on erythromycin 500 mg p.o. q.i.d. in lieu of the trimethoprim/sulfamethoxazole.

CASE 161

1. Adenocarcinoma of the stomach remains a significant oncologic problem in the United States, and is the ninth most common malignancy among males and fifteenth among females. However, it is the sixth most common cause of cancer-related mortality in men and eighth most common in women. Approximately 24,000 new cases of gastric carcinoma were diagnosed in 1993, with an estimated overall 5-year survival rate of 16%. Most U.S. patients present with advanced disease, and because survival after resection is highly dependent on disease stage, overall survival has not improved during this period of declining incidence.

2. The incidence of stomach cancer increases progressively after age 35. In the United States, the risk for males is 2.2 times greater than that of females. American blacks of either sex have a 3-fold greater risk than whites. Although genetic traits have been associated with increased risk, they cannot be clearly separated from environmental influences. Dietary factors are strongly associated with stomach cancer. Dietary nitrates found in preserved foods (pickled, salted, or smoked) when ingested are converted to nitrites and then to nitrosamines, which are potent carcinogens. Fresh fruits and vegetables containing vitamins A and C inhibit the conversion of dietary nitrates to nitrosamines and are associated with a decreased risk of gastric adenocarcinoma. Prior history with pernicious anemia, gastric polyps, chronic gastric ulcers, and previous ulcer surgery also increased the risk of developing gastric adenocarcinoma.

3. Stomach cancer produces few signs and symptoms until late in the disease, and when symptoms do occur, they are generally nonspecific. *Local manifestations* include: weight loss (80%), abdominal pain (69%), emesis (43%), change of bowel habits (40%), anorexia (30%), dysphagia (17%), massive hemorrhage (10%), and early satiety (5%) are common findings. *Systemic manifestations* include: weakness (19%), hepatic mass (10%); abdominal or bony pain; jaun-

dice; ascites; rectal urgency or obstruction; supraclavicular, axillary, or periumbilical adenopathy; and pulmonary, ovarian, or central nervous system (CNS) masses.

4. Although screening for stomach cancer is not feasible in the United States because of its low incidence, mass screening with upper GI x-rays and endoscopy in Japan has increased the detection of early mucosal lesions from 3.8% in 1955 to 34.5%. Patients with early-stage disease have a 5-year survival rate of greater than 90%.

5. The most frequent sites of metastatic spread from advanced gastric adenocarcinoma are: liver (45%), peritoneum (25%), lungs (20%), adrenals (12%), pancreas (10%), bone (5%), GI tract (5%), spleen (2%), CNS (2%), and GU tract (< 1%).

6. Surgery remains the only therapy with curative potential for gastric malignancies. Even in the presence of metastatic disease, resection of the primary lesion improves the patient's quality of life and duration of survival and therefore should be contemplated in selected patients. However, resection is not indicated in patients with widely metastatic disease, malignant ascites, or a brief life expectancy. Unresected gastric malignancies can cause bleeding, perforation, obstruction, and pain. Two major procedures have been used in the surgical treatment of gastric carcinoma. The choice of which type to use is determined by the size, location, histology, extent of the primary tumor, and the surgeon's preference. 1) *Subtotal gastrectomy* involves removal of the distal 50–85% of the stomach, including a 5–6cm margin of normal stomach around the lesion, the first part of the duodenum, and omentum. In addition, extensive lymph node dissections are performed in the areas of the porta hepatis and celiac lymph node groups. The speen is generally not removed unless obvious involvement occurs. 2) *Radical total gastrectomy* involves resection of the entire stomach, distal esophagus or proximal duodenum (depending on the location of the primary tumor), omentum, and frequently the spleen. In addition, lymph node dissection of the porta hepatis and celiac axis is also performed. Occasionally, extended total gastrectomy is performed which involves the dissection of the distal pancreas, peripancreatic nodes, and colon. Total gastrectomy is most often used for lesions involving the proximal stomach, a large portion of the gastric corpus, or both.

CASE 162

1. Early detection of breast cancer may lead to improved outcome. The American Cancer Screening Guidelines recommend both clinical examination and mammography as necessary in breast cancer screening. Screening for breast cancer should begin at age 35–40 years for all women with annual examinations and mammography at 1–2 year intervals. At age 50, both clinical examinations and mammography should be done yearly. In a high-risk population, more frequent examinations and screening may be needed. Women are encouraged to take an active role in early detection and learn about breast self-examination (BSE).

2. While mammography is an excellent tool for detecting breast tumors before they cause symptoms or can be felt, it cannot detect every abnormal area in the breast. Another important step in early detection is for women to have their breasts examined regularly by a physician or nurse. Between visits to the physician, women should learn about breast self-examination (BSE) and learn to examine their breasts every month. Patients should become familiar with how their breasts usually look and feel. If the patient still menstruates, the best time to do BSE is 2 or 3 days after her period ends. During this time period, her breasts are least likely to be swollen or tender. If the patient no longer menstruates, pick a certain day (such as the first day of each month) to do BSE. Below are 7 easy-to-follow steps (written in language for the patient) on how to do a breast self-examination (BSE):

1) Stand in front of a mirror that is large enough for you to see your breasts clearly. Check each breast for anything unusual. Check the skin for puckering, dimpling, or scaliness. Look for a discharge from the nipples. Do steps 2 and 3 to check for any change in the shape or contour of your breasts. As you do these steps, you should feel your chest muscles tighten.

2) Watching closely in the mirror, clasp your hands behind your head and press your hands forward.

3) Press your hands firmly on your hips and bend slightly toward the mirror as you pull your shoulders and elbows forward.

4) Gently squeeze each nipple and look for a discharge.

5) Raise one arm. Use the pads of the fingers of your other hand to check the breast and the surrounding area firmly, carefully, and thoroughly. Some women like to use lotion or powder to help their fingers glide easily over the skin. Feel for any unusual lump or mass under the skin. Feel the tissue by pressing your fingers in small, overlapping areas about the size of a dime. Be sure you cover your whole breast, paying special attention to the area between the breast and the underarm, including the underarm itself. Check the area above the breast, up to the collarbone and all the way over to your shoulder. Take your time and follow a definite pattern: lines, circles, or wedges.

   Lines: Start in the underarm area and move your fingers downward little by little until they are below the breast. Then move your fingers slightly toward the middle and slowly move back up. Go up and down until you cover the whole area.

   Circles: Beginning at the outer edge of your breast, move your fingers slowly around the whole breast in a circle. Move around the breast in smaller and smaller circles, gradually working toward the nipple. Don't forget to check the underarm and upper chest areas, too.

   Wedges: Starting at the outer edge of the breast, move your fingers toward the nipple and back to the edge. Check your whole breast, covering one small wedge-shaped section at a time. Be sure to check the underarm area and the upper chest.

6) Repeat step 5 while you are lying down. Lie flat on your back, with one arm over your head and a pillow or folded towel under the opposite shoulder. This position

flattens the breast and makes it easier to check. Check each breast and the area around it very carefully using one of the patterns described above.

7) Some women repeat step 5 in the shower. Your fingers will glide easily over soapy skin, so you can concentrate on feeling for changes underneath.

If you notice a lump, a discharge, or any other change during the month (whether or not it is during BSE), contact your physician.

3. Clinical staging of breast cancer is based on tissue sampling (biopsy), physical examination, chest x-ray, liver enzymes, alkaline phosphatase, and in some cases, abdominal CT and a bone scan to exclude liver and bone metastases. The most common sites of metastatic spread (by autopsy studies) are the following organs: regional lymph nodes (40–50%), lung (59–69%), liver (56–65%), bone (44–71%), pleura (23–51%), adrenal glands (31–49%), central nervous system (9–22%), and skin (7–34%).

4. Tamoxifen was approved by the FDA in 1978 for treatment of metastatic breast cancer in postmenopausal women. Currently, tamoxifen is used as first-line treatment for breast cancer therapy in premenopausal as well as postmenopausal women with estrogen-receptor positive tumors. The antiestrogenic effect of tamoxifen is evidenced by the 25% reduced rate of disease recurrence and 17% reduced annual risk of death in women receiving the drug as adjuvant therapy for breast cancer, with the greatest reductions in disease recurrence and in annual rate of death seen in women with estrogen-receptor positive tumors. Regression of tumor size also has been seen in women receiving the drug for metastatic breast disease. Common tamoxifen dosage of 20mg PO QD or 10mg PO BID are used. Duration of therapy is 3–5 years. Side effects from tamoxifen include: menopausal-like symptoms, atrophic vaginitis, occasional uterine bleeding, and thrombophlebitis.

5. Taxol (Paclitaxel®) was recently approved by the FDA for treatment of breast cancer after failure of combination chemotherapy for metastatic disease or relapse within 6 months of adjuvant chemotherapy. Preliminary data showed high rate of objective responses to taxol in heavily pretreated patients, and in patients who are refractory to prior standard chemotherapy. The recommended dosage is 175mg/m² administered intravenously over 3 hours every 3 weeks. All patients receiving taxol should be premedicated to prevent severe hypersensitivity. Such premedication may consist of: 1) dexamethasone 20mg PO approximately 12 and 6 hours prior to taxol, 2) diphenhydramine 50mg IV 30–60min prior to taxol, 3) cimetidine (300mg) or ranitidine (50mg) IV 30–60min prior to taxol. In addition, taxol is formulated in a vehicle known as Cremophor EL (polyoxyethylated castor oil) which has been found to leach the plasticizer DEHP from polyvinyl chloride infusion bags or administration sets. Diluted taxol solutions should preferably be prepared and stored in bottles (glass, polypropylene) or plastic bags (polypropylene, polyolefin) and administered through polyethylene-lined administration sets. Common toxicities include: (>10%) dose-limiting bone marrow suppression (primarily neutropenia), dose-depen-

dent peripheral neuropathy, and alopecia; (1–10%) bradycardia, and severe cardiovascular events.

CASE 163

1. Fatigability, abdominal discomfort, and blood in the stool

2. CEA is a tumor marker. An increase from the baseline is consistent with an increase in tumor progression. Conversely, a decrease would signify that the treatment was effective.

3. Disagree. This chemotherapy regimen should not produce a profound neutropenia.

4. a. Stomatitis/mucositis is defined as inflammatory responses of the oral mucosa and introital soft tissue structures to the cytotoxic effects of chemotherapy. The problem may be caused by nonspecific action of the chemotherapeutic agent on the rapidly dividing cells of the epithelium. It is primarily seen with antimetabolites such as 5-FU.

   b. Signs and symptoms include mild erythema and edema, dryness, and mild burning. Onset is about 5–14 days after administration of chemotherapy, with healing of the inflamed areas (unless secondarily infected) within 3–4 weeks after the last dose.

   c. • Candidiasis ("thrush") is the most common fungal infection and appears on the tongue and buccal mucosa.
   • Herpes simplex is the most common viral infection and appears on lips first.
   • Gram-negative bacterial infections (*Pseudomonas*, hemophilic) are common, serious, and can appear anywhere in the mouth.
   • Gram-positive bacterial infections (staphylococcal and streptococcal) are less common.

   d. Prevention of stomatitis/mucositis involves:
   • Daily oral assessment.
   • Oral regimen that should be done within 30 min after eating and every 4 hr while awake.
   • Flossing twice daily (unwaxed dental floss).
   • Brushing teeth (soft nylon bristle toothbrush). Should use a nonirritating dentifrice such as baking soda. Avoid lemon and glycerin (promotes dryness and irritation of mucous membranes).
   • Rinsing the mouth thoroughly with one of the following:
     a. Hydrogen peroxide with saline or water (1:2);
     b. Baking soda and water (1 tsp in 500 ml);
     c. Salt (1/2 tsp), baking soda (1 tsp), and water (1000 ml).
   • Drinking plenty of water (3000 ml), unless contraindicated.
   • Avoiding tobacco, alcohol, and foods that are spicy or physically irritating.
   • Determination of proper fit for denture wearers.

5. No. AV has several reasons for having an elevated platelet count, including hemorrhage and anemia. See mnemonic below.

Causes of Elevated Platelets

H-I P-L-A-T-E-L-E-T-S

*H*emorrhage (acute)—The mechanism of thrombocytosis here appears to be overproduction rather than lengthening of survival time. In response to acute hemorrhage, however, there may be the additional release of platelets from the spleen or the lungs.

*I*nflammatory disorders (such as rheumatoid arthritis, rheumatic fever, inflammatory bowel disease, sarcoid, osteomyelitis) cause increased production of platelets, possibly mediated by a platelet-stimulating factor.

*P*olycythemia vera—The bleeding tendency seen in polycythemia vera is due to both abnormal platelet aggregation and a distended vasculature secondary to increased blood volume.

*L*eukemia—In acute leukemia, the platelet count is usually moderately or greatly decreased. However, in the myeloproliferative syndrome, chronic granulocytic leukemia, half the patients will have platelet counts above 450×10^9 (450×10^3).

*A*nemia (iron deficiency)—Thrombocytosis occurring with iron deficiency anemia is corrected by iron therapy. Hemolytic anemia is also associated with elevated platelet counts.

*T*umor—Elevated platelet counts are commonly seen with many carcinomas and occasionally precede the diagnosis of malignancy.

*E*ssential thrombocythemia, a myeloproliferative disorder, is characterized by normal erythrocyte and leukocyte counts, and very high platelet counts. Bleeding and thrombotic complications are frequent.

*L*ymphoma—Hodgkin's disease and other lymphomas, like carcinoma, can be associated with high platelet counts.

*E*pinephrine and *E*xercise, like acute hemorrhage, cause release of platelets from storage areas. Postoperative thrombocytosis other than postsplenectomy cases is probably caused by this mechanism.

*T*oxin or recovery from *T*oxic state (vincristine, alcohol withdrawal).

*S*plenectomy results in thrombocytosis that commences within 2 weeks of surgery and lasts approximately 3 months.

CASE 164

1. ML is hypokalemic secondary to fluid replacement without potassium replacement. Normal potassium daily maintenance requirements are 75–100 mEq. BUN:Cr ratio is decreasing slightly, secondary to rehydration. Sodium and chloride concentrations remain at the high end of the normal range. Therefore, ML probably needs more free water at this time as well as potassium replacement.

   Change IV fluids to D51/4NS with KCl 30 mEq/liter and continue at 150 ml/hr. Monitor: daily electrolytes, BUN and Cr levels, urine output.

2. Calculate the total "on-demand" hydromorphone usage for the last 24 hr. Add this amount to the 24-hr basal rate. Continue with an "on-demand" availability for breakthrough pain. Reevaluate pain control and "on-demand" usage in 24 hr. Further adjustments may be required at that time.

   On-demand use per 24 hr:

0.5 mg every 30 min × 24 hr = 24 mg/24 hr

Therefore, increase basal rate to 1.5 mg/hr, continue 0.5 mg every 30 min on demand as needed for breakthrough pain. Reevaluate in 24 hr.

3. ML has stage IV pancreatic cancer, which is not curable. The median survival of patients with stage IV pancreatic cancer is less than 6 months from the time of diagnosis. In addition, ML has failed to respond to what are considered the most active agents currently available for this disease (leucovorin + 5-fluorouracil). It appears that his performance status is declining fairly rapidly. Taking all these factors into consideration, it is unlikely that ML will survive more than a few weeks to months. Supportive care is very important, to provide the best quality of life possible during his remaining time.

4. The combination of leucovorin plus 5-fluorouracil would be expected to be more toxic than 5-fluorouracil alone. The usual 5-fluorouracil side effects will be slightly more severe in ML. Expected side effects include:

   Mild nausea/vomiting
   Mild neutropenia/thrombocytopenia
   Mild alopecia
   Moderate mucositis (more severe with continuous infusion than with bolus dosing)
   Mild to moderate diarrhea

   Less-common side effects include:

   Hyperpigmentation of skin on face/hands
   Maculopapular rash
   Acute cerebellar syndrome (ataxia, headache, visual disturbances)

   ML reported nausea/vomiting, which was probably multifactorial. The chemotherapy may have exacerbated the nausea/vomiting, secondary to the tumor and other medications.

   ML had mild erythema of the oral cavity, but severe gastritis on upper endoscopy. Mucositis does not only occur in the oral cavity and may extend along the entire gastrointestinal tract. The gastritis seen on upper endoscopy was probably due in part to the chemotherapy.

   ML did not exhibit any evidence of neutropenia/thrombocytopenia in his current laboratory study results. If this were going to occur, you would expect to see the nadir (lowest) counts approximately 7–10 days after the administration of 5-fluorouracil, with recovery to baseline within 14–18 days.

   Diarrhea is very common with 5-fluorouracil administration. ML did not report any diarrhea, but this may have been partially prevented by the pain medication he was taking. The constipation induced by narcotics may have decreased bowel motility enough to prevent diarrhea.

   Alopecia tends to be relatively mild with 5-fluorouracil, usually consisting of some hair thinning but not overt alopecia. ML did not report any alopecia.

5. If ML's pain is not adequately controlled despite maximizing oral medications, one may consider either of the following options:

   Continuous IV narcotics using a hospice or home

healthcare agency to help with patient teaching, monitoring, and administration.

Celiac plexus nerve block may be done by an experienced practitioner. The injection of the celiac plexus with 50–100% ethanol is effective (>75% of patients) in significantly reducing abdominal pain. This may allow oral administration of narcotic agents for residual pain.

6. Nonpharmacologic methods to help prevent/treat constipation include maintaining adequate hydration (which is already being done) and increasing activity. If pain control is adequate, encourage ambulation.

Pharmacologic intervention in a patient who cannot/will not take anything orally is relatively limited:

Enemas (soap/H_2O, saline) may facilitate stool passage by increasing the water content of the stool and increasing the volume of stool in the rectum, thereby stimulating evacuation.

Suppositories that stimulate peristaltic activity of the intestine through local irritation of the mucosa may increase bowel motility (bisacodyl 10 mg rectally, may be repeated if no results within 1 hr).

Hyperosmotic laxatives (glycerin, sorbitol) may be given rectally by suppository or rectal solution. They work by drawing water from the surrounding tissues into the feces and reflexly stimulating evacuation. They should be administered only at infrequent intervals in single doses. The usual rectal dose of glycerin for adults is 2–3 g as a suppository or 10–15 ml of a 25–30% solution as an enema. The usual rectal dose of sorbitol for adults is 120 ml of a 20–30% solution.

CASE 165

1. Antiemetic therapy is extremely important to increase patient comfort and to prevent the patient from refusing to continue therapy due to extreme discomfort. It is important to control nausea and vomiting on the first course of chemotherapy, or it will be more difficult to control with subsequent chemotherapy due to anticipatory N/V. Cisplatin is one of the most emetogenic drugs, with prolonged N/V up to 24 hr or longer. Ondansetron is the first of a new class of antiserotonin antiemetics that is very effective in reducing cisplatin-associated N/V. It is also easier to administer and does not have the side effects associated with other antiemetic regimens (e.g., metoclopramide and dexamethasone). Give ondansetron 0.15 mg/kg (11 mg for LL) IV 30 min prior to cisplatin and at 4 and 8 hr after the beginning of the cisplatin infusion.

2. Calculate body surface area using nomogram or formula: BSA = Wt $(kg)^{0.5378}$ × Ht $(cm)^{0.3964}$ × 0.024265. LL's BSA = 1.73 m². Dose of cisplatin is 100 mg/m² × 1.73 m² = 173 mg. Dose of cyclophosphamide is 1000 mg/m² × 1.73 m² = 1730 mg. Give 170 mg of cisplatin and 1700 mg of cyclophosphamide.

3. Hemorrhagic cystitis is a common side effect. It is caused by the acrolein metabolite causing direct toxicity to the bladder mucosa. Toxicity can be avoided by maintaining adequate hydration and good urine output, which will reduce the contact time of acrolein in the bladder. A urinalysis should be routinely performed before each dose of cyclophosphamide to check for microhematuria. The patient should be given at least 2 liters of fluid by mouth (or IV in LL's case because of cisplatin therapy) in the 24 hr preceding the dose. If urine output is inadequate or if micro- or macrohematuria is detected, reducing or delaying the cyclophosphamide dose should be considered. Patients predisposed to hemorrhagic cystitis are those with evidence of previous toxicity and dehydrated patients.

4. Cisplatin is renally excreted, and the dose should be reduced or alternate therapy should be considered in patients with a creatinine clearance below 0.83 ml/sec (50 ml/min). Increased toxicity will occur if the cisplatin is administered in patients with renal impairment, including nephro- and ototoxicity.

5. Taxol is an investigational compound that is only indicated in patients who have failed standard therapy and have demonstrated a lack of response to platinum compounds. Cisplatin and cyclophosphamide are the treatment of choice for initial therapy in advanced epithelial ovarian cancer, and taxol would not be appropriate for LL at this time.

CASE 169

1. Patients with profound neutropenia, such as patients undergoing certain chemotherapy regimens or with late-stage AIDS, run a high risk for infection from bacteria, fungi, and viruses. The most common causes of bacterial infection in the neutropenic host are the gram-negative rods (*E. coli, K. pneumoniae, P. aeruginosa*) and the gram-positive cocci (*S. epidermidis*). The most common fungal pathogens in the neutropenic host include *Candida* and *Aspergillus* species. Most practitioners will wait to give the neutropenic patient prophylactic antibiotics until the patient has a febrile episode (38.5°C); some practitioners believe that prophylactic antibiotics should be initiated at the onset of neutropenia. At this point, prophylactic antibiotics are normally started immediately to cover gram-positive cocci (usually using vancomycin) and two antibiotics ("double coverage") with activity against gram-negative rods. Many combinations may be used, but most combinations include the aminoglycoside tobramycin, as it has superior activity against *Pseudomonas*, in combination with another antipseudomonal antibiotic (piperacillin, ticarcillin, ceftazidime, imipenem, or aztreonam). Prophylactic antibiotics are required for a minimum of 7 days. For patients who are clinically stable and afebrile after the first week of therapy, but continue to have ANC<500, most clinicians will either continue antibiotics for an additional 5–7 days or will continue antibiotics until the ANC >500. GC is neutropenic, but has not yet experienced fever, so prophylactic antibiotics are not necessary at this point. GC must be followed very carefully for any signs or symptoms of infection, including frequent monitoring of her temperature and daily CBCs.

2. BSA = Wt $(kg)^{0.5378}$ × Ht $(cm)^{0.3964}$ × 0.024265
GC's BSA = $(53)^{0.5378}$ × $(152)^{0.3964}$ × 0.024265
= 8.45 × 7.33 × 0.024265 = 1.5 m²
Cyclophosphamide dose = 1000 mg/m² = 1502 mg
Doxorubicin dose = 45 mg/m² = 67.5 mg

Etoposide dose = 50 mg/m² = 75 mg

3. GC has a serum calcium level of 2.1 (8.5). However, her albumin is also low at 30 (3.0). Serum calcium is partially bound to plasma proteins; the serum concentration of calcium is dependent upon the concentration of plasma proteins, especially albumin. A corrected value for serum calcium can be estimated by one of the following means: 1) For each 10 gm/liter change in the serum albumin concentration, total serum calcium will change 0.2 mmol/liter in the same direction; or 2) For each 1.0 gm/dL decrease in serum albumin, serum calcium will decrease by 0.8 mg/ dL. GC's corrected serum calcium can be estimated as 0.8(4.0 – 3.0) + 8.5 or 9.3 mg/dl. Therefore, she is not truly hypocalcemic and does not require a calcium supplement.

4. GC's current body weight is 53 kg (down 5.45 kg). She is still above her IBW for a woman of her height, but her albumin level is only 30 (3), which indicates decreased body protein stores. Also, GC has had 3 weeks of anorexia, and her chemotherapy regimen is likely to worsen her already poor appetite. For GC, the treatment options include nutritional supplements such as Ensure® or Sustacal® as long as she is able to take nourishment orally. If she becomes unable to tolerate oral products, she should be placed on total parenteral nutrition (TPN) while she is neutropenic. If she is not neutropenic, nutritional supplements may be administered via nasogastric (NG) tube.

5. Cigarette smoking is associated with an increased risk of peptic ulcer formation, delayed ulcer healing, and increased recurrence. Nicotine itself is thought to harm the gastric and duodenal mucosa by reducing pancreatic bicarbonate secretion, increasing the rate of gastric acid flow into the duodenum, and by promoting reflux of bile and duodenal contents into the stomach. Since GC has cut down her use of the nicotine gum from 25 to only 4 pieces per day, indicating a decrease in her urge to smoke (patients are instructed to chew one piece of nicotine gum at the onset of an urge to smoke), and since the nicotine in the gum might promote gastric mucosal damage, it would be prudent to wean her off the gum completely.

SECTION 17

PEDIATRIC AND NEONATAL THERAPY

CASE 176

1. There are two basic types of serologic tests for syphilis, the treponemal and the nontreponemal tests. The nontreponemal tests measure the nonspecific antibody against the tissue-treponemal proteins (reagin); these are useful in screening or for follow-up of known cases, and are useful in assessing response to therapy as titers become non-reactive within 1–5 years after treatment (depending on the stage of syphilis). The VDRL (Venereal Disease Research Laboratory) and the RPR (rapid plasma reagin) tests are nontreponemal titers often used for screening purposes, but positive results must be confirmed using treponemal tests. Since syphilis is caused by the *Treponema pallidum*, the more reliable tests are those that measure the specific antitreponemal antibody. A commonly used test for confirmation of syphilis is the FTA-abs (fluorescent treponemal antibody absorbent test). Although the FTA-abs is more specific, it remains positive in 75% of all patients for the duration of their lifetime; thus it is not useful in determining acute responses to therapy.

2. Rhinitis with purulent discharge from the mucous membranes is often the first sign of syphilis in a neonate. Dermatologic manifestations usually begin as a diffuse maculopapular rash, and can develop into epithelial sloughing. Bones can be affected, with areas of bone destruction caused by osteochondritis and perichondritis. The liver may develop hepatitis or overt liver failure resulting in death. The lungs may present with pneumonia or pulmonary hemorrhage. The most worrisome is the potential for neurosyphilis, which cannot always be ruled out in the differential diagnosis and would obligate the neonate to be treated with a full 10-day course of penicillin.

3. Since the likelihood of chronic HBV infection varies inversely with the age at the time of exposure, neonates have the highest rate of becoming infected. Eighty to ninety percent of untreated infants with HBsAg-(+) mothers acquire the infection and become chronic HBsAg carriers. Neonates rarely develop clinical hepatitis, but chronic HBsAg carriers are subsequently at higher risk of developing chronic active hepatits and hepatic carcinoma. Since most vertical transmissions occur during the perinatal or postnatal periods rather than in utero, HBIG and HBV play an important role in preventing the transmission of the virus.

4. Varicella (chicken pox) is a highly communicable disease in children, adolescents, and adults. Peak incidence occurs in children age 5–9. The rate of infection following household infection in healthy susceptible children was shown

to be 87%. If GJ's health care provider chooses to vaccinate her against varicella, this vaccine should be deferred until she is at least 12 months of age. Varicella vaccine is indicated for vaccination against varicella (chicken pox) in individuals ≥ 12 months of age. In children age 1–12, a single 0.5 mL dose should be administered SQ. Currently, booster doses are not indicated for children age 1–12. In adults and adolescents ≥ 13 years of age, a 0.5 mL dose should be administered SQ at the date recommended by the patient's health care provider and followed by a booster dose 4–8 weeks later.

CASE 177

1. Poisindex, available from Micromedex, Inc. provides information on over 400,000 toxic and nontoxic substances, including management information and treatment protocols. Substances may be indexed by brand name, manufacturer's name, generic/chemical name, "street" or slang terminology, botanical/common names, and also by commonly misspelled words.

2. Manifestations in infancy of cow's milk and soy protein allergy include vomiting, diarrhea, hematochezia, rhinitis, or skin allergy. Older infants may develop a protein-losing enteropathy syndrome. Other infants may only present with failure to thrive and frequent infections, without more specific signs of an allergic response. If the diagnosis of this allergy is delayed in infants with diarrhea, villus atrophy may develop as a complication. In most infants, the condition of cow's milk or soy protein allergy is self-limiting and tolerance appears at 1–2 years of age. For infants with cow's milk allergy, soy protein formulas may be tolerated, including Isomil, Nursoy, Prosobee, and RCF formulas. Infants unable to tolerate soy protein should receive a trial of an elemental formula such as Pregestimil, Nutramigen, and Portagen. Infants unable to tolerate either type of formula may require parenteral nutrition to support adequate growth and development until tolerance develops.

3. Yes. Systemic absorption from topical corticosteroids may produce reversible HPA-axis suppression. Topical application to large surface areas, prolonged use, and the addition of occlusive dressings promote systemic absorption. Infants and children may absorb proportionally larger amounts of topical corticosteroids and be more susceptible to HPA-axis suppression than adults. Patients at increased risk of systemic absorption resulting in HPA-axis suppression should have periodic measurement of urinary free cortisol and ACTH stimulation testing.

4. No. Systemic corticosteroids are generally not required for the treatment of atopic eczema in infants and children except in the most severely affected patients. Systemic treatment may be effective at clearing the skin, but withdrawal may result in reactivation of the eczema, and systemic steroids may cause many adverse effects including impairment of growth and development in infants and children after prolonged use.

CASE 178

1. Although it is always important to assess the immunization status of children in developing a differential diagnosis, it is not particularly helpful in identifying the pathogen in otitis media. This is because the two most likely culprits are *S. pneumoniae* and *H. influenzae* (non-typable). The vaccines that children normally receive do not include pneumococcal vaccine (which is reserved mainly for patients at high risk for complicated infection, i.e., patients with sickle-cell anemia, S/P transplant, HIV, and malignancies). Moreover, the *Hemophilus influenzae* type b vaccine that is a component of the immunization schedule in children does not prevent patients from getting the non-typable *H. flu*.

2. Failure of the signs and symptoms of otitis media to defervesce in light of treatment with amoxicillin indicates that a β-lactamase-producing organism may be infecting the ear. Antibiotic therapy *must* be altered in this case due to treatment failure (and not because of a hypersensitivity response to amoxicillin). In fact, the addition of a β-lactamase inhibitor such as clavulanate (with the combination amoxicillin / clavulanate) would be adequate if JB was not opposed to the possibility to continued self-limited rash. Otherwise, other alternatives as discussed in the SOAP notes could be selected.

3. Otitis media can become problematic if left untreated or if inadequately treated because of several complications. Fluctuating or persistent hearing loss may impact normal cognitive, language, and emotional development of the child. The tympanic membranes can perforate, and if not healed may lead to recurrent infections. Infection of the mastoid muscle and possibly bone may require surgical intervention. Other complications include facial paralysis, abscesses, and meningitis. Thus it is important to ensure adequate treatment for acute otitis media.

4. When used frequently, β₂-agonists may cause a down-regulation of the receptors in the lungs, thereby causing tachyphylaxis with increased usage. Paradoxical bronchoconstriction has also been reported with repeated and excessive use of the β₂-agonists. It is also possible that the bronchoconstriction is due to an immediate hypersensitivity response (thought to be caused by an inactive ingredient in the inhaler), but this is difficult to distinguish from the paradoxical effect. In order to maintain the potency of the β-agonists, they should be given only as symptoms arise (as needed) rather than as a maintenance dose (scheduled).

CASE 180

1. Numerous organ systems can be involved with CF. Because of this, CF is often characterized as a syndrome. However, the pulmonary and gastrointestinal complications predominate. Patients with CF may develop liver involvement, which usually takes the form of focal biliary cirrhosis. This can ultimately result in the complication of portal hypertension. Often, patients will have paranasal sinus complications resulting in chronic sinusitis. Patients with chronic sinusitis may complain of nasal congestion, rhinorrhea, headaches, or facial pain. The cardiovascular system may become in-

volved; this may progress to pulmonary hypertension or cor pulmonale. The reproductive tract of males and females is affected as well. Often males are sterile, while females demonstrate decreased fertility. It will be important to monitor LM throughout the course of her life for these potential complications.

2. DNase (Pulmozyme®) is a recombinant human DNA enzyme. Patients with CF have abnormally visous mucus secondary to chronic pulmonary infection and colonization. Theory states that during acute pulmonary infections, inflammatory cells are attracted to the site of infection. The destroyed neutrophils, macrophages, and bacteria then release DNA into the surrounding area. This extracellular release of DNA increases the mucus viscosity resulting in impaired mucus clearance, which leads to an accumulation of purulent sputum within the airways. DNase is the enzyme capable of breaking down the extracellular DNA in order to decrease the viscosity of the mucus. DNase is indicated for use in patients with CF in conjunction with standard therapy once their disease has progressed to the point that they are unable to clear the viscous sputum in their lungs with chest PT. Practitioners must weigh the benefits they expect to achieve with the cost of the medication; currently, DNase costs approximately $10,000 annually. The recommended dose is 2.5 mg daily via aerosol inhalation. Adverse effects to monitor include sore throat, dyspnea, voice changes, facial edema, pharyngitis, hemoptysis, rhinitis, and wheezing.

3. The use of fluoroquinolones in pediatric patients is controversial. It is especially important to explore this issue when considering patients with CF. Fluoroquinolones are the only class of oral antibiotics with reasonable activity against *Pseudomonas* spp. This is important as most CF patients become colonized or infected with *Pseudomonas* later in the course of their disease. The use of fluoroquinolones in children has been limited due to their potential role in irreversible cartilage damage; this data was first revealed while studying juvenile animals. Data suggests that quinolones may induce arthropathy in immature animals primarily in the major weight-bearing synovial joints; this damage occurred over days to weeks. Several small studies have explored the use of quinolones in children. In these studies, the majority of children were free from cartilage abnormalities. In these studies, small numbers of patients have complained of arthralgia and joint swelling while receiving quinolone therapy. With the few studies that have been performed, it is difficult to say with any certainty that quinolones result in cartilage toxicity in pediatric patients. While quinolones should never be the first-line agents for infections in children (not only because of the risk of cartilage toxicity, but also because of the issue of inducing resistant organisms), they may be used with caution. Appropriate indications would include a treatment failure to first-line antimicrobials or the development of resistance to standard antibiotics.

4. Currently, many medications are used in pediatric patients for which there is no published safety or efficacy information. To date, pharmaceutical companies have not been required to test medications for use in pediatric patients as this population is relatively small. These regulations have been reviewed and are now changing. Now, for medications that are to be used in treating disease states that affect children, companies must provide safety data that reflects how the medication will be handled in children, taking into account both safety and efficacy. Within two years, manufacturers must submit applications to comply with this new regulation. For those medications that do not qualify for pediatric use, the company may be required to perform clinical trials in order to supply the necessary safety and efficacy data.

5. It is important for LM's mother to be aware of over-the-counter (OTC) medications that should be avoided. LM's mother should read all labels carefully looking specifically for sugar- and alcohol-free products. As a general rule, capsules and tablets often contain less sugar and alcohol compared to liquid preparations. It is important to avoid sugar-containing products as they have the potential to elevate blood glucose. Conversely, alcohol may decrease the blood glucose in patients taking insulin. It is also important to avoid any medications containing sympathomimetics (examples include pseudoephedrine, phenylephrine, ephedrine, and phenylpropanolamine) as they may elevate blood glucose as well as blood pressure.

CASE 181

1. Several theories have been put forth to explain the mechanism of meningeal inflammation associated with meningitis. Cytokines and tumor necrosis factor (TNF) may play a role in the inflammation; furthermore, inflammation is thought to occur after initiation of antimicrobial therapy. A number of studies have examined the role of dexamethasone in diminishing the neurologic sequelae associated with meningitis, and their results been quite varied. Several trials administered dexamethasone as adjuvant therapy in children with meningitis, and results demonstrated that it decreased neurosensory hearing loss as well as the incidence of neurologic sequelae (mental retardation, seizures, and focal deficits), primarily in patients with meningitis caused by *H. influenzae*. The most recent trial addressing this issue found conflicting results: dexamethasone demonstrated no significant differences in neurologic sequelae, developmental assessment, or in unilateral or bilateral moderate or severe hearing loss. However, when this analysis was examined by infecting species, those patients infected with *H. influenzae* type b who received dexamethasone demonstrated significantly less bilateral moderate or severe hearing loss. Currently, there are no established guidelines for the use of dexamethasone in meningitis; therefore, the decision to treat with dexamethasone should be made on a patient-specific basis. Important patient-specific variables to consider include suspicion of *H. influenzae* as the infecting organism, concomitant disease states, and contraindications to corticosteroid therapy. If the decision to use dexamethasone is made, the recommended dose is 0.6 mg/kg/day IV divided QID for a duration of four days.

2. Infections with *H. influenzae* often occur in clusters, and spread via day care centers is a particular concern. Any persons having close contact with a child who has an infection caused by *H. influenzae* (such as family members or day care attendees) should receive prophylactic antibiotics. The purpose of prophylaxis is to eradicate the organism from the upper respiratory tract of those persons who have come into close contact with the infected patient. It is important to observe close contacts for symptoms of infection. The patient is given prophylaxis as well to prevent recolonization after the active infection has been treated. The drug of choice for *H. influenzae* prophylaxis is rifampin 20 mg/kg/day (maximum 600 mg) orally QD for 4 days. Thus, JD and his family should receive prophylaxis. As JD does not attend the day care that his sisters do, none of the children at day care need prophylactic therapy.

3. The cause of JD's seizure activity most likely results from meningeal inflammation and his fever. Febrile seizures arise after an elevation in body temperature in 2–4% of children between the ages of 6 months and 7 years. Febrile seizures are most often tonic-clonic in nature. JD will not be diagnosed with febrile seizures based on this one seizure; however, it will be important to observe JD for signs of seizure activity during his next febrile episode. Prophylactic anticonvulsant therapy is not standard practice after a single seizure secondary to meningitis. However, anticonvulsant therapy may be required should JD develop recurrent seizures after his fever and infection have been controlled. The choice of anticonvulsant would be based upon the seizure type JD might develop. The anticonvulsant of choice for febrile seizures is phenobarbital. For children less than one year old, the dose of phenobarbital is 5–6 mg/kg/day given QD or BID.

4. Recurrent episodes of OM (defined as three episodes of OM in six months, four episodes in twelve months or six in eighteen months) can be common; therefore, it is important to determine the underlying cause. Factors contributing to recurrence include treatment failure, noncompliance, and exposure to a day care center. The microbiology of chronic, recurrent OM is different from that outlined above in acute OM. Anaerobes are the most common organism in chronic OM, followed by *M. catarrhalis* and *H. influenzae*. Therapy for an OM in a child with chronic recurrence should cover these common organisms. Augmentin 25–50 mg/kg/day divided TID for ten days is an appropriate treatment. Prophylaxis against recurrent OM can significantly decrease the number of episodes of OM per year. Prophylaxis is given usually during the winter and early spring for a 3-month duration, or until failure occurs. The most common agents for prophylaxis include amoxicillin 25 mg/kg/dose QHS or trimethoprim/sulfamethoxazole 4 mg/kg/dose (trimethoprim component) QHS. The child should be evaluated every four weeks for acute OM.

5. It is important that JD's mother be able to recognize the signs and symptoms of dehydration. Signs of mild dehydration include thirst, restlessness, and moist mucous membranes. Signs of moderate dehydration include thirst, restlessness, lethargy, sunken eyes, and dry mucous membranes. Signs of severe dehydration include drowsiness, grossly sunken eyes, and very dry mucous membranes. If JD has mild dehydration (less than 5% weight loss), he can be treated at home with an oral rehydration regimen such as Pedialyte®. JD will need at least 20 ounces of fluid daily to maintain adequate hydration status; normally with mild dehydration, the child will regulate intake appropriately secondary to the thirst mechanism. It is important that electrolytes, especially Na, K, Cl, and HCO_3, are included in the oral rehydration solution to maintain an electrolyte balance, and that carbohydrates, in the form of glucose, are provided for caloric support.

SECTION 18

OB-GYN DISORDERS

CASE 182

1. If metronidazole 500 mg p.o. b.i.d. × 7 days fails to cure SK, she and/or her partner(s) (whoever remains symptomatic) should be treated with another course of metronidazole 500 mg p.o. b.i.d. for 7 more days. If this fails, a single 2-gm dose should be given daily for 3–5 days. Cases in which there are additional culture-documented treatment failures and in which reinfection has been excluded should be managed in consultation with an expert who can determine the susceptibility to metronidazole.

2. Aspirin 650 mg p.o. every 4 hr probably would not help SK's primary or secondary dysmenorrhea symptoms. Salicylates work poorly in the prevention of endometrial prostaglandin synthesis. It is unnecessary for SK to take aspirin 2 days before menses, since prostaglandins have half-lives of usually less than 1 min. The history of two episodes of pelvic inflammatory disease and the failure of both ibuprofen and naproxen in this patient are not promising for the efficacy

of aspirin in SK. It should be remembered that both ibuprofen and naproxen sodium are available without a prescription.

3. Since SK has heavy flow, any IUD may increase the amount of bleeding. She also has moderately severe dysmenorrhea, a component of which is probably primary dysmenorrhea, which is worsened by IUDs. Having multiple sex partners is another reason for not using IUDs, since the incidence of pelvic inflammatory disease may be increased in IUD users, and SK has already had 2 episodes. An exponential increase in infertility rates occurs as the number of episodes of PID increases (i.e., 12% after the first episode, 23% after the second, and 54% after the third). It is desirable to retain whatever reproductive potential SK has, since she has no children at this time.

4. If SK's history of 4 glasses of wine with dinner for 12 years is accurate, and she fears becoming an alcoholic, she probably is not an alcoholic. However, she suffers from bipolar disorder and is taking (successfully) protriptyline. Disulfiram may decrease the hepatic metabolism of protriptyline, and this combination may be associated with a high frequency of acute organic brain syndrome. Since we have to give SK metronidazole, disulfiram should be avoided because there is a high frequency of acute psychosis when the two drugs are taken together. The opioid-receptor antagonist naltrexone HCL could safely be used by SK, who has normal liver function and a negative history of narcotic abuse in the last 10 days. Although she is taking acetaminophen with codeine, she is not addicted and should not have withdrawal symptoms. It must be remembered that the analgesic effect of codeine will be neutralized by naltrexone. The 50 mg po once-daily dose induces mild and transient nausea in approximately 10% of patients taking the drug. SK may take metronidazole safely while taking naltrexone.

5. Cyclothymic disorder is a chronic mood disturbance lasting more than 2 years, involving numerous periods of depression and hypomania (mild mania). Symptoms are of shorter duration and of less severity than bipolar disorder. Normal mood intervals last for months at a time. Psychotic symptoms do not develop, hospitalization is rarely required, and drug treatment is only occasionally required. These patients often become substance abusers in an attempt to self-treat their mood fluctuations. Cyclothymic disorder is frequently found in relatives of bipolar patients, and it may represent a subaffective or abortive form of bipolar disorder. (See Chapter 52, "Mood Disorders.")

CASE 183

1. The typical failure rate in the U.S. during 1 year of use for COCs is 2–3%; for diaphragm plus spermicide it is 18%.

2. The most important COC pills to inhibit ovulation are the first 5–7 in each cycle. Ovulation for this cycle has probably been inhibited. However, she should be instructed to use another method of birth control throughout the remainder of this cycle. She should take 2 pills each day for the next 2 days until the missed pills are taken.

3. HD should be rechecked, so that at least 3 consecutive BP readings are in this range. If so, another method of birth control should be recommended because an obvious increase in BP has occurred.

4. Because of the drug interaction between COCs and oral antibiotics (see Chapter 91, "Contraception and Infertility"), caution should be used. At this time no one knows the exact relationship between effect and dose or which antibiotic may have the least effect on enterohepatic recycling of hormone. Low-dose cotrimoxazole has not been known to result in unwanted pregnancies in patients taking COCs and may be used with care.

CASE 187

1. JR's previous UTIs were all successfully treated with Septra. Treatment failure may have occurred due to the predominance of enterococcal bacteria. The ability to use exogenous folate limits the effectiveness of Septra against enterococcal bacteria.

2. JR's allergy precludes the use of penicillin antibiotics. Fluoroquinolones such as ciprofloxacin would provide adequate enterococcal coverage. Ciprofloxacin 500mg po bid for ten to fourteen days following intravenous antibiotic therapy should be sufficient. Bacterial susceptibility testing should be performed to ensure therapeutic efficacy.

3. The female anatomy predisposes women to the development of UTIs. The female urethra is much shorter than the male, allowing bacterial access to the bladder. In addition, men secrete antimicrobial substances from the prostate gland, which decreases risk of infection. Foreign devices such as diaphragms and cervical caps can also harbor bacteria if they are not properly cleaned and stored. This, in turn, may lead to an increased risk of UTIs.

4. Many antimicrobials interfere with the enterohepatic recycling of exogenous estrogens and progestin. JR should be advised to use additional protection (e.g., condoms) since she will be taking ciprofloxacin and prophylactic nitrofurantoin. In addition, JR should be told to consult with her pharmacist or physician regarding new medications and any possible drug interactions with her birth control pills.

5. With prolonged use of birth control pills, the formation of endometrial tissue is decreased. This, in turn, decreases prostaglandin formation, which is a leading cause of dysmenorrhagic symptoms.

SECTION 19

GERONTOLOGY

CASE 189

1. Almost any medical change could affect the mental status of an elderly, demented patient. Possible causes of acute decline include infections such as urinary tract infections and pneumonia, which are common in nursing homes. Often the first symptoms noticed in demented patients are mental status changes or increased confusion. Metabolic disturbances, especially those due to electrolyte imbalance, can cause changes. Impaction could also result in central nervous system changes. Drugs such as digoxin and prednisone could also be responsible for CNS changes.

2. U/A with C + S, thyroid function, iron, B_{12}, folic acid, repeat digoxin and electrolyte level determinations.

3. Medications will not help confusion and memory loss. More medications may in fact exacerbate these problems. Would not recommend the use of psychoactive agents, which may cause further deterioration in mental status functioning. Do not use any psychotropic agents such as antipsychotics or antianxiety medications for patient's occasional upset and repetitive talking. Try behavior interventions such as reassuring patient and putting her in an area where she will have contact with people.

   Flurazepam should be discontinued due to its extremely long half-life. Could judiciously (not every night) use a shorter-acting hypnotic such as triazolam, lorazepam, or temazepam. But need to minimize the use of CNS-sedating medications.

4. This patient should have adjustments in her medication regimen, which may increase her level of functioning. There are no cures, and little benefit is seen from therapeutic drugs currently tried for AD. When there are positive responses to drugs, they usually occur in mild-to-moderately impaired patients. With close control of her medical problems, EM will still suffer from severe dementia. She has already lost most of her ability to function. She will progress and probably die from an infectious process such as pneumonia or sepsis or an acute exacerbation of a medical problem in the near future.

5. Anticoagulation is often recommended in a patient with atrial fibrillation and a history of valvular heart disease or cerebral embolism to a level of 1.2–1.5 times the control prothrombin time. However, this is an elderly, demented patient at high risk for side effects such as subdural hematoma from gait instability (possible falls) and of spontaneous bleeding. Weighing the risks versus benefits in this patient, anticoagulation would not be recommended at this time.

6. EM is too demented to make her own healthcare decisions. If she had a living will or had established a durable power of attorney, she could have specified what measures she wanted taken to extend her life or who could make those decisions for her if she was unable to make them herself. The extent of care during an emergency situation must be determined. Areas of concern are whether to code a patient or put her on a respirator or maintain comfort measures. These decisions can be made by the physician, family, and conservator. May need to consider the placement of a nasogastric or gastric tube if she is not able to maintain adequate fluids and nutrition. This becomes a dilemma for a severely demented patient with a very poor quality of life. Should these means be used merely to prolong life? These issues will probably need to be addressed in the near future.

CASE 190

1. The duration of hormonal therapy in a post-menopausal patient is controversial. Hormones are effective in retarding bone loss if they are initiated post-hysterectomy or during the first five years of menopause. After age 70, loss of calcium from the bone appears to plateau, so benefit versus risk should be reassessed. Ten years' duration is considered the minimum effective time to prevent osteoporosis, with more and more clinicians favoring use to age yo or even for a lifetime if no contraindications are present. Major risk factors are a history or presence of estrogen-secreting tumors, abnormal bleeding, thromboembolic disease, or active liver disease.

2. Initial therapy with levothyroxine in geriatric patients and/or those with cardiac disease should be at 0.025 mg per day, which can be increased in 0.025-mg increments every 3–4 weeks; usual maintenance dose in a geriatric patient is 0.1 mg daily. Side effects to monitor include tachycardia (pulse), insomnia, and chest pain. Cautious use is recommended in patients with hypertension, congestive heart failure, angina pectoris, or any cardiac arrhythmia. See Chapter 16, "Thyroid and Parathyroid Disorders."

3. There is controversy on the issue of "tight" versus "loose" control of adult onset diabetes in a geriatric patient. Depending on other risk factors such as hypertension and hypercholesterolemia, many clinicians favor a somewhat looser control as long as the patient remains asymptomatic, to reduce the risk of hypoglycemia and mental confusion. Most microvascular complications take 20–30 years to develop; treatment generally will delay rather than prevent

these complications. See Chapter 17, "Diabetes" and Chapter 90, "Geriatric Drug Therapy."

4. With age, the renal threshold for glucose [normally 9.9 (180)] will increase, so that urine sugars may be negative even though blood sugars may be in excess of 11 (200). The Clinistix should be discontinued, and TY should be counseled on the proper use of a home blood glucose monitor that will more accurately determine diabetes control. See Chapter 90, "Geriatric Drug Therapy" and Chapter 17, "Diabetes Mellitus."

5. Prostaglandins are needed to maintain renal blood flow and glomerular filtration rate in patients with compromised renal function and/or volume depletion. All NSAIDs inhibit prostaglandin synthesis, resulting in azotemia and oliguria from decreases in RBF and GFR in patients with compromised renal function. Sulindac may have less inhibition of prostaglandin synthesis, leading to its claims of being the "renal-sparing" NSAID; in patients with moderate-to-severe renal impairment, there is probably no difference among existing NSAIDs. Pharmacists should monitor for proteinuria, changes in serum potassium, creatinine and BUN, as well as evidence of edema (weight gain). See "Geriatric Drug Therapy," Chapter 90.

6. The medical literature does not recommend routine antimicrobial prophylaxis for international traveler's diarrhea due to the risk of adverse drug reactions. Prophylaxis is restricted to high-risk patients visiting high-risk areas for extended lengths of time.

SECTION 20

CRITICAL CARE

CASE 193

1. FF should receive a 15 mg/kg load of phenobarbital. There are several treatment options if seizures persist after the administration of phenobarbital. FF may receive additional phenobarbital doses to increase the serum blood level into the high therapeutic range. Lidocaine 100 mg IVP may be administered, or general anesthesia should be initiated.

2. Delayed cerebral vasospasm occurs in 30% of patients with subarachnoid hemorrhage. Vasospasm occurs between 3 and 10 days after the event and may result in worsening of the neurologic deficit. Nimodipine is a calcium-channel blocker that produces cerebral vasodilation at doses that do not produce substantial systemic hypotension. This is due to its high lipid solubility and affinity for cerebral vasculature. Nimodipine in doses of 60 mg q4h will decrease the incidence and severity of delayed ischemic neurologic deficits. The drug should be started 72–96 hr after the onset of subarachnoid hemorrhage and continued for 21 days.

3. The use of diazepam and phenobarbital may cause respiratory depression. Hypotension may be due to the effects of phenytoin, phenobarbital, and nitroprusside. Initial treatment would be to decrease the nitroprusside dosage. The use of the H-2 blocker, cimetidine, may decrease phenytoin elimination. Close monitoring of phenytoin levels is necessary.

4. Dexamethasone administration will decrease ICP elevation associated with brain tumors. Dexamethasone administration will not decrease the ICP elevation caused by a subarachnoid hemorrhage.

5. Patients with neurologic insults have profound metabolic stress. In addition, they are at risk for developing stress-induced gastrointestinal erosions. The administration of tube feedings may help prevent sustained nitrogen loss. However, placement of a feeding tube will increase the ICP and should be delayed. Moreover, phenytoin oral absorption is reduced substantially when administered through the NG tube with the nutritional feedings.

CASE 194

1. If the blood pressure has been stabilized and the cardiac index remains low, then several other hemodynamic variables must be examined. If the pulmonary capillary wedge pressure (preload) and systemic vascular resistance remain elevated, then the cardiac index will be impeded. Thus, an agent that "unloads" the heart is desirable. Nitroprusside is a direct-acting vasodilator that dilates both venous and arterial vessels, and reduces preload and afterload. Nitroprusside also reduces the pulmonary capillary wedge pressure and ventricular filling pressures, which will ultimately improve pulmonary edema. Nitroprusside is an alternative agent to be combined with dopamine at this point and may be initiated at a dose of 0.25 µg/kg/min.

2. The major risk of using nitroprusside in DK is further reducing the mean arterial blood pressure. This may result in reduced coronary perfusion pressure and myocardial ischemia. Nitroprusside must be used cautiously and the hemodynamic effects balanced with dopamine. In addition, thiocyanate accumulation will occur if DK's renal function continues to deteriorate. In the blood, sodium nitroprusside is converted to cyanide, which is hepatically metabolized to thiocyanate and excreted renally. Thiocyanate toxicity usually occurs in patients with renal failure who receive prolonged infusion (>48 hr). Signs and symptoms include confusion, psychosis, weakness, hyperreflexia, seizures, and coma. Although toxicity may not be an immediate concern in DK, renal function should be monitored closely.

3. Dobutamine is a very effective inotropic agent that also possesses "unloading" effects on the heart. In DK, dobutamine may be combined with dopamine as an alternative to nitroprusside. Dobutamine, in doses of 2.5–15 µg/kg/min, increases cardiac output and decreases pulmonary capillary wedge pressure and systemic vascular resistance. Since dobutamine has minimal direct vasodilating effects, hypotension may be less of a problem than with nitroprusside. When compared with dopamine, dobutamine has equal or greater inotropic action. Evidence suggests that dobutamine may have less chronotropic effects than dopamine at lower infusion rates. If tachycardia becomes a problem with dopamine, combining the two agents may enable the clinician to augment the cardiac output while slowly reducing the dose of dopamine.

4. The management of agitation in DK first requires careful evaluation. Sedatives or skeletal muscle relaxants should not be administered without the exclusion of treatable causes of agitation. The blood glucose concentration should be determined immediately. If the agitation is temporally related to the administration of insulin or if a change in intravenous fluid orders has resulted in less dextrose administration, 25 ml of 50% dextrose should be immediately administered intravenously. Agitation could result from hypoxemia. Physical examination of the chest for new findings and arterial blood gas determination is essential. Pain could cause the development of agitation. Postoperative pain could con-

tribute to DK's agitation. If hypoglycemia and hypoxemia have been eliminated as causes of DK's agitation, pharmacologic treatment may proceed. Morphine sulfate should be administered in 2-mg increments every 5 min until the patient is calm. Thereafter, morphine may be administered in doses of 2–5 mg every 1–2 hr. The blood pressure and pulse must be monitored prior to administration of each dose. Hypotension may be managed with a fluid challenge. Respiratory depression may be managed with 0.4 mg of naloxone. Naloxone administration will ameliorate the analgesic effects of morphine.

CASE 195

1. The transplanted heart is denervated and is no longer under the cholinergic influence of the autonomic nervous system, and it cannot respond quickly to increased demands. It does respond normally to circulating catecholamines. During exercise, the heart rate increases slowly, reaches maximal level only after several minutes, and declines gradually after cessation of exercise. Patients should be instructed to increase their activity level slowly during any exercise. In addition, patients will notice that the resting heart rate for their newly transplanted heart will be higher than before.

2. Because of his immunosuppressed state, CL is at risk for developing several types of infections. Early in the posttransplant period, bacterial infections due to Gram-positive or Gram-negative bacteria may occur. Later, opportunistic infections, viral (CMV), fungal (*Candida, Aspergillus*), and protozoal (PCP, toxoplasmosis), may occur. Chemophylaxis with TMP/SMX and oral nystatin or clotrimazole have been shown to decrease the incidence of PCP and fungal infections, respectively.

a. The decrease in digoxin concentration could be due to discontinuance of the diltiazem, which may have previously decreased the clearance of digoxin. In addition, the previously elevated cyclosporine levels may have caused some degree of nephrotoxicity, which has now resolved.

b. The new expected digoxin steady-state concentration can be estimated as follows:

$$Cl = \frac{SF \times MD}{Css,ave} = \frac{(0.7)(125 \ \mu g/day)}{(0.7 \ \mu g/ml)}$$

$$= 125 \ liter/day$$

$$Css, ave = \frac{SF \times MD}{Cl} = \frac{(0.7)(250 \ \mu g/day)}{(125 \ liter/day)}$$

$$= 1.4 \ \mu g/ml \ (1.8 \ nmol/liter)$$

4. The AHA guidelines for antimicrobial prophylaxis for prevention of bacterial endocarditis should be followed for CL. Give 3 g amoxicillin p.o. 1 hr before the procedure and 1.5 g 6 hr later.